CLINICAL HANDBOOK of ADOLESCENT ADDICTION

CLINICAL HANDBOOK of ADOLESCENT ADDICTION

Edited by

RICHARD ROSNER MD, DLFAPA, FACPsych, FASAP, FAAFS
(Psychiatry and Behavioral Science)

Clinical Professor of Psychiatry and Former Director,
Forensic Psychiatry Residency Program,
New York University School of Medicine;
Former Medical Director, Forensic Psychiatry Clinic,
Bellevue Hospital Center, New York, NY, USA

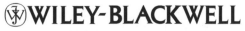

A John Wiley & Sons, Ltd., Publication

Library of Congress Cataloging-in-Publication Data

Rosner, Richard.
  Clinical handbook of adolescent addiction / Richard Rosner.
    p. cm.
  Includes bibliographical references and index.
  ISBN 978-0-470-97234-2 (cloth)
  1.   Compulsive behavior in adolescence–Handbooks, manuals, etc. 2.   Teenagers–Substance use–Handbooks, manuals, etc.
3.   Compulsive behavior–Handbooks, manuals, etc.   I. Title.
  RJ506.D78R66 2012
  616.85'8400835–dc23

                                                                                              2012010943

A catalogue record for this book is available from the British Library.

Wiley also publishes its books in a variety of electronic formats. Some content that appears in print may not be available in electronic books.

Chapter 1 – "The Scourge of Addiction: What the Adolescent Psychiatrist Needs to Know". Previously published in Adolescent Psychiatry, Volume 29, Analytic Press, Hillsboro, NJ, 2005, and reprinted here with their kind permission.

Chapter 27 – Rational Emotive Therapy. Previously published as "Albert Ellis' Rational-Emotive Behavior Therapy" in Adolescent Psychiatry, Volume 1, pages 82–87, Bentham, 2011, and reproduced here with their kind permission.

Chapter 28 – Relapse Prevention. Previously published in in Adolescent Psychiatry, Volume 2, Bentham, 2011, and reprinted here with their kind permission.

Chapter 33 – What's Old is New: Motivational Interviewing for Adolescents. Reprinted with kind permission from Adolescent Psychiatry, Vol 30, pages 117–127. © Francis and Taylor, 2008.

Chapter 41 – Introduction to Forensic psychiatry for adolescent psychiatrists. Previously published as "Forensic Psychiatry for Adolescent Psychiatrists: an Introduction" in Adolescent Psychiatry, Volume 24, Analytic Press, Hillsboro, NJ, 1999, and reprinted her with their kind permission.

Chapter 47 – Saving Adolescents. Previously published as "Essays on Saving Adolescents", in Adolescent Psychiatry, Volume 30, Analytic Press, Hillsboro, NJ, 2008, and reprinted here with their kind permission.

Cover image: Jeune homme nu assis au bord de la mer – Etude by Flandrin Hippolyte (1809–1864). Photo credit © RMN (Musée du Louvre) / Daniel Arnaudet.

Set in 9.25/11pt, Times by Thomson Digital, Noida, India.
Printed and bound in Singapore by Markono Print Media Pte Ltd.

First Impression 2013

*This book is dedicated to those from whom the editor
has learned most about addiction: my teachers, my students,
and my patients, especially Bay and Charles.*

Section Editors

Stephen Bates Billick
Department of Psychiatry, New York College of
Medicine, New York, NY, USA

Dean De Crisce
New York University School of Medicine,
Brooklyn, NY, USA

Timothy W. Fong
Semel Institute for Neuroscience and Human
Behavior at UCLA; UCLA Addiction Psychiatry
Fellowship; UCLA Addiction Medicine Clinic,
Los Angeles, CA, USA

Robert Lloyd Goldstein
College of Physicians and Surgeons of Columbia
University, New York, NY, USA

Manuel Lopez-Leon
New York University School of Medicine;
New York University Child Study Center,
New York, NY, USA

Avram H. Mack
Georgetown University School of Medicine,
Washington, DC, USA

Richard Rosner
Forensic Psychiatry Residency Program, New York
University School of Medicine; Forensic
Psychiatry Clinic, Bellevue Hospital Center,
New York, NY, USA

Charles L. Scott
Department of Psychiatry & Behavioral Sciences
University of California, Davis Medical Center,
Sacramento, CA, USA

Robert Weinstock
University of California Los Angeles, Los Angeles,
CA, USA

Contents

List of Contributors

Tahira Akbar University of Dundee Medical School, Dundee, UK

Ara Anspikian Semel Institute for Neuroscience and Human Behavior at UCLA, Los Angeles, CA, USA

Alex Baldacchino University of Dundee Medical School, Dundee, UK

Malena Banks Georgetown University Hospital, Washington DC, USA

Eraka Bath Department of Psychiatry, UCLA Neuropsychiatric Institute, Los Angeles, CA, USA

Matthew Biel Georgetown University Hospital, Washington DC, USA

Stephen Bates Billick Department of Psychiatry, New York College of Medicine, New York, NY, USA

Asad Bokhari Chesapeake Treatment Centers; Mountain Manor Treatment Center, Baltimore, MD, USA

Michael Boucher David Geffen School of Medicine, University of California at Los Angeles, Los Angeles, CA, USA

Mary Lynn Brecht Integrated Substance Abuse Programs, UCLA, Los Angeles, CA, USA

Michael Brendler Georgetown University School of Medicine, Washington DC, USA

Ann Bruner Johns Hopkins University Student Health and Wellness Center; Mountain Manor Treatment Center, Baltimore, MD, USA

Gregory C. Bunt Department of Psychiatry, New York University School of Medicine; Daytop Village, Inc., New York, NY, USA

Matthew J. Carpenter Department of Psychiatry and Behavioral Sciences; Hollings Cancer Center, Medical University of South Carolina, Charleston, SC, USA

Ellen Chang Department of Psychiatry and Bio-behavioral Sciences, UCLA, Los Angeles CA, USA

Le Ondra Clark California State Senate, California State Capitol, Sacramento, CA, USA

Jan Copeland National Cannabis Prevention and Information Centre, University of New South Wales, Sydney, NSW, Australia

Ilana Crome Department of Psychiatry, Keele University Medical School, Keele, UK

Dean De Crisce New York University School of Medicine, Brooklyn, NY, USA

Marlene Dobkin De Rios University of California, Irvine; California State University, Fullerton, CA, USA

Marc Fishman Department of Psychiatry and Behavioral Sciences, Johns Hopkins University School of Medicine; Mountain Manor Treatment Center, Baltimore, MD, USA

Lois T. Flaherty University of Maryland School of Medicine, Baltimore, MD, USA

Timothy W. Fong Semel Institute for Neuroscience and Human Behavior at UCLA; UCLA Addiction Psychiatry Fellowship; UCLA Addiction Medicine Clinic, Los Angeles, CA, USA

Robert Lloyd Goldstein College of Physicians and Surgeons of Columbia University, New York, NY, USA

Rachel Gonzales Integrated Substance Abuse Programs, University of California Los Angeles, Los Angeles, CA, USA

Jack A. Gottschalk Seton Hall University, Stillman School of Business, Livingston, NJ, USA

Kevin M. Gray Department of Psychiatry and Behavioral Sciences; Hollings Cancer Center, Medical University of South Carolina, Charleston, SC, USA

Daniel P. Greenfield Seton Hall University School of Health and Medical Sciences, Millburn, NJ, USA

Charles S. Grob Harbor-UCLA Medical Center, Torrance, CA, USA

John Gunn, Institute of Psychiatry, King's College London, London, UK

Andia Heydari Department of Psychiatry and Biobehavioral Sciences, UCLA, Los Angeles, CA, USA

John Howard National Cannabis Prevention and Information Centre, University of New South Wales, Sydney, NSW, Australia

Yasmin Jilla Department of Psychiatry, Georgetown University Hospital, Washington DC, USA

Abigail M. Judge Harvard Medical School, Massachusetts Avenue, Cambridge, MA, USA

Ari Kalechstein Baylor College of Medicine, The Menninger Department of Psychiatry, Houston, TX, USA

Reef Karim The Control Center For Addictions, Beverly Hills, CA, USA

Michal Kunz Kirby Forensic Psychiatric Center; New York University School of Medicine, New York, NY, USA

Roxanne M. Lewin University of Medicine & Dentistry of New Jersey, NJ, USA

Hallie A. Lightdale Georgetown University Counseling and Psychological Services; Georgetown University School of Medicine, Washington, DC, USA

Manuel Lopez-Leon New York University School of Medicine; New York University Child Study Center, New York, NY, USA

Julie Y. Low New York Medical College, New York, NY, USA

Avram H. Mack Georgetown University School of Medicine, Washington, DC, USA

Eve Maram Licensed Psychologist, Orange, CA, USA

Daniel A. Martell Semel Institute for Neuroscience and Human Behavior, David Geffen School of Medicine at UCLA, Los Angeles, CA, USA

Jeremy Martinez UCLA Addiction Medicine Clinic, Los Angeles, CA, USA

Maria E. McGee Georgetown University School of Medicine, Washington, DC, USA

Kathleen McKenna Child and Adolescent Psychiatry Fellowship; UCLA; Harbor-UCLA Medical Center, Department of Psychiatry, Torrance, CA, USA

Karen Miotto Department of Psychiatry and Biobehavioral Sciences, UCLA, Los Angeles, CA, USA

Christopher William Racine New York University School of Medicine, New York, NY, USA

Adam Raff New York University Medical Center, New York, NY, USA

Jesse A. Raley Adult, Child & Adolescent, and Forensic Psychiatrist, Columbia, SC, USA

Richard A. Rawson Integrated Substance Abuse Programs, UCLA, Los Angeles, CA, USA

Lara A. Ray Department of Psychiatry and Bio-behavioral Sciences, UCLA, Los Angeles, CA, USA

Lauren Reba-Harrelson University of Southern California, Institute of Psychiatry, Law, and Behavioral Science; Keck School of Medicine, Los Angeles, CA, USA

Karen B. Rosenbaum Woodhull Hospital Center; New York University Medical Center; Voluntary Faculty, New York Presbyterian Hospital, Cornell; Clinical and Forensic Psychiatrist in Private Practice, New York, NY, USA

Richard Rosner Forensic Psychiatry Residency Program, New York University School of Medicine; Forensic Psychiatry Clinic, Bellevue Hospital Center, New York, NY, USA

Charles L. Scott Department of Psychiatry & Behavioral Sciences University of California, Davis Medical Center, Sacramento, CA, USA

Fabian M. Saleh Harvard Medical School; Sexual Violence Prevention & Risk Management Program (SVP&RMP), Beth Israel Deaconess Medical Center, Boston, MA, USA

Preetpal Sandhu David Geffen School of Medicine at UCLA, Los Angeles, CA, USA

Diane Scheiner Department of Psychology, Fordham University, New York, NY, USA

Dionne Smith Coker-Appiah Georgetown University School of Medicine,Washington, DC, USA

Virginia A. Stanick Daytop Village, Inc., New York, NY, USA

Molly Tartter Department of Psychiatry and Biobehavioral Sciences, UCLA, Los Angeles, CA, USA

Pamela J. Taylor School of Medicine, Cardiff University, Wales; Abertawe Bro Morgannwg University Health Board

Patrick S. Thomas Department of Psychiatry and Biobehavioral Sciences, UCLA, Los Angeles, CA, USA

Christopher R. Thompson UCLA Department of Psychiatry, Child and Adolescent Division, Los Angeles, CA, USA

Tiffany G. Townsend Georgetown University School of Medicine, Washington, DC, USA

Tiffany Tsai, UCLA-Kern Department of Psychiatry, Bakersfield, CA, USA

John W. Tsuang Dual Diagnosis Treatment Program; Department of Psychiatry, UCLA; Harbor-UCLA Medical Center, Department of Psychiatry, Torrance, CA, USA

Himanshu P. Upadhyaya Department of Psychiatry and Behavioral Sciences; Eli Lilly and Company, Indianapolis, IN, USA

Wilfred G. van Gorp Columbia University College of Physicians & Surgeons, Department of Psychiatry, New York, NY, USA

Eleanor Vo Psychiatric Screening Center, Department of Psychiatry; Capital Health Regional Medical Center, Trenton, NJ, USA

Laura A. Ward Criminal Court of the City of New York, New York, NY, USA

Robert Weinstock University of California Los Angeles, Los Angeles, CA, USA

Farzin Yaghmaie University of California Los Angeles, Department of Psychiatry and Biobehavioral Sciences, Los Angeles, CA, USA

Todd Zorick UCLA Department of Psychiatry; VA West Los Angeles Medical Center, Los Angeles, CA, USA

Preface

The 1995 report of the Carnegie Council on Adolescent Development, *Great Transitions: Preparing Adolescents for a New Century*, states in its Executive Summary that:

> Since 1960, the burden of adolescent illness has shifted from the traditional causes of disease to the more behavior-related problems, such as . . . abuse of drugs (alcohol and cigarettes as well as illegal drugs). Instilling in adolescents the knowledge, skills, and values that foster physical and mental health will require substantial changes in the way health professionals work and the way they connect with families, schools, and community organizations. At least three measures are needed to meet these goals. The first is the training and availability of health providers with a deep and sensitive understanding of the developmental needs and behavior-related problems of adolescents.

The need for such training is all the more compelling in light of recent estimates of prevalence. The National Institute on Drug Abuse's (NIDA) *2011 Monitoring the Future Survey* tracks illicit drug use and attitudes of 8th-, 10th-, and 12th-grade students; it reports that, in 2010, for 12th-graders:

- 23.8% of American adolescents had used an illicit drug during the past 30-day period;
- 38.3% of American adolescents had used an illicit drug within the past year; and
- 48.2% of American adolescents had used an illicit drug sometime during their life.

By the time teenagers are seniors in high school, their use of illegal substances has become statistically almost "normal." In terms of the monetary costs and the numbers of persons affected, this is a major public health issue in the United States; other data suggest it is a major public health issue worldwide.

At the same time, a review of the major textbooks on addiction medicine and addiction psychiatry reveals that relatively little attention has been directed to the special problems of diagnosing and treating adolescent addicts. Similarly, a review of the major textbooks on general and child and adolescent psychiatry demonstrates that relatively little attention has been directed to the issues surrounding adolescent addiction. There is an "information gap" in the main textbooks that currently exist, that is, there is insufficient attention paid to addicted adolescents.

The *Clinical Handbook of Adolescent Addiction* is one response to the challenge of meeting the mental health needs and behavior-related problems of addicted teenagers. The work has been edited as an independent project by members of the American Society for Adolescent Psychiatry (ASAP), the oldest professional organization of psychiatrists devoted solely to the mental health care and treatment of teenagers in the United States. The ASAP endorsed the project in 2003 with the hope that, by putting the *Clinical Handbook of Adolescent Addiction* in the hands of those who help adolescents, a practical tool would be provided to those who need it most.

The *Clinical Handbook of Adolescent Addiction* is directed to practitioners of family medicine, general psychiatrists, child/adolescent psychiatrists, adolescent psychiatrists, addiction psychiatrists, non-psychiatric physicians specializing in addiction medicine, forensic psychiatrists, psychologists, clinical social workers, and mental health administrators, court/probation/ parole/correctional health workers; it may also be of interest and value to the parents and friends of adolescent substance abusers.

The editor gratefully acknowledges Robert Weinstock MD, Clinical Professor of Psychiatry at the University of California at Los Angeles, without whose sustained encouragement the current volume would not exist.

Richard Rosner MD

Bibliography

Carnegie Council on Adolescent, Development. *Great Transitions: Preparing Adolescents for a New Century; Concluding Report*. New York: Carnegie Corporation of New York, 1995.

National Institute on Drug Abuse. *2011 Monitoring the Future Survey*. www.drugabuse.com.

Foreword

Who does not see that I have taken a road along which I shall go, without stopping and without effort, as long as there is ink and paper in the world?

Montaigne iii, 9 [1]

Montaigne wrote this as the third sentence of his rather anxious opening paragraph in an essay on vanity. Sarah Bakewell [2] interprets it as the spirit of a man who never reached the point at which he could lay down his pen, but had to keep writing as his thoughts and experiences continued to accumulate and develop. We highlight it for this meaning too, feeling most privileged to have been invited to draft the foreword for this book, a volume that is one more powerful step in Richard Rosner's progress. Since his undergraduate thesis on Montaigne's development of a technique of personality analysis, Richard has written extensively for professional journals and written and edited some of the most important texts on adolescence and on forensic psychiatry (e.g., refs [3–5]). Notwithstanding their US focus, they are read worldwide for the thoughtfulness and scholarship he brings to everything he does. The principles of forensic and adolescent psychiatric practice, with their scientific and ethical underpinnings, are for all of us. Only laws and nature of service provision sometimes separate us.

This volume is Richard Rosner's latest edited text, this time on the problems of mind-altering substances for young people, how to recognize and assess them, and how to work towards primary prevention; but it also offers a rich array of options for damage limitation and for treatment and rehabilitation. Some of the chapters are from his own pen, many, as befits his great wisdom in this field, are from other people whom he has commissioned for their special expertise in specific aspects of the work. It is timely. Although the second chapter highlights some reductions in both moderate and hazardous alcohol use in the United Kingdom, figures remain alarming. Around the world, adolescence is the highest period of risk for starting to abuse a range of substances, and the figure of around 90% of substance-abusing adults having started to do so in their teenage years keeps emerging.

Alcohol, nicotine cigarettes, and a range of other drugs are attractive to many human beings as they variously make them feel confident and happy, relieve anxiety, block out misery or trauma, or take them into a wealth of exotic experience they would not otherwise have. Most of them have the tremendous advantage of more-or-less immediately desirable effects, and most of them have the tremendous disadvantage of a plethora of damaging but delayed effects. The certainty of immediate gratification coupled with a perceived risk – not a perceived certainty – of harm far away into the future is what makes such substances so dangerous. Health-risking behaviors are generally at their most common during adolescence [6], but promotion of health-creating behaviors of any kind is much more complex than sometimes recognized [7]. Not only do such behaviors depend on access to relevant information and services, but also they are affected by demographic and social network characteristics as well as the cognitive capacities of each individual concerned. The assumptions that underpin public participation in the prevention of disease – whether influenced by substance misuse or not – are that individuals can make an accurate cost-benefit analyses of the likely outcome of differing courses of action, believe in their own capacity for control, and implement an appropriate course of action. That collection of abilities is not always apparent in adults, and it is a big ask of adolescents, particularly when the conjunction of such skills is with poverty in social networks. This book takes account of these issues, and of the pharmacology of drugs of addiction, which, it must be acknowledged, explains a large part of the variance here, but takes us on a much richer journey too.

Some chapters broadly cluster into factors that may increase the risks of turning to alcohol or other drugs in adolescence – family context for sure, but also intrinsic individual issues, possibly interrelated, from genetics through organic brain deficits or dysfunction to both primary externalizing disorders, such as attention-deficit/hyperactivity disorder (ADHD), and primary internalizing disorders, such as depression. Too often, genetics apart, the other conditions have been taken as merely collateral damage from the substance abuse, so it is refreshing to see their etiological role considered in depth. Establishing an association between problems is only the first step. Longitudinal pathway analysis has been vital to showing that primary disorder or damage increases risk, although this is often considerably influenced by context [8]; in the longitudinal English national comorbidity study the population-attributable risk – the maximum proportion of the outcome attributable to the exposure – of psychiatric illness attributable to substance misuse was 0.2%, but that of substance misuse to psychiatric illness was 14.2% [9]. Nevertheless, the wide ranging damage done by substance abuse is substantial, not least in our field where it is a major factor in both crime victimization and crime perpetration [10]. Richard Rosner's text includes another cluster of chapters on these adverse outcomes. Thus, this important book provides ample data for primary prevention points and reasons why this is so important and, in turn, the places where secondary and tertiary interventions are so needed.

The substantial section on screening and assessment is particularly welcome. An important difficulty that emerged in younger male prisoners, who in England and Wales are much more likely to be hazardous drinkers than problem illicit drug users, was that the young men did not recognize the alcohol problem for themselves, although given an opportunity to complete a screening tool by this means did in fact reveal not only problem drinking but likely dependence of which they appeared genuinely unaware [11]. At least in the United Kingdom, little is offered to such young offenders, with a notable dearth of alcohol treatment programs in prisons [12]; they do, though, get exposed there to older prisoners who have graduated to opiates. Failure to recognize the problem may be shared by offenders and authorities.

Perhaps Montaigne's association between his writing and vanity lay in a fear that writing alone has little impact on humanity's difficulties. This text promises to be one of the exceptions. The wealth of information is brought together by a consummate clinician who cares profoundly for the young people who have come to him – whether for court reports or treatment – and who is determined to make a difference. The clinical eye that chose the authors and edited the whole has provided just what politicians as well as clinical and criminal justice practitioners are so often calling for – an evidence base for appropriate action. It should be widely read by those practitioners but also influence policy and improve life prospects for many, many young people.

Pamela J. Taylor MBBS, MRCP,
FRCPsych, FMedSci
School of Medicine, Cardiff University,
Wales; Abertawe Bro Morgannwg
University Health Board

John Gunn CBE, MD, FRCPsych,
FMedSci
Institute of Psychiatry, King's College London

References

1. Montaigne M de. *The Complete Essays* [1533–92] Penguin Classics Edition. London: Penguin Books, 1997.
2. Bakewell S. *How to Live, or a Life of Montaigne*. New York: Other Press, 2010.
3. Rosner R. *Critical Issues in American Psychiatry and the Law*. Charles C. Thomas Publishers, Ltd, 1982.
4. Rosner R. *Textbook of Adolescent Psychiatry*. London: Edward Arnold, 2003.
5. Rosner R. *Principles and Practice of Forensic Psychiatry*, 2nd edn. Oxford: Oxford University Press: 2003.
6. Blaxter M. *Health and Lifestyles*. London: Tavistock, 1990.
7. Conner M, Norman P. *Predicting Health Behaviour*. Buckingham: Open University Press, 1996.
8. Saraceno L, Heron J, Monafo M, Craddock N, van den Bree MBM. The relationship between childhood depressive symptoms and problem alcohol use in early adolescence: findings from a large longitudinal population-based study. *Addiction* 2012;**107**:567–577.
9. Frisher M, Crome I, Macleod J, Millson D, Croft P. Substance abuse and psychiatric illness: Prospective observational study using the General Practice Research Database. *J Epidemiol Commun Hlth* 2005;**59**:847–850.
10. Gunn J, Taylor PJ (eds)., *Forensic Psychiatry. Clinical, Legal and Ethical Issues*, 2nd edn. London: Hodder Arnold (in press).
11. Plant G, Taylor PJ. Recognition of problem drinking among young adult prisoners. *Behav Sci Law* 2012; **30**:140–153.
12. HM Inspectorate of Prisons. Alcohol services in prisons: an unmet need. HM Inspectorate of Prisons, 2010. Available from: http://www.justice.gov.uk/downloads/publications/hmipris/thematic-reports-and-research-publications/Alcohol_2010_rps.pdf accessed 23 03 2012.

Section One

The Scourge of
Adolescent Addiction

Edited by Richard Rosner

1

The Scourge of Addiction: What the Adolescent Psychiatrist Needs to Know[1]

Richard Rosner

Forensic Psychiatry Residency Program, New York University School of Medicine;
Forensic Psychiatry Clinic, Bellevue Hospital Center, New York, NY, USA

Adolescent dual diagnosis and the scourge of teenage addiction are endemic in the United States. The use of alcohol and other drugs by adolescents in the United States has become so common that all adolescent psychiatrists must possess baseline levels of information about the diagnosis and treatment of dually diagnosed teenagers (i.e., adolescents who have mental disorders and are using alcohol or other drugs).

This chapter is an adaptation of the Presidential Address presented at the 2004 Annual Meeting of the American Society for Adolescent Psychiatry (ASAP), Los Angeles, California. It reviews the essentials of adolescent addiction psychiatry for general adolescent psychiatrists.

ADOLESCENT DUAL DIAGNOSIS

According to Daley and Moss [1], the 1996 National Comorbidity Study of more than 8000 respondents found that lifetime rates for the general population are 26.6% for substance use disorder and 21.4% for mental disorder. Among those with mental health disorders, 51% have a coexisting substance use disorder. Among those with substance use disorders, 41–66% (depending on the drug of choice) have coexisting mental disorders.

The federal government's National Institutes of Health conducts an annual survey of teenage drug abuse in the United States. The 2010 annual survey, published in 20011, revealed that the percentages of 12th-graders using illicit drugs were as follows: 23.8% had used an illicit drug during the past 30-day period,

38.3% within the past year, and 48.2% sometime during their life [2]. In 1992, the cost of alcohol abuse for all ages of alcohol users in the United States was estimated at $148 billion, and other drug abuse costs for all ages of drug users were estimated at an additional $98 billion [3].

In addition to the considerations that make use of alcohol and other drugs a matter of concern for all psychiatric patients, particular issues need to be considered when working with dually diagnosed teenagers. Among those special issues are considerations that relate to the biological, psychological, and social ways in which adolescents differ from adults in their vulnerabilities to drugs.

The biological differences include the fact that the adolescent brain is in a process of age-related growth and development. It is now common knowledge that it is dangerous to expose the brain of a fetus to many legal and illegal drugs. Unfortunately, it is not so well known that exposing the brain of a teenager to many such drugs is also dangerous. The biological processes that ideally lead to the development of executive functions of the brain may be compromised by exposure to exogenous chemicals, so that failure of normal cognitive development may occur in adolescents who frequently use or abuse drugs. Even if a teenager eventually attains a state of recovery from his or her substance abuse disorders, it is not clear whether or not chemically induced cognitive developmental problems will spontaneously resolve themselves. With adults, the question may be whether or not drug-induced cognitive impairments will return to pre-drug adult normal brain functioning. With teenagers, however, because of the interference with normal brain development, there may be no pre-drug normal

---

[1] This chapter is a revision and up-date of a previously published article: Rosner R. The scourge of addiction: What the adolescent psychiatrist needs to know. Adolescent Psychiatry 2005; volume 29: pages 19–31.

brain functioning to which to return. Whether the teen-aged brain can ever recover from a drug-induced developmental delay or arrest is unknown at this time.

The psychological vulnerabilities of adolescents – closely correlated with their biological vulnerabilities – relate to their still-developing capacity to control impulses, engage in rational decision-making, exercise wise judgment (rather than merely acquiring knowledge), and grasp the implications of facts (rather than merely learning the facts themselves). When the focus of an adolescent's attention is on drugs (obtaining drugs, using drugs, and recovering from the acute intoxication induced by drugs), insufficient time and effort are likely to be devoted to learning and mastering the psychological abilities needed to function effectively as an autonomous person (e.g., stable accurate positive identity, emotional self-regulation). Socially, when much of an adolescent's energy is devoted to the processes related to obtaining drugs, there is likely to be impairment in interpersonal effectiveness, in establishing a stable supportive social network, and in the acquisition of positively valued knowledge and skills.

Given teenagers' special vulnerabilities to the deleterious effects of alcohol and other drugs, it is particularly important that adolescent psychiatrists have basic knowledge about addiction. Substance abuse can mimic psychiatric disorders. For example, the effects of stimulants (and the side effects of withdrawal from sedatives) may be mistaken for anxiety disorders. The effects of sedatives (and the side effects of withdrawal from stimulants) may be confused with depression. Substance-induced psychoses may be misperceived as functional psychoses. In some instances, a psychiatric diagnosis can be made with relative certainty only after the adolescent has been in a truly drug-free milieu for one or more months.

At a minimum, adolescent psychiatrists should know the answers to the following questions:

1. What screening tests are available to detect adolescent substance abusers?
2. What factors may be protective in reducing the risk of adolescent substance abuse?
3. What factors may predispose adolescents to alcohol and other drug use and abuse?
4. What warning signs suggest that an adolescent may have problems with drugs?
5. What treatment options are available to adolescent addicts?
6. What factors may reduce the risk of relapse?

What Screening Tests Are Available to Detect Adolescent Substance Abusers?

Among the rapid-screening instruments for substance abuse by teenagers are the Problem-Oriented Screening Instrument for Teenagers (POSIT) [4], the Alcohol Use Disorders Identification Test (AUDIT) [5], and the CRAFFT Screening for Substance Use Problems [6,7]. Because the CRAFFT uses an acronym for its six questions, they are especially easy to remember:

C   Have you ever ridden in a car driven by someone (including yourself) who was high or had been using alcohol or drugs?
R   Do you ever use alcohol or drugs to relax, feel better about yourself, or fit in?
A   Do you ever use alcohol or drugs while you are alone?
F   Do you ever forget things you did while using alcohol or drugs?
F   Do your family or friends ever tell you that you should cut down on your drinking or drug use?
T   Have you ever gotten into trouble while you were using alcohol or drugs?

Two or more positive responses on the CRAFFT identifies teenagers whose alcohol and/or drug use warrants further assessment. The psychiatrist must be aware of the fact that the CRAFFT only works if the adolescent provides honest answers to its questions; it is invalidated by deceit.

Any teenager who is suspected of substance abuse should have a urine drug screening. It is a challenge to present the request for a urine specimen in a manner that does not harm the adolescent's rapport with the psychiatrist. It may be useful to put the request for a urine specimen in the most positive frame: for instance, by stating that it is an opportunity for the adolescent to demonstrate objectively that he or she is not currently abusing drugs. (The psychiatrist should be aware that most drugs are undetectable in urine more than 3 days after the drug has been used.) If an adolescent has no substance abuse to hide, he or she has every reason to provide a urine sample. Teenagers who refuse to provide urine specimens for drug screening should be regarded as at higher risk for using drugs. The more vociferous the adolescent's refusal and the greater his or her indignation, the higher should be the psychiatrist's level of suspicion.

Adolescent psychiatrists should be familiar with the special precautions to be taken with substance-abusing teenagers to ensure that the urine sample obtained is actually from the specific patient from whom it was sought. Substance-abusing teenagers are often sophisticated in methods to avoid being detected on urine screening tests. Substitution of someone else's clean urine sample is common. So is dilution of a urine sample so that the concentration of the drugs is too low to be detected. Claiming to have urinated so recently that there is no urine left to provide for an immediate sample is another dodge. Most commercial laboratories and most pediatricians are not trained to routinely address, let alone avoid, these urine collection problems. Patients should provide a urine sample under the direct observation of a health professional (if necessary, after being given two ordinary glasses of water to drink and after sufficient time has elapsed for a urine sample to be obtainable). The possibility that the drug-abusing teenager (often much more knowledgeable about these matters than the psychiatrist) has deliberately ingested some food or other legal substance to mask the presence of an illegal substance should also be considered. Drug-abusing youths may claim that a urine test has produced a false positive; all positive findings on routine high-sensitivity urine screenings for drugs should automatically be retested using more highly selective tests.

What Factors May Reduce the Risk of Adolescent Substance Abuse?

According to MacNamee [8], protective factors include the following:

1. strong ties to family and community;
2. involvement in church or religious groups;
3. parents who set limits, provide supervision, and make clear their explicit expectations that alcohol and drugs will not be used;
4. personal traits of optimism, self-esteem, and risk avoidance; and
5. residence in a stable community without drug trade or street violence.

What Factors May Predispose Adolescents to Alcohol and Other Drug Use and Abuse?

As cited by Bates and Hendren [9], these factors include:

1. parental attitudes toward substance abuse, such as permissiveness;
2. genetic vulnerability to substance abuse;
3. participation in a peer culture in which others use drugs; and
4. individual characteristics such as low self-esteem, aversion to conformity, lack of religious and school involvement, and sensation-seeking.

Generally, a teenager with two or more of these predisposing factors may be regarded as at relatively increased risk for substance abuse.

What Warning Signs Suggest Adolescent Problems with Alcohol and Other Drugs?

A high index of suspicion is warranted in the presence of other psychiatric disorders, notably attention-deficit/hyperactivity disorder, conduct disorder, depressive disorders, or anxiety disorders [10]. Warning signs cited by MacNamee [8] include the following:

1. Problems at school (e.g., unexplained drop in grades, unexplained drop in performance, irregular attendance).
2. Problems with health (e.g., accidents; frequent "flu" episodes; chronic cough, chest pains, and allergy symptoms).
3. Problems with the family (e.g., decreased interest in family activities, not bringing friends home, unexplained delays in returning home after school, unaccounted-for personal time, evasive responses about activities, unexplained disappearance of possessions in the home, mistreatment of younger siblings).
4. Problems with peers (e.g., old friends are discarded, new friends are acquired, preference for parties at which parental adults are not present, strange phone calls).

What Treatment Options Are Available to Adolescents Who Abuse Alcohol and Other Drugs?

These include (i) self-help organizations such as Alcoholics Anonymous (AA), Narcotics Anonymous (NA), and Self-Management and Recovery Training (SMART Recovery®[2]); (ii) individual, group, and family outpatient therapies; (iii) day treatment centers; (iv) intensive outpatient treatment programs; (v) residential treatment centers; and (vi) psychiatric hospitalization.

In considering which patients should be treated on an outpatient basis, Bates and Hendren [9] suggest that the indications for outpatient treatment include the adolescent's acceptance of having a substance abuse problem and acceptance of the need for help; willingness to abstain from all substances of abuse; cooperation with random urine drug screens to ensure compliance; and ability to commit to regular attendance at therapy and support groups. They further state that teenagers should not be treated on an outpatient basis if they have acute medical or psychiatric problems requiring an intense level of supervision, chronic medical problems that

---

[2] SMART Recovery® is an alternative to AA, NA and 12-step programs, using cognitive behavioral therapy (CBT) principles and a secular approach. Detailed information is available at www.smartrecovery.org.

preclude outpatient treatment, continued association with substance-abusing peers, lack of motivation for treatment, or history of prior failure of outpatient treatment. Other contraindications to outpatient treatment include significant resistance to authority, major family dysfunction, and inability to function without strong outside support [9].

What Factors May Reduce the Risk of Relapse?

In reviewing treatment outcome studies, Bates and Hendren [9] found that relapse rates ranged from 35% to 85% overall, and that positive outcome is associated with constructive peer influences and family and religious support, active family involvement in the treatment, court pressure (especially during the early phase of treatment), and voluntary participation in treatment.

How Does One Learn to Treat Adolescents with Addiction Problems?

Most adolescent psychiatrists are not trained in addiction psychiatry. Such training may be obtained by participation in postresidency continuing medical education programs, such as those provided by the American Society for Addiction Medicine (ASAM) and the American Academy of Addiction Psychiatry (AAAP) and by reading any of the major textbooks on addiction psychiatry. The US government, through the National Institute of Drug Abuse (NIDA) and the National Institute of Alcohol Abuse and Alcoholism (NIAAA), provides some excellent reading materials related to addiction. For example, in Project MATCH, NIAAA funded a multicenter research project involving more than 1700 alcohol-abusing patients [11,12]. This project studied the comparative efficacy of three treatment approaches: motivational enhancement therapy, a modification of motivational interviewing; cognitive behavioral therapy; and 12-step facilitation. All three types of treatment were found to be of essentially equal effectiveness. One of the most useful outcomes of Project Match was the development of its training manuals for the three types of treatment. Therapists who wish to learn these specific psychotherapeutic approaches can obtain the manuals from NIAAA and train themselves in the theory and practice of each of the techniques (see the NIAAA webpage at http://www.niaaa.nih.gov/publications/publications. htm, for a list of publications).

Which Therapy is Appropriate for Whom?

The therapeutic intervention that should be used depends on the stage of substance use of the individual adolescent. There are four stages of substance use:

1. *Experimentation or casual use.* Teenagers who are experimenting or casually using alcohol or other drugs may respond to education about the risks of substance abuse, and brief counseling.
2. *Regular use.* Teenagers who regularly use alcohol or other drugs may respond to education and counseling, to individual or group psychotherapy, to family therapy, and to implementation of abstinence contracts.
3. *Abuse.* Teenagers who are abusing alcohol or other drugs may respond to such individual outpatient therapies as motivational interviewing, cognitive behavioral therapy, or 12-step programs. Those who do not respond to such individual outpatient therapies may respond to intensive outpatient treatment, to partial hospitalization, or to inpatient treatment in a residential treatment center or a hospital.
4. *Dependence.* Teenagers who are dependent on alcohol or other drugs may respond to inpatient treatment in a residential treatment center or a hospital with aftercare at an intensive outpatient treatment program or a halfway house, or to multisystemic therapy as developed by Pickrel and Henggeler [12].

It is essential, when recommending treatment, to consider the adolescent's stage of readiness for change. The therapist's efforts are most likely to be effective when they are consistent with the adolescent's stage of readiness. Prochaska and DiClemente have developed a transtheoretical model (TTM) of intentional change, a model that focuses on decision-making [14]. This model integrates key constructs from other theories to describe how people modify a problem behavior or acquire a positive behavior. It involves emotions, cognitions, and behavior, and takes into account the fact that individuals vary in their readiness to change. Prochaska and DiClemente note that relapse may occur repeatedly and at any stage of change. The following are their stages of readiness for change.

- *Precontemplation.* The adolescent has not considered changing or has no thought of changing during the coming 6 months. An adolescent at the precontemplation stage may be willing to consider facts about the risks of substance use but almost certainly will not be willing to accept any proffered treatments.
- *Contemplation.* The adolescent has considered changing or has thought of changing sometime in the coming 6 months. An adolescent at the contemplation stage may be willing to consider the advantages and disadvantages of changing but is also unlikely to be willing to commit to any specific treatment.
- *Preparation.* The adolescent is planning specifically how and what to change. An adolescent at the preparation state may be willing to consider what

types of treatments are available and their costs, convenience, and efficacy but is not likely to respond to pressure to commit to treatment.

- *Action.* The adolescent is implementing a specific change or changes. An adolescent at the action stage may respond to referral to specific treatments but is unlikely to be ready to address relapse prevention strategies.
- *Maintenance.* The adolescent is continuing the change or changes. An adolescent at the maintenance stage may respond to relapse-prevention training.

When the therapist's efforts with the adolescent are not consistent with the adolescent's stage of readiness, then the therapist's efforts are not likely to be effective. The therapist needs to determine the stage of readiness for change of the specific adolescent patient in order to have any hope of moving the teenager from an earlier stage to the next stage.

Motivational Interviewing

One of the individual psychotherapeutic approaches that is suited to the TTM conceptualization of stages of change is motivational interviewing [15], which focuses on exploring and resolving ambivalence. In motivational interviewing, the therapist avoids telling patients what to do; rather, the focus is on assisting the patient in resolving ambivalences constructively and engaging in self-determined courses of action.

The spirit of motivational interviewing is based on four core approaches to patients: expression of empathy for the patient; development of discrepancies between the patient's current situation and the patient's aspirations; finding ways around the patient's resistances; and supporting the patient's efforts at self-efficacy. Miller and Rollnick [15] regard motivational interviewing as a systematically respectful philosophical approach to patients, rather than as a set of techniques that can paternalistically be applied to manipulate patients into changing. Their approach is derived in part from Carl Rogers' client-centered therapy [16]. Although motivational interviewing involves reflective listening, it is more focused and goal-directed than Rogers' nondirective counseling. Among the hallmarks of motivational interviewing are the following:

Open-ended questions. Motivational interviewers ask questions that require discursive responses. (Miller and Rollnick [15] suggest that no more than three questions be asked in a row before engaging in reflection or summarization.)
Reflective listening. Motivational interviewers selectively inquire about facets of the patient's discursive responses.

Affirming and supporting the patient. Motivational interviewers are empathically encouraging and supportive of the patient's constructive aspirations.
Summarizing the patient's own statements. Motivational interviewers periodically link elements of the patient's discursive responses to summarize the themes and meaningful content of the patient's utterances.
Eliciting change talk. Drawing on the patient's ambivalence regarding the costs and benefits of continued use of alcohol or other drugs, motivational interviewers encourage patients to consider their options (e.g., what might be changed, what are the advantages and disadvantages of changing or not changing, how change might occur, how to overcome obstacles to change, and how to sustain change).

There are reasons to think that motivational interviewing might be especially effective with adolescents, who often are unwilling to take direction from adult authorities. Unlike cognitive behavioral therapists or 12-step facilitating therapists, motivational interviewers do not tell patients what to do, do not tell patients what is right and wrong, and do not assume a superior interpersonal stance in their work with patients. Rather, motivational interviewers work with the patient's own ambivalence about substance use and, through selective reinforcement of the patient's own discursive remarks, assist the patient in developing the motivation to move along the stages of change from precontemplation to contemplation, to preparation, to action, to maintenance. Motivational interviewers regard the patient's resistance to change as a technical problem to be constructively addressed by continuing to work with the patient in a non-confrontational manner. According to Zweben and Zuckoff [17], motivational interviewing can be constructively adapted for use with the adolescent population with practical therapeutic success.

CONCLUSION

Given the ubiquity of alcohol and other drugs in our society, and given the data on the prevalence of adolescents' experimentation with substances of abuse, adolescent psychiatrists must have baseline levels of information about addiction psychiatry. It is appropriate that the American Society for Adolescent Psychiatry (ASAP) devoted fully one-third of its annual scientific program in 2004 in Los Angeles to issues related to adolescent addiction. It is consistent with ASAP's dedication to the health of all teenagers that ASAP is taking a leadership role in bridging the knowledge gap between specialists in adolescent psychiatry and specialists in addiction psychiatry. In the future, it is hoped that every adolescent psychiatrist will possess competence in the diagnosis and treatment of teenagers with substance abuse problems.

Acknowledgement

This chapter is a revision and up-date of a previously published article: Rosner R. The scourge of addiction: What the adolescent psychiatrist needs to know. Adolescent Psychiatry 2005; volume 29: pages 19–31.

References

1. Daley D, Moss H. *Dual Disorders: Counseling Clients with Chemical Dependency and Mental Illness*, 3rd edn. Center City, MN: Hazelden, 2002.
2. The National Institute on Drug Abuse. *Monitoring the Future Survey 2010*. NIDA, 2011. Available at: http://www.drugabuse.gov/.
3. National Institute on Drug Abuse and National Institute on Alcoholism and Alcohol Abuse. *The Economic Costs of Alcohol and Drug Abuse in the United States 1992*. Rockville, MD: NIAAA, 1998.
4. Gruenewald PJ, Klitzner M. Results of preliminary POSIT analyses. In: Radhert E (ed.), *Adolescent Assessment Referral System Manual*. DHHS Publication No. (ADM) 91-1735, reprint 1994. Rockville, MD: National Clearinghouse for Alcohol and Drug Information, 1991.
5. Saunders JB, Aasland OG, Babor TF, de laPuente JR, Grant M. Development of the Alcohol Use Disorders Screening Test (AUDIT): WHO collaborative project on early detection of persons with harmful alcohol consumption, II. *Addiction* 1993;**88**:791–804.
6. Knight JR, Sherritt L, Shrier LA, Harris SK, Chang G. Validity of the CRAFFT substance abuse screening test among adolescent clinic patients. *Arch Pediatr Adolesc Med* 2002;**156**:607–614.
7. Knight JR, Sherritt L, Harris SK, Gates EC, Chang G. Validity of brief alcohol screening tests among adolescents: A comparison of the AUDIT, POSIT, CAGE, and CRAFFT. *Alcohol Clin Exp Res* 2003;**27**:67–73.
8. MacNamee H. Adolescents. In: Kinney J (ed.), *Loosening the Grip: A Handbook of Alcohol Information*. New York: McGraw-Hill, 2003; pp. 351–378.
9. Bates M, Hendren R. Adolescent substance abuse. In: Rosner R (ed.), *Textbook of Adolescent Psychiatry*. London: Edward Arnold, 2003; pp. 328–340.
10. Paoletti D, Stewart K, DiClemente R. Alcohol and substance abuse among adolescents: Prevention and intervention. In: Rosner R (ed.), *Textbook of Adolescent Psychiatry*. London: Edward Arnold, 2003; pp. 101–111.
11. Project MATCH Research Group. Project MATCH (Matching Alcoholism Treatment to Client Heterogeneity): Rationale and methods for a multisite clinical trial matching patients to alcoholism treatment. *Alcohol Clin Exp Res* 1993;**17**:1130–1145.
12. Project MATCH Research Group. Matching alcoholism treatments to client heterogeneity: Project MATCH three-year drinking outcomes. *Alcohol Clin Exp Res* 1998;**22**:1300–1311.
13. Pickrel SG, Henggeler SW. Multisystemic therapy for adolescent substance abuse and dependence. *Child Adolesc Psych Clin N Am* 1996;**5**:201–212.
14. DiClemente C, Velazquez M. Motivational interviewing and the stages of change. In: Miller W, Rollnick S (eds), *Motivational Interviewing: Preparing People for Change*, 2nd edn. New York: Guilford Press, 2002; pp. 201–216.
15. Miller W, Rollnick S. *Motivational Interviewing: Preparing People for Change*, 2nd edn. New York: Guilford Press, 2002.
16. Rogers CR. *Client-Centered Therapy: Its Current Practice, Implications, and Theory*. Boston: Houghton Mifflin, 1951.
17. Zweben A, Zuckoff A. Motivational interviewing with adolescents and young adults. In: Miller W, Rollnick S (eds), *Motivational Interviewing: Preparing People for Change*, 2nd edn. New York: Guilford Press, 2002; pp. 299–319.

2

Adolescent Addictions in the United Kingdom

Tahira Akbar,[1] Alex Baldacchino,[1] and Ilana Crome[2]

[1] University of Dundee Medical School, Dundee, UK
[2] Department of Psychiatry, Keele University Medical School, Keele, UK

EPIDEMIOLOGY

Context

Over the last two decades there has been an increasing realization that substance problems in teenagers are a reality and may be associated with formidable social, psychological, and physical problems. Substance use trends worldwide are derived using a variety of methodologies and population samples, therefore establishing differing global trends can be difficult.

In general terms, teenage confers the highest risk for the development of substance use disorders. Those with the most severe substance disorders are likely to suffer psychiatric and physical comorbidity. However, even though there may be a reduction of substance use during adulthood, the consequences may linger as it is estimated that about 90% of adults who are dependent started to use during adolescence, and half initiated substance use before the age of 15. It is beyond the scope of this chapter to discuss the symptomatology of medical and psychiatric consequences in detail (see other relevant chapters in this book), so selected relevant findings from the recent UK literature pertaining to the epidemiology of substance misuse, associated risk factors and the relationship to policy and practice are presented.

In the United Kingdom alone substance use trends are measured within a number of national surveys [1–5]. The European School Survey Project on Alcohol and other Drugs (ESPAD) and the Health Behaviour in School-aged Children (HBSC) survey are examples of standardized surveys reporting substance use trends among young people across Europe and countries worldwide [6,7]. Limitations for all of the above surveys are, however, acknowledged; most notable is that data collection is frequently made from easily accessible populations, including school students, therefore individuals at highest risk are underrepresented in the statistics, namely the homeless, people in prison, or those housed within institutional settings. Moreover, the key national household surveys in England and Wales (British Crime Survey), Scotland (Scottish Crime and Justice Survey), and Northern Ireland (Northern Ireland Crime Survey) present trends and prevalence derived from private households and will therefore exclude young people living in student accommodations. These surveys will also report behaviors over at least three time periods: lifetime use, last year use and last month use. Whilst last month use is noted to be an indicator of recent behaviors it is also recognized that last month use is subject to seasonal variations and, when compared with last year use, is a weaker statistic. In terms of drug-related behaviors the national surveys will frequently report illicit drug use patterns and therefore omit unlegislated drugs currently unidentified in the drug classifications (Misuse of Drugs Act 1971). For example, the use of increasingly popular drugs termed "legal highs" are not currently reported in UK household surveys. The schools surveys are also largely comparable in terms of methodologies, measures, and definitions although there is some variability across countries; for example, the Scottish Schools Adolescent Lifestyle and Substance Use Survey (SALSUS) survey in Scotland has a number of questions pertaining to known risk factors, such as family attitudes and influence on behaviors. Thus, not all the information presented in these surveys can

Clinical Handbook of Adolescent Addiction, First Edition. Richard Rosner.

be compared across countries. Currently in the United Kingdom, prescription drug misuse is not measured in either the household or school surveys.

Alcohol

In comparison with other countries, UK consumption of alcohol is rising, especially in women and young people. It is both the quantity of alcohol and pattern of drinking that lead to harm and to dependence, and that need to be considered. "Binge drinking" in young people has become a particular source of concern in some countries. Although this behavior does not necessarily persist into adult life, there are concerns that damage accrued during this period may impact upon long-term health. There is considerable interest around the "risk" of harm; for example, heavy alcohol intake may lead to cirrhosis but "moderate" consumption may reduce the risk of coronary artery disease.

Younger drinkers are more likely to suffer accidents, assaults, and acute intoxication. It is estimated that 30 000 hospital admissions per year are due to alcohol dependence syndrome, and 150 000 are related to alcohol misuse, whereas 20 000 alcohol misusers die prematurely. At a conservative estimate, this costs the UK's National Health Service 1.9 billion GBP, and this excludes the inestimable cost to families and communities, partly due to alcohol-related crime and public order offences, for which the cost is calculated at 7.3 billion GBP. Unemployment and decreased productivity are additional consequences and costs. The wider, and more difficult to quantify, social harms cannot be ignored. Family relationships, stability, and income diminish, with an estimated one million children affected by alcohol misuse in the family.

England

During 2009, 51% of 11–15-year-olds in England reported consumption of at least one alcoholic drink in their lifetime (a decline from 61% in 2003), and the number of pupils reporting no alcohol consumption rose from 39% in 2003 to 49% in 2009. Alcohol consumption within the previous week had also declined from 26% in 2001 to 18% in 2009, with older pupils drinking more than younger ones (3% of 11-year-olds compared to 38% of 15-year-olds). The mean weekly alcohol consumption was 11.6 units for 11–15-year-olds, with no significant difference between boys and girls (11.0 vs 11.3 units, respectively). Boys were, however, more likely to consume beer, lager, or cider in the last week than girls, who drank more alcopops, wine, and spirits. White pupils were more likely to have consumed alcohol within the previous week than pupils from Mixed or Asian ethnic backgrounds [8].

An estimated 10 000 children and young people, under the age of 18, were reportedly admitted to hospital each year as a result of their drinking [9]. Where problematic use is concerned, the number of under-18s receiving help for alcohol use in specialist treatment services was observed to decline by more than 6% to 8227 during 2009–10 in England (a reduction of 572 since 2008–09). Similar to drug use trends, young patients are less likely to be represented in specialist treatment services. Alcohol is almost equally represented as the primary drug of concern across the younger age ranges (from 40% at age 12 and under to 34% at 17–18 years) [10].

Scotland

Alcohol consumption trends in Scottish school children have been measured since 1990. The most recent survey results from 2008 reported that 66% of 12–16-year-olds had "ever had an alcoholic drink," representing a reduction from previous self-reported data. This population is divided into two distinct age groups (13 years and 15 years) in order to maintain comparability with previous classroom surveys. No gender difference was apparent between the two age groups although, at "15 years," girls were slightly more likely than boys to have ever had an alcoholic drink (83% vs 80%, respectively). In contrast, "15-year-old boys" consumed significantly greater amounts of alcohol than "15-year-old girls" (21 units vs 15 units, respectively). When choosing which alcohol product to consume the greatest difference reported was that boys were more likely to consume beer, lager, cider, and shandy (beer mixed with non-alcoholic drink) whereas girls had a preference towards alcopops in both age groups. From the pupils who reported having ever consumed alcohol, half of "13-year-olds" reported having been "really drunk" at least once, rising to 72% for "15-year-olds." At "15 years" girls were more likely to report having been "really drunk" than boys, with no significant gender difference with younger respondents. For the period 2004–08 reports of being "really drunk" have remained relatively stable [1].

Another of the measures reported in the SALSUS are self-reported effects of alcohol consumption. The two most common complaints reported were vomiting and having an argument. Boys were more likely than girls to be involved with police. Incidents of hospitalization or visiting the emergency department (A&E) were more common amongst "15-year-olds" although overall relatively uncommon (5%) [1].

During 2009, Scottish victims of violent crimes reported the offender(s) involved had been under the influence of alcohol in 62% of cases. This figure was higher than the equivalent reported in England and Wales during the same period (50%). A further 30% of Scottish victims of violent crime reported they themselves had consumed alcohol immediately prior to the incident [3].

Wales

During the period 2005–06, 4% of girls and 7% of boys aged 11 years in Wales reported consuming alcohol at least once a week. By age 13 years weekly alcohol consumption had increased to 20% of girls and 23% of boys, and by 15 years of age 38% of girls and 51% of boys drank alcohol on a weekly basis. No significant gender difference was indicated for all these ages; however, high family affluence was significantly associated with higher rates of drinking in boys. When asked about the age at which they first experienced drunkenness, 21% of girls and 25% of boys in Wales responded at age 13 years or younger. When asked if they had been drunk at least twice, no significant difference was apparent between the genders at ages 13 years and 15 years, although prevalence did substantially increase with age (4% of girls and 8% of boys at age 13 years and 26% of girls and 27% of boys aged 15 years). Weekly alcohol consumption in 13-year-olds was higher in Wales than in England and Scotland, and Wales had the third highest percentage amongst 13-year-old girls when compared with all countries taking part in this international study [6].

During 2009–10 alcohol was identified as the main concern for treatment; 218 referrals were indicated for individuals aged under 15 years (101 male; 117 female) and 1031 for those aged 15 to 19 years (643 male, 388 female). The number of annual hospital admissions attributed to alcohol use is consistently higher in females aged 14 years or younger when compared with boys; however, the number of admissions has consistently declined in females (110 in 2008 to 95 in 2009) whereas in boys an increase was observed between the last two surveys (58 during 2008 to 68 in 2009). For 15–19-year-olds, an initial increase in hospital admissions between 2005 and 2006 has since continued to decline (118 admissions for males during 2009 compared with 91 for females) [4].

Northern Ireland

Just over half (54%) of 11–16-year-olds in Northern Ireland report they have consumed alcohol, of which over three-quarters (76%) were aged 13 years or younger when they had their first drink. One-fifth of these pupils no longer drink, and two-fifths (38%) report drinking alcohol within the previous week [5]. On 1 March 2010 a total of 644 young people aged under 18 years were seeking treatment from drug and alcohol services in Northern Ireland. Half of these young people (49.5%) accessing health services were seeking treatment for alcohol use alone, and 23.9% sought treatment for alcohol and drug use [11].

Illicit Drug Use

England and Wales

According to the 2009/10 British Crime Survey, 40.7% of 16–24-year-olds in England and Wales were estimated to have ever used illicit drugs (approximately 2.7 million young people). Of this population 20.0% had used illicit drugs over the previous year (an estimated 1.3 million people) compared with higher figures reported in the past (29.7% in 1996 and 22.6% in 2008–09). Cannabis remained the most common drug, used by an estimated one in six adults (16.1%; an estimated 1.1 million young adults) followed by powder cocaine (5.5%) and ecstasy (4.3%). Within the same population, the age of first use had lowered with respect to cannabis (16 years) and cocaine (18 years) whereas age of first use of ecstasy had reportedly stabilized (18 years) [2].

England Alone

A survey of 11–15-year-olds in England during 2009 reported a continuing decline in overall drug use, from 29% in 2001 to 22% in 2009, with boys more likely to have taken drugs than girls in the last year (16% and 14% respectively). The most common drugs used included cannabis (8.9%) or volatile substances such as glue, gas, aerosols or solvents (5.5%). Drug use also directly correlated with age, with 5% of 11-year-olds using drugs over the previous year rising to 30% of 15-year-olds. The reported trends in relation to age of first use showed those aged 12 years or younger were more likely to have used volatile substances whereas respondents who reported age of first use as 13 years or older were more likely to have consumed cannabis. Moreover, the pattern of drug use was also linked to the type of drugs students used. The younger users using volatile substances were less likely to describe frequent drug use when compared to older students using Class A drugs including cocaine [8].

The treatment trends for substance use amongst young people in England have seen figures more than double in the last 5 years; however, recent reports indicate the numbers are stabilizing, with 23 528 under-18s identified in specialist substance misuse services – a reduction of 525 from 2008–09. The majority of young people will experience problems with cannabis (53%), 2% will seek help with problematic heroin or crack use, less than 2% will seek assistance with cocaine use (a reduction of 43% over the last 2 years), and less than 0.5% will seek help with ecstasy use (a reduction of 79% over the last 2 years). The number of young people seeking help is also directly correlated with age, and those who are younger are less likely to be seen in treatment services. Moreover, in the under-12 age range no individual was treated for Class A drug use although a small number did require support for cannabis, alcohol, and solvent use [10].

Wales Alone

Reported lifetime cannabis use amongst 15-year-olds during 2005–06 was 32% amongst girls and 30% amongst boys. Recent cannabis use (within the last 30 days) was 12% amongst boys and 11% amongst girls [6].

Welsh statistics for 2009–10 provide further information regarding admissions to healthcare services for drug- and alcohol-related concerns across the population. Where substance use was identified as a main concern, 180 referrals were aged 15 years or younger and 1222 were between 15 and 19 years. Amongst the under-15-year-olds, five referrals were identified for heroin-related treatment, 121 for cannabis, three for amphetamines, and two cases for cocaine use. For the 15–19-year-olds, 218 referrals were reportedly for heroin-related concerns, 698 for cannabis, 36 for amphetamines, 77 for cocaine, and six for crack cocaine [4].

From referrals made during 2009–10 for individuals aged under 20 years, 1760 (75.1% of individuals) were not previously known to services; however, 1099 had been seen on an earlier occasion and 516 had been seen during the previous year [4].

Further statistics reported for young people during 2009–10 included those aged 16 years or younger who had been excluded from school. From the 19 247 exclusions reported, substance misuse was identified in 14.1% ($n = 30$) of permanent exclusions, 2.2% ($n = 384$) of fixed term 5 days or less, and 4.3% ($n = 70$) were for fixed term exclusions of 6 or more days. Whilst overall numbers for all exclusions have declined over past surveys, the proportion linked with substance misuse increased by 14.1% from 2006–07 to 2007–08 and by 15.2% from 2007–08 to 2008–09 [4].

Scotland

The 2009/10 Scottish Crime and Justice Survey (SCJS) reported the incidence of drug use correlating with age and the lowest age ranges surveyed reporting the highest use. Drug use within the previous year was reported by 20.2% of 16–24-year-olds compared with 0.2% of those

aged 60 and over. Drug use in the month prior to survey found 11.7% of 16–24-year-olds had used drugs compared with 0.1% of those aged 60 or over. When questioned about age of first use most reported 16–19 years (52%), and 25.2% indicated they were less than 16 years old. The majority of users (78.3%), regardless of age, reported cannabis as their first drug used [12].

In a survey of the younger Scottish population, drug use was observed to increase with age (23% of 15-year-olds reporting drug use compared with 7% of 13-year-olds). The reported trends for drug use show that the figures in Scotland have stabilized since 2006, with the only reduction observed in 13-year-old boys (from 4% to 3%). In the past boys were more likely to report drug use than girls; however, in 2008 a significant difference was only reported amongst 15-year-olds (25% of boys vs 22% of girls). The majority of students reported cannabis as their drug of choice (13% of 15-year-old boys, 10% of 15-year-old girls and 2% for both 13-year-old girls and boys) [1].

Social housing was also correlated with age of first use: those living in social rented accommodation were more likely to have first tried a drug when aged under 16 compared with those in private rented accommodation (36.6% vs 25.8%, respectively). This trend was also evident with those living in the 15% most deprived areas of Scotland, who more likely to first try drugs aged under 16 when compared with the rest of the population (36.6% vs 23.1%, respectively) [12]. The most frequently reported locations of drug use in Scotland, were outdoors (46% of 15-year-olds and 47% of 13-year-olds) and at someone else's home (36% of 15-year-olds and 24% of 13-year-olds). Girls were more likely than boys to take drugs at someone else's home [1].

The SCJS 2009/10 victims of violent crimes reported the offender(s) involved had been under the influence of drugs in just over one in four (26%) cases. The figure for Scotland was higher than the equivalent figure for England and Wales for the same period (20% of violent crimes) [3].

Northern Ireland

In Northern Ireland a survey of 6902 school pupils aged 11–16 years during 2007 determined that 15% had been offered solvents. Whilst 8% of pupils had inhaled solvents, over half (55%) indicated they were no longer using. Twenty-four percent of pupils surveyed reported they had been offered drugs (excluding solvents) of which fewer than half (49%) had used drugs at any time. The most common drugs tried included cannabis (9%), poppers (6%), ecstasy (3%), and cocaine (3%). Questions in relation to frequency of use for the most common drug determined that one in four (26%) used cannabis at least a few times a month, one in four (26%) used less than a few times a year, and two out of five (41%) were not current users [5]. On 1 March 2010 a census in Northern Ireland identified that 5846 individuals were enrolled in treatment programs offered by drug and alcohol treatment agencies. Of these, 73% were male and 27% female, and the majority were over 18 years of age (89%). Six hundred and forty-four individuals aged under 18 years were treated of whom 80% were male. A total of 1294 individuals presented for treatment in relation to drug use alone and of these 13% (171 individuals) were under 18 years. From the 1224 individuals presenting for both drug and alcohol misuse, 13% were under 18 years [11].

Smoking

England

Three in ten (29%) students aged 11–15 years in England during 2009 reported having tried smoking at least once. Six percent of students reported regular smoking at least once a week with girls more likely to do so than boys (7% vs 5%, respectively). Prevalence was reported to increase with age, from less than 0.5% to 15% in 11- and 15-year-olds respectively, although overall the trends for prevalence had declined from previous annual surveys. Other factors associated with higher likelihood of smoking included ethnicity (White pupils were more likely to smoke than pupils of Black or Mixed ethnicity), being in receipt of free school meals, and coming from a low income family. Regular smoking was linked to alcohol consumption, drug use, and truancy and exclusion from school [8].

For the period 2005–06, 15-year-old girls were significantly more likely to have smoked at age 13 years or less (34% of girls compared with 26% of boys). When weekly smoking habits were analyzed over a range of years no significant age difference was apparent in 11-year-olds (1% of boys and girls smoked weekly). By age 13 years, a significant difference was determined, with girls more likely to report smoking weekly (12% of girls compared with 6% of boys). At 15 years this significant difference between genders was sustained, with 23% of girls smoking at least once a week compared with 12% of boys. Lower family affluence was significantly associated with both early smoking initiation and reporting weekly smoking in girls surveyed. This association was not apparent in boys [6].

Scotland

In Scotland the legal age for smoking was increased from 16 to 18 years during October 2007. The most recent trends, published in 2008, reported prevalence of smoking increasing with age, with 4% of 13-year-olds smoking regularly and 4% smoking occasionally, compared with 15% and 6% respectively of 15-year-olds. There was no gender difference amongst 13-year-olds; however, 15-year-old girls were less likely to have never smoked than boys (47% vs 55%, respectively) [1].

In Scotland, most school students surveyed reported that family played a significant role in stopping them smoking or persuading them to smoke. Where families were aware of smoking behaviors regular smokers were more likely to be allowed to smoke at home. Deprivation was also associated with smoking, with a greater association observed amongst 13-year-olds when compared with 15-year-olds. The ages of friends was also shown to vary by smoking status, with smokers more likely to have friends of mixed ages when compared with non-smokers [1].

Wales

During 2005–06 girls were significantly more likely to report first smoking at age 13 years or younger (34% of girls compared with 26% of boys). At age 11 years 1% of girls and boys reported smoking at least once a week. By age 13 years, girls reported significantly higher rates of weekly smoking (12% of girls compared with 6% of boys). This significant difference was sustained up to the age of 15 years, when 23% of girls and 12% of boys reported smoking at least once a week. The findings show early experience of smoking and higher levels of weekly smoking amongst girls was significantly associated with lower family affluence in Wales [6].

Northern Ireland

During 2007 just under a quarter of 11–16-year-olds in Northern Ireland reported having smoked tobacco, of whom four-fifths indicated starting at age 13 years or younger. Sixty-four percent of those who had smoked reported no longer doing so and a quarter reported smoking every day. Four-fifths of pupils who smoked at least once a week indicated a desire to quit [5].

Prescription Drugs

In Britain many of the national resources for indicating drug use prevalence and trends do not provide information regarding prescription drug use. The SCJS explicitly excludes data in relation to prescription drug use; similarly, SALSUS, British Crime Survey and General Lifestyle Survey do not report prescription drug use trends.

Across Europe, figures for use of non-prescribed tranquilizers or sedatives can be derived from the 2009 ESPAD survey for respondent countries across Europe. The reported trends varied from 0 to 2% in Armenia, Austria, Russia, and the United Kingdom to 15% in Poland, Lithuania, France, and Monaco. Overall figures for gender differences indicated girls reported higher levels of prescription drug use (8% vs 5%) although no difference was found in half of all countries.

RISK AND RESILIENCE

There are a host of "reasons" why people use substances, and of factors, or interaction of factors, that may influence their decisions. These may include increasing availability, low price, promotion of drinks aimed at a particular group, peer pressure, a culture that encourages "drinking to get drunk," early onset of substance misuse, parental divorce, poor parental supervision, parental substance misuse, age, sex, region of the country, genetic predisposition, and personality type. Associations or correlations between some of these so-called risk factors do not equate to causality, thus decreasing or eliminating one or more might not result in any reduction of incidence of misuse (see [13–15]).

There is a substantial epidemiological literature on factors associated with increased risk of illicit drug use among young people [14]. The nature of the evidence is complex, with high-risk groups identified such as the homeless, those looked after by local authorities, prostitutes, truants, those excluded from school, young offenders, children from families with substance-abusing parents or siblings, and young people with conduct or depressive disorder. The detailed review undertaken by Frisher et al. [14] further explored these issues and identified some inconsistencies and contradictions. The following summary not only outlines that review but highlights some of the complexities in the analysis and interpretation of the findings as well as the implications for treatment and for policy.

The strongest and most consistent evidence links family interaction to drug use. The key elements of family interaction are parental discipline, family cohesion, and parental monitoring. Modification of parental monitoring may be effective in reducing adolescent drug use. Some aspects of family structure are linked to adolescent drug use. There is also consistent evidence linking peer drug use and drug availability to adolescent drug use. These factors probably explain the consistent findings that age is strongly associated with prevalence of drug use. There is also limited evidence linking self-esteem and hedonism to drug use. Where the current evidence for a relationship with drug is less clear, additional categories include gender, mental health,

parental substance use, attention deficit-hyperactivity disorder (ADHD), stimulant therapy, religious involvement, sport, health educator-led interventions, school performance, early onset of substance use, and socioeconomic status. No evidence was found linking adolescent drug use in the United Kingdom to ethnicity, language, or place of birth. This does not mean that such links do not exist, only that the review did not consider any relevant studies.

The evidence points to associations between a diverse group of risk factors for drug use. These factors include parental discipline, family cohesion, parental monitoring, peer drug use, drug availability, genetic profile, self-esteem, hedonistic attitudes, reasons for drug use, and the ratio of risk/protective factors. There is less consistent evidence linking drug use to mental health, parental substance use, ADHD/stimulant therapy, religious involvement, sport, health educator-led interventions, school performance, early onset of substance use, and socioeconomic status.

Where the causal nature of these associations has been tested in intervention trials, effects have generally been small. This could be because the factors are not readily amenable to intervention, because the associations are not causal, because the influence of individual factors is small, because findings in one population do not generalize to others, or for a combination of these reasons.

Risk factors have differential predictive values throughout adolescence. Some factors may occur at birth (or before) while others occur at varying times throughout adolescence. Some factors may persist for long periods of time while others are short lived. Different factors may be associated with the initiation and continuation, or even cessation, of drug use, although this distinction is not always clear in the literature. Risk factors are not discrete entities and their complex interactions are difficult to conceptualize, let alone analyze. The distinction between early- and late-onset risk factors is important as preventive measures may need to differentiate and to focus on particular age groups.

The psychosocial developmental stage and associated cognitive, social, and biological risk factors may influence both the development of comorbidity and the way it is manifest in a clinical situation. For example, impulsivity may feature prominently since decision-making and appreciation of risk have not fully developed. An appreciation of this complexity should inform interpretation of further studies and surveys.

England

A survey of young people in England during 2009 determined a number of risk factors associated with drug use, smoking, and alcohol consumption. Demographics that were determined to be associated with the likelihood of trying drugs included gender (boys more likely than girls), age (use became more common with age), and ethnicity (increased likelihood with Mixed, Asian, and Black ethnicity when compared with White ethnicity). Different types of drugs used also influenced the pattern of drug use: for example, pupils experimenting with volatile substances or solvents were typically younger than those taking other drugs; however, those using volatile substances were less likely to report frequent drug use. Family attitudes toward drug use significantly influenced drug use, with students' behaviors paralleling expected family attitudes. Drug use within the previous year was also more likely with students who reported regular smoking and recent drinking, exclusion from school, and truancy from school.

Smoking was also linked to gender and ethnicity but followed the opposite trends to drug use: girls were more likely to smoke regularly than boys, and White pupils were more likely to smoke than those of Black or Mixed ethnicity. Like drug use, prevalence was linked with age, drinking alcohol, drug use, exclusion from school, and truancy. In addition pupils in receipt of free school meals (indicator of low family affluence) were more likely to smoke.

A gender difference was not as apparent where alcohol consumption over the previous week was reported. The link to ethnicity followed the same trends as smoking, that is, White pupils were more likely to have drunk alcohol recently than Mixed or Asian ethnicities. Other similar patterns included age, regular smoking, recent drug use, exclusion from school, and truancy.

Pupils who reported one of either smoking, drinking, or drug use were more likely to have done one or both of the others [8]. Frequency of alcohol consumption has been shown to be associated with poly-substance use in other surveys of slightly older young people aged 16 to 19 years. Here visiting nightclubs and age were the strongest indicators of poly-substance use; however, the young adults (16 to 19 years) were more likely to have been poly-drug users within the previous year than older respondents surveyed [2].

Global Findings

The findings for Wales are reported in the HBSC survey, which also reports associations for gender, age categories, and family affluence. Associations will vary across countries and geographical regions. During 2005–06, in one-third of all countries boys were more likely than girls to start smoking at a young age; low family affluence was also an identified indicator although

more typically reported in girls in northern Europe. Weekly smoking rates were observed to increase between the ages of 11 and 15, with the greatest increase observed between 13 and 15 years. Where gender was identified as a risk factor, boys were more likely to smoke weekly when compared with girls. Geographically, rates of weekly smoking were lowest in Canada and the United States, and highest in eastern Europe. Higher rates of smoking were associated with lower family affluence although more strongly in girls in northern Europe. Age and gender were also identified as risk factors for weekly drinking rates and the associations were identical to those for smoking. Overall boys in northern Europe reported low rates of weekly drinking, although the United Kingdom was an exception to this. Higher family affluence was also strongly associated with higher rates of weekly drinking particularly in boys but less so in girls. Age, gender, and family affluence were also associated with reports of drunkenness. Geographically, high rates of drunkenness were more common in northern Europe and more strongly linked with girls than boys.

The only drug use measured in the HBSC survey is cannabis use and where lifetime cannabis use is concerned the data present findings from the 15-year-old age range alone therefore no association with age can be determined within these parameters. Cannabis use was more prevalent in boys compared with girls (where a significant difference between the genders was apparent); however, it must be noted that no gender difference was apparent in many of the countries. Geographically the highest rates were reported in the United States, Canada, and northern and eastern European countries. Whilst associations with family affluence were determined these were mixed between low and high family affluence depending on geographical region. Generally high family affluence was associated with cannabis use in eastern European countries [6].

Prescription Drugs

Whilst risk factors for prescription drug use are notably absent from many of the national surveys, a number of scientific studies are recognized to provide evidence of association, albeit contradictory in a number of instances [16]. One study using data from the National Survey on Drug Use and Health (NSDUH) in the United States reported the findings for risk factors associated with prescription drug use in adolescents aged 12 to 17 years. The significant predictors were determined to be poorer academic performance, past-year depression, past-year mental health treatment, risk-taking preference, and use of cigarettes, alcohol, marijuana, and cocaine and/or inhalants [16].

SPECIALIST SERVICES FOR ADOLESCENTS

A framework for an integration of epidemiological methods and provision of service has been conceptualized by Frisher *et al.* [14]. Those young people whose use/misuse was established in general population or school surveys such as ESPAD were likely to require Tier 1 services, whilst those who had "regular" use/misuse were likely to require Tier 2 provision. However, once the young people had progressed to harmful use, reported in, for example, drug misuse databases, and who presented in general medical, criminal justice, and social services, the components of a Tier 3 service were required. The most severely affected, namely those with dependence and who attended specialist clinical services, were likely to need intensive Tier 4 services.

As noted above, as young people who are at risk of poor health outcomes are the least likely to approach services, integration of agencies can promote entry, and avoid duplication and gaps. While these agencies include the health services (including addiction, child and adolescent and adult psychiatry, general medicine, obstetrics, pediatrics, midwifery, health visitors, and others), other statutory, and increasingly non-statutory, agencies, such as social services (for education, training, employment, housing), criminal justice, and the voluntary sector, are essential components [17]. Protocols and pathways, although conforming to NICE (National Institute for Health and Clinical Excellence) guidelines where feasible and encompassing national policies (e.g. National Treatment Agency, the Children's and Young People's National Service Framework), must allow for flexibility and sustainability. Therefore, resources for staffing, facilities, and training are vital components [18–20].

What the appropriate goals and outcomes for adolescents are is a question for debate – as many normally functioning young people are using substances, abstinence may not be perceived as appropriate. Offending is commonplace among the most severely affected young drug users, often in the context of parental substance misuse and/or mental illness, family conflict, school exclusion, mental illness in the young, self-harming, poor housing, and social service involvement. For this reason, the "Pathways to Problems" report [21] recommended that ". . . the NTA should continue to promote and monitor the development of accessible services for young people with serious tobacco, alcohol or drug-related problems, and to take active steps that these services are coordinated with other initiatives that engage with vulnerable young people." The perceptions, views, and experiences of practitioners are also important [22].

A triage or stepped approach has been conceptualized to manage multi-provider, multi-agency, and multi-disciplinary services. The structure of services for adolescents is very different from that for adults. The Health Advisory Service reports (1996, 2001) identified a four-tier framework similar to that described for child and adolescent services. The functions of each tier rather than the professional discipline involved are the focus [18,19]. A key issue is that interventions for those young people whose substance misuse is serious enough to require specialist help are not isolated but integrated with other medical and social services so that continuity is established and maintained. Whilst recognizing that different models and configurations have developed in different regions due to a variety of factors including the prevalence of substance misuse, the general level of affluence or deprivation, existing services, and leadership in service development and innovation, the following outlines the conceptualization of UK addiction services [18,19].

- **Tier 1: Universal, generic, and primary services.** This tier is aimed at all young people. It provides information and advice, health promotion, and support to all young people, parents, families, and carers. At this level, vulnerable individuals with risk factors including child protection issues may be identified. Staff in such generic and mainstream services should be aware of the need for a destigmatizing, non-confrontational, empathic approach to substance issue and be equipped to identify where more complex interventions may be required.
- **Tier 2: Specialist services.** This tier is directed at vulnerable children who are in contact with children's services such as Child and Adolescent Mental Health Services (CAMHS), Youth Offending Team (YOT), pediatrics, child psychology, and voluntary services and who are potentially vulnerable to the use of substances. Staff should be skilled in the comprehensive assessment of children and young people and appreciate the context of developmental issues. Implementation of advice and counselling, crisis management, outreach, interventions with family, as well as competence in "brief interventions" or motivational enhancement treatments for substance misuse are part of the role. Collaboration with agencies in the formulation of care planning so that interventions are integrated – and substance misuse interventions are not delivered in isolation – is a key component.
- **Tier 3: Specialist addiction services.** This tier comprises a multi-disciplinary team to deliver a complex range of interventions for young people who have harmful and potentially serious substance misuse

problems and dependence on substances. Close collaboration with CAMHS, youth justice, voluntary agencies, and medical services is needed in the delivery of these complex care plans. These services should be integrated with children's services and should cater for the needs of young people and not be based on adult models. Staff should be competent in the delivery of the range of pharmacological and individual, group, and family psychological treatments that are available for the treatment of dependent substance use. Staff also need to be trained in the intricacies of the relationship between mental, physical, and social problems and substance misuse in this age group so that appropriate links can be forged between the diverse agencies in the locality or region.

- **Tier 4: Very specialized services.** These are intensely focused interventions of a pharmacological and psychological nature that need to be implemented in a residential or inpatient setting or in a structured day program due to the severity of the problems. Since there are no residential units for adolescent substance misusers at present, units such as inpatient CAMHS, forensic, or pediatric units might be appropriate for different stages of the care plan. Inpatient detoxification for alcohol dependence or titration of opiate substitution treatment are examples of medical interventions requiring inpatient treatment. Intense daily psychological support may only be achieved in an inpatient CAMHS unit or a structured day program. Coordination of support for accommodation, education, and other social needs may also require crisis and fostering placements in order to achieve stability and safety in critical situations rather than the professional groups involved in provision of care.

Children and young people may need a range of services from a number of tiers at different times. Tiers 3 and 4 should not be involved without support from Tiers 1 and 2. Tiers 1 and 2 are key to the development of a broader base, a more comprehensive approach, and the establishment of credibility and trust. Continuity of care from Tier 1, particularly in health and education, is crucial. Where possible the intervention should be coordinated and managed within Tier 1. This should reduce the stigmatization and attempt to "normalize" the child and his/her family. For those young people not connected with Tier 1, any other services involved should seek to ensure reintegration and provision of services at Tier 1. Tiers 3 and 4 act as a base for specialist opinion and focused interventions. Thus, adolescents with comorbid disorders are most likely to be treated in Tiers 3 and 4.

The main elements that contribute to quality and effectiveness are assessment, a comprehensive approach, family involvement, developmental appropriateness, engagement and retention, qualified staff, gender and cultural competence, and outcomes [23,24]. Of note is the finding that treatment quality was significantly greater in programs offering intensive levels of care. This is relevant since mental illness makes the likelihood of relapse greater even after remission [25].

POLICY

In recent years UK substance misuse policy has prioritized young people and has attempted to utilize evidence to underpin recommendations where possible. Amongst the policy initiatives that have evolved are: *Hidden Harm* [26]; *Hidden Harm: Three Years On* [27]; *Every Child Matters* [28]; the National Service Framework for Children, Young People and Maternity Services [29]; *Every Child Matters: Change for Children, Young People and Drugs* [30]; the updated *Working Together to Safeguard Children* [31], with its updated and revised models of care for drug treatment [32]; *Pathways to Problems* and the implementation of its recommendations [21]; and the report of the most recent National Confidential Inquiry into Maternal and Child Health (2007), *Saving Mothers' Lives* [33].

Governments around the world have attempted to deal with alcohol-related problems. Babor rated the UK Strategy according to a set of guidelines he and others had developed [34]. Almost 90% of the recommendations were "untested" or "ineffective" policy options. Five areas were well supported by research (e.g. early identification of problem drinkers, server training). In some of the areas supported by the Strategy, there was evidence that these would not be effective (e.g. product labels, responsible drinking messages, designated driver programs). Other areas had insufficient research evidence (e.g. good policing, information dissemination).

Drugs

In the UK the most recent drug strategy was published in 2010 setting out the three key responses to illicit drug use: reducing demand, restricting supply, and building recovery and the move toward more local powers to take direct actions in response to local needs. Young people are featured more prominently where reducing demand is reported and the key responses highlighted include education and advice and early intervention. The strategy also highlights the need for a more concerted response to alcohol and drug use given the normalization of poly-substance use and increasing numbers of people presenting to services with complex treatment needs. The key treatment concern highlighted within the strategy was mental health issues, with the acknowledged literature demonstrating that mental illness starts before adulthood and that those experiencing mental illness are at higher risk of substance misuse. Since most young people are unlikely to present to services with substance dependence issues the need for services to adapt to their unique needs is identified [35].

In the United Kingdom NICE is a major national resource for clinicians and agencies seeking guidance with regard to health improvement and treatment. The current guidelines include a number addressing mental health and behavior that provide information on alcohol, drug use, and smoking in young people [36]. The summaries provided here are derived from completed documents; however, a number of others currently under development are also available from the NICE website.

For drug use treatment in the general population, NICE have published guidance for opioid detoxification and psychosocial interventions although neither of these are recommended when considering a population younger than 16 years [37,38]. The guidance, which has been specifically developed for young people, highlights the need to identify vulnerable groups within the population of those aged 25 or younger. Specific recommendations highlight the need for local policy development, the use of existing assessment and screening tools, a coordinated response that includes all relevant agencies and stakeholders, the use of family-based therapy programs, utilization of group-based behavioral therapy where appropriate (high-risk 10–12-year-olds), inclusion of parents/carers in interventions, and the use of motivational interviewing in older children (those attending secondary or further education) [39].

Alcohol

From the general guidance on prevention and treatment of alcohol misuse/abuse, young people are consistently reported as a unique population with specific needs; the age range considered is typically 10 years or above with the exception of one piece of guidance informing school-based interventions on alcohol. In the United Kingdom there are no recommended consumption levels for children and young people and the focus for school-based interventions is underpinned by the prevention model, which seeks to encourage nil consumption or to delay the age at which young people start drinking. Different countries, however, do have different approaches to alcohol education within this age group. Whilst the "harm reduction" approach is typically favored for young people in the United Kingdom by contrast in the United States, where most of the research on school-based interventions comes from, abstinence is encouraged among children and young people. The three key recommendations are aimed at ensuring that alcohol-related interventions are embedded within the school curriculum, are comprehensive, include parent/carer support packages, promote awareness among teaching staff to recognize and respond to risks, work in partnership across services, ensure appropriate referrals are made when required, and follow best practice on child protection, consent, and confidentiality. A number of factors that influence alcohol consumption in children and young people are identified among a range of sources including drug use, family conflict, parenting, poor school attendance/attainment, pre-existing behavioral problems, and living circumstances (e.g. living with single or step-parent, being in care, homelessness) [40].

The current guidance for prevention of harmful or hazardous alcohol consumption is underpinned by two approaches – at the population level and at the individual level. Specific recommendations from the national policy include action taken to address the cost of alcohol, the availability of alcohol (licensing regulations), alcohol advertising, improved server training and enforcement of current regulations, screening for alcohol-related problems in those aged 16 years or over, and supporting those at risk aged 10 to 15 years. The evidence supporting each of these recommendations can be accessed from the guidance. However, it is highlighted that much of the evidence is derived from studies with adults and therefore, in some instances, is inappropriate for a young population (e.g. understanding, emotional development) [40].

The increased risks that apply with those younger than 18 years are further acknowledged by the recommendation that lower thresholds be used in assessment and referrals for treatment although the unlikelihood of an individual presenting with harmful alcohol consumption levels at these ages is also acknowledged. These recommendations are further extended to other vulnerable populations including those who have cognitive impairment or multiple comorbidities, lack of social support, or learning difficulties. The lack of evidence available for young people was noted [41].

In the United Kingdom, owing to the limitations within the current knowledge base, there is no robust alcohol dependence assessment tool available for use with young people. The current guidelines recommend use of the Alcohol Use Disorders Identification Test (AUDIT) amongst 10–16-year-olds with a caution to adopt lowered thresholds considering the higher risks in this population. The use of a more comprehensive validated assessment tool is recommended when a need for treatment is identified, with the examples given including the Adolescent Diagnostic Interview (ADI) or Teen Addiction Severity Index (T-ASI). The limitations of these tools are also acknowledged, and the inclusion of data from parents or carers wherever possible is recommended. For those aged between 10 and 17 years two first-line treatment models are described: (i) individual cognitive therapy for those with limited comorbidities and good social support; and (ii) multi-component programs for those with significant comorbidities and/or limited social support. The goal for all treatments directed toward this age range should be to achieve abstinence in the first instance. Where multi-component therapy proves ineffective the use of drug treatment alongside cognitive therapy is recommended. For this age range no drug is currently recommended for use in the United Kingdom. However, in 2000 the Royal College of Paediatrics and Child Health issued a policy statement about the use of unlicensed medicines in children and young people where professional opinion is identified and there are no suitable alternative treatments. NICE guidelines recommend the use of acamprosate or naltrexone [42].

On an international level, Anderson in 2004 noted the evidence for three types of effective policy [43]:

1. Population-based, including taxation, advertising, regulation of density of outlets, hours and days of sale, drinking locations and minimum drinking age.
2. Problem-directed policies (e.g. drunk driving).
3. Interventions aimed at individual drinkers (e.g. primary care-based brief interventions).

A World Health Organization (WHO) report further underlines the fact that taxes are the most cost-effective option in terms of preventing ill health or premature death. However, brief interventions prevent more ill health and death, although at a greater cost [44].

Smoking

In the UK during 1998 the "Smoking kills" White Paper set targets to reduce the number of children aged 11–15 who were regularly smoking, from 13% in 1996 to 9% by 2010 [45]. In 2007 further legislation was introduced to make public places smoke-free and during the same year the legal age for tobacco sales was increased from 16 to 18 years. In recent years the Health Act 2009 has resulted in the banning of prominent tobacco displays in shops by 2013, and a further tobacco control strategy was published in 2010. In terms of specific public health guidance the strategies employed at a population level should include the utilization of mass media to raise awareness of the harms of smoking and point-of-sale measures located where tobacco is sold and acting as a deterrent to illegal sales [46]. Within the school setting five key recommendations drive the efforts to ensure those aged 19 years or under receive the appropriate messages within educational institutions:

- development of comprehensive and widely publicized policies across establishments;
- adult-led interventions embedded within the teaching curriculum;
- peer-led interventions with special reference to those that are evidence-based – e.g. A Stop Smoking in School Trial (ASSIST);
- appropriate training and development opportunities for those delivering interventions; and
- coordinated action that includes local action groups [47].

The first-line treatment for those seeking smoking cessation services is the provision of information, advice, and support preferably through local smoking cessation services. Since 2005, the Medicines and Healthcare Regulatory Authority (MHRA) in the United Kingdom has approved the use of nicotine replacement therapy (NRT) amongst young people aged 12 to 17 years. NRT alone is not, however, recommended and it should be considered alongside appropriate behavioral support. Other treatments, such as varenicline or bupropion, are not offered to young people under the age of 18 in the United Kingdom [48].

CONCLUSION

Young populations are still excluded in terms of availability and accessibility of services [49,50], and are sometimes excluded from NICE guidance [38,51–53]. Accessibility, social acceptability, and the legal framework not only influence the development of substance misuse but also associated comorbid conditions, and therefore also treatment options. In the United Kingdom social and cultural differences across national boundaries must be considered when devising policy. Thus it is a difficult task to formulate policy based on evidence partly because the evidence is not available.

There are many potential preventive and treatment "interventions," which include political, social, medical, psychiatric, and economic measures. Some may be implemented before the substance misuser ever experiences a "problem," in many different settings, whereas some may apply at acute crisis points. Currently it is acknowledged that those substance misusers who access the health system are the more severely affected, and some, for example binge drinkers, may be subject to criminal justice measures; and yet the entire population could benefit from educational interventions and market forces, for example with regard to supply and pricing. Thus any policy needs to be sustainable,

coherent, long-term, and pragmatic. Finally consideration must be given to how to formulate action across
international boundaries because substance use, perhaps
especially in the case of young people, is an increasingly
global phenomenon.

In 2008 the key elements of the services being
provided were outlined [20]. Providers were energetic
senior professionals working proactively and respon-
sively. The young people whom they served had multiple complex needs and risks and were disadvantaged and
vulnerable. A comprehensive assessment was required
as were a cohesive range of interventions. It was
acknowledged that one service model was not the solution. The question as to which medical or other professional was most appropriate to manage this group was
not answered, and none were excluded. However, the
experience in the United Kingdom then was that addiction psychiatrists and child and adolescent psychiatrists
were the ones who were actually seeking out the role and
undertaking the difficult but rewarding job. The report
ended as follows: "Everything that is done to help
troubled and distressed children should be informed
by a sense of history, a reflective awareness of current
value systems, economic and social factors, and by a
mature balanced judgement of what is or what is not
possible. Unfortunately, one of the enduring myths
about substance misuse is that treatment is generally
ineffective. Well-led, integrative, multiagency treatments addressing a range of crucial aetiological factors
have the potential to dispel myths, helplessness and
stigma, engender a culture of therapeutic optimism
and salvage some young lives."

APPENDIX 2.1: EPIDEMIOLOGY DATA FOR THE UNITED STATES

Alcohol

During 2009 the national Substance Abuse and Mental
Health Services Administration (SAMHSA) survey
reported current alcohol use amongst young people.
The proportions drinking alcohol were 3.5% of 12- or
13-year-olds, 13.0% of 14- or 15-year-olds, 26.3% of
those aged 16 or 17 years, 49.7% of 18–20-year-olds,
and 70.2% of 21–25-year-olds. Amongst older age
groups this trend was reversed to declining alcohol
use. Binge drinking was reported amongst 1.6% of
12- or 13-year-olds, 7.0% of 14- or 15-year-olds,
17.0% of 16- or 17-year-olds, and 34.7% of 18–20-
year-olds. The reported rates above were similar to those
for 2008 indicating a stabilization in alcohol consumption patterns. Amongst young people aged 12 to 17 years
gender did not significantly affect their likelihood to
consume alcohol (15.1% of males and 14.3% of females

were current drinkers). Ethnicity was determined to be
an influencing factor for current alcohol use, with the
lowest rates found in Asians (6.5%), followed by black
youths (10.6%), American Indian/Alaska Native
(11.9%), Hispanic (15.2%), and white youths
(16.1%). Of youths who reported two or more races,
16.7% were current drinkers. The key difference
between the SAMHSA survey and other comparable
national surveys is the greater range of ethnicities
defined. Furthermore, the majority of US states will
have a higher minimum purchase age (typically 21
years) when compared with many European countries
(typically 18 years). In 2009, an estimated 10.4 million
persons in the United States aged 12 to 20 years,
reported under-age alcohol use within the last month
(27.2% of the population), 6.9 million (18.1%) were
binge drinkers, and 2.1 million (5.4%) were heavy
drinkers. Previous published findings reported a decline
in these figures between 2002 and 2008; however, the
findings between 2008 and 2009 are comparable [52].

For the period 2005–06 the HBSC survey provides
self-reported evidence of alcohol consumption at least
once a week amongst 11-, 13-, and 15-year-olds in the
United States. Two percent of girls and 4% of boys aged
11 years reported drinking alcohol, rising to 6% of girls
and 7% of boys at age 13 years, and 12% of girls and
14% of boys at age 15 years. Moreover, 9% of girls and
13% of boys aged 15 years indicated they had first
experienced drunkenness at age 13 years or younger.
There was no significant difference between the genders
for all age groups. Repeated incidence of drunkenness
was also investigated in the three key age groups (11, 13,
and 15 years). At age 11 years, girls were significantly
less likely to report being drunk on at least two occasions
(<0.5% compared with 2%). The difference between the
genders was not apparent at age 13 years (5% of boys
and girls reported being drunk at least twice) or 15 years
(20% of boys and girls reported being drunk at least
twice) [6].

Illicit Drug Use

In 2009 the reported numbers of illicit drug users were
lower in the 12–17-year (2.5 million) and 18–25-year
(7.1 million) age categories when compared with people
aged 26 years or older (12.2 million). However, when
asked about current drug use, adults aged 26 years or
older were less likely to be current users when compared
with 12–17-year-olds and 18–25-year-olds (6.3% vs
10.0% and 21.2%, respectively). Moreover, when compared with the previous year's survey, the rate of past
month illicit drug use had increased amongst both
12–17-year-olds (from 9.3% to 10.0%) and 18–25-
year-olds (19.6% to 21.2%) [52].

During 2005–06 the United States, alongside England, Wales, Scotland, and Ireland, were amongst the top 12 countries where 15-year-olds reported having used cannabis during their lifetime. International findings indicate boys are more likely than girls to report using cannabis at this age; however, in countries with the highest rates this gender difference is typically less significant. In the United States the figures for lifetime cannabis use were 31% for both boys and girls, and for recent use (within last 30 days) 15% of boys and 12% of girls [6].

Smoking

During 2005–06, 16% of 15-year-old boys and girls surveyed in the United States reported first smoking at age 13 years or younger. Higher levels of weekly smoking were significantly associated with lower family affluence in both boys and girls. At age 11 years, boys were significantly more likely to report smoking at least once a week (3% of boys compared with 1% of girls). By age 13 years 4% of girls reported smoking at least once a week compared with 3% of boys; however, the difference was not significant. Fifteen-year-olds in the United States had the lowest levels of weekly smoking levels compared with all countries taking part; at age 15 years 9% of girls and 7% of boys reported weekly smoking with no significant difference between the genders [6].

Prescription drug use

In the United States the prevalence of prescription drug abuse can be derived in part from the annual SAMHSA survey, which reports non-medical psychotherapeutic drug use including use of pain relievers, tranquilizers, stimulants, and sedatives. In 2009, 3.1% of 12–17-year-olds reported non-medical prescription drug use [52]. The prevalence trends indicated prescription drug use was most popular within the 12–13-year age range and thereafter was superseded by marijuana use in the 14–17-year age groups. The longer-term trends for non-medical use of prescription drugs in 12–17-year-olds show a decline from 2002–03 (4.0%) and a stabilization over the last two years of data available. The figures for young adults aged 18 to 25 years from 2002 to 2009, however, provide evidence of increasing prescription drug use (psychotherapeutic drug use increased from 5.5% to 6.3% and use of pain relievers from 4.1% to 4.8%) [52]. A US study of self-reported behaviors in 12–17-year-olds across the country identified 36% of those who had used prescription drugs as describing a detectable adverse effect, including tolerance, lost time as a result of seeking, using, or recovering from use, and withdrawal. An estimated 17.4% of prescription drug users met the criteria for substance abuse or substance dependence, and the majority (63.5%) were attributed to opioid medications, 21.5% were exhibiting problems resulting from multiple prescription drugs, 6.5% were attributed to tranquilizers alone, 6.4% to stimulants, and 2.1% to sedatives. The study found the strongest risk factors for prescription misuse were: being 15 years or older, having poor academic performance, past-year major depressive episode, past-year mental health treatment, risk-taking preference, and past-year cigarette, alcohol, marijuana, or cocaine and/or inhalant use [14].

References

1. Black C, MacLardie J, Mailhot J, Murray L, Sewel K. Scottish Schools Adolescent Lifestyle and Substance Use Survey (SALSUS) National Report. Smoking, drinking and drug use among 13 and 15 year olds in Scotland in 2008. ISD Scotland, 2009.
2. Hoare J, Moon D. Drug misuse declared: findings from the 2009/10 British Crime Survey. England and Wales. Home Office Statistical Bulletin. London: Home Office, 2010.
3. Page L, MacLeod P, Kinver A, Iliasov A, Yoon P. 2009/10 Scottish Crime and Justice Survey: main findings. Edinburgh: Scottish Government, 2010.
4. Welsh Assembly Government (2010) Substance misuse in Wales 2009-10. Welsh Assembly Government, 2010. Available from: http://wales.gov.uk/docs/dsjlg/publications/ commsafety/101020submisuse0910en.pdf.
5. Northern Ireland Statistics & Research Agency. Young Persons' Behaviour and Attitudes Survey Bulletin October 2007 – November 2007. Northern Ireland Statistics & Research Agency, 2008.
6. Currie C, Gabhainn SN, Godeau E, et al. (eds). Inequalities in Young People's Health: HBSC International Report from the 2005/2006 Survey. Copenhagen: World Health Organization Regional Office for Europe, 2008.
7. Andersson B, Hibell B, Beck F, Choquet M, Kokkevi A, Fotiou A. Alcohol and Drug Use Among European 17-18 Year Old Students. Data from the ESPAD Project. Stockholm: Swedish Council for Information on Alcohol and Other Drugs, 2007.
8. Fuller E, Sanchez M (eds). Smoking, Drinking and Drug Use Among Young People in England in 2009. London: NHS Information Centre for Health and Social Care, 2010.
9. National Institute for Health and Clinical Excellence. Alcohol-use disorders: preventing the development of hazardous and harmful drinking. NICE public health guidance 24. London: NICE, 2010.
10. National Treatment Agency for Substance Misuse. Substance misuse among young people: the data for 2009-10. London: NTA, 2010.
11. Northern Ireland Statistics & Research Agency. Census of Drug and Alcohol Treatment Services in Northern Ireland: 1st March 2010. Statistical Bulletin PHIRB 3/ 2010.
12. MacLeod P, Page L. 2009/10 Scottish Crime and Justice Survey: Drug Use. Edinburgh: Scottish Government Social Research, 2011.
13. Crome IB, Baldacchino A. The young person's perspective In: Cooper DB (ed.), Responding in Mental Health – Substance Use. London: Radcliffe Publishing, 2011, pp. 48–60.

14. Frisher M, Crome I, Macleod J, Bloor R, Hickman M. *Predictive Factors for Illicit Drug Use among Young People: A Literature Review*. London: Home Office, 2007.

15. Beckett H, Heap J, McArdle P, *et al. Understanding Problem Drug Use Among Young People Accessing Drug Services: a Multivariate Approach Using Statistical Modelling Techniques*. London: Home Office, 2004.

16. Schepis TS, Krishnan-Sarin S. Characterizing adolescent prescription misusers: a population-based study. *J Am Acad Child Adolesc Psychiat* 2008;**47**:745–754.

17. Crome I, Chambers P, Frisher M, Bloor R, Roberts D. The relationship between dual diagnosis: substance misuse and dealing with mental health issues. In: *SCIE Research Briefing 30*. London: Social Care Institute for Excellence, 2009, pp. 9–10.

18. Crome IB. Comorbidity in young people: perspectives and challenges. *Acta Neuropsychiatr* 2004;**16**:47–53.

19. Crome IB, Gilvarry E. Young people and substance misuse. In: Williams R, Kerfoot M (eds), *Child and Adolescent Mental Health Services: Strategy, Planning, Delivery, and Evaluation*. New York: Oxford University Press, 2005; pp. 299–314.

20. Mirza K, McArdle P, Crome I, Gilvarry E (eds). *The Role of CAMHS and Addiction Psychiatry in Adolescent Substance Misuse Services*. London: National Treatment Agency for Substance Misuse, 2008.

21. Advisory Council on the Misuse of Drugs. *Pathways to Problems: Hazardous Use of Tobacco, Alcohol and other Drugs by Young People in the UK and its Implications for Policy*. London: ACMD, 2006.

22. Molesworth S, Crome I. What is so special about young people? Views from practitioners. *Mental Health and Substance Use* 2011;**4**:83–92.

23. Knudsen H. Adolescent-only substance abuse treatment: Availability and adoption of components of quality. *J Subst Abuse Treat* 2009;**36**:195–204.

24. Brannigan R, Schackman BR, Falco M, Millman RB. The quality of highly regarded adolescent substance abuse treatment programs: results of an in-depth national survey. *Arch Pediatr Adolesc Med* 2004;**158**:904–909.

25. Xie H, Drake R, McHugo G. Are there distinctive trajectory groups in substance abuse remission over 10 years? An application of the group-based modeling approach. *Adm Policy Ment Health* 2006;**33**:423–432.

26. Advisory Council on the Misuse of Drugs (ACMD). *Hidden Harm – Responding to the Needs of Children of Problem Drug Users*. London: Home Office, 2003.

27. Advisory Council on the Misuse of Drugs (ACMD). *Hidden Harm – Three Years On: Realities, Challenges and Opportunities*. London: Home Office, 2007. Available from: http://www.homeoffice.gov.uk/acmd1/HiddenHarm20071.pdf?view=Binary.

28. Department for Education and Skills. *Every Child Matters*. London: The Stationery Office, 2003.

29. Department of Health and Department of Education and Skills. *National Service Framework for Children, Young People and Maternity Services*. London: Department of Health, 2004.

30. Department for Education and Skills, Home Office, Department for Health. *Every Child Matters: Change for Children – Young People and Drugs*. Nottingham: Department for Education and Skills, 2005.

31. Department for Health, Home Office, Department for Education and Skills. *Working Together to Safeguard Children: A Guide to Inter-Agency Working to Safeguard and Promote the Welfare of Children*. London: The Stationery Office, 2006.

32. HM Government. The updated and revised models of care for drug treatment. 2006.

33. Confidential Enquiry into Maternal and Child Health (CEMACH). *Saving Mothers' Lives: Reviewing Maternal Deaths to Make Motherhood Safer - 2003–2005*. London: CEMACH, 2007.

34. Babor T, Caetano R. *Alcohol: No Ordinary Commodity – Research and Public Policy*. Oxford: Oxford University Press, 2003.

35. HM, Government., Drug strategy 2010: reducing demand, restricting supply, building recovery. Supporting people to live a drug free life. London: Home Office, 2010.

36. National Institute for Health and Clinical Excellence (NICE). *Mental Health and Behavioural Conditions*. London: NICE, 2011.

37. National Collaborating Centre for Mental Health. Drug misuse: psychosocial interventions (NICE clinical guideline 51). London: NICE, 2007.

38. National Collaborating Centre for Mental Health. Drug misuse: opioid detoxification (NICE clinical guideline 52). London: NICE, 2007.

39. National Institute for Health and Clinical Excellence (NICE). Community-based interventions to reduce substance misuse among vulnerable and disadvantaged children and young people (NICE public health intervention guidance 4). London: NICE, 2007.

40. National Institute for Health and Clinical Excellence (NICE). Interventions in schools to prevent and reduce alcohol use among children and young people (NICE public health guidance 7). London: NICE, 2007.

41. National Clinical Guideline Centre. Alcohol use disorders: diagnosis and clinical management of alcohol-related physical complications. Clinical Guideline 100. London: NICE, 2010.

42. National Collaborating Centre for Mental Health. Alcohol-use disorders. Diagnosis, assessment and management of harmful drinking and alcohol dependence (NICE clinical guideline 115). London: NICE, 2011.

43. Anderson P. State of the world's alcohol policy. *Addiction* 2004;**99**:1367–1369.

44. World Health Organization. *Alcohol and Mental Health*. Copenhagen: WHO Regional Office for Europe, 2004.

45. Department of Health. *Smoking Kills: A White Paper on Tobacco*. London: The Stationery Office, 2010.

46. National Institute for Health and Clinical Excellence (NICE). Mass-media and point-of-sales measures to prevent the uptake of smoking by children and young people (NICE public health guidance 14). London: NICE, 2008.

47. National Institute for Health and Clinical Excellence (NICE). School-based interventions to prevent the uptake of smoking among children and young people. NICE public health guidance 23. London: NICE, 2010.

48. National Institute for Health and Clinical Excellence (NICE). Smoking cessation services in primary care, pharmacies, local authorities and workplaces, particularly for manual working groups, pregnant women and hard to reach communities (NICE public health guidance 10). London: NICE, 2008.

49. Hodges C-L, Paterson S, Taikato M, McGarrol S, Crome I, Baldacchino A. *Co-morbid Mental Health and Substance Misuse in Scotland*. Edinburgh: Scottish Executive, 2006.

50. Five year report of the national confidential inquiry into suicide and homicide by people with mental illness.

Avoidable Deaths. Manchester: National Confidential Inquiry into Suicide and Homicide by People with Mental Illness, 2006.

51. National Institute for Health and Clinical Excellence (NICE). Psychosocial interventions in drug misuse (Clinical Guideline CG51). London: NICE, 2007.

52. National Institute for Health and Clinical Excellence (NICE). Methadone and buprenorphine for the management of opioid dependence (NICE technology appraisal guidance 114). London: NICE, 2007.

53. National Institute for Health and Clinical Excellence (NICE). Naltrexone for the management of opioid dependence (NICE technology appraisal guidance 115). London: NICE, 2007.

54. Substance Abuse and Mental Health Services Administration. Results from the 2009 National Survey on Drug Use and Health: Volume I. Summary of National Findings (Office of Applied Studies, NSDUH Series H-38A, HHS Publication No. SMA 10-4856Findings). Rockville, MD: SAMHSA, 2010.

Section Two

Assessment of the Substance-Abusing Adolescent

Edited by Robert Weinstock and Manuel Lopez-Leon

3

Clinical Assessment of Addiction in Adolescents

Farzin Yaghmaie[1] and Robert Weinstock[2]

[1]*University of California Los Angeles, Department of Psychiatry and Biobehavioral Sciences, Los Angeles, CA, USA*
[2]*University of California Los Angeles, Los Angeles, CA, USA*

INTRODUCTION

Every year, approximately one in five adolescents engages in abusive, dependent, or problematic use of illicit drugs or alcohol [1,2]. While the vast majority of adolescent experimentation and use of psychoactive substances does not progress to substance use disorders, studies suggest that adolescents generally exhibit higher rates of experimental use and substance use disorders than older populations [3,4]. Similarly, potential behavioral addictions, such as problematic gambling, video gaming, and internet use, have been shown to occur at higher prevalences in younger than older populations [5–8]. In addition, addictive disorders identified in adults most commonly have onset in adolescence or young adulthood [9,10], and earlier onset of substance use predicts greater addiction severity and morbidity [10–13].

Early intervention reduces the severity and persistence of addictive disorders and helps prevent the development of secondary disorders, like substance-induced mood, anxiety, or psychotic disorders. Identifying and treating addiction in adolescence, during critical periods in cognitive, personality, and social development, also reduces the risk for developing maladaptive personality traits and poor coping skills later in life. Furthermore, because the risk for substance use increases markedly in adolescents with pre-existing or co-occurring conditions like attention-deficit/hyperactivity disorder (ADHD), bipolar disorder, depression, or anxiety, and in those with history of trauma or abuse; recognizing addiction can serve as the proverbial "canary in the coal mine," and alert physicians to other conditions or issues that would benefit from further evaluation and treatment. Thus, targeting adolescent populations for addiction

screening and assessment is a prudent strategy that can yield important clinical data.

Given this, addiction screening should be an institutional priority and including the assessment of addiction as a component of every clinical encounter with adolescents should be considered the standard of care. This chapter summarizes current knowledge regarding the assessment of addiction in adolescents in outpatient clinical settings. Strategies for the general approach to evaluating adolescents and an overview of the "red flags," signs, and symptoms of common substance use disorders and behavioral addictions seen in adolescents are provided here.

TERMS USED IN THIS CHAPTER

Adolescence: The state of development, between puberty and maturity, encompassing most of the changes associated with the transition from childhood into adulthood. Adolescence is a critical period of cognitive, personality, and social development. Adolescence is broadly defined here as the time of life from 11 to 21 years of age. Adolescents are a heterogeneous population that includes individuals at various stages of development and therefore exhibiting a wide range of physical, emotional, and mental capacity. Because adolescence represents a critical time in neuro-development, the brains of adolescents are especially sensitive to the effects of psychoactive substances. Exposure to psychoactive substances in adolescence can impact neural circuitry in maladaptive ways that can reverberate well into adulthood.

Severity of use: For the purpose of assessment, it is helpful to view adolescent substance use along a

Clinical Handbook of Adolescent Addiction, First Edition. Richard Rosner.
© 2013 John Wiley & Sons, Ltd. Published 2013 by John Wiley & Sons, Ltd.

continuum of severity, which extends from experimentation with alcohol and drug use through non-problematic use, problematic use, and finally disorders of abuse and dependence [13,14].

Experimentation: The first use of psychoactive substances, most commonly alcohol, marijuana, inhalants, and diverted prescription medications. While not all experimentation leads to problematic use, early experimentation with some substances is thought to serve as a predictor of subsequent substance use disorders. Because experimentation amongst adolescents is so common, some view it as "normal" behavior in older adolescents and even a sign of mental health when it is limited experimentation with more socially acceptable substances, such as alcohol or nicotine. Similarly, total abstinence from experimentation with psychoactive substances in adolescence may in fact be a marker of potential psychopathology. Alternatively, any experimentation with certain illicit substances, such as heroin, and via certain modes of administration, such as intravenous, is considered maladaptive and should raise clinical suspicion for current or future substance misuse, abuse, or dependence.

Non-problematic use: Sporadic use, usually with peers, without negative consequences.

Problematic use: Use with the first appearance of adverse consequences such as accidents, injury, truancy, decline in school performance, or interpersonal conflicts with parents or peers.

Substance abuse: Adapted from the American Psychiatric Association's *Diagnostic and Statistical Manual of Mental Disorders, Fourth Edition* (DSM-IV) [14]; defined here as a pattern of substance use meeting one or more of the following four criteria and occurring repeatedly over the course of the previous 12 months, but not meeting criteria for diagnosis of dependence:

- substance-related problems at school, work, or home;
- use of substance in hazardous situations, such as driving a car or riding a bicycle;
- substance-related legal problems;
- continued use despite problems or arguments with friends or family.

Substance dependence: Adapted from DSM-IV [14], defined here as a pattern of substance use meeting any three of the seven following criteria during the previous 12 months:

- tolerance or diminution of response to the substance after repeated use;
- withdrawal, which may be either physiological or psychological;
- using more of a substance or using for longer periods of time than intended;

- unsuccessful attempts to quit or cut down on use of substance;
- spending a great deal of time obtaining, using, or recovering from effects of a substance.

Of note, the appropriateness of applying substance use-related diagnostic nomenclature designed for adults to adolescents is the subject of much discussion [15,16]. While in general the use of DSM-IV criteria for diagnosing substance use disorders in adolescents is acceptable and sufficient, because adolescents report fewer physiological symptoms of withdrawal than adults and on average have had shorter time periods to use substances compared to adults, fewer adolescents meet strict criteria for dependence. This has led some to suggest combining DSM-IV abuse and dependence criteria into a single category for adolescents, in which abuse and dependence are differentiated by the number rather than the type of criteria experienced [17]. Similarly, the DSM-V, projected to be published in 2012–13 and still in draft at the time of this writing, has sought to diagnose substance use disorders based on a range of severity indicated by the number of symptoms endorsed [18].

Phase of abuse: In addition to severity of use, identifying the phase of active substance abuse is helpful to establish an accurate assessment. The phases of active substance abuse include current intoxication, current withdrawal, early abstinence, sustained abstinence, or recent relapse.

Motivation for use: An adolescent's motivation or reported reason for substance use is crucial for facilitating treatment and should always be established during assessment. Adolescents use substances for a variety of reasons. Commonly reported reasons for use are for recreation; to enhance social interactions; to enhance academic performance; to regulate or enhance mood or experiences; to boost self-confidence; and to relax or cope with negative affective states like anxiety or depression.

Motivation for change: An adolescent's willingness or readiness to stop substance use is his or her motivation for change. Five stages of change have been identified [19], through which addicts are thought to progress before sustained abstinence and recovery are achieved:

1. *Precontemplation:* The first stage of change in which addicts lack insight and have no wish to change their addictive behavior.
2. *Contemplation:* The second stage of change during which addicts are aware of and thinking about changing their addictive behavior but have not committed to change.
3. *Preparation:* The third stage of change during which patients have decided to change and are preparing to do so.

4. *Action:* The fourth stage of change during which patients actively modify their addictive behavior and may cease substance use.

5. *Maintenance:* The fifth and final stage of change during which patients maintain abstinence from addictive behaviors and continuously work at preventing relapse into substance use.

Screening: A brief procedure, in which standardized questionnaires are administered to estimate the probability of the presence of a problem and identify the need for further evaluation. Screening does not establish definitive diagnosis of an addictive disorder but is used to identify adolescents that need further assessment. Screening can also provide insight into an adolescent's awareness of a problem, his/her thoughts on it, and his/her motivation for changing addictive behavior.

Clinical assessment: A comprehensive evaluation process conducted by physicians to determine the nature and complexity of an adolescent's problems and to establish the severity of use and diagnosis of addiction.

SCREENING TOOLS

Screening instruments are more accurate in identifying adolescent risk level than a clinician's impression alone. They provide a standardized and reliable protocol with which to initiate communication with adolescents about addiction and supplement clinical assessment. Furthermore, because many adolescents are unlikely to answer substance use questions truthfully aloud in the presence of a parent or an adult; self-rated, paper and computer-based screening has been shown to elicit more accurate answers from adolescents, than direct verbal questioning.

Screening tools provide relatively rapid risk stratification and when applied at regular intervals can be an important tool in both prevention and monitoring. Screening can be used at the onset of care and to monitor escalation of use or treatment outcomes. In effect, a good screening tool provides a snapshot of addiction risk at a given point in time, from which the need for further evaluation can be determined and baseline activity can be documented and monitored.

Treatment providers may choose to repeat the same screening measures administered initially and/or adjust the instructions of the measures to address more limited time frames (i.e., rather than assessing substance use in the last 12 months, assess use in the past 4 weeks). Repeating this on multiple visits can assess changes in substance use patterns and pathology. For adolescents at high risk for substance use disorder, a negative screen should be followed up with re-evaluation at regular intervals, at least every 4 months.

Screening focuses primarily on adolescent substance use consumption patterns and the impact of use on associated factors such as mental health status, educational functioning, legal problems, and living situation. Many different screening tools have been developed specifically for adolescent populations and are available for use. Several studies have reviewed various screening tools developed specifically for adolescents, and compare relative reliability and validity [20,21]. Both written and oral assessments have their respective advantages and disadvantages related to time, privacy, and content. Physicians should take the time to review different screening instruments and choose those that best meet their needs and preferences. Specific screening tools developed for use in adolescent populations can be reviewed in more detail in Table 3.1.

When using questionnaires, it is advisable to have the adolescent read aloud the instructions that accompany the test to ensure he or she understands what is expected

Table 3.1 Screening instruments for adolescent alcohol and substance use.

Screening tool	Length	Method	Focus	Reference
AUDIT[a]	10 items 5 minutes	Written assessment	Substance abuse, mental health, behavioral disorders	[22]
CRAFFT[b]	6 items 5 minutes	Interview format	Alcohol and substance abuse severity	[23]
Adolescent Drinking Inventory (ADI)	24 items 5 minutes	Interview format	Psychological, physical and social symptoms of alcohol abuse	[24]
Rutgers Alcohol Problem Index (RAPI)	23 items 10 minutes	Interview format	Measures consequences of alcohol use related to social, familial, psychological and physical problems, and delinquency	[25]

[a]Alcohol Use Disorders Identification Test.
[b]CRAFFT is a mnemonic acronym of the first letters of key words in the six screening questions.

and to judge whether an adolescent's reading comprehension is appropriate for the testing situation.

Lack of confidentiality can strongly inhibit minors from disclosing sensitive information and create barriers that prove counteractive to measures aimed at serving the young patient and their parents. Given this, before using a screening instrument or initiating more comprehensive assessment, it is important to first ask parents to leave the room and to explain confidentiality policies one-on-one with the adolescent. An explanation of confidentiality is essential in creating a trusting and productive physician-patient relationship. Adolescents must be reassured that their answers will be kept confidential but be made aware of specific situations, such as information that may suggest a safety risk for themselves of others, that can be grounds for breaching confidentiality.

CLINICAL ASSESSMENT

The goal of comprehensive clinical assessment of adolescent addiction is to accurately identify signs and symptoms of problematic substance use so that prevention and early intervention can take place. Unlike screening, clinical assessment is a more comprehensive process in which the diagnosis of substance use disorders and other comorbid psychiatric conditions is established via clinical interview, focused physical examination, and if consent is provided, lab testing and collateral information from past medical records,

other clinicians, and elicited from parents or other people who know the adolescent.

Several structured and semi-structured interviews for evaluation of substance abuse are available that can identify substance abuse problems with greater validity than a non-structured clinical assessment [26–28]. Despite this, because structured interviews can sometimes misinterpret special situations and miss important details better identified in a comprehensive clinical interview, it is important to supplement structured interviews with more in-depth clinical inquiries and interviewing.

A comprehensive evaluation of adolescent substance use should address the following major domains of content:

- *History of substance use*: Adolescents should be asked about every major category of substance use (a list of the major categories of substance use can be reviewed in Table 3.2). For each substance the pattern of use should be established, including the first onset of use; duration or length of use; most recent use; frequency and severity of use; and mode of ingestion. In addition, the motivations for use, preoccupation with use, social and legal consequences of use, subjective loss of control with use, and substance abuse treatment history should be elicited.
- *History of problematic behaviors*: Adolescents should be asked about engaging in potentially problematic behaviors like gambling, video gaming,

Table 3.2 Major categories of commonly abused drugs.

Category	Examples
Cannabinoids	Marijuana, hashish
Alcohol	
Gamma-hydroxybutyrate (GHB)	
Benzodiazepines	Diazepam (Valium), alprazolam (Xanax), chlordiazepoxide (Librium), triazolam (Halcion), lorazepam (Ativan)
Amphetamines	Clandestine methamphetamine ("speed"), pharmaceutical methamphetamine (Desoxyn) and amphetamine (Adderall, Dexedrine)
Methylphenidate (Ritalin)	
Nicotine	
Caffeine	
Cocaine	
Hallucinogens	LSD (D-lysergic acid diethylamide), mescaline, DMT (dimethyltryptamine), DOM (2,5-dimethoxy-4-methylamphetamine), PCP (phencyclidine hydrochloride), psilocybin/psilocin, MDA (methylene dioxyamphetamine), MDMA (methylene dioxymethamphetamine)
Opioids and morphine derivatives	Morphine, heroin, codeine, meperidine (demerol), methadone, fentanyl, opium
Dissociative anesthetics	Ketamine (Ketalar SV), phencyclidine (PCP)
Inhalants	Solvents (paint thinners, gasoline, glues), gases (butane, propane, aerosol propellants, nitrous oxide), nitrites (isoamyl, isobutyl, cyclohexyl)

and internet use. Excessive preoccupation with and excessive time spent gambling, gaming, or on the internet warrants additional inquiry for a possible addiction to those activities. Patterns of problematic gaming, gambling, or internet use, including first onset, frequency, and duration of activity, should be assessed. The social, financial, and legal consequences, the subjective loss of control, and any treatment history should be assessed. Specific information about pathological gambling should be elicited, including returning to gambling to win back previous losses, growing debts, or borrowing or stealing money to cover debts.

- *Psychiatric history*: Prior or current history of mental illness, including depression, suicidal ideation, suicide attempts, self-injurious behavior, anxiety disorders, psychotic disorders, attention-deficit disorders, and behavioral or impulse control disorders. Past history of evaluation and treatment of mental health problems, including emergent psychiatric evaluation and inpatient and outpatient psychiatric treatment history, should be elicited. Baseline mental health before initiation of substance use or during extensive periods of sobriety should be elicited, as should psychiatric history during periods of substance use, in part to distinguish premorbid mental illness from substance-induced psychiatric problems.
- *Medical history*: Prior and current history of illness; including infections or infectious diseases, recurrent fever, ulcers or gastrointestinal symptoms, chronic cough, rhinorrhea, sinusitis or other respiratory symptoms, nosebleeds, poor nutritional status, poor exercise tolerance, fatigue, weight loss, and sleep disturbances should be elicited. Past history of emergency room visits, inpatient hospitalization, and outpatient treatment of medical problems should be established. In part this is important to distinguish side effects of drug use or physical signs of substance withdrawal, from independent unrelated physical symptomatology. In addition, some medical problems such as cardiac pathology could make abuse of stimulants especially risky and serve as a basis for psychoeducation and prevention.
- *Physical and mental status examination*: Acute signs and symptoms of intoxication and withdrawal are reviewed elsewhere, but any of the following should be noted on physical or mental status exam: conjunctival injection, mydriasis, miosis, rhinorrhea, xerostomia, excessive diaphoresis, lethargy, tremulousness, psychomotor agitation or retardation, restlessness, nervousness, confusion, or slurred speech. A focused physical examination for signs and symptoms consistent with the mode of administration or ingestion of substances should be included as part of a comprehensive evaluation for addiction. The odor from clothes or breath may reveal recent cannabis, tobacco, or alcohol use; respiratory exam may reveal bronchitis or chronic cough consistent with inhalation; runny nose, nosebleeds, or damage to the nasal mucosa or nasal cavity may be consistent with insufflation; signs of cellulitis, abscess or injection sites may be consistent with intravenous (i.v.) or subcutaneous administration of drugs; perioral or nasal rash, burns, solvent stains, paint or correction fluid on clothing or the face may be consistent with inhalant abuse. Similarly, a focused physical examination of general body habitus can reveal signs and symptoms consistent with substance abuse or behavioral addictions. Obesity and/or physical deconditioning may be signs of excessive video gaming or internet use; anorexia and excessive weight loss may be signs of prescription or illicit stimulant abuse; gynecomastia may be a sign of cannabis abuse.

- *Sexual history*: Elicit information about past and current sexual activity, sexual orientation, history of rape or sexual abuse, sexually transmitted diseases (STDs), and history of high STD/HIV risk behaviors such as past and current unprotected sex, prostitution, exchanging sex for drugs, and sharing needles for i.v. drug use. Substance abuse in adolescence may also disinhibit and impair judgment increasing the risk of engaging in dangerous sexual behaviors.
- *Family history*: The past and current history of substance use in parents, legal guardians, siblings, and extended families can reveal heritable and environmental risk factors for substance use that can inform both evaluation and treatment.
- *Home environment and peer relationships*: A description of the current living situation should be elicited, including the neighborhood, type of home, and with whom the young patient lives. Is tobacco, alcohol, or drug use in the home common? It is important to explore whether permissive parents, family addiction, or disruptive family relationships are present. Current or past history of social services or welfare agency involvement, homelessness, or history of running away should also be noted as these associated factors inform both assessment and treatment planning.
- *Developmental issues, trauma/abuse history*: Information about learning problems, developmental disorders, attention-deficit disorders; history of trauma and post-traumatic stress disorder (PTSD); and any history of sexual, physical, or emotional abuse should be elicited.
- *Academic and vocational history*: Past and current academic performance, paid or volunteer employment, attendance record, and disciplinary/behavioral issues should be assessed.

- *Legal history*: History of juvenile delinquency and legal problems, including the type and repercussions of legal activity; history of gang involvement, and physical aggression or violence should be elicited. In addition, the young patient's general attitude regarding illegal behavior, and whether they believe substance use played a part in illegal behavior or misconduct, should be elicited.
- *Motivation and capacity for change*: Insight into problematic use, willingness or readiness to stop substance use, and the stage of motivation should all be assessed. Self-esteem, coping skills, inter-personal skills, community and social support systems, and financial resources should also be explored to inform treatment planning.

Several factors influence the accuracy of addiction assessment in the adolescent, including the presence of comorbid psychiatric conditions, the severity of sub-stance use, the phase of substance use, and the motiva-tion of the adolescent for change. In addition, the clinical setting, confidentiality, and interviewing style and atti-tude of the eliciting physician have a major impact on the validity of an assessment. Developing rapport with the adolescent is essential if a valid history is to be obtained. Establishing trust is crucial since many ado-lescents fear punishment or negative consequences if they are honest about the extent of their drug use. An interactive interviewing approach is more important to develop rapport with an adolescent than with older patients since adolescents are more likely to mistrust an adult interviewer.

Setting

The adolescent interview must take place in a private setting. The adolescent's concern over whether responses are overheard should be addressed. Every effort should be made to provide a setting in which adolescents can feel secure and comfortable. Adequate time should be allotted for the evaluator to explain confidentiality, establish rapport, and to allow for the adolescent to explain, in his or her own words, the pattern of use and perceived impact of use.

Confidentiality

In the United States, laws governing confidentiality vary from state to state. Regardless, lack of confidentiality can be an insurmountable barrier to eliciting sensitive information from adolescents. Breaching confidentiality can prove counteractive to measures aimed at serving minors and their parents. Parents must agree to not

receiving the details of treatment and not having fre-quent contact with the doctor, even if in a state where they are legally entitled to that information. In drug treatment there are also special federal protections for confidentiality that can supersede state laws, as discussed below.

A thorough explanation of the clinician's definition of confidentiality is essential to establishing rapport and creating a trusting and productive therapeutic relation-ship with adolescents. Adolescents must be reassured that their answers will be kept confidential but be made aware of specific situations, such as information that may be a safety risk for themselves or others, that can be grounds for breaching confidentiality to parents or if applicable, school officials. If confidentiality cannot be offered in a specific situation or if there are limitations to it, that should be made clear at the outset. For example, if a school or institution or juvenile detention facility or jail limits confidentiality, that should be made clear at the outset. Adolescents should always be informed if self-reported drug use or results from drug testing will be reported to parents, school officials, or other institution authorities. This may be especially important to school athletes, for whom a positive drug screen may result in exclusion from competitions. In jurisdictions where the family may be entitled to treatment information, it is advisable to set up an agreement with parents in advance, with the aim of protecting confidentiality for the adolescent except for dangerous situations.

Clinicians should establish an interviewing process that prioritizes and protects confidentiality. If other people, such as parents or family members, are present, the clinician should first ask the parents to leave and interview the adolescent in private, then the parents in private, then the group as a whole. Each person should be informed that all information provided will be held in confidence in order to maximize valid responses. Although family involvement is important, it is impor-tant not to violate the adolescent's confidentiality in such meetings. Although there are situations in which it is best for the same therapist to continue to treat the adolescent and the family, to prevent conflicts of interest and divided loyalties it is most prudent to have different therapists play these roles in order to minimize potential complications. Despite this, during the initial evaluation of addiction, family assessment is important for collat-eral information and to establish the parameters of when the family will be informed of positive drug tests or evidence of dangerous behaviors.

It is also important to be aware that in clinical settings with federal funding, additional legal protection for the confidentiality of drug treatment information and records may apply. In some circumstances, even if otherwise valid requests or subpoenas by others to obtain substance abuse treatment records are made, federally protected confidentiality for the records of drug treatment may outweigh the validity of the requests. Compliance with requests to breach confidentiality should not occur without a ruling from a judge of competent jurisdiction, declaring that an exception should be made to federal protections.

Style and Attitude

The degree to which a clinician gains the trust of an adolescent and establishes rapport directly influences the validity of the substance use history elicited. In addition to expressing a commitment to confidentiality and privacy, maintaining an open and non-judgmental attitude is essential to cultivating trust and rapport. If the evaluating clinician is perceived as judgmental or punitive, adolescents are less likely to provide reliable information. Conversely, if the interviewing clinician is perceived as being accepting and genuinely interested in who they are and what interests them, beyond the scope of assessing addiction potential, adolescents are more likely to self-report and respond accurately to questioning. Realistically, however, until an adolescent gets to know a clinician over time, suspicion of the adult doctor will remain and this needs to be taken into account.

Starting the interview with less sensitive questions about leisure time activities, hobbies, school or vocational performance, and medical history, can help establish rapport and patient comfort before addressing more sensitive issues. Using open-ended and non-judgmental questions also aids in obtaining more accurate information. A more active approach may be needed to develop rapport with an adolescent than with an adult. It might help to ask what interests an adolescent and talk about that. Unlike with adults, where traditional interviews may suffice, with the adolescent it might even help to take a walk, go outside, or even engage in an activity the adolescent likes in an effort to create rapport.

Clinicians should make an effort to learn about local drug use trends and slang for commonly used drugs. Avoiding the use of stilted language and instead using appropriate slang when asking about substance use can help the young patient feel you are aware or experienced in drug culture. A working knowledge of common drug paraphernalia and modes of administration is also very helpful. However, trying to act like an adolescent can be counterproductive and correctly perceived as phony by an adolescent.

In addition, a clinician's personal biases and preconceived ideas about the type of adolescent that would or wouldn't abuse drugs, can hinder accurate assessment. As in adults, addiction afflicts adolescents from every socioeconomic class, culture, race, and background. By remaining objective and open, a good clinician should let the assessment shape the diagnosis not his or her own prejudices. It is common for most patients to deny or minimize the extent of their substance abuse. Adolescents are no exception.

Collateral Information

Eliciting collateral information is essential for a comprehensive evaluation of addiction in the adolescent. Sources of collateral information include family members, school officials, past medical providers, or past medical records. Clinicians should explicitly request consent to communicate with others and to request confidential medical records from outside institutions. Once consent has been granted, eliciting collateral information should be a top priority and must be elicited for accurate assessment.

Collateral information can provide valuable data on adolescent substance use patterns, history of use, and consequences of use. It can also provide data about the effects of substance use on close relationships and help identify maladaptive family dynamics or associated factors that can increase risk for use or complicate assessment and subsequent treatment. Collateral information can also provide specific evidence about the harm caused by drug use that can help persuade an adolescent to diminish or stop such use and form a therapeutic alliance.

Parents should be asked about any family history of addiction, and current alcohol or drug use by other family members, and be encouraged to express their perception of the adolescent's substance use history. Parents or other sources of collateral information should be asked about objective evidence of substance use, including:

- Finding alcohol, illicit drugs, nicotine, prescription medications, or commonly abused inhalants or volatile substances, such as empty spray paint cans or glues, in the adolescent's possession.
- Finding drug paraphernalia or any equipment, product, or material used in preparing, injecting, ingesting, inhaling, or otherwise introducing a controlled substance into the human body.
- Witnessing intoxication or withdrawal episodes, or red flags such as acute intermittent disturbances or fluctuations in behavior, perception, mood, anxiety, appetite or sleep patterns; disciplinary problems or poor academic performance; borrowing or stealing money.

The interviewing clinician should also note the reliability of the collateral information source and document this. Parents may be unwilling or resistant to provide accurate information about the current living situation fearing repercussions for lack of supervision, permissive attitudes about alcohol or substance use, or their own personal history of substance use.

Past medical records and chart review are also a valuable source of information that can provide an indication of the progression of symptoms and problem severity. Despite this, records must also be viewed critically for objective evidence justifying past diagnoses. Because many young patients conceal their substance use, any emergent psychiatric hospitalizations for acute mood, psychotic, or behavioral issues must be viewed as potential episodes of substance-induced mood or psychotic disorders. There is a risk of misdiagnosing adolescents and giving them an erroneous diagnosis of bipolar disorder or psychotic disorders to explain acute or episodic signs and symptoms resulting from substance-induced disorders or substance withdrawal syndromes. Failure to recognize that symptoms are being caused by substance abuse is a common occurrence. Similarly, antisocial acts perpetrated by an adolescent to obtain drugs are not necessarily an indication of a developing antisocial personality in the adolescent.

LABORATORY SCREENING

A detailed review of laboratory screening is beyond the scope of this chapter but substance detection is an important tool in both assessment and treatment of addiction. Laboratory testing, however, must be conducted with informed consent and in a manner protecting confidentiality. Despite this, random drug toxicology screens are often necessary to monitor some adolescents. Parental permission alone is not sufficient for testing in an adolescent, and involuntary or covert testing is ill advised, illegal in many states, and can irreversibly poison the therapeutic relationship. If random drug testing is planned, it should also be done with the adolescent's consent. Even if the law in a particular jurisdiction does not consider an adolescent competent to give informed consent because of age, it is advisable to seek the adolescent's consent for lab testing. Similarly, in jurisdictions where parents have the legal right to make decisions for the adolescent, it is still advisable to seek assent for drug testing. In other jurisdictions, adolescents may have the cognitive capacity to give consent tempered by immaturity even if lacking legal capacity and almost certainly the capacity to assent, so it is always important to know the law on these matters in your jurisdiction and act accordingly.

Drug testing can help identify or confirm a substance abuse problem that has been overlooked, or minimized or concealed by adolescents, or a relapse into drug use.

Like screening, it can be conducted at regular intervals to establish baseline patterns of drug use and monitor escalation or treatment effect. The results of drug testing should always be reported to the adolescent in a manner that protects confidentiality, and the implications of results should be discussed.

Clinicians should also be aware of the limitations of drug testing and proper collection techniques. Adolescents may deliberately engage in excessive hydration to dilute their urine, use the urine of others, or tamper with or adulterate samples with such substances as lemon juice, vinegar, and salt, all of which may interfere with detection. Given this, the collection of samples should be observed and attention to the temperature, volume, and sample color should be noted. Measuring urine pH, specific gravity, and creatinine clearance can also help detect aberrant tests or adulterated samples. Additionally, there can be false positives. In some cases further testing is needed to confirm or determine the cause of a positive test result.

Commercially available point of care urine drug tests exist for common classes of misused drugs. However, many substances of abuse are not detected with routine screening and require special testing that may be cost prohibitive. For example, methylphenidate, a commonly abused prescription stimulant used to treat ADHD, is not detectable when screening for amphetamines and requires special testing.

Drug testing should be viewed as a snapshot of substance use and cannot rule out prior use. Detection time of substances in urine varies depending on dose, route of administration, metabolism, fat solubility, urine volume, and pH. The detection time of most drugs in urine is 1 to 3 days but long-term use of fat-soluble drugs such as marijuana or phencyclidine hydrochloride (PCP) may extend the window of detection to weeks.

DOCUMENTATION

Because addiction is a chronic, relapsing, and remitting disorder, an accurate record of assessment at a given point in time can help establish baseline and/or escalating use, which can inform current and subsequent treatment planning. A detailed electronic or written record of addiction assessment should include, as accurately as possible, data elicited from the patient interview, physical exam, mental status exam, collateral sources of information, and results from laboratory testing. Adolescent consent, assent, or refusal should be documented, as should the perceived reliability of adolescent responses and the reliability of collateral information. Because medical records can follow a young patient for years, it is important not to include descriptions or diagnosis from past reports that are perceived as currently inaccurate or unreliable. In addition to documenting diagnostic impressions, motivation for use, motivations for change, and any associated factors that may facilitate or hinder treatment should be clearly noted.

References

1. Johnston LD, O'Malley PM, Bachman JG, Schulenberg JE. *Monitoring the Future National Results on Adolescent Drug Use: Overview of Key Findings, 2010.* Ann Arbor: Institute for Social Research, University of Michigan, 2011.
2. Substance Abuse and Mental Health Services Administration. *Results from the 2009 National Survey on Drug Use and Health: Volume I. Summary of National Findings* (Office of Applied Studies, NSDUH Series H-38A, HHS Publication No. SMA 10-4586Findings). Rockville, MD, 2010.
3. Warner LA, Kessler RC, Hughes M, Anthony JC, Nelson CB. Prevalence and correlates of drug use and dependence in the United States: results from the National Comorbidity Survey. *Arch Gen Psychiatry* 1995;**52**:219–229.
4. Anthony J, Helzer J. Syndromes of drug abuse and dependence. In: Robins LN, Regier DA (eds), *Psychiatric Disorders in America: The Epidemiologic Catchment Area Study.* New York: Free Press, 1991; pp. 116–154.
5. Gentile DA. Pathological video-game use among youth ages 8 to 18: a national study. *Psychol Sci* 2009;**20**:594–602.
6. National Research Council. *Pathological Gambling: A Critical Review.* Washington, DC: National Academy Press, 1999.
7. Gupta R, Derevensky J. Adolescent gambling behavior: A prevalence study and examination of the correlates associated with excessive gambling. *J Gambl Stud* 1998;**14**:319–345.
8. Moreno MA, Jelenchick L, Cox E, Young H, Christakis DA. Problematic internet use among US youth: a systematic review. *Arch Pediatr Adolesc Med* 2011;**165**:797–805.
9. Wagner FA, Anthony JC. From first drug use to drug dependence; developmental periods of risk for dependence upon marijuana, cocaine, and alcohol. *Neuropsychopharmacology* 2002;**26**:479–488.
10. Kandel DB, Yamaguchi K, Chen K. Stages in progression in drug involvement from adolescence to adulthood: further evidence for the gateway theory. *J Stud Alcohol* 1992;**53**:447–457.
11. Anthony JC, Petronis KR. Early-onset drug use and risk of later drug problems. *Drug Alcohol Depend* 1995;**40**:9–15.
12. Taioli E, Wynder E. Effect of the age at which smoking began on frequency of smoking in adulthood. *N Engl J Med* 1991;**325**:968–969.
13. American Academy of Pediatrics Committee on Substance Abuse. Indications for management and referral of patients involved in substance abuse. *Pediatrics* 2000;**106**:143–148.
14. American Psychiatric Association. *Diagnostic and Statistical Manual of Mental Disorders*, 4th edn, Text Review. Washington, DC: American Psychiatric Publishing, Inc., 1994.
15. Winters KC (Revisions Consensus Panel Chair). *Screening and Assessing Adolescents for Substance Use Disorders.* Rockville, MD: US Department of Health and Human Services, 1999.
16. Mikulich SK, Hall SK, Whitmore EA, Crowley TJ. Concordance between DSM-II-R and DSM-IV diagnosis of substance use disorders in adolescents. *Drug Alcohol Depen* 2001;**61**:237–248.
17. Ridenour TA, Bray BC, Cottler LB. Reliability of use, abuse, and dependence of four types of inhalants in adolescents and young adults. *Drug Alcohol Depen* 2007;**91**:40–49.
18. American Psychiatric Association. DSM-5 Development. Available from: http://www.dsm5.org/.
19. Prochaska JO, DiClemente CC, Norcross JC. In search of how people change: Applications to addictive behaviors. *Am Psychol* 1992;**47**:1102–1114.
20. Farrow JA, Smith WR, Hurst MD. *Adolescent Drug and Alcohol Assessment Instruments In Current Use: A Critical Comparison.* Washington State Division of Alcohol and Substance Abuse, 1993.
21. Knight JR, Sherritt L, Harris SK, Gates EC, Chang G. Validity of brief alcohol screening tests among adolescents: a comparison of the AUDIT, POSIT, CAGE, and CRAFFT. *Alcohol Clin Exp Res* 2003;**27**:67–73.
22. Santis R, Garmendia ML, Acuna G, Alvarado ME, Arteaga O. The Alcohol Use Disorders Identification Test (AUDIT) as a screening instrument for adolescents. *Drug Alcohol Depend* 2009;**103**:155–158.
23. Knight JR, Sherritt L, Shrier LA, Harris SK, Chang G. Validity of the CRAFFT substance abuse screening test among adolescent clinic patients. *Arch Pediatr Adolesc Med* 2002;**156**:607–614.
24. Harrell A, Wirtz PW. *Adolescent Drinking Index: Professional Manual.* Odessa: Psychological Assessment Resources, 1989.
25. White HR, Labouvie EW. Towards the assessment of adolescent problem drinking. *J Studies Alcohol* 1989;**50**:30–37.
26. Winters K, Henly G. *Adolescent Diagnostic Interview (ADI) Manual.* Los Angeles, CA: Western Psychological Services, 1993.
27. Cottler LB. *Composite International Diagnostic Interview – Substance Abuse Module (SAM).* St Louis, MO: Department of Psychiatry, Washington University School of Medicine, 2000.
28. Boyle MH, Offord DR, Racine Y, Sanford M. Evaluation of the Diagnostic Interview for Children and Adolescents for use in general population samples. *J Abnorm Child Psychol* 1993;**21**:663–681.

4

Emergency Room and Medical Evaluation

Christopher William Racine[1] and Stephen Bates Billick[2]

[1] New York University School of Medicine, New York, NY, USA
[2] Department of Psychiatry, New York College of Medicine, New York, NY, USA

INTRODUCTION

Emergency and medical evaluation of the adolescent substance abuser is a topic that warrants particular attention given the far-reaching effects that addiction can have on the physical and emotional well-being of adolescents and their family, peers, and others. Substance-related mortality is an especially troubling concern in the adolescent population, and awareness of potentially lethal medical issues surrounding substance abuse is essential for any practitioner who interacts with this population. The emergency room has become a particularly important location for diagnosis and initial treatment for adolescent substance users. Due to unique biological and environmental factors, it is important to separately consider adolescents as a subpopulation that is distinct from adults and must be treated as such. The goal of this chapter, therefore, will be to review the medical and emergency room evaluation of substance-abusing adolescents.

MEDICAL EVALUATION

Full medical evaluation is an essential, yet often overlooked, portion of a complete work-up of adolescent patients who are suspected to have an addictive disorder. Thorough and complete medical evaluation of the adolescent suspected to have a substance use disorder is the most important job of the provider who evaluates such patients. Often, providers assume that the young patient is physically healthy and fail to complete a full medical examination. However, even in young patients, many known medical abnormalities are secondary to substance use itself. Adolescents who abuse substances are also at higher risk of presenting with comorbid injury, illness, and other maladies. An astute provider will need to consider these factors during their assessment. Triage, diagnosis, and future direction of treatment will naturally follow from the initial and follow-up medical evaluations. The evaluation should begin with a complete review of systems followed by a full physical exam. Based on this information, clinicians can make informed decisions about further laboratory and imaging tests. The intent of this section is not to review the entirety of medical assessment of patients with substance use disorders. It is, however, meant to review pertinent findings that may aid in the evaluation of patients with suspected substance use disorders, with special emphasis on the adolescent population.

Clinical Evaluation of Adolescents

Adolescents who are using substances may present with unpredictable and wide-ranging clinical variations. The substance that has been used, the time since use, and amount of drug that has been consumed will all influence how a patient will appear. While adolescent substance abusers will frequently present in an intoxicated state, or with signs of significant drug tolerance, they are less likely than adult substance users to present with symptoms of dependence or withdrawal [1]. Diagnosis is often complicated by the fact that adolescents with addictive disorders are more likely to be abusing more than a single substance. In addition to careful history-taking, familiarity with the clinical signs and symptoms of substances commonly used by adolescent patients is important in making a diagnosis, which can then be used to guide treatment decisions.

Alcohol

The clinical presentation of adolescents who have been abusing alcohol can take on various forms. As with adult patients, adolescents who have abused alcohol will have very different clinical symptoms based on their level of

Clinical Handbook of Adolescent Addiction, First Edition. Richard Rosner.
© 2013 John Wiley & Sons, Ltd. Published 2013 by John Wiley & Sons, Ltd.

habituation to the drug. These may range from mild, nearly undetectable clinical symptoms all the way to respiratory arrest and coma. Adolescent patients may present with or without a distinct smell of alcohol on their breath. Young alcohol consumers are known to combine alcohol with energy drinks in order to enhance their ability to remain awake and "party," counteracting the sedating effects of alcohol [2]. This is of particular concern given that the ingestion of carbonated beverages speeds the rate of alcohol absorption, leading to more rapid and profound intoxication [3].

In general, symptoms of acute alcohol intoxication correspond to blood alcohol levels. In turn, blood alcohol levels are influenced by the rapidity at which alcohol is consumed and eliminated. At levels below 0.08%, adolescents may have mild changes in mood or personality, such as feeling disinhibited or euphoric. Adolescents in particular are vulnerable to increased risk-taking behaviors at this level of intoxication. Some adolescents may also have mild coordination problems even at "low" blood alcohol concentrations [4]. At blood alcohol levels in the moderate range, from 0.1 to 0.2%, coordination becomes more severely impaired and ataxia becomes pronounced. Patients may also experience blurry vision, memory deficits, sedation, and difficulty comprehending their environment. Speech may become slurred. At levels higher than 0.2% to 0.25%, patients typically display signs of severe intoxication including amnesia, diplopia, nystagmus, nausea, vomiting, hypothermia, staggering gait, and almost complete incoherence. At levels higher than 0.4%, patients at all ages can have respiratory depression and coma that may potentially lead to death. Clinical signs that a level of potentially fatal intoxication has been reached include decreased muscle reflexes, cessation of pupillary response, anesthesia, and bradycardia. While withdrawal symptoms are less likely to be seen in the adolescent population, they do at times occur and should be monitored for in patients with a history or suspected history of heavy and sustained alcohol use. Initial withdrawal symptoms include tachycardia, hypertension, hyperthermia, sweating, hyperreflexia, tremor, vomiting, diarrhea, and tongue fasciculation. These may progress to confusion, psychosis, seizures, delirium, and even death.

Chronic alcohol consumption in adolescence may also lead to clinically detectable negative sequelae. Neurocognitive deficits in teens who have heavily abused alcohol have been detected. Deficits in vocabulary, general information, and memory tests were increased in a select group of young alcohol users when compared with non-users [5]. Severe sleep cycle disruption may be noted, and can even mimic many symptoms of depression. Although not clinically relevant in establishing a diagnosis, it is important to remember that chronic alcohol use in this population may disrupt maturation by affecting the neuroendocrine system, including disruption of growth hormone release [6].

Cannabis (Marijuana)

Delta-9-tetrahydrocannabinol (THC) is the active metabolite in marijuana that is suspected to produce intoxication, including the mild euphoria and sense of well-being that is often sought by adolescent users. Signs of acute THC intoxication include conjunctival injection, tachycardia, loss of coordination, slowed reaction time, and even perceptual disturbances. Distortions of time are commonly reported by young marijuana users. Frank paranoia may result, especially in marijuana users who are new to the substance. Cognition may also be impaired, with memory, learning, attention, and problem-solving difficulties noted [7]. In users, THC may also have sedative, analgesic, anxiolytic, and appetite-enhancing effects. Acute effects are relatively short-lived, with an average half-life of 1.6 hours. However, intoxication effects can often be felt for up to 8 hours by some users [8]. Furthermore, in youths with heavy, chronic marijuana use followed by abrupt cessation, a withdrawal syndrome may be seen. While this syndrome and its characteristics are still being debated, symptoms may include anger and aggression, decreased appetite, irritability, nervousness, restlessness, shakiness, sleeping difficulty, stomach pain, strange dreams, sweating, and weight loss [9,10]. Increasingly, adolescents are turning to synthetic cannabinoid-based designer drugs such as K2 or "spice," which can be purchased legally in many US states. These designer cannabinoids produce effects that are purportedly similar to those obtained from marijuana use. While study of these compounds and their effects is still underway, it is important to note that most of these designer cannabinoids are not detected by commercial urine screens [11].

Cocaine and Amphetamines

Cocaine and amphetamines, although different in many respects, may be considered as a single class for the purpose of medical evaluation. The increasing availability of illicit amphetamines and methamphetamines necessitates that the modern-day provider become familiar with the signs and symptoms of non-medical use of these drugs. Signs of intoxication on physical exam are similar for both cocaine and amphetamines. These include, but are not limited to, tachycardia, tachypnea, hyperthermia, hypertension, diaphoresis, tremor, flushing, and mydriasis. Patients may further report or exhibit anorexia, stereotyped movements, increased energy, disrupted or decreased need for sleep, psychosis, aggression, and increased interest in sexual activity. When symptoms are pronounced or known large quantities have been used, providers must be aware that there exists a higher risk for seizure. Large quantities also have the potential to induce cardiovascular collapse, requiring that adequate screening and monitoring of cardiovascular status be undertaken. Prolonged use of methamphetamines in young patients can lead to consequences that require medical attention, including memory loss, aggression, violence, and psychotic behavior [12]. Providers must also be aware of the "crash," or withdrawal phase, that may be seen in youths who have used significant amounts of cocaine or illicit amphetamines. The withdrawal syndrome may last from 9 hours to 4 days and includes psychomotor slowing, increased appetite, depression, hypersomnolence, anergia, and even suicidal thinking. Evaluation must consider the risk of suicide when assessing such patients in emergency and other settings.

Opiates

Opioid use, including illicit use of prescription medication, is becoming more frequently encountered by medical practitioners who treat adolescent patients. In particular, a screening for use of additional substances is especially important, as adolescent opiate users are significantly more likely to have additional comorbid substance use diagnoses as compared to those who use other substances [13]. Completion of a comprehensive physical evaluation is also especially important given the high incidence of medical comorbidity. This is particularly true in patients who engage in intravenous opiate use. Chronic and intravenous opiate users are more susceptible to cardiac infections, cellulitis at injection sites, abscess formation, pneumonia and pneumonitis, liver disease (in particular hepatitis C infection), and increased incidence of HIV infection.

Clinical findings in adolescent opiate users vary according to the specific opiate that was used and the route by which it was administered. Characteristic of this class, all opiates are analgesic and typically induce a sense of euphoria sought by abusers. At low doses, opiates are typically activating, while becoming increasingly more sedating at higher doses. Features of acute intoxication include facial flushing and itchiness, a sense of warmth, dry mouth, bradycardia, hypotension, and pupil constriction. As intoxication becomes more severe, areflexia, pronounced hypotension, reflex tachycardia, respiratory depression, and death may result.

Commonly, adolescent users will present for treatment in the setting of opiate withdrawal, as many may be unfamiliar with the signs and symptoms associated with this condition. Accurate identification of the opiate withdrawal syndrome through medical evaluation is important in this setting, as this affords a unique opportunity for the medical provider to potentially intervene and alter the course of an abuse pattern that is associated with delinquent or criminal behavior, difficulties in school, and rapid psychosocial decline [14]. Characteristics of withdrawal include tachycardia, hypertension, joint and muscle aches, abdominal cramping, diarrhea, vomiting, photophobia, insomnia, piloerection, restlessness, and anxiety. Accurately assessing the severity of withdrawal symptoms in these patients will inform treatment decisions.

MDMA

3,4-Methylenedioxymethamphetamine (MDMA), or "ecstasy" as it is commonly known, has physical manifestations that resemble both the stimulant effects of amphetamines and the hallucinogenic effects that resemble lysergic acid diethylamide (LSD) and other hallucinogens. Physical symptoms do not fit a typical pattern like that seen in many other substances of abuse. Symptoms are disparate and may include hypertension, tachycardia, trismus, muscle tightness, nausea, blurred vision, tremors, dizziness, chills, ataxia, and diaphoresis. After acute MDMA intoxication has passed, users will often describe a period characterized by lethargy, irritability, anxiety, depression, and insomnia [15]. In certain instances, through unclear mechanisms, MDMA has been known to lead to malignant hyperthermia in adolescent users that can potentially be fatal [16]. Additional reports of renal failure, hyperpyrexia, disseminated intravascular coagulation, hepatitis, subarachnoid hemorrhage, and sudden cardiac death have also been reported in those having recently used recreational MDMA.

Inhalants

Caution must be utilized in conducting the medical evaluation of adolescents who have used or are suspected of using the gases and fumes of volatile organic compounds for the purpose of getting "high," as these are amongst the most toxic of psychoactive substances. In general, acute intoxication resembles that seen in alcohol, with an initial period of euphoria and disorientation followed by drowsiness and central nervous system (CNS) depression. Intoxication is short-lived, typically lasting only minutes. Key signs of inhalant abuse include stains on clothing or skin, sores in and around the mouth, conjunctival injection, rhinorrhea, chemical odor on the breath, and a dazed appearance [17]. Symptoms are often non-specific and may include dizziness, irritability, tiredness, loss of appetite, headache, photophobia, or cough [18]. Patients should be monitored closely as many recreationally abused inhalants can lead to unconsciousness and death. In adolescents who have chronically abused inhalants, evaluation should include a comprehensive neurological exam to evaluate for known toxicity, including memory loss, psychotic symptoms, slurred speech, ataxic or otherwise abnormal gait, nystagmus, and sensory loss including hearing, vision, or sense of smell.

Steroids

Anabolic steroid use for the purpose of athletic performance enhancement continues to be a growing problem amongst the adolescent population [19]. Steroids are typically taken to enhance muscle development in the setting of exercise. Illicitly purchased steroids may come in many forms and are typically administered in cycles. When used, anabolic steroids may lead to damage in many organ systems, which clinicians should evaluate for when treating an adolescent with suspected steroid use. Adverse effects may include hepatotoxicity and liver cancer, tachycardia, cardiomegaly, acne, and reproductive system abnormalities. Use may lead to testicular atrophy, increased voice pitch, and gynecomastia in young men. In young women, clitoral hypertrophy, hirsuitism, menstrual abnormalities, decreased breast mass, and a male pattern balding can result. Psychiatric manifestations such as mood swings and increased aggressiveness often lead patients and their families to seek treatment, and steroid abuse should be considered when these are presenting symptoms. Dependence may occur in the context of heavy use, and cessation of steroid use is associated with a withdrawal syndrome characterized by fatigue, anorexia, insomnia, and mood swings. Although somewhat counterintuitive given that these patients may be overly concerned with their appearance and health, evidence shows that adolescent steroid abusers are actually more likely to user other illicit substances, and so screening for comorbid use is an essential part of evaluation in this population [20].

Nicotine (Tobacco Products)

Medical problems secondary to tobacco use are rare during the adolescent period, as more severe health consequences are not typically seen until much later in life. However, adolescents who smoke, chew, or "dip" tobacco products may present for evaluation in many other contexts. Nicotine produces CNS stimulation that lasts approximately 30 minutes. This CNS stimulation is associated with increased arousal and improved concentration. Nicotine commonly produces a psychological and physiological dependence syndrome, even in adolescents. After approximately 24 hours of abstinence, chronic users may experience a withdrawal syndrome that is characterized by irritability, difficulty concentrating, anxiety, depressed mood, and increased aggression. In an emergency room evaluation, adolescents should always be questioned regarding tobacco use and encouraged to pursue a smoking cessation referral.

Caffeine

Caffeine is an often overlooked substance of abuse during adolescence. When presenting for treatment in an emergency room or primary care setting, more immediate issues are often addressed as caffeine use is often considered normative behavior in this age group. However, up to one-fifth of teenagers are physiologically dependent on caffeine [21]. Caffeine intake in adolescent patients produces dose-dependent vital sign changes similar to those seen in adult patients including decreased heart rate and increased diastolic blood pressure [22]. Small doses of caffeine produce an enhanced sense of well-being, increased arousal, increased energy, and improved concentration. Higher doses can lead to anxiety, "jitteriness," nausea, and fidgetiness. While adults typically do not experience these unpleasant symptoms until they have consumed greater than 400 mg of caffeine, adolescents may have unpleasant symptoms at doses as low as 100 mg [23,24]. This is roughly equivalent to two cans of caffeinated soda or one large cup of coffee. Tolerance to caffeine may occur in adolescent patients and abrupt cessation can lead to withdrawal symptoms including headache, fatigue, and drowsiness.

Other Substances

Phencyclidine (PCP), lysergic acid diethylamide (LSD), psilocybin (hallucinogenic mushrooms), gamma-hydroxybutyrate (GHB), and dextromethorphan (cough syrup) use can also be seen in the adolescent population. Accurate and early detection using associated clinical symptoms is important. A review of associated signs and symptoms associated with these drug classes can be found in Table 4.1 .

Laboratory and Radiological Examination

Detection of substance use and evaluation for associated medical abnormalities through laboratory tests remains an important component of the medical evaluation of adolescent substance abusers. Serum, saliva, sweat, and

Table 4.1 Clinical features of substances of abuse in adolescents.

Substance of abuse	Key clinical symptoms
Dextromethorphan	Dissociation, perceptual disturbances, nausea, drowsiness, hyperthermia, hypertension, respiratory depression, diarrhea, urinary retention, mydriasis
GHB (gamma-hydroxybutyrate)	Nausea, drowsiness, respiratory depression, amnesia, death
LSD (lysergic acid diethylamide)	Mydriasis, hyperthermia, hypertension, tachycardia, insomnia, dry mouth, tremor, anorexia
PCP (phencyclidine)	Ataxia, nausea, blurred vision, hypotension, bradycardia, flushing, sweating, loss of muscle control, respiratory depression, agitation, perceptual disturbance
Psilocybin	Mydriasis, hyperreflexia, tachycardia, drowsiness, perceptual disorders

hair detection tests are now commercially available for many of the substances of abuse. In addition, many settings are increasingly utilizing breathalyzer tests for detection of alcohol. However, urine detection remains the most common and practical means of evaluating for recent substance use, particularly in emergency room and primary care settings where adolescent users are most likely to present. Typically, providers will order a urine drug "panel" to screen for substance use when there is clinical suspicion of abuse. This is particularly important as adolescents are unlikely to be forthcoming in disclosing their substance abuse. Clinicians should also be aware that the specific substances for which a screening test evaluates may differ by manufacturer and setting in which it is being used. Typical drug screening tests evaluate for all or a combination of the major drugs of abuse: marijuana, heroin, methadone, cocaine,

Table 4.2 Typical urine detection periods of illicit substances.

Substance	Urine detection time
Alcohol	6–10 hours
Amphetamine/methamphetamine	1–3 days
Anabolic steroids	Oral up to 3 weeks, injected up to 3 months
Benzodiazepines	6–72 hours
Cannabis	2–30+ days based on amount used
Cocaine	1–4 days
Codeine/morphine	1–3 days
Heroin	1–3 days
PCP	2–8 days
Psilocybin	2–8 days
LSD	8 hours to 5 days

methamphetamines, PCP, and benzodiazepines. Typically, specific blood or urine tests to detect recent use of MDMA, hallucinogens, or GHB must be sent separately and are not detected by commercial screening tests. The utility of urine drug screening is further limited by the fact that many major substances of abuse are only detectable in urine if used within a few days of testing (Table 4.2). Thus, negative results on drug tests do not necessarily suggest the absence of abuse, especially when clinical suspicion is high. Moreover, positive testing on urine drug screening is unable to distinguish between casual use, abuse, and dependence. Again, testing should be supplemented and aided by historical and clinical information whenever available.

In addition to detection of drug use, laboratory tests can be judiciously utilized to identify medical abnormalities that may be comorbid with, or secondary to, substance use in adolescents. Laboratory tests may be utilized to aid in diagnosis or confirm clinical suspicion of abuse; an example is elevated serum aminotransferase levels in alcohol abuse. They may also be used to detect medical abnormalities that may be secondary to substance use, such as the detection of abnormal fasting lipid levels in adolescents who abuse anabolic steroids [25]. Finally, laboratory tests can be utilized to detect conditions that adolescent substance users are at high risk of acquiring. For instance, adolescent substance users are at higher risk of becoming pregnant and acquiring sexually transmitted diseases [26]. Therefore, testing for pregnancy, HIV, gonorrhea, chlamydia, and other sexually transmitted diseases should be considered in adolescents who present having used or abused illicit substances.

EMERGENCY ROOM EVALUATION

Over the past several decades, emergency departments in the United States have expanded their traditional role of treating only serious, acute medical illness.

Marginalized populations, including those who abuse and are addicted to illicit substances, have increasingly utilized the emergency room as a gateway to receipt of medical care [27]. Adolescent substance abusers may present for care in an emergency room for various reasons. Some are specifically seeking treatment for substance abuse or dependence. However, many adolescents who present to the emergency room will not list substance use as their primary reason for coming to the emergency service. Some will present with comorbid psychiatric symptoms that have been exacerbated by substance use. Others may be experiencing unwanted or unexpected effects from the use of illicit drugs. Still others may present as a result of medical illness or accident that was suffered as a result of intoxication, abuse, or dependence on illicit substances. Thus, emergency rooms have become increasingly vital in the identification of youths with substance use disorders. Moreover, emergency settings have increasingly been utilized to initiate treatment in youths who have, or are at high risk of developing, a substance use disorder. The goal of this section is to aid practitioners in the emergency room in the identification and management of adolescents who present with substance use.

The Emergency Room Interview

The emergency room (ER) interview of an adolescent patient, as reviewed above, offers the unique opportunity to intervene in the course of a substance use disorder. However, the urgent care setting may not always serve as the ideal place to conduct an in-depth patient interview. Many distinctive challenges face the emergency room interviewer. By the very nature of emergency care, practitioners will almost never have encountered their patients prior to meeting in the ER. To many patients and their families, the emergency room may look like organized chaos, making them reluctant to address major personal challenges with a practitioner they are unfamiliar with. Physical space is often limited in emergency room settings, threatening both privacy and confidentiality. However, despite these challenges, a skilled and thoughtful clinician can maximize the potential benefit of the emergency room setting. Previous chapters have examined the interview of adolescent patients who are suspected to have an addictive disorder. Here, we briefly review and highlight the psychiatric interview as it relates to the emergency room.

Whenever possible, adolescent patients should be interviewed in a private setting, offering them the opportunity to share freely without fear of being overheard by others. This may be achieved by choosing a more secluded area within the ER or identifying a designated area outside of the ER that still offers the protections and services available in the ER. First interviews with adolescent patients should be conducted alone, unless otherwise specifically requested by the adolescent patient. If family members or friends have accompanied the patient to the emergency room, they should be interviewed separately, also in a private setting. Furthermore, in young patients with possible addiction, collateral contact should extend beyond those contacts who are present in the emergency room. Adolescents will often under-report or fail to report substance use [28]. Key risk factors for adolescent substance use, including chaotic home environment, parental substance abuse, poor parenting, and poor social coping, may not be apparent upon interview with the patient or family members present in the ER. Thus, accurate assessment hinges on obtaining multiple sources of collateral information from parents, teachers, case workers, and even peers [29,30].

Unlike youths with medical conditions or many psychiatric conditions, adolescents seeking treatment for substance use disorders may be doing so only at the prompting of others. During ER evaluation, more so than in other settings, it is important to first engage patients in a non-threatening line of questioning prior to asking directly about substance abuse. Establishing a therapeutic alliance, although challenging amidst the chaos of the ER during a first meeting with a new patient, moves the interviewer towards his or her goal of obtaining accurate information that will be used to guide decision-making regarding disposition and treatment.

Key elements of the psychiatric interview merit specific focus during the emergency evaluation of adolescents who may have used substances. Because safety is of primary concern in the emergency setting, a complete evaluation for risk of suicide and violence should be undertaken. In the same vein, evaluation for comorbid psychiatric illness should not be overlooked amidst the substance use disorder. For instance, substance use is almost twice as common in adolescents with major depressive disorder compared with other adolescents [31]. Risk factors for substance abuse can be addressed either informally during interview or formally through use of a screening test.

Rating scales and screening tests may also be helpful in assessing adolescents with suspected substance use disorders. While not mandatory for use in emergency settings, scales and screening exams may be helpful in establishing a diagnosis when information is incomplete or unclear. Typical adult rating scales have generally not been validated amongst adolescent patients. For instance, the CAGE Questionnaire, which serves as the most rapid screening test amongst adults for problem drinking, has been normed for adults over the age of 16 only [32] and is not recommended for use in adolescent patients [33]. Over the past decade, however, advances have been made in development of rapid screening tests for the evaluation of substance use in the adolescent population.

The six-item CRAFFT screen, which is short enough for use in the emergency room setting, was developed specifically for the adolescent population and has been validated [34]. CRAFFT screening questions include queries that are targeted to a younger population:

1. C – Have you ever ridden in a car driven by someone (including yourself) who was "high" or had been using alcohol or drugs?
2. R – Do you ever use alcohol or drugs to relax, feel better about yourself, or fit in?
3. A – Do you ever use drugs while you are by yourself, alone?
4. F – Do you ever forget things that you did while using alcohol or drugs?
5. F – Do your family or friends ever tell you that you should cut down on your drinking or drug use?
6. T – Have you ever gotten into trouble while you were using alcohol or drugs?

Positive responses are counted as one point and an overall score of greater than two points signifies that further evaluation is necessary [35]. While the CRAFFT is brief and well validated, other screening tests that may potentially be of use in screening adolescents for substance abuse in the emergency setting include the 10-item AUDIT (Alcohol Use Disorders Identification Test) [36], 16-item Simple Screening Instrument for Alcohol and Other Drugs (SSI-AOD) [37], and 17-item POSIT (Problem Oriented Screening Instrument for Teenagers) [38]. The reliability of such screens is dependent upon cooperation and the honest answering of screening questions, limiting their utility in certain populations of antisocial or oppositional youths.

Emergency Room Interventions

As stated before, the emergency room serves as a pivotal setting in which to diagnose and assess for adolescent substance abuse. More recently, it has also been increasingly utilized as the location in which to provide patient education and initiate brief interventions targeted at promoting behavior change. The potential to enact major, life-altering change is large in substance-using youth populations. For instance, each year that drinking onset can be delayed in adolescents, the risk for development of alcohol dependence goes down by 14% [39]. This is no minor finding, as emergency rooms have been increasingly utilized as primary care settings and serve as the gateway to continued psychiatric and medical care.

A rash of literature has recently evaluated the utility of motivational interviewing to enact behavioral change in adolescent patients who present to the ER. As motivational interviewing is targeted to address patients at different stages of change, this technique is particularly helpful in ER settings because it can be universally applied [40]. The data are particularly strong for motivational interviewing in adolescents presenting to emergency rooms with alcohol use disorders. Research has shown that a single, brief motivational interviewing session with a trained clinician can lead to decreased alcohol consumption in adolescents as far out as 12 months after the initial interview [41]. In addition to lowered alcohol consumption, motivational interviewing has also been shown to significantly lower the incidence of drinking and driving, traffic violations, alcohol-related injuries, and alcohol-related medical problems in older adolescents [42]. Studies have also shown significant reductions in cigarette and marijuana use after brief motivational interviewing sessions in emergency settings [43,44]. While motivational interviewing takes more time and training than traditional emergency room evaluation, cost-effectiveness estimates approximate large societal savings from use of this technique [45].

SPECIAL TOPIC: MEDICAL MANAGEMENT OF SUSPECTED OVERDOSE IN ADOLESCENT PATIENTS

Adolescents will at times present for medical attention, typically in an emergency room setting, after overdosing on substances of abuse. Accurate detection and management of suspected overdose of these patients may be critical to minimizing morbidity and preventing possible mortality. Clinical diagnosis can be made even more difficult when overdose victims are obtunded and unable to give an accurate clinical history. In this case, clinicians must be able to identify signs and symptoms of abuse presented above in order to guide a clinical investigation. The medical signs and symptoms of the major substances of abuse are reviewed above. The goal of this section is to give providers a practical guide to the identification and management of youths who may present to the ER after acute substance intoxication.

Identification and Toxidromes

There are innumerable different substances on which adolescents presenting to the emergency room may

Table 4.3 Toxidromes commonly seen after overdose of illicit substances.

Toxidrome	Substances	Vital signs	Signs/symptoms	Serious adverse consequences
Adrenergic	Cocaine, amphetamine, methamphetamine	HR↑ BP↑ Temp.↑ RR↑	Mydriasis Increased BS Diaphoresis Agitated/anxious	Cardiac dysrhythmia Seizure Coma
CNS depressant	Heroin, morphine, methadone, oxycodone, hydroxycodone	HR↓ BP↓ Temp. Nl RR↓	Miosis Decreased BS Slowed mentation	Respiratory arrest Coma
Sedative-hypnotic	Alcohol, benzodiazepines, barbiturates	HR Nl/↓ BP Nl/↓ Temp. Nl/↓ RR↓	Slowed mentation Variable pupil, skin, and BS changes	Coma Respiratory arrest Seizure

BP, blood pressure; BS, bowel sounds; HR, heart rate; Nl, normal; RR, respiratory rate.

have overdosed on. The clinical picture in adolescent patients will commonly be complicated by the fact that young substance abusers are more likely to have used more than one particular substance prior to presentation. In order to simplify identification of which substance or combination of substances a patient may have overdosed on, one approach is to classify substances into groups based on clinical features. Doing so may help guide initial management decisions to prevent further injury or death. Thus, identification of the major toxic syndromes, or "toxidromes," is important in the initial management of the adolescent patient who has potentially overdosed. In the overdose and poisoning literature, five major toxidromes have been identified: (i) adrenergic, (ii) anticholinergic, (iii) cholinergic, (iv) CNS depressant, and (v) sedative-hypnotic [46,47]. Anticholinergic and cholinergic toxidromes are not typically seen after overdose of substances of abuse, and are more commonly associated with accidental or intentional overdose of prescription and over-the-counter medications. However, in evaluating potential substance abuse overdose, knowledge of adrenergic, CNS depressant, and sedative-hypnotic toxidromes is useful. Table 4.3 reviews the illicit substances that may be associated with and the clinical features of each associated toxidrome [48].

General Overdose Management

Initial management of overdose in adolescents should begin with a primary survey that is standard of care for other patients who present to the emergency room with a serious medical condition. The ABCDs of emergency management serve as a practical guide to the initial

evaluation to assess for immediate need for life-sustaining intervention: Airway, Breathing, Circulation, and Disability in the adolescent should be assessed and treated. Whether respiratory support will be necessary should be especially considered in adolescents who may have overdosed on illicit substances. After such, a complete set of vital signs should be performed, as they may direct a clinician into suspecting one of the toxidromes above. When possible, a secondary survey to assess for physical signs and symptoms associated with overdose should be performed, focusing on skin changes, pupil abnormalities, bowel sounds, and mental status changes. Intravenous access should be established and cardiac monitoring – 12-lead electrocardiogram (ECG) or continuous cardiac monitor – should be performed. Based on clinical scenario, lab tests including urine toxicology, urinalysis, complete blood count (CBC), serum electrolytes, and liver function testing should be performed.

In patients presenting to acute care settings with alterations in consciousness, including adolescents who may have overdosed on illicit substances, some emergency room providers have advocated the empirical use of several medications that may be of most benefit without significant risk of side effects. This "coma cocktail" calls for the use of supplemental oxygen (100% at flow rates 8–10 L/min), dextrose 50% in water (D50W; 25–50 mL), naloxone (0.1–0.2 mg starting dose followed by repeat dosing), and thiamine (100 mg i.v.) [49]. With the advent of rapid finger glucose testing, empirical glucose is typically not necessary and no longer considered an essential empirical therapy in these cases [46]. Previously, the "coma cocktail" has also included empirical flumazenil to treat benzodiazepine overdose. However, this agent has been known to provoke withdrawal seizures and is no longer recommended during empirical treatment in unresponsive patients [50].

In the past, various methods had been used in emergency room settings to purge or minimize the impact of potential toxic ingestion of substances in patients known to have overdosed. In the case of adolescent substance-abusing patients, ingested substances of particular concern are alcohol, prescription opiates, MDMA, prescription benzodiazepines, and other pills of abuse. Various methods, including induced vomiting using ipecac and gastric lavage, have largely fallen by the wayside as patients were noted to be at risk for serious side effects with unclear benefits [51,52]. In modern emergency room practice, use of activated charcoal to prevent gastrointestinal absorption of toxic substances remains the primary method used to prevent toxicity from overdose. Typically, activated charcoal is administered in a single dose of 25–100 g in adolescents [46]. The utility of activated charcoal in ingested overdoses is highly dependent upon the time from ingestion and the compound that has been ingested. In particular, alcohol is poorly absorbed by activated charcoal. Activated charcoal is also associated with significant risks including aspiration, particularly in patients who are unable to protect their own airways due to altered mental status. Thus, while it remains the key method to prevent morbidity from overdose, activated charcoal use remains of unclear benefit, particularly in the care of those who have overdosed on illicit substances [53].

Management of Overdose in Known Substances of Abuse

In some cases, the substance that has been used is known and treatment can be specifically targeted toward management of known consequences. Here follows a brief review of the management of the adolescent patient who may have overdosed on substances that commonly lead to emergency room presentation.

Opiate Overdose

When treating an adolescent with suspected opiate overdose, the most important, life-threatening problem typically encountered is that of respiratory depression. Assessment of respiratory status and appropriate intervention is the key consideration when first approaching a patient. If apoxia is suspected or confirmed, initial management is typically with 100% oxygen and use of a bag-valve-mask device. Oral and nasopharyngeal devices, while they may be helpful, are typically used with caution as they have the potential to induce vomiting, which may lead to aspiration. In cases of severe hypoxia, site-specific respiratory emergency procedures should be followed and intubations should be performed.

In cases of adolescent overdose, an opiate antagonist, naloxone initially at a dose of 0.1–0.4 mg, is recommended. Intravenous, intramuscular, endotracheal, and intralingual formulations of naloxone are available. This dose is targeted to minimize symptoms of respiratory depression while minimizing risk of withdrawal [54]. If this dose fails to produce a response, it is recommended that clinicians administer repeated, escalating doses of naloxone based on clinical response up to a 10 mg dose. If a 10 mg dose fails to produce a response, there is a very low possibility that opiates are responsible for the patient's altered mental status. If successfully treated, practitioners must be aware that the half-life of naloxone is approximately 60 minutes [55]. In the case of long-acting opiate overdose, successful treatment of an adolescent must be followed by prolonged monitoring as there is the risk of relapsing into respiratory depression due to continued presence of long-acting opiate in serum after naloxone has been metabolized.

Seizure is possible as a result of opiate overdose, but typically this is a response to hypoxia, as opposed to being provoked by opiate use itself. Management follows that which is typical for seizures, based on age of the adolescent. Opiate overdose also carries the risk of severe cardiovascular abnormalities. An electrocardiogram should be obtained to evaluate for QRS prolongation followed by continuous cardiac monitoring during the acute intoxication period. Finally, because many prescription opiates also contain acetaminophen (paracetamol), many opiate overdoses are accompanied by concomitant acetaminophen overdose. Management should include obtaining an acetaminophen level and use of a nomogram to determine if intervention is necessary to prevent hepatotoxicity.

Cocaine Overdose

Serious symptoms of cocaine overdose in adolescents are typically those that result from the adrenergic "toxidrome" (see Table 4.3). Associated with this toxidrome is extreme hyperthermia, manifested in temperatures that may escalate to over 108 °F (42.2 °C), leading to delirium, rhabdomyolysis, kidney failure, and death [56]. Associated vasoconstriction can also lead to end-organ damage, particularly in the brain. Immediate intervention is crucial, as the events leading to death progress rapidly in adolescents with severe cocaine intoxication syndrome. Initial management includes fluid resuscitation with intravenous saline, supplemental oxygen, and aggressive cooling measures with ice-water baths or cooling blankets. Pharmacological management is with benzodiazepines, preferably administered intravenously, which provide a dual benefit of prophylaxis against seizures [57]. Other pharmaceutical interventions have failed to show benefit in acute cocaine overdose.

Although often overlooked in the adolescent population, serious cardiac manifestations including myocardial infarction are possible in acute cocaine overdose in younger patients. Myocardial infarction and dilated cardiomyopathy have been reported in patients as young as 18 years old [58]. ECG, continuous cardiac monitoring, and cardiology consultation are recommended when cocaine-induced abnormalities are suspected. Consideration should be given to obtaining cardiac enzymes. In addition to standard management of acute cardiac events, benzodiazepines may also be useful for associated cardiac pain. Beta-blocking agents are absolutely contraindicated in suspected cocaine overdose, as unopposed alpha-adrenergic stimulation may lead to increased vasoconstriction, hypertension, and worsened clinical outcomes.

Inhalant Overdose

The clinical presentation of inhalant overdose is almost never typical given the wide range of inhalants that are abused. Treatment is largely supportive and should be targeted at manifestations of the overdose. Acute direct causes of death from inhalant use are typically caused by "sudden sniffing death syndrome," which has largely been attributed to methemoglobinemia [59]. In suspected cases of overdose, methylene blue may be administered [46]. Inhalant users are also prone to myocardial sensitization, which may lead to ventricular fibrillation and death. When ventricular fibrillation is the presenting symptom, epinephrine (adrenaline) use should be avoided and other antiarrhythmics including lidocaine and beta-blockers should be used as first-line agents [46]. Careful cardiac monitoring thus remains an important part of the evaluation process. In addition, laboratory evaluation should include evaluation for the presence of metabolic acidosis, as some volatile inhalants including methanol may present in such a manner.

SUMMARY

Medical work-up is an important part of the evaluation of adolescent patients in whom substance use is suspected. Knowledge of the signs and symptoms of use, abuse, and withdrawal can provider diagnostic clarity and guide treatment decision-making. Combined with clinical and historical data, informed use of laboratory testing can further guide treatment. The emergency

room setting is increasingly utilized as the location where the adolescent substance-using population is being cared for. Adolescents may come to the emergency room specifically seeking substance abuse treatment, but often will present for other reasons, requiring clinicians to have a low threshold for substance abuse screening. Clinicians in emergency settings who are evaluating adolescents must remember that they may be reluctant reporters of the true severity of their own actual substance abuse. Unfortunately, adolescents will far too often come into the emergency department after overdose on illicit substances. While the urgent care setting offers many unique challenges, it also offers rich opportunities to alter the course of addictive illness through therapeutic techniques such as motivational interviewing and pertinent and timely referrals for definitive treatments.

References

1. Cheung K. Substance use disorders. In: Cheng K, Myers KM (eds), *Child and Adolescent Psychiatry: The Essentials*, 1st edn. Philadelphia: Lippincott Williams & Wilkins, 2005; pp. 90–109.
2. Bigard AX. Risks of energy drinks in youths. *Arch Pediat Adol Med* 2010;**17**:1625–1631.
3. Paton A. Alcohol in the body. *Brit Med J* 2005;**330**:85–87.
4. Maldonado JR. An approach to the patient with substance use and abuse. *Med Clin North Am* 2010;**94**:1169–1205, x-i.
5. Brown SA, Tapert SF, Granholm E, *et al.* Neurocognitive functioning of adolescents: effects of protracted alcohol use. *Alcohol Clin Exp Res* 2000;**24**:164–171.
6. Upadhyaya HP, Brady KT, Liao J, *et al.* Neuroendocrine and behavioral responses to dopaminergic agonists in adolescents with alcohol abuse. *Psychopharmacology (Berl)* 2003;**166**:95–101.
7. Harvey MA, Sellman JD, Porter RJ, *et al.* The relationship between non-acute adolescent cannabis use and cognition. *Drug Alcohol Rev* 2007;**26**:309–319.
8. Toennes SW, Ramaekers JG, Theunissen EL, *et al.* Pharmacokinetic properties of delta9-tetrahydrocannabinol in oral fluid of occasional and chronic users. *Kauert GFJ ANAL Toxicol* 2010;**34**:216–221.
9. Budney AJ, Hughes Jr., The cannabis withdrawal syndrome. *Curr Opin Psychiatry* 2006;**19**:233–238.
10. Kouri EM, Pope HG. Abstinence symptoms during withdrawal from chronic marijuana use. *Exp Clin Psychopharmacol* 2000;**8**:483–492.
11. Seely KA, Prather PL, James LP, *et al.* Marijuana-based drugs: innovative therapeutics or designer drugs of abuse? *Mol Interv* 2011;**11**:36–51.
12. Monterosso JR, Aron AR, Cordova X, *et al.* Deficits in response inhibition associated with chronic methamphetamine abuse. *Drug Alcohol Depen* 2005;**79**:273–277.
13. Hopfer CJ, Mikulich SK, Crowley TJ. Heroin use among adolescents in treatment for substance use disorders. *J Am Acad Child Adolesc Psychiatr* 2000;**39**:1316–1323.
14. Hopfer CJ, Khuri E, Crowley TJ, *et al.* Adolescent heroin use: a review of the descriptive and treatment literature. *J Subst Abuse Treat* 2002;**23**:231–237.

15. Davidson D, Parrott A. Ecstasy (MDMA) in recreational users: self-report psychological and physiological effects. *Hum Psychopharmacol* 1997;**12**:221–226.

16. O'Leary G, Nargiso J, Weiss RD. 3,4-methylenedioxyme-thamphetamine (MDMA): a review. *Curr Psychiatry Rep* 2001;**3**:477–483.

17. Anderson CE, Loomis GA. Recognition and prevention of inhalant abuse. *Am Fam Physician* 2003;**68**:869–874.

18. Kurtzman TL, Otsuka KN, Wahl RA. Inhalant abuse by adolescents. *J Adolesc Health* 2001;**28**:170–180.

19. Mulcahey MK, Schiller JR, Hulstyn MJ. Anabolic steroid use in adolescents: identification of those at risk and strategies for prevention. *Phys Sportsmed* 2010;**38**:105–113.

20. Bahrke MS, Yesalis CE, Kopstein AN, *et al.* Risk factors associated with anabolic and androgenic steroid use among adolescents. *Sports Med* 2000;**29**:397–405.

21. Bernstein GA, Carroll, ME, Thuras PD, *et al.* Caffeine dependence in teenagers. *Drug Alcohol Depend* 2002;**66**:1–6.

22. Temple JL, Dewey AM, Briatico LN. Effects of acute caffeine administration on adolescents. *Exp Clin Psychopharmacol* 2010;**18**:510–520.

23. Garret BE, Griffiths RR. The role of dopamine in the behavioral effects of caffeine in animals and humans. *Pharmacol Biochem Behav* 1997;**57**:533–541.

24. Bernstein GA, Carroll ME, Crosby RD, *et al.* Caffeine effects on learning, performance, and anxiety in normal school-age children. *J Am Acad Child Adolesc Psychiatry* 1994;**33**:407–415.

25. Glazer G. Athrogenic effects of anabolic steroids on serum lipid levels. *Arch Intern Med* 1991;**151**:1925–1933.

26. Cook RL, Comer DM, Weisenfeld HC, *et al.* Alcohol and drug use and related disorders: an underrecognized health issue among adolescents and young adults attending sexually transmitted disease clinics. *Sex Transm Dis* 2006;**33**:565–570.

27. McGeary KA, French MT. Illicit drug use and emergency room utilization. *Health Serv Res* 2000;**35**:153–169.

28. Gray KM, Upadhyaya HP, Deas D, *et al.* Advances in diagnosis of adolescent substance abuse. *Adolesc Med* 2006;**17**:411–425.

29. Carroll KM. Methodological issues and problems in the assessment of substance use. *Psychol Assessment* 1995;**3**:349–358.

30. Sobell LC, Sobell MB, Litten RZ, *et al.* Timeline follow-back: a technique for assessing self-reported alcohol consumption. In: Litten RZ, Allen JP (eds), *Measuring Alcohol Consumption: Psychosocial and Biochemical Methods.* Totowa, NJ: Humana Press, 1992; pp. 41–72.

31. Substance Abuse and Mental Health Services Administration, Office of Applied Sciences. *The NSDUH report: depression and the initiation of alcohol and other drug use among youth aged 12 to 17.* Rockville, MD: SAMHSA, 2007.

32. Ewing JA. Detecting alcoholism: The CAGE questionnaire. *JAMA* 1984;**252**:1905–1907.

33. Chung T, Colby S, Barnett N, *et al.* Screening adolescents for problem drinking: performance on brief screens against DSM-IV alcohol diagnoses. *J Stud Alcohol* 2000;**61**:579–587.

34. Knight JR, Sherritt L, Shier LA, *et al.* Validity of the CRAFFT substance abuse screening test among adolescent clinic patients. *Arch Pediatr Adolesc Med* 2002;**156**:607–614.

35. Knight JR, Shier L, Bravender T, *et al.* A new brief screen for adolescent substance abuse. *Arch Pediatr Adolesc Med* 1999;**153**:591–596.

36. Saunders JB, Aasland OG, Barbor TF, *et al.* Development of the alcohol use disorders identification test (AUDIT): WHO collaborative project in early detection of persons with harmful alcohol consumption. *Addiction* 1993;**88**:791–804.

37. Winters K, Zenilman J. *Simple screening instruments for outreach for alcohol and other drug abuse and infectious diseases: Treatment Improvement Protocol (TIP) series,* Vol. 11. Rockville, MD: US Department of Health and Human Services, 1994; pp. 94–209.

38. Knight JR, Goodman E, Pulerwitz T, *et al.* Reliability of the problem oriented screening instrument for teenagers (POSIT) in adolescent medical practice. *J Adolesc Health* 2001;**29**:125–130.

39. Grant BF, Dawson DA. Age at onset of alcohol use and its association with DSM-IV alcohol abuse and dependence: results from the National Longitudinal Alcohol Epidemiologic Survey. *J Subst Abuse* 1997;**9**:103–110.

40. Miller WR, Rollnick S. *Motivational Interviewing: Preparing People to Change Addictive Behavior,* 2nd edn. New York: Guilford Press, 2002.

41. Monti PM, Barnett NP, Colby SM, *et al.* Motivational interviewing versus feedback only in emergency care for young adult problem drinking. *Addiction* 2007;**102**:1234–1243.

42. Monti PM, Colby SM, Barnett NP, *et al.* Brief intervention for harm reduction with alcohol-positive older adolescents in a hospital emergency department. *J Consult Clin Psychol* 1999;**67**:989–994.

43. Colby SM, Monti PM, O'Leary TT, *et al.* Brief motivational intervention for adolescent smokers in medical settings. *Addict Behav* 2005;**30**:865–874.

44. Magill M, Barnett NP, Apodaca TR, *et al.* The role of marijuana use in brief motivational intervention with young adult drinkers treated in an emergency department. *J Stud Alcohol Drugs* 2009;**70**:409–413.

45. Neighbors CJ, Barnett NP, Rohsenow DJ, *et al.* Cost-effectiveness of a motivational intervention for alcohol-involved youth in a hospital emergency department. *J Stud Alcohol Drugs* 2010;**3**:384–394.

46. Haynes JF. Medical management of adolescent drug overdoses. *Adolesc Med* 2006;**17**:353–379.

47. Nice A, Leikin JB, Maturen A, *et al.* Toxidrome recognition to improve efficiency of emergency room urine drug screens. *Ann Emerg Med* 1988;**17**:676–680.

48. Radis MI, Keyes C. Toxidromes: an approach to the poisoned patient. In: Aghababian RV (ed), *Emergency Medicine: The Core Curriculum.* Philadelphia: Lippincott Williams & Wilkins, 1998; pp. 984–997.

49. Bartlett D. The coma cocktail: indications, contraindications, adverse effects, proper dose, and proper route. *J Emerg Nurs* 2004;**30**:572–574.

50. Hoffman RS, Goldfrank KR. The poisoned patient with altered consciousness: controversies in the use of the coma cocktail. *JAMA* 1995;**274**:562.

51. Lapus RM, Slattery AP, King WD. Effects on a poison center's (PC) triage and follow-up after implementing the no Ipecac use policy. *J Med Toxicol* 2010;**6**:122–125.

52. American Academy of Clinical Toxicology and European Association of Poison Centers and Clinical Toxicologists. Position paper: whole bowel irrigation. *J Toxicol Clin Toxicol* 2004;**42**:843–854.

53. American Academy of Clinical Toxicology and European Association of Poison Centers and Clinical Toxicologists.

Position paper: single-dose activated charcoal. *J Toxicol Clin Toxicol* 2005;**43**:61–87.

54. Buylaert WA. Coma induced by intoxication. *Acta Neurol Belg* 2000;**100**:221–224.

55. Fassoulaki A, Theodoraki K, Melemeni A. Pharmacology of sedation agents and reversal agents. *Digestion* 2010;**82**:80–83.

56. Catavas JD, Waters JW. Acute cocaine intoxication in the conscious dog: studies on the mechanism of lethality. *J Pharmacol Exp Ther* 1981;**217**:350–356.

57. Brody SL, Slovis CM, Wrenn KD. Cocaine-related medical problems: consecutive series of 233 patients. *Am J Med* 1990;**88**:325–331.

58. Isner J, Estes N, Thompson PD, *et al.* Acute cardiac events temporally related to cocaine abuse. *New Engl J Med* 1986;**315**:1438–1443.

59. Williams JF, Strock M, Committee on Substance Abuse and Committee on Native American Child Health. *Inhalant abuse. Pediatrics* 2007;**119**:1009–1017.

5

Psychological Assessment

Lauren Reba-Harrelson[1] and Daniel A. Martell[2]

[1] *University of Southern California, Institute of Psychiatry, Law, and Behavioral Science;
Keck School of Medicine, Los Angeles, CA, USA*
[2] *Semel Institute for Neuroscience and Human Behavior, David Geffen
School of Medicine at UCLA, Los Angeles, CA, USA*

Identifying mental illness and associated features is the initial step in providing or referring adolescents to tailored treatment services. Prior to an evaluation of an adolescent, mental health professionals are faced with the challenge of deciding their approach. This may be based on many factors, including the referral question, the stage of illness or context in which one is encountering the adolescent, the availability or existence of previously collected data (e.g., an initial screening, evaluation, or relevant mental health records), and the minor's age, cultural identity, cognitive capacity, or language spoken. In some cases, a thorough clinical interview of the adolescent and reviewing information from collateral sources may provide enough information to facilitate a diagnosis or answer other relevant questions. However, in many cases, the use of psychological testing can be an integral tool to obtaining all the data necessary to make a comprehensive diagnosis or answer specific referral questions.

This may be particularly true in the context of disorders of addiction in adolescents, for which comorbid psychiatric illnesses and complex, contributing environmental, behavioral, and other factors are the rule rather than the exception. The American Society of Addiction Medicine in its 2011 Policy Statement Report [1], in contrast to the *Diagnostic and Statistical Manual of Mental Disorders, Fourth Edition, Text Revision* (DSM-IV-TR), defines addiction as a condition that can extend beyond substance use disorders:

> Addiction is a primary, chronic disease of brain reward, motivation, memory and related circuitry. Dysfunction in these circuits leads to characteristic biological, psychological, social and spiritual manifestations. This is reflected in an individual pathologically pursuing reward and/or relief by substance

use and other behaviors. Addiction is characterized by inability to consistently abstain, impairment in behavioral control, craving, diminished recognition of significant problems with one's behaviors and interpersonal relationships, and a dysfunctional emotional response. Like other chronic diseases, addiction often involves cycles of relapse and remission. Without treatment or engagement in recovery activities, addiction is progressive and can result in disability or premature death.

Moreover, in the case of adolescents who abuse substances, over 70% may present with at least one comorbid psychiatric disorder, and around half are diagnosed with three or more conditions. Co-occurring illnesses may include conduct disorder, attention-deficit/hyperactivity disorder (ADHD), mood disorders, anxiety, post-traumatic stress, psychotic disorders, as well as eating disorders, self-harm, and other impulsive behaviors, such as gambling [2,3]. This is consistent with the position of the National Institute on Drug Abuse (NIDA), that non-drug-related behaviors and disorders are important to consider in understanding substance dependence [4] Further, based on the argument that impulse control disorders (ICDs) should fall under the addictive disorders umbrella [5], psychological testing can be a useful means to identify personality traits such as impulsivity, and rule out the impact of possible neuropsychological or cognitive factors on inhibition. Moreover, in time-limited or crisis situations, a brief screening measure may be an efficient diagnostic tool for referral.

This chapter aims to provide an overview of the most commonly implemented, valid and reliable psychological tests for use in adolescent populations across various domains. This will include tests of broad psychopathology, personality characteristics, behavior and functioning, substance abuse and dependence, neuropsychological symptoms, and crisis assessment, as well as a brief overview of projective testing, intelligence, and achievement tests. The chapter will also present guidelines to help the reader determine when it may be useful to include psychological measures in an evaluation, which measures to include, and when to make a referral to a psychologist.

OVERVIEW OF PSYCHOLOGICAL ASSESSMENT MEASURES

Definitions of Psychological Tests and Assessment

In the literature, various semantic distinctions have been made in defining the terms "psychological test" and "psychological assessment" [6]. A psychological test may be considered to be one standardized measure used within a psychological assessment, or a more complex, in-depth process that integrates data from various sources. In its *Report of Test User Qualifications*, the American Psychological Association defines a psychological test as a measurement procedure for assessing psychological characteristics in which a sample of an examinee's behavior is obtained and subsequently evaluated and scored using a standardized process [7]. In contrast, a psychological assessment was defined as a process that "integrates test information with information from other sources; a process for evaluating behavior, psychological constructs, and/or characteristics of individuals or groups for the purpose of making decisions regarding classification, selection, placement, diagnosis, or intervention" [7].

Psychological tests may take many forms, including brief screening instruments, such as those used in the triage process, or more detailed pencil-and-paper or computer-based psychometric measures. Another method of testing is the use of an empirically established, structured or semi-structured interview. Psychological measures address multiple domains, including broad psychopathology, personality, cognitive ability, and malingering, and are usually completed by the patient or collateral sources, such as a parent/caregiver or teacher.

Validity and Reliability in Psychological Testing

Psychological tests are grounded in psychometric theory, in which raw test scores (often across a variety of subscales) are compared to scores of a large population sample on which the test has been normed and that is representative of the specific test-taker based on demographic, clinical, or other factors. The quality of a standardized psychological test is measured through methodology addressing *reliability* and *validity*.

Reliability refers to the consistency of the measure, both within the measure (e.g., among items), between its parts (e.g., alternate forms, different parts of the same measure), in performance over time (test-retest), and the ability of two different examiners to obtain the same score. Types of reliability include internal consistency, test-retest reliability, inter-rater reliability, and parallel forms reliability [8,9]. Reliability may be influenced by characteristics of the test taker, the test itself (length, heterogeneity of questions, etc.), the test administrator, the testing environment and procedures, and the stability of the intended use of the scores [10]. A test's standard measurement error is another important factor related to a test's reliability, providing an estimate of the range of scores consistent with the individual's level of performance [9]. These factors are integral to consider in determining whether a test is useful in general, or appropriate for use based on the specific characteristics of the assessment at hand [7].

Validity refers to a test's ability to accurately measure the construct of interest (construct validity) and/or assess the domain of interest, comparing the performance of the test at hand to other measures tapping the same construct [9]. There are several different types of validity including construct, content, concurrent, predictive, criterion, face, convergent, and discriminate factors, each of which help to establish that the test accurately measures what it intends to measure.

When considering a type of test to use, beyond the reliability and validity of a specific measure, the strengths and weaknesses of a general test format should be considered in relationship to the testing situation at hand. For example, self-report inventories often include multiple items designed to sample specific domains of functioning. Tests using these formats may have extensive data to support construct validity and be useful for tapping into domains of functioning, and underlying states, feelings, and psychological issues that are not captured by other techniques or direct patient report [9,10]. However, limitations of self-report measures include the reading level of the test-taker; the impact of item wording, format, or order on responses; the possibility of response bias or distortion (e.g., socially desirable responding); and contextual or assessment conditions (e.g., reactivity, setting) [9].

Structured and semi-structured interviews present their own set of issues regarding reliability and validity. It has been argued that structured and semi-structured interviews have advantages over unstructured interviews in reducing the interviewer bias that comes from unique interactional processes (e.g., the "halo effect," confirmatory bias, and the primacy effect) and that significantly decreases reliability and validity [11]. Other strengths of structured interviews include the development of reliable ratings, reduced information variance, and the use of consistent diagnostic criteria [12]. Further, compared to standardized tests, standardized interviews have the benefit of rapport building, and a flexible, person-centered approach that allows for observation of factors unique to the interviewee that could otherwise be missed. However, limitations of structured or semi-structured interviews have also been noted, such as requiring a long time to administer and relying on criteria for diagnoses that might be controversial (e.g., not in the current DSM-IV-TR or up for debate for DSM-V). Moreover, research is not conclusive regarding their utility for assessing treatment selection or response [11]. Further details on research methodology related to psychological assessments may be found elsewhere (see refs [5–9]).

Overview of Psychological Tests Across Domains

As with any approach to assessment, a single psychological test cannot functionally provide enough data to appropriately make a diagnosis or facilitate a case conceptualization. Regardless of the type of psychological measures chosen, it is imperative to keep in mind that scores of any psychometric test cannot stand alone. Rather, results provide additional data points that must be integrated into the context of other information sources, such as history, other test results, observations, etc., to enrich the case conceptualization. Specifically in the case of children and adolescents, this may also include additional behavioral observations (included as part of some psychological tests), caregiver or teacher reports, or a battery of psychological testing. This section will focus on the most commonly used, individual psychological tests that may be chosen in the evaluation of adolescents to answer specific questions regarding psychopathology, personality traits, behavior, and functioning. A focus will be placed on usefulness of various tests in relationship to addictive disorders.

PSYCHOLOGICAL TESTS

Broad Psychopathology and Personality Factors

Some of the most empirically established psychological tests that allow for the broad evaluation of clinical disorders and personality traits include the Minnesota Multiphasic Personality Inventory –Adolescent (MMPI-A) [13], the Millon Adolescent Clinical Inventory (MACI), and the Millon Adolescent Personality Inventory (MAPI) [14].

Minnesota Multiphasic Personality Inventory – Adolescent Version

Since its development in 1940 by Hathaway and McKinley at the University of Minnesota, the Minnesota

Multiphasic Personality Inventory (MMPI) and subsequent versions – the revised MMPI-2 [15] and Minnesota Multiphasic Personality Inventory – Adolescent (MMPI-A) [13], have become the most commonly used inventories of clinical and personality factors. The MMPI-A has been extensively empirically supported by the literature and normed in a population of adolescents aged 14 to 18 years. (Of note, the MMPI-2 has also been normed with a 16 to 18-year-old population, but the MMPI-A has been noted to be a preferable test for use with adolescents [11].) Like its predecessors, the MMPI-A is a standardized, pencil-and-paper questionnaire that elicits a wide range of self-descriptions scored to provide a quantitative dimensional profile of an individual's overall emotional adjustment and test-taking attitudes. It comprises 478 true/false items, which make up 10 clinical and personality scales that assess psychiatric, psychological, neurological, and physical symptoms. Based on the adolescent's ability to complete this number of items, the test may be shortened by administering only the first 350 items (which provide enough data to allow for a valid interpretation). Clinical Scales include:

- Scale 1, Hypochondriasis (HS)
- Scale 2, Depression (D)
- Scale 3, Hysteria (Hy)
- Scale 4, Psychopathic Deviate (Pd)
- Scale 5, Masculinity-Femininity (Mf)
- Scale 6, Paranoia (Pa)
- Scale 7, Psychasthenia (Pt)
- Scale 8, Schizophrenia (Sc)
- Scale 9, Hypomania (Ma)
- Scale 0, Social Introversion (Si).

The MMPI-A also includes seven validity scales:

- VRIN – Variable Response Inconsistency
- TRIN – True Response Inconsistency
- F1 – Infrequency of responses 1
- F2 – Infrequency of resonses 2
- F – Infrequency of responses
- L – Lie
- K – Correction.

These scales are integral in assessing the test-taker's approach to responding, including whether they were exaggerating or minimizing symptoms. These scales are also important in determining whether the test's results are interpretable.

While the MMPI was originally designed to distinguish normal from abnormal behavior, results currently are considered to be more useful when individual scale scores are interpreted as clusters of personality traits. Multiple subscales have also been validated to produce a more nuanced interpretation, including Content scales, Content Component scales, Harris–Lingoes subscales, Critical items, and other Supplementary scales.

The MMPI-A can be scored and interpreted through various methods. These include hand-scoring, as well as the more recent options of paying a fee to obtain an interpretive report or extensive score report through the test's publisher, or purchasing software such as the Q^{TM} Local Software, which enables one to obtain a printout of computer-generated interpretation by entering each item response into the program [16]. Regardless of the scoring method used, the MMPI-A produces results based on an analysis of elevated item responses in comparison to the norm group of interest. This occurs through the transformation of raw scores from the test profile to standardized T-scores, which map the peaks and valleys across test scales. However, beyond simply interpreting these scale and subscale scores in relationship to relevant cut-offs of clinical significance (which is on average a T-score of 65), it is imperative to consider the overall configuration of scales, demographic factors of the adolescent, and behaviors noted during the administration. Based on the latter factor (and the importance of ensuring that the test is completed by the appropriate party), it is recommended that test administrators be present throughout the administration of the MMPI-A.

Regarding interpretation of the MMPI-A, the scales, regardless of their names, are not representative of specific diagnostic categories and cannot be interpreted individually. For example, Scale 8 (Schizophrenia) does not reflect DSM-IV criteria for this disorder alone; elevation on this scale can capture other traits including alienation and social estrangement, as well as constricted emotional responsivity. In turn, the clinician interpreting the MMPI-A must be knowledgeable of the two- and three-point code systems that have been extensively empirically validated to accurately reflect the personality traits of the test-taker, as well as other clinical factors associated with the responder.

Adolescents commonly have elevated scores on Scale 4, which may reflect developmentally normative factors such as identity formation and achieving independence [11]. However, very high scores on this scale may alternately reflect pathological levels of antisocial behavior (described through interpretation of the Conduct Problem scales) or alcohol or drug use (reported in addiction-related subscales, described below) [11,13].

The assessment of substance abuse problems has been well researched in the context of the MMPI-A. Subscales have been developed to specifically address drug and alcohol problems, including the MacAndrew Alcoholism Scale-R (MAC-R) [15], Alcohol-Drug Problem

Acknowledgments Scale (ACK) [17], and the Alcohol Drug Proneness Scale (PRO). The MAC-R captures traits common in substance-abusing adolescents, including impulsiveness, risk-taking and sensation seeking, assertiveness, and self-indulgence. The ACK is a useful subscale in determining an adolescent's awareness and willingness to report substance-related problems, as well as addressing problem use, use as a coping skill, and the impact of drug or alcohol use on other harmful behavior. In contrast, rather than focusing on current drug- or alcohol-related problems, the PRO scale measures personality and lifestyle patterns associated with addiction, which may also aid in determining the presence of other addictive behaviors. This scale is similar to Alcohol Proneness Scale (APS) [17] on the MMPI-2.

Millon Adolescent Clinical Inventory (MACI) and Millon Adolescent Personality Inventory (MAPI)

The Millon Adolescent Clinical Inventory (MACI) [14] and Millon Adolescent Personality Inventory (MAPI) [14] are measures of symptoms of psychopathology and associated personality characteristics that have been well validated and are commonly used with adolescents [18,19]. Both are based on Theodore Millon's theory of personality, which conceptualizes personality styles as not mutually exclusive [11,20,21] and underlines the nature of the instruments' structures and interpretation. Details regarding Millon's personality theory can be found elsewhere [20,21].

The MACI is a 160-item, self-report, true/false inventory, normed for adolescents aged 13 to 19 in clinical and non-clinical settings. It consists of 31 scales in three domains of psychopathological functioning – personality patterns, expressed concerns, and clinical syndromes – as well as modifying indices that capture test-taking attitudes and response patterns, and a validity scale. Personality and Clinical scales are reflective of DSM-IV-TR Axis I and Axis II disorders (common in adolescents), respectively. (See the *Manual for the Millon Adolescent Clinical Inventory* for further description of scale components [14].)

However, in assessing for disorders of addiction in adolescents, it is relevant to note that the Clinical Scales include measures of Eating Dysfunctions, Substance-Abuse Proneness, and Impulsive Propensity. Moreover, the Expressed Concerns scales capture factors that may be commonly associated with addiction in adolescents, including Identity Confusion, Peer Insecurity, and Family Discord. Further interpretations of elevations on the Personality Pattern scales can also be found in the Grossman Facet Scales, which describe personality processes (e.g., temperament, mood, sense of self).

Designed to supplement the MACI, the MAPI measures adolescent personality characteristics in 13–18-year-olds, and was originally normed in a non-clinical population. Although again a 160-question true/false format with a validity index, and three broad domains including personality styles and expressed concerns, the MAPI differs from the MACI in that it contains 22 scales and a third domain that assesses for behavioral correlates rather than clinical syndromes. Behavioral subscales include factors common in adolescents: Impulse Control, Social Conformity, Scholastic Achievement, and Attendance Consistency.

For both the MACI and MAPI, scale scores are obtained by transforming raw scores into base rates (BR). The conversion provides a basis for establishing valid scale cut-off points by considering the relative prevalence rates of scale attributes. Scale score cut-off points representing prominence of traits range from 75 to 85 [14]. Interpretation of the MACI and the MAPI is akin to approaches described for the MMPI-A, including hand-scoring, as well as the aforementioned computerized and mail-in options to the publisher [22].

Regarding mental health issues in pre-adolescents, the Millon Pre-Adolescent Clinical Inventory (M-PACI) was developed in 2005 to assess psychological issues in children aged 9 through 12 years. Rather than focusing on single diagnostic areas, this instrument aims to provide a synthesized view of developing personality and clinical characteristics that may be associated with DSM-IV-TR disorders. However, with less literature available on this instrument, carefully monitoring research supporting its validity in populations of interest is imperative to ensure appropriate usage.

As with all psychological tests, the MMPI-A and the Millon Inventories possess assets and limitations that are important to consider in deciding if either is a good fit for the assessment at hand. While neither test should be used in isolation to provide diagnoses, both are useful in assessing both personality patterns and clinical symptoms relevant to Axis I and Axis II disorders. Moreover, both are grounded in substantive research supporting their reliability and validity in assessing complex relationships between personality patterns and clinical symptoms. This is particularly important in that it provides information on more enduring and problematic personality traits that may be missed in clinical interviews, which may focus more on diagnostic symptoms. This is particularly relevant in adolescents for assessing characterological traits that may be associated with maladaptive behaviors other than those admitted to during an interview. For example, an adolescent with known drug use may not admit to promiscuous sexual behavior or disordered eating, but patterns of impulse control problems, social difficulties, and poor self-

esteem captured on aforementioned tests may help to identify the presence or development of such problem behaviors, with strong implications for future treatment.

Assets and limitations must be considered in relationship to the individual adolescent one is evaluating. One major benefit of the MACI and MAPI over other instruments of psychopathology and personality is their shorter length, useful for those who may not have the attention span to complete a full MMPI-A. In contrast to the MMPI-A, which generally takes around one hour to complete, the Millon instruments can be completed by many adolescents in around 20 to 30 minutes [22]. However, the MMPI-A has a larger body of clinical scales. While both the MMPI-A and MACI have been supported by literature in juvenile justice populations, suggesting they may be validly used in a forensic setting [19], the MMPI-A also has a larger overall body of research supporting its validity and reliability across populations. As with all tests, appropriate use must be considered in relationship to cultural factors. Both the MMPI-A and Millon instruments have been translated into multiple languages and normed in associated populations. For example, the MMPI-A can be found in Croatian, Dutch, French, Italian, Korean, and Spanish (for Mexican, South American, Central America, and US dialects) versions, as well as other languages. However, one's own language limitations and knowledge of variations of scores based on a test-taker's cultural identity must be considered in appropriate administration and interpretation of these, and all tests [23].

Other Approaches to Assessing Psychopathology in Adolescents

Myriad psychological tests exist to assess more specifically psychopathology in youths. One of the most widely used instruments is the Child Behavior Checklist for Ages 4–18 (CBCL/4–18) [24], a measure of childhood internalizing (e.g., anxious/depressed symptoms, withdrawal, somatic complaints) and externalizing (attention problems, intrusiveness, aggressiveness, delinquent behavior) symptoms and behaviors. This measure comprises a multiaxial, empirically based set of measures for assessing children from parent report (CBCL), teacher report (Teacher Report Form – TRF), and youth self-report (YSR).

Another approach to assessing mental illness in children and adolescents includes the use of semi-structured or structured interviews. While this approach has been traditionally used in a research context to standardize and increase inter-rater reliability in diagnosing disorders, it may also provide a useful tool in a clinical setting as a guideline for DSM-IV diagnoses. Commonly used semi-structured interviews include the

Kiddie-Schedule for Affective Disorders and Schizophrenia – Present Lifetime Version (K-SADS-PL) [25] and the Diagnostic Interview for Children, Fourth Version (DISC-IV) [26].

The K-SADS-PL [25] is a semi-structured psychiatric interview that ascertains both lifetime and current diagnostic status based on DSM-IV criteria. This test includes an introductory interview to collect background information, and a screen interview that includes 82 symptoms across 20 diagnostic areas, and diagnostic supplementary areas, including (i) affective disorders, (ii) psychotic disorders, (iii) anxiety disorders, (iv) disruptive behavior disorders, and (v) substance abuse, tic disorders, eating disorders, and elimination disorders. The K-SADS is administered first to the caregiver to obtain a screening interview score, then to the child alone by the same administrator to obtain a second score. Using both clinical judgment and summary scores, a summary rating is made that captures diagnostic symptoms [27].

Due to its development for use in research settings, the DISC-IV and its predecessors can be administered by a lay interviewer to assess for over 30 diagnoses mostly commonly found in children and adolescents covered by the DSM-IV and the *International Classification of Diseases, Tenth Revision* (ICD-10) [26]. Current and lifetime diagnoses are found in six domains: Anxiety Disorders, Mood Disorders, Disruptive Disorders, Substance-Use Disorders, Schizophrenia, and Miscellaneous Disorders (similar to those covered in the aforementioned fifth domain of the K-SADS-PL). The DISC comprises both parent (DISC-P) and child (DISC-Y) versions, to be administered to caregivers of children aged 6 to 17 and to youths aged 9 to 17, respectively. Regarding the assessment of substance abuse addiction on this measure, one study found that the DISC was highly sensitive in correctly identifying youths who had received a hospital diagnosis of any substance use disorder [28]. A computerized version of the DISC (C-DISC) has also been developed and can either be interview administered or self-administered using computerized voice-files. Both produce a diagnostic report describing symptoms and diagnoses [26] An internet version of the DISC-IV parent report has also been created with the main purpose of administering it at home without an interviewer [29]; however, more research is needed to assess the validity and reliability of this version.

Other notable instruments have been developed that assess specific psychopathology, including the Beck Depression Inventory (BDI and BDI-II) [30,31]. The BDI-II [31] is a brief, multiple-choice, self-report screening instrument developed for both adults and adolescents aged 13 years and older. The original BDI tool was developed in 1961, and both the BDI-II and its predecessor have become widely used measures for assessing depression, as well as other symptoms of mental illness. The BDI-II is a 21-item measure scored on a scale from 0 to 3, and provides cut-off scores that measure depression on a continuum from mild to severe symptoms. In validity studies assessing the BDI-II's usefulness in relationship to clinical interview and other notable instruments, including the Hamilton Depression Rating Scale, good inter-rater agreement and high internal consistency have been shown [32–34]. The BDI has also been noted to be a useful screening instrument with moderate to high psychometric properties in assessing major depressive disorder in adolescents with comorbid substance use disorders [35].

Other well-established, valid, and reliable tests and interviews exist to measure specific psychopathology in adolescents. These include brief screening tools designed to identify symptoms of psychopathology or crisis situations that warrant follow-up assessment. Two commonly used screening tools include the Symptom Checklist 90-R (SCL-90-R) and its shortened version, the Brief Symptom Inventory (BSI). Assessing type and severity of self-reported symptoms, these instruments have been validated in adolescent populations and are commonly used due to their efficiency, relevance for a wide range of target groups, sensitivity to change, and simple administration process [23]. Description of details regarding other inventories, such as the Beck Anxiety Inventory, Yale–Brown Obsessive Compulsive Scale, and Hamilton Anxiety Scale can be found elsewhere [23,36].

Drugs and Alcohol Use

Many reliable and valid instruments exist for the assessment of substance abuse in adolescents. One recent study attempted to measure the quality of such instruments through various methods, including referencing measures in the University of Washington's Substance Use Screening & Assessment Instruments Database [37], deemed "widely used and have proven reliability and validity" [38]. These researchers also established whether instruments had either a published manual or a description in a peer-reviewed journal article, and were originally developed for an adolescent population. Tests meeting these criteria for adolescents include the Substance Abuse Subtle Screening Inventory (SASSI) [39], the Global Appraisal of Individual needs (GAIN) [40], and the Teen Addiction Severity Index (T-ASI) [41]. Moreover, subscales on the MMPI-A [13], MACI [22], K-SADS [27], and BDI [30] have also been found to be a useful tools in assessing for substance abuse in adolescents.

The SASSI has been developed in multiple versions, including one specifically targeting an adolescent population, the Adolescent Substance Abuse Subtle Screening Inventory – A2 (SASSI-A2) [42]. This pencil-and-paper screening tool measures both high and low probability of substance dependence and substance abuse disorders in adolescents aged 12 to 18 years across clinical settings. It identifies family and social risk factors, defensive responding, and consequences of substance use. Based on studies assessing validity and reliability, the SASSI-A2 has been found to have a moderate to high test-retest reliability and its results are not influenced by the test-takers level of functioning (e.g., scores skewed by the presence of other endorsed maladaptive behaviors) [43,44]. Face valid scales have also been found to have moderate utility for identifying substance dependence in a juvenile justice population, though some caution should be taken in using the subtle scales in this group [44]. It also has the benefit of being a brief screening tool, taking around 15 minutes to administer, and showing no significant differences in responses by the adolescent's ethnic identity [43].

Current thinking suggests that a comprehensive evaluation should include an assessment tool that addresses not only diagnostic characteristics but also factors related to treatment success, motivation, and readiness for change. One instrument that addresses these factors is the GAIN, version 5 [45], available in multiple formats, including a screen, a biopsychosocial intake, and a follow-up assessment battery. This measure can be used with individuals aged 11 and older; it has been well-studied and widely adapted to assess for substance use and comorbid symptoms and disorders in clinical, drug-treatment, and correctional contexts. The GAIN comprises eight main sections – Background, Substance Use, Physical Health, Risk Behaviors/Disease Prevention, Mental and Emotional Health, Environment and Living Situation, Legal, and Vocational – as they relate to the timeline of problems, severity, and treatment utilization, as well as motivation and treatment resistance. It further measures change over time and categorizes participants in terms of abuse, dependence, and problems/diagnosis by substance type. Large-scale studies of adolescents from outpatient and residential programs have found high internal consistency on GAIN scales, including the Substance Problem Scale, and its subscales: Substance Issues Index, Substance Abuse Index, Substance Dependence Scale, and Substance Use Disorder Scale [46]. Moreover, this measure has shown high internal consistency between the Substance Problem Scale, Internal Mental Distress Scale, Behavior Complexity Scale, and Crime/Violence Scale [45].

Another empirically supported measure of addiction includes the Teen Addiction Severity Index (T-ASI) [47], a semi-structured interview adapted from the adult-oriented Addiction Severity Index for use with adolescents aged 12 to 19. This measure assesses factors including medical, employment/support, drug and alcohol use, legal, family history, family/social relationships, and psychiatric problems. Administration can generally be completed in 30 to 50 minutes (contingent upon symptom severity and comorbid problems), during which severity ratings are made on a five-point scale across content areas [48]. Regarding use cross-culturally, the T-ASI has been translated into multiple languages including Spanish, Dutch, Portuguese, Arabic, Finnish, Hebrew, Italian, and Spanish, though further research is required to substantiate the validity of these translations from English [48].

Many brief screening tools have also been developed to identify substance use problems in adolescents as a first step toward a more detailed assessment. These include the Problem Oriented Screening Instrument for Teenagers (POSIT), created by NIDA as part of a more extensive assessment and referral system for use with adolescents to identify problems in the areas of substance abuse, mental and physical health, and social relations. Other screens validated for use in adolescents include the Alcohol Use Disorders Identification Test (AUDIT) [49], CRAFFT (Car, Relax, Alone, Forget, Friends, Trouble) [50], the Drug Use Screening Inventory-Revised (DUSI-R) [51], and the Personal Experience Screening Questionnaire (PESQ) [52]. A brief summary of multiple measures of substance abuse and associated research can be accessed in the University of Washington's Alcohol and Drug Abuse Institute's Substance Use Screening & Assessment Instruments Database [37].

Behavior and Adaptive Functioning

In children and adolescents, the assessment of behavior and adaptive function is important to detect present and future symptoms of mental illness and related problems. Over the past decade, these types of measures have begun to replace the use of projective instruments, which have received criticism for insufficient psychometric properties and their time-consuming nature [23]. Frequently used and well-studied measures of behavior and overall functioning include the CBCL [24], Conners' Rating Scales–Revised (CRS-R) [53], and the Vineland Adaptive Behavior Scales, second edition (VABS-II) [54].

The CRS-R is a measure of a broad spectrum of behaviors, emotions, and academic and social problems in children and adolescents. Available in both pencil-and-paper and computer-based formats, the CRS-R includes three versions – parent, teacher, and adolescent self-report – each of which have separate short- and long-form versions. While the parent and teacher reports can be administered in assessing children aged 3 to 17, the adolescent self-report can be given to youths aged 12 to 17. Beyond obtaining multiple perspectives on an adolescent's behavior, this test is helpful in providing a relatively brief assessment; the 80-item version takes around 20 minutes to complete, and the 27-item short form takes between 5 and 10 minutes [53]. The long version contains scales that capture a breadth of behavioral problems common in youths, including oppositional behavior, cognitive problems/inattention, hyperactivity, anxious-shy, perfectionism, social problems, and psychosomatic scales. The short form is based on a three-factor model, including the oppositional, cognitive problems/inattention, hyperactivity subscales of the longer form [53,55].

The VABS-II is a widely used survey of adaptive functioning in communication, daily living, and socialization. It can be administered via pencil-and-paper rating form or interview, and has been normed for use across the lifespan, from birth through age 90. The Communication Domain assesses receptive, expressive, and written language development. The Daily Living Skills Domain incorporates self-care as well as domestic and community functioning. The Socialization Domain contains items tapping interpersonal, play, and social coping skills. The VABS-II yields a Total Adaptive Behavior Composite Score, and quantifies adaptive functioning in each domain with standard scores. Each of the three domains is divided into subdomains with age-equivalents, including: Receptive, Expressive, and Written (Communication Domain); Personal, Domestic, and Community (Daily Living Skills Domain); Interpersonal Relationships, Play and Leisure Time, and Coping Skills (Socialization Domain). The VABS-II also includes an additional Motor Skills Domain and a Maladaptive Behavior Index, which can be particularly useful with adolescent clients. Like the CRS-R, the VABS-II has the benefit of obtaining data from multiple sources, across contexts, including four formats – a survey interview, expanded form, parent/caregiver rating form, and teacher rating form. However, administration time is generally longer, ranging between 20 and 90 minutes, contingent upon the form used.

Cognitive Abilities

Multiple tests exist under the broad category of cognitive assessment in adolescents, which can include intelligence and achievement testing. While neuropsychological testing may be rightly considered its own distinct form of psychological assessment, the major instruments in this area will also be briefly reviewed in this section.

Although intelligence tests are commonly conceptualized in relationship to educational abilities, it is important to underscore their specific utility in relationship to behavioral problems, including substance abuse in adolescents. Neuropsychological studies of adults and adolescents with substance use disorders have shown that cognitive deficits are correlated with low IQ [56,57]. Another study comparing adolescents with behavioral problems found a strong correlation between impaired cognitive processes and the ability to weigh rewards and penalties in decision-making tasks [58], which may increase one's vulnerability to impulse control problems, including substance use disorders.

Perhaps the most commonly encountered intelligence tests for children and adolescents are the Wechsler tests, including the Wechsler Intelligence Scale for Children, fourth edition (WISC-IV) [59]; and the Stanford–Binet Intelligence Scale, fifth edition (SB5) [60]. The WISC-IV evaluates cognitive functioning in youths aged from 6 years to 16 years 11 months; older adolescents can be assessed using the adult version of the WISC-IV, the Wechsler Adult Intelligence Scale (WAIS). The WISC-IV produces an overall IQ score, as well as domain standard scores (mean = 100, standard deviation = 15) and subtest scaled scores (mean = 10, standard deviation = 3), each of which allow the assessment of relative strengths and weaknesses across domains [59]. The primary domains evaluated by the WISC-IV are the Verbal Comprehension Index, Perceptual Motor Reasoning Index, Working Memory Index, and Processing Speed Index. The Verbal Comprehension Domain of the WISC-IV provides a measure of verbal reasoning ability, verbal fluency, and vocabulary. The Perceptual Reasoning Domain measures non-verbal reasoning, sequencing, and visual spatial skills. The Working Memory Domain assesses auditory short-term memory, concentration, and working memory. The Processing Speed Domain assesses visual processing speed, attention, and fine motor skill.

The SB5 is the most recent edition of a battery of intelligence measures that stem from the original development of the Binet–Simon Scale by Lewis Terman in 1916 [60]. Like the WISC, the SB5 assesses cognitive functioning of children and adolescents with a focus on both strengths and weaknesses. While research has supported its use as a reliable measure for assessing specific learning disabilities, it also more broadly assesses cognitive ability in five primary domains: Fluid Reasoning, Knowledge, Quantitative Reasoning, Visual-Spatial Processing, and Working Memory. The SB5 has been validated for use with individuals from the age of 2 through 85+, a larger range than in previous versions, and can be administered across settings. As well as many subscale and factor scores, the test produces a Full Scale IQ score, as well as two domain scales: Non-verbal IQ (NVIQ) and Verbal IQ (VIQ). The SB5 can be scored by hand or scored with a software program that includes a score report and brief narrative summary.

Other measures of cognitive functioning may be found in brief versions. These include the Test of Nonverbal Intelligence, Version 4 (TONI-IV) [61], the Wechsler Abbreviated Scales of Intelligence (WASI) [62], and the Kaufman Brief Intelligence Test, Version 2, (K-BIT-2) [63].

In contrast to intelligence testing, achievement tests measure specific areas of knowledge and skill relative to age or grade level. Through comparison with intelligence test results, achievement test scores are commonly used as one means to diagnose a learning disorder, and strengths and weaknesses in specific academic areas, such as reading, mathematics, written language, science, and social studies. In contrast, high achievement scores generally reflect a student's mastery and readiness for a more advanced educational level. Commonly used and well-validated achievement tests include the Wechsler Individual Achievement Test, Version II (WIAT-II) [64], the Woodcock–Johnson Tests of Achievement, Version III [65], and the Kaufman Test of Educational Achievement-II (KTEA-II) [66].

Substance use and addiction can have a strong impact on academic achievement. Multiple studies have found that adolescent substance use is associated with poor sustained engagement in academic pursuits, externalizing behavioral problems, and decreased likelihood of educational attainment or completion [67–70]. In turn, adolescents with poor school performance may be pigeonholed as have learning problems or disabilities, when in fact their academic difficulties are secondary to substance abuse and associated negative behaviors (e.g., behavioral problems, poor school attendance). Academic and achievement testing can play an important role in distinguishing students with true intellectual deficits from those whose educational problems are mediated by substance use and associated behavioral problems.

Neuropsychological testing can be a useful approach to better understanding language, memory, attention and concentration, behavior, motor skills, perception, abstraction, and learning abilities. Involving the performance of relatively simple tasks, multiple widely used neuropsychological tests have been empirically validated in adolescent populations. These include the Halstead–Reitan Neuropsychological Test Battery for Children (ages 9 to 14) and Halstead–Reitan Neuropsychological Test Battery for Adults (ages 15 and older), the Bender–Gestalt Test [71], Trail Making Test [72], and the Luria–Nebraska Neuropsychological Battery [73].

In relationship to disorders or addiction, the administration of neuropsychological tests may be particularly useful in elucidating cognitive risk factors, as well as potential cognitive impairment secondary to prolonged drug or alcohol use. Recent studies assessing cognitive factors associated with substance abuse in adolescents have used measures including the Continuous Performance Task (CPT), a measure of sustained and selective attention and impulsivity; and the Wisconsin Card Sorting Test (WCST) [74], a measure of flexibility as reinforcement patterns change. Successful completion relies upon attention, working memory, and visual processing. The Iowa Gambling Test, a measure of one's ability to balance immediate rewards against long-term consequences, is also considered a useful instrument in identifying impairments in individuals with maladaptive behaviors, such as substance use disorders, commonly associated with difficulty in delaying gratification [75].

Using these instruments, one study found that alcohol-dependent patients possess deficits related to motor, non-planning, and attentional components of impulsivity in the period immediately after acute alcohol withdrawal [76]. These results suggest that when compared to controls, alcohol-dependent patients show more commission errors on the CPT, make more disadvantageous choices on the Gambling Test, and made more perseverative errors on the Wisconsin Card Sorting Test [76]. Also using the Gambling Test, another study assessed differences in decision-making in adolescents with and without behavioral problems [58]. In contrast to healthy adolescents, teenagers with any behavior disorders were more likely to show deficits in decision-making and weighing short-term/long-term consequences, similar to deficits found in substance abusers [58]. Beyond their implications for treatment planning, these results underline the application of neuropsychological testing as a tool for identifying underlying cognitive characteristics associated with other maladaptive behaviors or impaired functioning.

DECISION-MAKING IN THE USE OF PSYCHOLOGICAL ASSESSMENTS

In determining whether to use a psychological assessment (or make a referral to a psychologist colleague for assessment), various issues should be considered:

1. the usefulness or need of a psychometric to answer the clinical question at hand;
2. the appropriateness of an assessment in relationship to a specific evaluee; and
3. one's ability to appropriately administer the assessment.

To determine whether a psychological test would be of use, first it is necessary to define the construct you are interested in measuring. For example, when evaluating the cognitive and social functioning of an adolescent with a history of substance dependence, one may consider frequency and impairment associated with history of substance use, familial, personality, and environmental factors, other maladaptive behaviors, as well as cognitive and adaptive abilities. With this in mind, the question arises how best to collect the information needed to address these areas. In considering the youth's cognitive abilities, beyond use of clinical interview with the adolescent and review of relevant data (e.g., school or treatment records), existing measures of intelligence could be useful. Further, measures of adaptive functioning, personality characteristics, and substance abuse may also be important to better understand the adolescent's functioning across contexts, contributing personality characteristics, and severity of substance abuse behavior.

Second, consideration of factors specific to the individual being evaluated, including various aspects of cultural identity, gender, age, and preferred language, must be carefully approached in making the decision to use any psychological test. Important factors to consider include construct equivalence (e.g., cultural equivalence) and test bias [7]. Knowledge of the literature regarding the validity and reliability of individual tests across various cultural groups is necessary not only to understand the limits or lack of applicability of the instrument to a specific adolescent, but also in choosing the correct group norms when interpreting scores. Other issues to consider include the impact of psychological characteristics on test performance (e.g., stereotype threat) and procedures for examining between-groups differences in test performance [7]. Other specific guidelines regarding cultural competency in administration of testing can be found in the American Psychological Association's Report of the Task Force on Test User Qualifications [7] and Guidelines for Psychological Practice with Girls and Women [77].

The determination of when to administer an assessment oneself versus when to make a referral to a qualified psychologist is a decision warranting careful consideration. The American Psychological Association's (APA's) Code of Ethics [78] presents guidelines regarding the administration of psychological assessments, found predominantly in Section 9. While these practice standards have been established for the profession of psychology, they may provide useful guiding principles for psychiatrists and other mental health professionals in determining when and how to implement psychological assessments. Regarding the use of assessments, the APA's Ethics Code underlines the importance of having knowledge of the state of the research regarding each instrument: "Psychologists administer, adapt, score, interpret, or use assessment techniques, interviews, tests, or instruments in a manner and for purposes that are appropriate in light of the research on or evidence of the usefulness and proper application of the techniques."

The Ethics Code also suggests that only assessments with established "validity and reliability" should be used "with members of the population tested . . . and if validity or reliability has not been established, psychologists describe the strengths and limitations of test results and interpretation." Other issues are also discussed regarding the use of psychological assessment, such as informed consent, release of data, test construction, interpretation of results, use by unqualified persons, obsolete and outdated test results, explaining results, and maintaining test security.

Section 9.09 of the APA's Ethics Code may also be particularly useful as reference when deciding when to use a psychological assessment and best practices in using "Test Scoring and Interpretation Services." Beyond the prerequisite of understanding the empirical basis and appropriate administration of an assessment, knowledge of the limitations of particular methods of scoring and interpretation is particularly important, especially in light of the many commercial services marketed for these purposes. Before using a scoring service (such as computerized or automated programs), it is essential to choose a service that provides data regarding its "purpose, norms, validity, reliability, and applications of the procedures and any special qualifications applicable to their use" [78]. Without this information, one cannot appropriately assess that the program's approach to scoring is valid. It is also important to consider that the interpretations provided by these services are a product of an automated algorithm based on the test-taker's response pattern. In turn, such interpretations may be limited in their ability to address unique individual factors explaining why a particular test-taker responded in a particular manner. Hence blind reliance on computerized interpretations can be inappropriate and the results misleading.

Acknowledgement of the scope of one's knowledge regarding the constructs operationalized by a given test is important to ensure a valid interpretation of scores. Knowing labels or rote definitions of a specific scale is not sufficient. For example, cut-off scores, such as "less than 70" for a full-scale intelligence quotient (FSIQ), or "above 65" on a Minnesota Multiphasic Personality Inventory, Adolescent (MMIP-A) scale can be misleading in suggesting that a score falling in the described range has a straightforward meaning or interpretation. However, these scores can be complex and influenced by a variety of contributing factors, such as cultural identity, test-taking environment, and relationship to other subscales. In turn, an honest acknowledgement of the extent of one's understanding of a given measure is important to ensure appropriate and ethical implementation.

As with all approaches to evaluation, results must be considered as a single data point to be used in conjunction with all information collected during a thorough evaluation process. In the end, as stated in the APA Ethics Code, the test-taker retains "responsibility for the appropriate application, interpretation, and use of assessment instruments, whether they score and interpret such tests themselves or use automated or other services" [78]. The best practice is generally to consult with a qualified psychologist or neuropsychologist to ensure proper test selection, administration, and interpretation.

CONCLUSION

Given the complex interplay of personality, cognitive, and psychosocial factors and varied presentations of addictive disorders in adolescents, psychological testing can be a useful tool in the assessment process. Regardless of one's knowledge of administration, scoring, and interpretation of various psychological measures, familiarity with the breadth of available instruments and what they test can help one make an informed choice in conducting a comprehensive clinical assessment.

References

1. The American Society of Addiction Medicine. *Public Policy Statement: Definition of Addiction (Short Version)* American Society of Addiction Medicine, Inc., 2011.
2. Kaminer Y, Bukstein OG. *Adolescent Substance Abuse: Psychiatric Comorbidity and High-Risk Behaviors*. New York: Taylor & Francis, 2007.
3. Kaminer Y, Bukstein O. *Adolescent Substance Abuse: Dual Diagnosis and High Risk Behaviors*. New York: Routledge/Taylor & Francis, 2008.
4. National Institute on Drug Abuse (NIDA), National Institute of Mental Health (NIMH), National Institute of Diabetes and Digestive and Kidney Diseases, (NIDDK). Reward and decision-making: opportunities and future directions. *Neuron* 2002;**36**:189–192.
5. Potenza MN. Should addictive disorders include non-substance-related conditions? *Addiction* 2006;**101** (Suppl. 1):142–151.
6. Matarazzo JD. Psychological assessment versus psychological testing. Validation from Binet to the school, clinic, and courtroom. *Am Psychol* 1990;**45**:999–1017.
7. American Psychological Association Council of Representatives. Report of the Task Force on Test User Qualifications. APA, 2000. Available from: www.apa.org/science/programs/testing/qualifications.pdf.
8. Anastasi A, Urbina S. *Psychological Testing*, 7th edn. Upper Saddle River: Prentice Hall, 1997.
9. Kazdin AE. *Methodological Issues and Strategies in Clinical Research*, 3rd edn. Washington DC: American Psychological Association, 2003.
10. Kazdin AE. *Research Design in Clinical Psychology*, 4th edn. Needham Heights, MA: Allyn & Bacon, 2003.
11. Groth-Marnat G. *The Handbook of Psychological Assessment*, 4th edn. Hoboken, NJ: John Wiley & Sons, Ltd, 2003.
12. Summerfeldt LJ, Antony MM. Structured and semistructured diagnostic interviews. In: Antony MM, Barlow DH (eds) *Handbook of Assessment and Treatment Planning for Psychological Disorders*. New York: Guilford Press, 2002; pp. 3–37.
13. Butcher JN, Williams CL, Graham JR, *et al.Minnesota Multiphasic Personality Inventory-Adolescent Version (MMPI-A): Manual for Administration, Scoring and Interpretation*. Minneapolis, MN, University of Minnesota Press, 1992.
14. Millon T, Millon C, Davis R, Grossman S. *Manual for the Millon Adolescent Clinical Inventory*. Minneapolis, MN: National Computer Systems, 1993.
15. Butcher JN, Dahlstrom WG, Graham JR, Tellegen A, Kaemmer B. *The Minnesota Multiphasic Personality Inventory-2 (MMPI-2): Manual for Administration and Scoring*. Minneapolis, MN: University of Minnesota Press, 1989.
16. Butcher JN, Dahlstrom WG, Graham JR, Tellegen A, Kaemmer B. Minnesota Multiphasic Personality Inventory-Adolescent (MMPI-A). Psychcorp; 2011 [cited 2011 May 28]. Available from: http://psychcorp.pearsonassessments.com/HAIWEB/Cultures/en-us/Productdetail.htm?Pid=PAg522.
17. Weed NC, Butcher JN, McKenna T, Ben-Porath YS. New measures for assessing alcohol and drug abuse with the MMPI-2: The APS and AAS. *J Pers Assess* 1992;**58**:389–404.
18. Cashel M. Child and adolescent psychological assessment: Current clinical practices and the impact of managed care. *Prof Psychol-Res Pract* 2002;**33**:446–453.
19. Baum L, Archer R, Forbey J, Handel RW. A review of the Minnesota Multiphasic Personality Inventory-Adolescent (MMPI-A) and the Millon Adolescent Clinical Inventory (MACI) with an emphasis on juvenile justice samples. *Assessment* 2009;**16**:384–400.
20. Millon T, Davis R. *Personality Disorders in Modern Life*. New York: John Wiley & Sons, Ltd, 2000.
21. Millon T, Davis R. *Disorders of Personality: DSM-IV and Beyond*. New York: John Wiley & Sons, Ltd, 1996.
22. Millon T, Millon C, Davis R, Grossman S. Millon Adolescent Clinical Inventory. 2011 [cited 2011 May 29]; Available from: http://psychcorp.pearsonassessments.com/HAIWEB/Cultures/en-us/Productdetail.htm?Pid=PAg501.
23. Groth-Marnat G. *The Handbook of Psychological Assessment*, 5th edn. Hoboken, NJ: John Wiley & Sons, Ltd, 2009.
24. Achenbach T. *Manual for the Child Behavior Checklist/4–18*. Burlington: University of Vermont, 1991.
25. Kaufman J, Birmaher B, Brent D, *et al.Schedule for Affective Disorders and Schizophrenia for School-Age Children-Present and Lifetime Version (K-SADS-PL): initial reliability and validity data. *J Am Acad Child Adolesc Psychiatry* 1997;**36**:980–988.
26. Shaffer D, Fisher P, Lucas C, Dulcan M, Schwab-Stone M. NIMH Diagnostic Interview Schedule for Children

version IV (NIMH DISC-IV): description, differences from previous versions, and reliability of some common diagnoses. *J Am Acad Child Adolesc Psychiatry* 2000;**39**:28–38.

27. Kaufman J, Birmaher B, Brent DA, Ryan ND, Rao U. K-Sads-Pl. *J Am Acad Child Adolesc Psychiatry* 2000;**39**:1208.

28. Fisher PW, Shaffer D, Piacentini JC, et al. Sensitivity of the Diagnostic Interview Schedule for Children, 2nd edition (DISC-2.1) for specific diagnoses of children and adolescents. *J Am Acad Child Adolesc Psychiatry* 1993;**32**:666–673.

29. Steenhuis MP, Serra M, Minderaa RB, Hartman CA. An Internet version of the Diagnostic Interview Schedule for Children (DISC-IV): correspondence of the ADHD section with the paper-and-pencil version. *Psychol Assess* 2009;**21**:231–234.

30. Beck AT, Ward CH, Mendelson M, Mock J, Erbaugh J. An inventory for measuring depression. *Arch Gen Psychiatry* 1961;**4**:561–571.

31. Beck A, Steer R, Brown G. *Manual for the Beck Depression Inventory-II*. San Antonio, TX: Psychological Corporation, 1996.

32. Storch EA, Roberti JW, Roth DA. Factor structure, concurrent validity, and internal consistency of the Beck Depression Inventory-Second Edition in a sample of college students. *Depress Anxiety* 2004;**19**:187–189.

33. Beck AT, Steer RA, Ball R, Ranieri W. Comparison of Beck Depression Inventories -IA and -II in psychiatric outpatients. *J Pers Assess* 1996;**67**:588–597.

34. Steer RA, Cavalieri TA, Leonard DM, Beck AT. Use of the Beck Depression Inventory for Primary Care to screen for major depression disorders. *Gen Hosp Psychiatry* 1999;**21**:106–111.

35. Subramaniam G, Harrell P, Huntley E, Tracy M. Beck Depression Inventory for depression screening in substance-abusing adolescents. *J Subst Abuse Treat* 2009;**37**:25–31.

36. Achenbach T, Rescorla L. *Multicultural Understanding of Child and Adolescent Psychopathology: Implications for Mental Health Assessment*. Guilford Press, 2006.

37. Alcohol and Drug Abuse Institute. Substance use screening & assessment instruments database. Seattle: University of Washington, 2006. Available from: http://lib.adai.washington.edu/instruments/.

38. Gans J, Falco M, Schackman BR, Winters KC. An in-depth survey of the screening and assessment practices of highly regarded adolescent substance abuse treatment programs. *J Child Adolesc Subst Abuse* 2010;**19**:33–47.

39. Miller GA. *The Substance Abuse Subtle Screening Inventory (SASSI) Manual, Second Edition*. Springville, IN: The SASSI Institute, 1999.

40. Dennis M. Global Appraisal of Individual Needs (GAIN): Administration guide for the GAIN and related measures. Chestnut Health Systems, 1999. Available from: www.chestnut.org/li/gain/gadm1299.pdf.

41. McLellan AT, Luborsky L, Woody GE, O'Brien CP. An improved diagnostic evaluation instrument for substance abuse patients. The Addiction Severity Index. *J Nerv Ment Dis* 1980;**168**:26–33.

42. Miller FG, Lazowski LE. *The Adolescent Substance Abuse Subtle Screening Inventory-A2 (SASSI-A2) Manual*. Springville, IN: The SASSI Institute, 2001.

43. Lazowski LE, Miller FG. *Estimates of the Reliability and Criterion Validity of the Adolescent SASSI-A2*. Springville, IN: The SASSI Institute, 2001.

44. Sweet RI, Saules KK. Validity of the Substance Abuse Subtle Screening Inventory-Adolescent version (SASSI-A). *J Subst Abuse Treat* 2003;**24**:331–340.

45. Dennis ML, White MK, Titus JC, Unsicker JI. *Global Appraisal of Individual Needs (GAIN): Administration Guide for the GAIN and Related Measures (Version 5)* Bloomington, IL: Chestnut Health Systems, 2006.

46. Dennis ML, Funk R, Godley SH, Godley MD, Waldron H. Cross-validation of the alcohol and cannabis use measures in the Global Appraisal of Individual Needs (GAIN) and Timeline Followback (TLFB; Form 90) among adolescents in substance abuse treatment. *Addiction* 2004;**99**(Suppl. 2):120–128.

47. Brodey BB, McMullin D, Kaminer Y, et al. Psychometric characteristics of the Teen Addiction Severity Index-Two (T-ASI-2). *Subst Abus* 2008;**29**:19–32.

48. Kaminer Y. The Teen Addiction Severity Index around the globe: the Tower of Babel revisited. *Subst Abus* 2008;**29**:89–94.

49. Babor TF, de laFuente JR, Saunders J, Grant M. *Audit: The Alcohol Use Disorders Identification Test Guidelines for Use in Primary Care*, 2nd edn. Geneva: World Health Organization, 2001.

50. Knight JR, Sherritt L, Shrier LA, Harris SK, Chang G. Validity of the CRAFFT substance abuse screening test among adolescent clinic patients. *Arch Pediatr Adolesc Med* 2002;**156**:607–614.

51. Tarter RE. Evaluation and treatment of adolescent substance abuse: a decision tree method. *Am J Drug Alcohol Abuse* 1990;**16**:1–46.

52. Winters KC. Development of an adolescent alcohol and other drug abuse screening scale: Personal Experience Screening Questionnaire. *Addict Behav* 1992;**17**:479–490.

53. Conners CK. *Conners' Rating Scales – Revised*. Toronto, ON: Multi-Health Systems Inc., 1997.

54. Sparrow SS, Balla DA, Cicchetti DV. *Vineland Adaptive Behavior Scales*. Circle Pines, MN: American Guidance Service, 1984.

55. Kumar G, Steer RA. Factorial validity of the Conners' Parent Rating Scale-revised: short form with psychiatric outpatients. *J Pers Assess* 2003;**80**:252–259.

56. Bolla KI, Cadet JL, London ED. The neuropsychiatry of chronic cocaine abuse. *J Neuropsychiat Clin Neurosci* 1998;**10**:280–289.

57. Nnadi CU, Mimiko OA, McCurtis HL, Cadet JL. Neuropsychiatric effects of cocaine use disorders. *J Natl Med Assoc* 2005;**97**:1504–1515.

58. Ernst M, Grant SJ, London ED, Contoreggi CS, Kimes AS, Spurgeon L. Decision making in adolescents with behavior disorders and adults with substance abuse. *Am J Psychiatry* 2003;**160**:33–40.

59. Wechsler D. *The Wechsler Intelligence Scale for Children – Fourth Edition*. London: Pearson Assessment, 2004.

60. Roid GH. *Stanford-Binet Intelligence Scales, Fifth Edition: Technical Manual*. Itasca, IL: Riverside Publishing, 2003.

61. Brown L, Sherbenou RJ, Johnsen SK. *Test of Nonverbal Intelligence-Fourth Edition (TONI-4) Examiner's Manual*. Austin, TX: PRO-ED, 2010.

62. Wechsler D. *Wechsler Abbreviated Scale of Intelligence (WASI)*. San Antonio, TX: Harcourt Assessment, 1999.

63. Kaufman AS, Kaufman NL. *Kaufman Brief Intelligence Test, Version 2 (K-BIT-2)* Circle Pines, MN: AGS, 2004.

64. Wechsler D. *Wechsler Individual Achievement Test 2nd Edition (WIAT II)* London: The Psychological Corporation, 2005.

65. Woodcock RW, McGrew KS, Mather N. *Examiner's Manual: Woodcock-Johnson III Tests of Achievement*. Itasca, IL: Riverside Publishing, 2001.

66. Kaufman AS, Kaufman NL. *KTEA II: Kaufman Test of Educational Achievement Comprehensive Form Manual (KTEA II)* Bloomington, MN: AGS Publishing, 2004.

67. King KM, Meehan BT, Trim RS, Chassin L. Marker or mediator? The effects of adolescent substance use on young adult educational attainment. *Addiction* 2006;**101**:1730–1740.

68. Godley SH, Passetti LL, White MK. Employment and adolescent alcohol and drug treatment and recovery: an exploratory study. *Am J Addict* 2006;**15**(Suppl. 1):137–143.

69. Harrington Godley S. Substance use, academic performance and the village school. *Addiction* 2006;**101**:1685–1688.

70. Lynskey M. Substance use and educational attainment. *Addiction* 2006;**101**:1684–1685.

71. Reitan RM, Wolfson D. *The Halstead–Reitan Neuropsychological Test Battery: Theory and Clinical Interpretation*, 2nd edn. Tucson, AZ: Neuropsychology Press, 1993.

72. Davies ADM. The influence of age on trail making test performance. *J Clin Psychol* 1968;**24**:96–98.

73. Golden CJ, Freshwater SM. Luria-Nebraska Neuropsychological Battery. In: Dorfman WI, Hersen M (eds), *Understanding Psychological Assessment: Perspectives on Individual Differences*. New York: Kluwer Academic/Plenum Publishers, 2001; pp. 59–75.

74. Psychological Assessment Resources. Computerised Wisconsin Card Sort Task, Version 4 (WCST). Psychological Assessment Resources, 2003.

75. Bechara A, Dolan S, Denburg N, Hindes A, Anderson SW, Nathan PE. Decision-making deficits, linked to a dysfunctional ventromedial prefrontal cortex, revealed in alcohol and stimulant abusers. *Neuropsychologia* 2001;**39**:376–389.

76. Salgado JV, Malloy-Diniz LF, Campos VR, *et al.*Neuropsychological assessment of impulsive behavior in abstinent alcohol-dependent subjects. *Rev Bras Psiquiatr* 2009;**31**:4–9.

77. American Psychological Association. *Guidelines for Psychological Practice with Girls and Women*. Washington DC: APA, 2007.

78. American Psychological Association. American Psychological Association ethical principles of psychologists and code of conduct 2002. Available from: http://www.apa.org/ethics/code2002.html.

6

Cultural Assessment

Karen B. Rosenbaum,[1] and Roxanne M. Lewin[2]

[1]*Woodhull Hospital Center; New York University Medical Center; Voluntary Faculty, New York Presbyterian Hospital, Cornell; Clinical and Forensic Psychiatrist in Private Practice, New York, NY, USA*
[2]*University of Medicine & Dentistry of New Jersey, NJ, USA*

Culture is defined as "the behaviors and beliefs characteristic of a particular social, ethnic, or age group, *i.e. the youth culture; the drug culture*" (Dictionary.com). In addition to understanding that adolescence is inherently culturally different from adulthood, recognizing ethnic, racial, and religious differences among the adolescent population when assessing substance issues in adolescents is equally important. These behaviors and beliefs can include thoughts, styles of cosmmunicating, and ways of interacting in relationships, values, practices, and customs. Adolescence, a phase in life with few responsibilities and expectations, became widespread throughout the world in the middle of the twentieth century after the Industrial Revolution. For the first time, teenagers no longer needed to work to support their families, and also parents were busy at work, leaving adolescents more time to mature on their own. As a consequence, adolescence became a time filled with self-doubt, anxiety, and unclear role identity.

In order to alleviate this anxiety, often teenagers turn to their peers and as a group, experiment with alcohol and drugs. Young people often turn outward from their family and are less subjected to parental control. Insecure or anxious boys or girls might then turn to alcohol or drugs and may later in life have a difficult time coping without these substances. This could potentially lead to crime, dropping out of school, and making money at unskilled jobs in order to support their drug use. Therefore, substances can become detrimental to teenagers entering adulthood and coping with the realities of adult life [1].

Different cultures and social groups use substances and alcohol in various ways – recreationally, medicinally, and even ritualistically – and different cultures may sanction different drugs for these various uses. Because the United States is so culturally diverse, it is important for the clinician to become culturally competent when assessing adolescent substance use, abuse, or dependence. When clinicians can use cultural context to better understand their patients, they will become more effective in the assessment and treatment of medical and psychiatric disorders including substance use disorders.

Understanding a wide variety of cultural norms and practices is important for clinicians to better assess their young patients' risk factors for alcohol and drug use and abuse. In 1978, the US Department of Commerce, under a Statistical Policy Directive No. 15, declared four primary racial categories, which included American Indian/Alaska Native, Asian/Pacific Islander, African American or Black, and White. These classifications have been criticized by many as failing to acknowledge the growing diversity of the US population and failing to recognize subtle distinctions between groups within these four major categories [2]. In her article "Three is Not Enough" in *Newsweek* in 1995, Sharon Begley illustrates the reasons and science behind why fitting great diversity into three major race categories is no longer meaningful biologically [3].

In 1998, the US Department of Health surveyed the country and estimated the prevalence of the past month drug use broken down by age, sex, and race/ethnicity. The five race/ethnicities it surveyed included: White, non-Hispanic; Black, non-Hispanic; American Indian/ Alaska Native; Asian/Pacific Islander; and Hispanic. The survey found that among children aged 12–17, the highest percentage of any illicit drug consumed was by the American Indian/Alaska Native group. This held true when examining the individual substances of marijuana, cocaine, alcohol, heavy alcohol, and tobacco cigarettes. The Hispanic group contained the next highest users of cocaine.

Clinical Handbook of Adolescent Addiction, First Edition. Richard Rosner.
© 2013 John Wiley & Sons, Ltd. Published 2013 by John Wiley & Sons, Ltd.

However, for each of the other listed substances, the White, non-Hispanic group comprised the next highest consumers among this age group. These results were consistent with results found by Bachman *et al.* in 1991 when they examined racial/ethnic differences in smoking, drinking, and illicit drug use among high-school seniors between 1976 and 1989 in the United States [4].

It is important to understand ethnic, cultural, and gender differences when assessing and treating adolescents for possible substance abuse and dependence. One study compared White and African American girls on several alcohol use variables and found that African American girls generally reported less alcohol use and related consequences, and more internalizing and externalizing problems than White girls. It found four typologies for White girls including abstainers, experimenters, moderate drinkers, and heavy drinkers. For African American girls, the study found only three groups including abstainers, experimenters, and problem drinkers. Compared with White girls, a higher percentage of African American girls were abstainers. Also, African American problem drinkers reported having lower rates of driving drunk and drinking while using, than both groups of White problematic drinkers, and higher rates of carrying a weapon while drinking than both groups of Whites [5].

Krupinski *et al.* observed that in Australia, immigrants and refugees tend to have low rates of substance abuse during their first few years of immigration [6], but after several years of relocation, rates of substance abuse begin to increase. Three other features following migration have emerged among ethnic groups. It has been shown that immigrants are at risk for abusing the substance or substances that were abused in their countries of origin. For example, adolescents from Chile might be more apt to abuse cocaine [7]. In addition, young immigrants are more likely to begin abusing substances that are abused in their new country. Because the substances may be unfamiliar to them, they may not realize the dangers associated with them. Because their families may be unfamiliar with these substances, they may not be able to guide their children appropriately in avoiding these substances.

Immigrants may seek ways to assimilate into their new society and may seek illegal means to support themselves. Because many immigrants speak two languages and may have contacts in countries in which drugs are produced, it may be easier for them to become involved with illegal trafficking of drugs.

Borges *et al.* found that although the prevalence of alcohol and drug use, abuse, and dependence has historically been lower in Mexico than in the United States, this gap may be closing due to migration and acculturation [8]. These authors looked at the association between migration to the United States, substance use, and substance use disorders in three urban areas of northern Mexico. They looked at northern Mexico because of its proximity to the United States and prior evidence that alcohol and drug use is about twice as common in this region compared with other areas in Mexico. They found that the prevalence of alcohol, marijuana, cocaine, and other drug use was higher among migrants and relatives of migrants compared with other Mexicans. The lifetime prevalence of any drug use and of using multiple drugs was also higher for both the return migrants and relatives of migrants, but more so for return migrants. Current year alcohol use, heavy drinking and drug use, alcohol dependence, drug dependence, and any substance dependence were all elevated among return migrants compared to other Mexicans. They concluded that migrants to the United States were more likely to be initiated with substances, and patterns of use and abuse persisted after they returned to Mexico. They found that risk for alcohol and drug use in this population may be related to certain types of work, the length of stay in the United States, and experiences of discrimination and associated stress. Preventive measures to help cope with these factors are important and should be put into place on both sides of the US-Mexican border.

Rush *et al.* examined the client profile of youths seeking addiction treatment in Chile [7]. Compared with data from the United States, which showed that for clients 14 to 19 years old, the prevalence of cocaine abuse and dependence was 2.2%, it was 42.8% for Chilean youth [7,9]. For inhalants, the data were 1.6% for youths in the United States compared with 2.5% for Chile. Because of the high rates of substance use, abuse, and dependence for Chilean youths, the authors concluded that there must be an adequate supply of more intensive services especially in areas where people may not be able to access treatment easily. Often this is where there are people who are most in need of treatment. In the United States it is important for clinicians to understand that adolescents who immigrated from countries such as Chile where drug use is prevalent and commonplace may be more at risk for substance use disorders, and more in need of preventive services.

Similarly, there is extensive literature on the increased drug use of American Indian adolescents living on reservations. Beavais *et al.* administered anonymous surveys to 7th through 12th grade students in Indian reservation schools [10]. They found that although there was a drop in drug use from 1981 to 1985, 53% of Native American youths were still classified as "at risk" in their drug involvement compared with 35% of non-Native American adolescents. They attributed this difference to unemployment, prejudice, poverty, and lack of optimism about the future. The authors did not believe that the high levels of drug and alcohol use resulted from anything inherent in the history or culture of Native Americans. They theorized that the likely reason for the higher rates of substance abuse was the effects of the disruption of culture, not the elements of culture itself. Native Americans have historically been the most economically and socially disadvantaged cultural group in the United States. In addition, people living on reservations have tended to be geographically isolated from major cities. Binion et al. suggested that there is a need for strong cultural and social supports and teaching of coping skills to deal with negative affect such as boredom, worry, nervousness, and anger that can occur in daily living in isolated environments such as Native American reservations [11]. A more recent study looked at the development of substance use and psychiatric comorbidity in White and Native American adolescents aged 9–15 as part of the Great Smoky Mountains Study [12]. The authors found that in these adolescents, alcohol use was associated with increased risk of later tobacco and illicit drug use. They also found that rates of recent use of alcohol and "hard" illicit drugs were similar for Native American youths and other adolescents living in the same rural area in southern Appalachia. However, they found that rates of marijuana and tobacco use were higher among Native Americans compared with Whites.

There have been many studies showing that individual characteristics of neighborhoods can be even stronger predictors of alcohol-related problems than the population's racial or ethnic background [13,14]. Alaniz reviewed research revealing that "alcohol availability and advertising are disproportionately concentrated in ethnic minority communities" [14]. Research has shown that alcohol-related problems are proportional to the density of bars and liquor stores in a given neighborhood, and that this density is disproportionally higher in communities consisting of African-American and other non-Caucasian residents [15]. Hackbarth et al. conducted an elegant study looking at the quantity of tobacco and alcohol billboards in 50 Chicago neighborhoods [14]. They found that 86% of these billboards were located in minority wards, despite the fact that these wards comprise only 66% of the population. They found that the mean number of billboards per ward in minority wards was 150 compared to 50 in White wards. The authors illustrated that billboard advertisements were more dangerous to children in the community than other types of advertisements because there is no way to protect children from seeing them while in the car, walking to school, etc. [9,16]. Data generated by this study have since been used to influence public policy and helped reduce billboards advertising alcohol and cigarettes in minority communities.

In a study by Kuntsche et al., the authors tested the theory of "gender and cultural convergence in drunkenness among adolescents from 23 mostly European and North American countries." They showed that in 2005–06, 15-year-old adolescents had on average been intoxicated by alcohol two to three times. Their results showed that over an 8-year span, youths in Eastern European and Western countries became more similar in terms of drunkenness frequency. The study was done because decades ago, adolescents from Eastern European countries had reported less frequent drunkenness than did adolescents from Western countries. The authors speculated that the recent convergence among Eastern and Western countries was attributed to alcohol advertising and marketing practices. Eastern European countries, and particularly their youths, have increasingly become targeted by global alcohol marketing strategies [17,18].

In addition to sociological factors in minority communities, family structure is also important when considering cultural differences in adolescent substance use. In a study that examined family structure and adolescent risk-taking behavior among Mexican, Cuban, and Puerto Rican communities [19], the authors found that Mexican adolescents living in female-headed households had higher rates of alcohol and drug use, and overall risk-taking behaviors, than adolescents living with both parents. However, Puerto Rican adolescents living in female-headed households had higher rates only on the overall risk-taking behaviors compared with those living with both parents. In contrast, the study found that Cuban family structure was unrelated to adolescent risk-taking behaviors. Gender differences were also found in risk-taking behaviors among Mexicans and Puerto Ricans, with males reporting higher rates of alcohol, drugs, and overall risk behaviors than females. Cuban males had higher rates of alcohol use than females, but there were no gender differences in drug use or overall risk behaviors. Family structure only explained risk-taking behaviors among Mexicans. This study is another example of why it does not make sense to group all Hispanics together.

Cultural groups that value abstinence of alcohol and substances tend to have lower rates of substance abuse, at least as long as the individuals remain within that group. If they leave that group and associate with another cultural group, then the risk of substance abuse increases especially if the new group has higher rates of substance abuse [20].

Cultural groups that sanction or ritualize substance use also have lower rates of substance abuse. This socialization of substances often begins in childhood or early adolescence, involving rituals or ceremonies, and may involve multiple generations and celebratory meals. However, when peers teach each other to drink in secular settings that are not religious, and in a deviant, secretive manner as opposed to an open, culturally accepted setting, it can lead to substance abuse [20].

A group of researchers examined the differences in substance use, depression, peer relationships, and parental monitoring and practices among a matched sample of Hispanic and White adolescents between the ages of 13 and 17 years presenting for a brief alcohol intervention [21]. They found that across all substance use variables, there was only one significant difference. Hispanic adolescents reported smoking significantly fewer cigarettes per day than did their White non-Hispanic counterparts [22]. There were no significant differences between the two groups on alcohol use, marijuana use, or riding in a car with a driver who had been drinking alcohol or using drugs. White non-Hispanic adolescents perceived greater acceptance from their neighborhood environment than did Hispanic adolescents. The authors concluded that attention should be paid during counseling to help Hispanic adolescents cope with feelings of perceived neighborhood rejection. Also, according to the parents of the Hispanic sample, these adolescents were receiving less parental supervision compared with the White adolescents. Parental supervision has been shown to be protective against substance use problems. Therefore, these factors should be addressed when assessing and treating Hispanic adolescents for possible addictive disorders.

A review paper outlined disparities among ethnic/racial minority use in availability and quality of treatment for substance use disorders [23]. It showed that certain healthcare policies, such as restrictions on Medicaid or on the State Children's Health Insurance Program eligibility criteria, affect the African American and Hispanic population to a greater degree than White children. More than 60% of uninsured children are Hispanic or African American. Therefore, these restrictions cause difficulty for these children in obtaining treatment for substance use disorders.

Another significant paper showed that when only school data are available, such as in all self-report surveys of youths in school, "errors in estimating drug use among [ethnic] groups with high rates of school dropout can be substantial" [24]. The authors looked at rates of alcohol, marijuana, inhalant, stimulant, cocaine, and LSD use by students and dropouts (defined as 7th- through 12th-grade students who had a period of absence from school lasting for one month or longer with no excused absence or contact with the school) among Mexican Americans, non-Hispanic Whites, and Native Americans. The results showed that within the populations of the southwestern United States that they used, rates of lifetime substance use among school dropouts were much higher than rates for youths who remained in school. The students who dropped out were likely to have tried substances at rates from 1.3 to 3.0 times greater than those of students in school for all six of the above substances. As far as current use, the dropouts reported rates from 1.2 to 6.4 times greater than those reported by students in school. The authors found that when substance rates were corrected to include dropouts from minority groups that have high dropout rates, this could lead to large changes as well as differences in relative rates of use across ethnic groups. The higher proportion of dropouts in the Mexican American and Native American group in their study compared with the White group led to substantial shifts in drug use estimates when their weighted formula was used to correct estimates of substance use based on youths enrolled in school only. They concluded that without results for school dropouts, surveys are likely to provide poor estimates of rates of use for any group with a high school dropout rate.

Drug and alcohol use practices may vary between genders as well as cultures. Regarding gender differences, some authors suggest that adolescent boys had slightly heavier alcohol consumption rates and greater endorsement of problems related to drinking than girls [25]. However, girls were equally likely to endorse more social consequences of alcohol use. Physical fighting was a more severe item for girls than for boys. Dating problems due to drinking were more common for girls than for boys given the same level of alcohol involvement; the authors felt this indicated that girls may be more prone to alcohol's effect on romantic relationships. In contrast, a Dutch survey found no gender differences when examining the association between weekly alcohol use and mental health among adolescents [26]. Another study showed that although higher perceived scholastic competence was associated with less substance use in both genders, there were some gender differences. In boys, more support from teachers and to a lesser extent parents, was associated with less substance use. In girls, social support was unrelated to substance use except for support from classmates, which was associated with more cigarette and marijuana use [27]. However, in girls with low scholastic competence, more support from peers was associated with more substance use.

A study in Spain showed that while the level of use for all drug types was similar in boys and girls aged 12 to 14, the differences between the genders increased with age, reaching statistical significance for alcohol and cannabis among adolescents aged 15–17 [28]. The authors thought this could be related to the presence of female-specific protective factors that stop girls from progressing to substance use problems and disorders. They did not find gender differences for tobacco use.

One researcher found that males across race/ethnicities had more opportunity for first illicit drug use than did girls, but that once the opportunity for first illicit drug use occurred, girls and boys were at equal risk for actual drug use after the first exposure [29]. This finding held for Caucasian, African American, and Hispanic respondents, and for those living in the northeast, north central, southern and western United States, and for those inside and outside major cities at the time of the interview.

A study of lifetime psychoactive drug use among 1054 medical students in Rio de Janeiro, Brazil, found that alcohol abuse was more prevalent among male students from higher income families [30]. Tobacco, cannabis, and inhalant lifetime use was more prevalent among males, and tranquilizer use more prevalent among females. Students with divorced or dead parents were found to be more likely to use tobacco, cannabis, and tranquilizers. Inhalant lifetime use was also more prevalent among students from higher income families, while cocaine was more prevalent among male students from higher income families. Cannabis users were more likely to be students who had college-educated, divorced, or dead parents, or had lifetime tobacco, cocaine, or inhalant use. The authors found that substance use among medical students in Rio de Janeiro was not widespread compared to rates reported for more developed countries. They concluded that preventive efforts should focus on alcohol and cannabis use by medical students.

ASSESSMENT INSTRUMENTS

Because adolescent substance abusers are distributed across diverse racial, cultural, and socioeconomic backgrounds there is the need for the multidimensional assessment of the needs of adolescents that transcend all patient types [31]. Adolescent assessment relies heavily upon interviewer-driven processes, with the clinical interview being the cornerstone of the assessment and the therapeutic process. Comparative measures of adolescent self-report data are commonly obtained (family interview, historical documents) [17,32,33]. Adolescents are developmentally distinct from adults and differ in their substance use patterns and their mental health needs. This fact must be taken into account by the assessment instruments used [34]. Computer- or paper-based standardized assessment instruments are sometimes useful in the assessment of adolescent substance use. But, the clinician has the daunting task of choosing an appropriate instrument. A search for "adolescent" assessment instruments in the University of Washington's Substance Use Screening & Assessment Instruments Database reveals 207 screening and assessment instruments.

Using Standardized Instruments to Assess Adolescent Substance Use?

There are many problems associated with evaluating substance abuse in adolescents. To begin with, adolescents are administered standardized instruments normed on adults, which therefore are not specific to the adolescent population [35]. Additionally, inattention, lack of motivation, disinterest, and reading difficulties can minimize the collection of accurate questionnaire data [36–38]. To complicate things further, instruments that do not account for cultural variables can also lead to inaccurate data collection. There are encouraging data showing that when mental health treatment interventions are culturally modified, they are found to be significantly more effective. Meta-analytic reviews report that mental health treatment was four times more effective when they were culturally modified for a specific group and when attention was tailored to cultural context and values. A meta-analysis of 76 studies of culturally adjusted interventions reported a moderately strong benefit of culturally adapted interventions [39].

Szapocznik et al. have comprehensively described five representative issues, which transcend their work with multicultural populations [40]:

1. Back translation of instruments to ensure linguistic comparability.
2. Identification of clinically relevant cultural characteristics.
3. The comparability of measured constructs across diverse populations.
4. Assessment of acculturation and biculturation; assessment of transcultural and culture-specific dimensions of family functioning.

However, what is widely known is that standardized measurements used to assess adolescent psychopathology are not sufficiently validated in various racial and ethnic groups [36]. Huey and Polo identified the lack of culturally validated measurements for assessing and tracking substance use outcomes. Their review demonstrated that reliability and validity of measurements are not routinely assessed in cross-cultural intervention research [41].

Another problem for the clinician is that identifying racial and ethnic differences is not enough as this does not account for the degree of *acculturation* to the culture in the host country, and the nature of the acculturation stressors [42]. Acculturation is defined as the "dual process of cultural and psychological change that takes place as a result of contact between two or more cultural groups and their individual members [43]. As immigrants become more acculturated, a change in behavior can ensue as they adopt the attitudes and practices of the host country [44]. However, not all individuals undergo acculturation in the same fashion, as acculturation is a long-term process [43].

Huey and Polo also found that minority youths tend to be more acculturated than minority adults, and culturally sensitive adaptations/instruments will not work as well for acculturated youths as they may have already *integrated* or *assimilated* with the host culture [45].

Previous studies have found that acculturation to the US culture has been associated with a number of negative health outcomes for Latino adolescents, specifically a rise in use of alcohol and other drugs [22,46,47]. The Acculturation, Habits, and Interests Multicultural Scale for Adolescents [47] is a multidimensional acculturation scale that examines the degree of acculturation in the United States. It generates four subscores: United States Orientation (Assimilation), Other Country Orientation (Separation), Both Countries Orientation (Integration), and Neither Country Orientation (Marginalization).

SUMMARY

There are important considerations when choosing an instrument that will adequately account for ethnic and cultural differences:

1. Adolescent substance use instruments are not sufficiently validated across cultural and ethnic groups.
2. Race is not the important identifying factor. For example, the Hispanic population is a diverse group made up of people from many different countries with specific cultural and ethnic differences.
3. Second-language skills and cultural diversity vary among different ethnic groups. For example, an instrument that was developed and performed adequately for Hispanic youths in Miami may produce considerably more errors with Hispanic youths in New York City.
4. Before administering standardized scales, assess the patient's reading level and language proficiency.
5. The degree of acculturation to the culture in the host country and the nature of the acculturation stressors are specific to the individual. The patient's history should include the patient's immigration status and history, degree of acculturation, and nature of acculturation stressors.

References

1. Wu LT, Ringwalt CL. Use of alcohol treatment and mental health services among adolescents with alcohol use disorders. *Psychiatr Serv* 2006;**57**:84–92.

2. U.S. Department of Health and Human Services. *Drug Use Among Racial/Ethnic Minorities*. National Institute on Drug Abuse, Division of Epidemiology, Services & Prevention Research, 2003; pp. 1–188.
3. Begley S. Three is not enough. *Newsweek* 1995; 13 Feb.
4. Bachman JG, Wallace JM, Patrick MO, Johnston LD, Kurth CL. Neighbors HW, Racial/ethnic differences in smoking, drinking, and illicit drug use among American high school seniors 1976-1989. *Am J Public Health* 1991;**81**:372–377.
5. Dauber S, Hogue A, Paulson JF, Leiferman JA. Typologies of alcohol use in white and African American adolescent girls. *Subst Use Misuse* 2009;**44**:1121–1141.
6. Krupinski J, Stoller A, Wallace L. Psychiatric disorders in Eastern European refugees now in Australia. *Soc Sci Med* 1972;**7**:31–45.
7. Rush B, Sapag J, Chaim G, Quinteros C. Client characteristics within the Chilean national youth addiction treatment demonstration system. *J Subst Abuse Treat* 2011;**40**:175–182.
8. Borges G, Medina-Mora ME, Orozco R, Fleiz C, Cherpitel C, Breslau J. The Mexican migration to the U. S. and substance use in Northern Mexico. *Addiction* 2009;**104**:603–611.
9. Chan YF, Godley MD, Godley SH, Dennis ML. Utilization of mental health services among adolescents in community based substance abuse outpatient clinics. *J Behav Health Serv Res* 2009;**36**:35–51.
10. Beavais F, Oetting ER, Edwards RW. Trends in drug use of Indian adolescents living on reservations: 1975–1983. *Am J Drug Alcohol Abuse* 1985;**11**:209–229.
11. Binion A, Miller CD, Beavais F, Oetting ER. Rationales for the use of alcohol, marijuana, and other drugs by eighth-grade Native American and Anglo Youth. *Int J Addictions* 1988;**23**:47–64.
12. Federman EB, Costello EJ, Angold A, Farmer EMZ, Erkanli A. Development of substance use and psychiatric comorbidity in an epidemiologic study of white and American Indian young adolescents. The Great Smoky Mountains Study. *Drug Alcohol Depen* 1997;**44**:69–78.
13. Alaniz ML. Alcohol availability and targeted advertising in racial/ethnic minority communities. *Alcohol Health Res W* 1998: Fall; 286–291.
14. Hackbarth DP, Silvestri B, Cosper W. Tobacco and alcohol billboards in 50 Chicago neighborhoods: market segmentation to sell dangerous products to the poor. *J Public Health Pol* 1995;**16**:213–230.
15. Botvin GJ, Griffin KW, Diaz T, Ifill-Williams M. Preventing binge drinking during early adolescence: one- and two-year follow-up of a school-based preventive intervention. *Psychol Addict Behav* 2001;**15**:360–365.
16. Sue S, Fujino DC, Hu L, Takeuchi D, Zane N. Community mental health services for ethnic minority groups. A test of the cultural responsiveness hypothesis. *J Consult Clin Psychol* 1991;**59**:533–540.
17. Center for Substance Abuse Treatment. Screening, assessment, and treatment planning for persons with co-occurring disorders. COCE Overview Paper 2. DHHS Publication No. (SMA) 06-4164. Rockville, MD: Substance Abuse and Mental Health Services Administration, and Center for Mental Health Services, 2006.
18. Kuntsche E, Kuntsche S, Knippe R, *et al.* Cultural and gender convergence in adolescent drunkenness; evidence from 23 European and North American countries. *Arch Pediatr Adolesc Med* 2011;**165**:152–158.

19. Sokol-Katz JS, Ulbrich PM. Family structure and adolescent risk-taking behavior: A comparison of Mexican, Cuban, and Puerto Rican Americans. *Int J Addictions* 1992;**27**:1197–1209.

20. Westermeyer, J. The role of cultural and social factors in the cause of addictive disorders. *Psychiatric Clin N Am* 1999;**22**:253–273.

21. Hernandez L, Eaton CA, Fairlie AM, Chun TH, Spirito A. Ethnic group differences in substance use, depression, peer relationships and parenting among adolescents receiving brief alcohol counseling. *J Ethn Subst Abuse* 2010;**9**:14–27.

22. Epstein JA, Doyle M, Botvin GJA. Mediational model of the relationship between linguistic acculturation and poly-drug use among Hispanic adolescents. *Psychol Rep* 2003;**93**:859–866.

23. Alegria M, Carson N, Goncalves M, Keefe K. Disparities in treatment for substance use disorders and co-occurring disorders for ethnic/racial minority youth. *J Am Acad Child Adolesc Psychiatry* 2011;**50**:22–31.

24. Swaim RC, Beavais F, Chavez EL, Oeting ER. The effect of school dropout rates on estimates of adolescent substance use among three racial/ethnic groups. *Am J Public Health* 1997;**87**:51–55.

25. Kahler CW, Hoeppner BB, Jackson KM. A Rasch model analysis of alcohol consumption and problems across adolescence and young adulthood. *Alcohol Clin Exp Res* 2009;**33**:663–673.

26. Verdurmen J, Monshouwer K, VanDorsselaer S, TerBogt T, Vollebergh W. Alcohol use and mental health in adolescents: interactions with age and gender – findings from Dutch 2001 health behavior in school-aged children survey. *J Stud Alcohol* 2005; September: 605–609.

27. Lifrak PD, McKay JR, Rostain A, Alterman Al, O'Brien CP. Relationship of perceived competencies, perceived social support, and gender to substance use in young adolescents. *J Am Acad Child Adolesc Psychiatry* 1997;**36**:933–940.

28. Diaz R, Goti J, Garcia M, *et al.* Patterns of substance use in adolescents attending a mental health department. *Eur Child Adolesc Psychiatry* 2011;**20**:279–289.

29. VanEtton ML, Anthony JC. Male-female differences in transitions from first drug opportunity to first use: searching for subgroup variation by age, race, region, and urban status. *J Women Health Gen-B* 2001;**10**:797–804.

30. Lambert Passos SR, Americano do Brasil PEA, Borges dos Santos MA, Costa de Aquino MT. Prevalence of psychoactive drug use among medical students in Rio de Janeiro. *Soc Psychiatry Psychiatr Epidemiol* 2006;**41**:989–996.

31. Meyers K. Critical issues in adolescent substance use assessment. *Drug Alcohol Depen* 1999;**55**:235–246.

32. Substance Abuse and Mental Health Services Administration. Screening and assessing adolescents for substance use disorders. Treatment Improvement Protocol, Series 31. U.S. Department of Health and Human Services, 2001.

33. U.S. Department of Justice. *Screening and assessing mental health and substance use disorders among youth in the juvenile justice system (NCJ 204956)*. Washington, DC: US Dept of Justice, 2004.

34. Winters KC. Screening and assessment instruments. Available from: http://www.drugstrategies.com/teens_screening.html.

35. Gans J, Falco M, Schackman BR, Winters KC. An in-depth survey of the screening and assessment practices of highly regarded adolescent substance abuse treatment programs. *J Child Adolesc Subst Abuse* 2010;**19**:33–47.

36. Blotcky AD. A framework for assessing the psychological functioning of adolescents. *Dev Behav Pediatr* 1984;**5**:74–77.

37. McLellan AT, Kushner H, Metzger DS, *et al.* The fifth edition of the Addiction Severity Index: Historical critique and normative data. *J Subst Abuse Treat* 1992;**9**:199–213.

38. Prout HT, Chizik R. Readability of child and adolescent self-report measures. *J. Consult Clin Psychol* 1988;**56**:152–154.

39. Griner D, Smith TB. Culturally adapted mental health intervention: a meta-analytic review. *Psychother Theory Res Pract Train* 2006;**43**:531–548.

40. Kurtines WM, Szapocznik J. Cultural competence in assessing Hispanic youths and families: challenges in the assessment of treatment needs and treatment evaluation for Hispanic drug-abusing adolescents. *Adolesc Drug Abuse Clin Assess Ther Interv* 1995;**156**:172–189.

41. Huey SJJr, Polo AJ. Evidence-based psychosocial treatments for ethnic minority youth. *J Clin Child Adolesc Psychology* 2008;**37**:262.

42. Gilvarry E. Substance abuse in young people. *J Child Psychol Psychiat* 2000;**41**:55–80.

43. Berry J. Acculturation: living successfully in two cultures. *Int J Intercult Rel* 2005;**29**:697–712.

44. Epstein JA, Botvin GJ, Dusenbury L, Diaz T, Kerner J. Validation of an acculturation measure for Hispanic adolescents. *Psychol Rep* 1996;**79**:1075–1079.

45. Betancourt JR. Cultural competency, providing quality care to diverse populations. *The Consultant Pharmacist* 2006;**21**:988–995.

46. Epstein JA, Botvin GJ, Diaz T. Linguistic acculturation and gender effects o smoking among Hispanic youth. *Prev Med* 1998;**27**:583–589.

47. Unger JB, Gallahen P, Shakib S, *et al.* The AHIMSA Acculturation Scale: a new measure of acculturation for adolescents in a multicultural society. *J Early Adolesc* 2002;**22**:225–251.

USEFUL WEB RESOURCES

National Institute on Drug Abuse: nida.nih.gov/nidahome.html

Substance Abuse and Mental Health Services Administration: samhsa.gov

7

Psychosocial Assessment of the Substance-Abusing Adolescent

Eve Maram

Licensed Psychologist, Orange, CA, USA

INTRODUCTION

Assessment uses diagnostic instruments and processes to determine an individual's needs and problems. It is an essential first step in detecting substance abuse problems, determining the possible causes of addiction for the individual, and developing the most appropriate treatment modality for his or her needs. Appropriate psychosocial assessment of the substance-abusing adolescent is timely and takes into consideration choosing the right instrument for the individual, the setting, the purpose, and the administrator of the test. Ineffective psychosocial assessment of the substance-abusing adolescent leads to poor treatment and discharge planning, repeated relapses, and increased rates of recidivism. Psychosocial assessment of the adolescent focuses upon social factors and influences, such as family dynamics, school, peers, risk behaviors, medical and physiological conditions, juvenile delinquency or dependency, and mental health. Influential factors to be considered include the presence of child abuse, domestic violence, chronic or severely dysfunctional family or living situations, and criminal behavior or tendencies [1,2].

A variety of instruments are available to measure psychosocial status in these areas, including standardized psychosocial screening tools, assessments, and questionnaires. Choosing the appropriate tool involves considering the setting, whether home, school, juvenile justice, medical, or social services institutions, or out-of-home care facilities. Effective psychosocial assessment of the substance-abusing adolescent requires determining the appropriate tool depending on the setting, the level and quality of individual functioning, whether or not the assessment is voluntary, who is conducting the assessment, and the intended purpose. The level of assessment may be either preliminary screening or more complete questionnaires or surveys for diagnostic or treatment planning purposes.

STRATEGIES, APPROACHES, AND SPECIAL CONSIDERATIONS

The defining characteristic of the adolescent period of development is a confounding variable in obtaining an accurate psychosocial assessment of substance abuse behavior among this population. Adolescence is a time of rebellion and experimentation, distrust of adults and authority figures, and resistance to authority. Most psychosocial assessments involve subjective, self-inventory, self-disclosing histories and questionnaires.

Barriers Specific to Adolescence

While a certain level of denial and minimization is typical even of adult responses to such tools, it is not only predictable but also in fact characteristic that adolescents' responses on such instruments are inevitably even less straightforward. This also means that an even greater importance may be attached to the setting and circumstances in which such an assessment takes place, as well as the assessor.

Most assessment tools designed to elicit information about adolescent substance abuse have in common a potentially contaminating factor of subjectivity, since the primary source of information is dependent on personal disclosure from the adolescent. The assessor and setting can mediate this to some extent. This may be subject to circumstances beyond the control of the participant, involving the juvenile justice system, the juvenile dependency system, or medical programs [3,4].

Assessor and Setting

If the adolescent is in a controlled, involuntary setting such as juvenile hall, a home for dependent children, or a hospital, for example, he or she is likely to be somewhat more cooperative. Extremely limiting circumstances such as incarceration may induce a level of desperation and make subsequent disclosure unlikely if left to the adolescent's own discretion. Adolescents who are in out-of-home care such as a foster or group home may be more receptive than if they feel they have a choice, depending on who is administering the assessment and the purpose. They may fear the consequences of not cooperating, which may include further restriction of their already jeopardized freedom. They may also be more inclined to participate because if they are forced to undergo the assessment instead of choosing it, they can project responsibility for having to do so on the assessor, thereby maintaining their adolescent self-image of rebellion and defiance to authority.

Building trust to solicit an honest assessment regarding substance-abusing behavior on the part of an adolescent who participates in such a process either voluntarily or through family or school referral, for example, may be daunting for most adults. Utilizing an adult who already has an established relationship with the adolescent or others who are viewed as safe may increase the likelihood of a valid self-report. Individuals who have some personal history of genuine connection with the adolescent, such as a trusted school counselor or certain peers, may maximize the possibility of genuine, open disclosure. For these reasons it is always helpful whenever possible to gather information from people who are close to the adolescent, who have observed his or her behavior and personality characteristics over time.

INDICATORS FOR ASSESSMENT

Substance abuse is not a selective illness; it is found among all segments of the population. Adolescence refers to the population between the ages of 11 and 17.

Adolescents of both genders, all racial and ethnic groups, and socioeconomic strata are subject to the destructive impact of alcohol and drug abuse and addiction. Thus, the identification of those who have a substance abuse disorder requires attentiveness and sensitivity to the range of complex indicators that might signal the need for assessment and possible treatment.

Risk Factors

There are many clues that can alert health professionals, educators, employers, family members, criminal and juvenile justice personnel, and others that the use of alcohol or other drugs is a problem for an individual. For example:

- a physician might become suspicious of frequent injuries, liver damage, weight changes, or a variety of other physical symptoms for which one explanation could be substance abuse;
- a teacher or employer might be alerted by changes in performance or attendance at school or on the job;
- family members, significant others, and peers might become concerned over changes in mood, familiar patterns of behavior, and relationships; or
- criminal or juvenile justice personnel might infer associations between substance abuse and criminal or delinquent behavior, such as income-generating crimes, including theft or prostitution, violent offenses, or drug-related criminal activity such as possession or sale of controlled substances.

There is often a precipitating event that brings alcohol- or drug-involved adolescents to the attention of those concerned about them. An automobile accident or Driving Under the Influence of a Controlled Substance (DUI) arrest, being fired from a job, an arrest for shoplifting, or a head injury from a fight or fall may result from the effects of alcohol or other drugs [4]. On the other hand, the indicators of problem drinking or drug use may be pieced together over time. For example, a teacher may notice a steady decline in a student's grades and social functioning, or an employer might notice changes in productivity. A parent, girlfriend, or boyfriend may notice that an individual's disposition has changed, and there may be increasing tensions and difficulties in the adolescent's relationships [5].

When these and other problems become apparent it is vital that the person be evaluated and referred for appropriate treatment if needed. A thorough assessment for substance abuse is important because it can identify not only chemical dependency, but also other medical, psychological, or psychiatric problems that may underlie the symptoms. Even if the primary problem is not substance abuse, it is just as vital that the individual receives other appropriate interventions, such as primary healthcare or human services [6].

Obtaining a useful psychosocial assessment of the substance-abusing adolescent is critical to developing appropriate treatment and achieving effective outcomes. Substance abuse may result from any number of psychosocial influences, including school problems, peer pressure, psychological stress, child abuse or neglect, and dysfunctional family dynamics, including alcoholism, marital difficulties, and domestic violence [7,8]. Conversely, once the problem of substance abuse is present, it becomes yet another barrier to psycho-social functioning, and will worsen the very problems that may initially have led to the abuse – as a means of avoiding those problems – thereby creating a self-perpetuating cycle.

SCREENING AND ASSESSMENT

A comprehensive assessment of the substance-abusing adolescent consists of at least five consecutive stages, including recognition of risk factors, initial screening, comprehensive assessment, appropriate interventions, and evaluation of process and outcome.

Screening

Screening refers to brief procedures used to determine the presence of a problem, substantiate that there is realistic concern, or identify the need for further eval-uation. Screening may occur in various community, institutional, or correctional settings [9]. Private medical practices, public health clinics, mental health programs, and schools are among those settings where screening adolescents for substance abuse might occur [10]. Within the criminal and juvenile justice systems, screen-ing is often done throughout the individual's contact. Adolescent substance use is the United States' number one public health problem according to the National Center on Addiction and Substance Abuse [8].

Interview techniques and screening instruments may be designed to attempt both to elicit and deliver infor-mation about substance abuse from/to alcohol- or drug-involved adolescents or their parents or caretakers. These self-reports may be helpful in determining if there is a need for assessment and intervention. Screening interviews might include a few brief questions asked during intake procedures that query the individual regarding his or her use of alcohol or other drugs. Screening instruments include brief tests, usually self-administered, that require individuals to provide infor-mation about their abuse of substances. In both cases, the alcohol- or drug-involved adolescent is asked to provide a self-report of his or her substance abuse.

Comprehensive Assessment

Assessment is a critical element of effective substance abuse treatment. It is the first stage of intervention with individuals who are chemically dependent. A compre-hensive appraisal of an adolescent's alcohol or drug problem and how it affects his or her health and func-tioning is vital for selecting treatment sources and modalities that best meet his or her needs. This includes a determination of many factors, including: the severity

of the problem; possible influences that have perpetu-ated chemical use, culminating in addiction; related difficulties; and the individual's perception and attitude toward treatment.

There are at least five objectives for conducting appropriate and comprehensive assessments of adoles-cents with substance use problems or chemical depen-dency. These include:

- identify those who are experiencing problems related to substance abuse and/or have progressed to addiction;
- assess the full spectrum of problems for which treatment may be needed;
- plan appropriate interventions;
- involve appropriate family members or significant others, as needed; and
- evaluate the effectiveness of the interventions that are implemented [11,12].

While screening is useful in differentiating adolescents who are alcohol- and drug-involved from those who abstain or participate in limited use without associated problems, assessment indicates a process to determine the nature and complexity of the adolescent's spectrum of drug abuse and related problems. An assessment uses extensive procedures that evaluate the severity of the substance abuse problem, gather information about rel-evant factors, and assist in developing treatment and follow-up recommendations.

Related Problem Areas

In addition to assessing substance abuse, a comprehen-sive psychosocial assessment will probe related problem areas. These might include medical status (including both general health conditions and infectious diseases such as tuberculosis, hepatitis, and sexually transmitted diseases); psychological status and possible psychiatric disorders; social functioning; family and peer relations; educational and/or job performance; criminal or delin-quent behaviors and legal problems; and socioeconomic status and associated issues.

Basic Steps and Sources

Three basic steps in the assessment process include information, data analysis, and treatment plan develop-ment. Sources of information that can be helpful in conducting a comprehensive psychosocial assessment of the substance-abusing adolescent include existing information, individual and collateral interviews, and testing instruments. Testing instruments can include standardized interviews, structured interviews, and/or self-administered tests.

Screening, assessment, and diagnosis are important in the treatment of any illness. The assessment of persons with drug or alcohol problems is very similar to the diagnosis of other disorders. The assessment process includes gathering information from a variety of sources. These may include the adolescent's statements, previous records, and significant others. When the information is collected, it is reviewed and evaluated by a trained professional. A variety of instruments have been developed as tools for the assessment process [13].

Standardized Assessment Instruments

Assessment instruments should be evaluated for validity (Do they measure what they say they measure?) and reliability (Do they consistently provide the same results?). When assessment instruments are used, it is important to ascertain that research has been conducted to determine their validity and reliability on populations similar to those on which the instrument will be used. For example, an instrument might be a valid and reliable tool for White adult males, but it may not necessarily be useful for assessing adolescent females.

An advantage of using standardized instruments is that information regarding their reliability and validity will be available. If the instrument has high validity and reliability, it will accurately measure what it intends to, and produce stable results; the test's outcome will not be significantly influenced by fluctuating or extraneous factors such as the adolescent's mood or the time of day.

In addition, the instrument should be normed, or validated, with similar populations to those being tested. An instrument used with adolescents should be normed on other adolescents. Even when the reliability and validity of standardized tests have been proven, assessment outcomes may be affected by other factors. These include attempts by individuals using them to slant the outcome by deliberately asking or answering questions accordingly, varying ability of individuals to read and understand the test items, relative motivation of the adolescent to take the test seriously, and the level of cultural sensitivity of the test.

Continuum of Severity

Accurately identifying the problem, thoroughly assessing it, and determining the appropriate assessment and recommendations regarding level of treatment for an adolescent are particularly challenging. In addition to factors normally considered when assessing an individual for a substance abuse disorder, such as severity of substance abuse, cultural background, and presence of coexisting disorders, assessment must also examine other variables such as age, level of maturity, and family and peer environment when working with adolescents.

Researchers and treatment professionals have found it useful to characterize adolescent substance use behavior on a continuum of severity, extending from the developmental variation of experimentation with substances through problem use, to the disorders of abuse and dependence. The degree of substance involvement is an important consideration for assessment, as are any coexisting disorders, the family and peer environment, and the individual's stage of mental and emotional development [14]. Any response to an adolescent who is using substances, including strategies for identification of the problem as well as choice of tools for screening and assessment, should be consistent with the severity of involvement.

Denial and Resistance

Denial is a common facet of substance abuse disorders, as individuals of all ages, as well as significant others in the person's life, tend to minimize both the nature and amount of their drug or alcohol use. Often individuals in denial are actually convinced that substance abuse is not a serious problem, though objective indicators suggest serious consequences, particularly during adolescence, when it is likely to be both egosyntonic and supported by peer pressure.

Individuals who are drug-involved may be more truthful about their use if they perceive the assessor, setting, and purpose as non-threatening. In these cases, reports from adolescents in treatment may be more credible than those from within the juvenile justice system. Assurance of confidentiality is an important factor that enhances self-reporting, whereas threats of prosecution and other sanctions may diminish disclosures. Although screening interviews and assessment instruments may not provide a true picture of drug and alcohol use in all cases, there are some individuals who will be truthful. Coupled with other methods, such as chemical tests, these measures help distinguish users from non-users [15].

PSYCHOSOCIAL ASSESSMENT PROCESS

A comprehensive psychosocial assessment of the substance-abusing adolescent generally consists of a multiple assessment model, including three main components: content, methods, and sources. Each pertains to specific evaluation goals.

The content domain refers to the important clinical variables of adolescent substance use and related problems. These include substance disorder severity, predisposing and perpetuating risk factors, coexisting psychiatric disorders, and response distortions, such as faking good and faking bad tendencies [16]. This assumes that substance use disorders are usually accompanied by other problems in an adolescent's life, such as school performance, peer and family adjustment, medical problems, and crime [17]. Furthermore, it is of utmost importance to determine at what stage of change the individual is situated [18].

The second component of this model refers to the methods used to measure the content. There are numerous available instruments using the methods of self-report questionnaires and interviews. However, direct observation and laboratory testing, such as blood and urine tests, are also relevant assessment methods to consider.

Finally, several information sources may be relevant when evaluating an adolescent's substance use. In addition to the client, other informants include parents, teachers, peers, employers, and significant others. These collateral sources cannot be contacted for information without the adolescent's written consent. Written reports and records from schools, previous treatment experiences, and juvenile courts also contain information that may be relevant to assessing the adolescent's substance use problems. Relying on any one source may lead to an overestimate or underestimate of the problem. Assessors need to evaluate the relative validity of the information from different sources and should not assume that the client's self-report is necessarily less valid than other information sources. While there is some evidence to the contrary, several instruments have documented the validity of adolescent self-report of drug involvement [19].

Information Gathering

A comprehensive psychosocial assessment includes existing information, individual and collateral interviews, and testing instruments.

Information from existing sources may include:

- drug history;
- medical history and current status;
- mental health history and current status;
- criminal or delinquency history;
- educational history and current status; and
- employment history and current status.

Interviews with individuals are more extensive than screening, and can reveal valuable details about the adolescent that complement other information to obtain an accurate evaluation of problems. An assessment interview can also make the foundation for a

positive, trusting working relationship during future interventions.

As with screenings, collateral interviews involve gathering information from others who are or have been involved with the person being assessed. Collateral sources should be asked to provide descriptive information rather than to make subjective judgments about the person. As with patient interviews, information received is not always accurate. Possible collateral sources include family members, peers, teachers, employers, and others who may have helpful information.

Information gathering may involve a single professional obtaining the information in all areas. However, an interviewer or case manager may request consultation with other professionals. For example, if the adolescent discloses that he or she is troubled by certain physical symptoms, and the assessor is not a physician, a referral is made for a medical examination. Similarly, it might be necessary to obtain psychological or psychiatric evaluation if it is determined that in-depth assessments are needed in these areas, and the assessor is from another discipline, such as a social worker or probation officer. For this reason, a multi-disciplinary team approach is recommended for obtaining the range of information needed for comprehensive assessment and treatment planning, whenever feasible.

Interviews should be adapted to the age and culture of the patient. Cognitive abilities can affect the interview; the assessor must be aware of the patient's cognitive ability level and structure the interview accordingly, or this may present another barrier in the assessment process. If the adolescent being assessed is not fluent in the language or culture of the assessment, then the options are either an assessor who shares the same language and culture or an experienced interpreter.

Testing instruments can include: standardized interviews; structured interviews; and/or self-administered tests. These techniques have been developed to assess individuals in multiple areas, including personality, aggressive tendencies, social skills, stress factors, risk for substance abuse, and intellectual capacity. Most of the instruments have been formally standardized through a systematic research and validation process [20]. The standardized interview differs from the structured interview in that it limits the interviewer to a prescribed style and list of questions. Using the standardized interview, the interviewer is restricted from freely probing beyond conflicting or superficial answers, sometimes considered a disadvantage of this technique. An advantage is that this interview may be more credible than the structured interview, an important consideration when results are used to support significant decisions such as treatment referrals or legal actions [21].

Areas of Assessment through Patient and Collateral Interviews

Content domains to be assessed in order to arrive at an accurate picture of a substance-abusing adolescent's problems can be measured by comprehensive instruments. These areas include the following.

- History of use of substances, including over-the-counter and prescription drugs, tobacco, and inhalants; age of first use; frequency, duration, and pattern of use; mode of ingestion; treatment history; and signs and symptoms of substance use disorders, including loss of control, preoccupation, and social and legal consequences.
- Strengths and resources to build on, including self-esteem, family, other community supports, coping skills, and motivation for treatment.
- Medical health history and physical examination, including previous illnesses, ulcers or other gastrointestinal symptoms, chronic fatigue, recurring fever or weight loss, nutritional status, recurrent nosebleeds, tremors or tics, infectious diseases, medical trauma, and pregnancies.
- Sexual history, including sexual orientation, sexual activity, sexual abuse, sexually transmitted diseases (STDs), and STD/HIV risk behavior status, including past or present use of injecting drugs, past or present practice of unsafe sex, and selling sex for drugs or food.
- Developmental issues, including possible presence of attention deficit disorders, learning problems, and influences of traumatic events, such as physical or sexual abuse.
- Mental health history, focusing on depression, suicidal ideation or attempts, attention deficit disorders, anxiety disorders, and behavioral disorders, as well as details regarding prior evaluation and treatment for mental health problems [22].
- Family history, including the parents', guardians', and extended family's history of substance use, mental and physical health problems and treatment, chronic illnesses, incarceration or illegal activity, child management concerns, and the family's ethnic and socioeconomic background and acculturation. This description of home environment should include family history of substandard housing, homelessness, time the adolescent has spent in shelters or on the streets, and running away from home. History of child abuse or neglect, involvement with a child welfare agency, and out-of-home placements, are also key considerations. The family's strengths should be noted as well.

- School history, including academic and behavioral performance and attendance problems.
- Vocational history, including paid and volunteer work.
- Peer relationships, interpersonal skills, gang involvement, and neighborhood environment.
- Juvenile justice involvement and delinquency, including types and incidence of behavior and attitudes toward that behavior.
- Social services agency program involvement, child welfare agency involvement, including number and duration of out-of-home placements in group homes or foster care, and residential treatment.
- Leisure time activities, including recreational activities, hobbies, and interests.

Involvement of other Sources

The adolescent's family is an important factor in assessing the adolescent's involvement in substance use disorders. Therefore, it is critical to form a therapeutic alliance with the family to the fullest extent possible and to involve the family in the assessment process [23]. If there is evidence that the adolescent is being abused at home, the family should still be questioned about the matter. It is important to pursue what is known about possible abuse from the parents, even the abusing parent, as well as siblings or other family members. The mandated reporting requirements for professionals regarding evidence of abuse must be disclosed to individuals being interviewed.

The assessment should not be considered complete unless there has been time to assess the traditionally defined family and others identified by the court as legal guardians who can speak for the best interests of the adolescent, as well as the individuals the adolescent defines as family. The assessor must determine who the "family" is as perceived by the adolescent as well as by legal or biological considerations.

The assessment of an entire family requires a specific set of skills in addition to those needed to assess an individual. Such assessments require professionals who are highly skilled and trained to interpret family dynamics, strengths, weaknesses, and social support systems. Assessors must also be able to identify key family structures and interrelationship patterns in which the adolescent's substance use disorder is enmeshed. It is also essential for the assessor to elicit previous treatment experiences, as well as previous attempts by the family to address the substance use problem. It is useful to determine the family's feelings about the adolescent, in particular whether their focus is upon helping the adolescent, or identifying the adolescent as the problem.

The absence of a traditional family can be a barrier for adolescents seeking treatment, and they may escape identification and assessment altogether. At-risk adolescents may be homeless or on the verge of homelessness. Some youths may go from shelter to shelter and have no address. In some states, a minor cannot gain access to any services unless an adult signs for him or her; potential assistance may be obtained only if the adolescent achieves emancipation or becomes a temporary ward of the state.

Key sources other than family members include adult friends, school officials, surrogate parent advocates in school-related issues, court officials, Court Appointed Special Advocates, social services workers, previous treatment providers, and previous assessors. Contacting these additional sources of information, with the client's consent, may be necessary to support or supplement the information that the adolescent provides in the comprehensive assessment.

SELECTION OF SCREENING AND ASSESSMENT INSTRUMENTS

Selection of screening and assessment instruments intended for use with adolescents must be guided by several factors: evidence for reliability and validity; the adolescent population(s) for which the instrument was developed and normed; the types of settings in which the instrument was developed; and the intended purpose of the instrument. Important features of screening and assessment instruments include:

- *High test-retest reliability.* There are similar results when the test is given again to the same adolescent after a brief interval, for example, a week.
- *Evidence of convergent validity with other instruments attempting to measure the same construct.* There is a strong relationship between the results obtained from this instrument and the results obtained from other instruments designed to look at the same kind of problem, for example, substance use disorder severity.
- *Demonstrated ability to measure outcomes that correspond to a criterion or standard for comparison.* The test has proven over time that it has helped to predict specific behaviors, such as performance in treatment, or clinical/diagnostic decisions, in the same or similar populations.
- *Availability of normative data for representative groups defined by age, race, gender, and type of settings.* The research has shown evidence of a test's reliability and validity among different populations of young people, such as males or females, in different kinds of settings, such as school, treatment programs, foster homes, or juvenile justice detention centers.
- *Sensitivity of the instrument to measure meaningful behavioral changes over time.* There is evidence that the tool reliably measures the changes in an adolescent's behavior and related thinking.

Test Features

In addition to the above criteria, it is important to consider several other features. The instrument should be relatively easy to administer and not burdensome in length. A detailed user's manual and appropriate scoring materials need to be available. Expertise and time required of staff to administer and score the test, as well as the cost of the materials for administering and scoring the instrument, should not be excessive. If training is required to administer and score the test, it must be available.

Other considerations include: the possibility of bias, either cultural or in administration of the test; the credibility of the test among members of the judiciary and treatment professionals; adaptation of the test to management information system input and retrieval; the availability of the test in languages other than English; the motivational level, and verbal and reading skills required of individuals to be assessed; and the propensity of the test to be manipulated.

Of great importance to the user is the author's description of how the test is to be administered, scored, and interpreted. Specific statements should include the purpose and aim of the test; for whom the test is and is not appropriate; whether the test can be administered in a group or only on an individual basis; whether it can be self-administered or if it must be given by an examiner; whether training is required for the assessor, and if so, what kind, how much, and how and where it can be obtained; and where the test can be obtained and what it costs.

Sources of Assessment Instruments

Proprietary instruments are developed and copyrighted by individuals or organizations. There is usually a cost for their use. Some instruments are developed by local agencies. They are often program-specific and may or may not be useful in other settings. Often they have not been validated to determine their accuracy. Many agencies are willing to share such instruments without a charge. Instruments developed by federal agencies are in the public domain and may be used without a fee. Validity and reliability studies for them are documented.

SUBSTANCE ABUSE ASSESSMENT INSTRUMENTS

Information about a sampling of available assessment instruments, both interviews and self-administered, is included at the end of this chapter. Inclusion on this list does not represent an endorsement of particular instruments. Rather, these are offered as a brief representative compilation of particular instruments located through literature review. The needs of various agencies and systems vary. Service providers and decision-makers should examine an array of instruments and select those best suited to their particular needs.

Psychosocial Assessment Instruments

Screening Instruments

Several adolescent substance abuse screening tests are available. These tools are useful because they can briefly estimate the severity of a youth's problem. Screening measures typically call for conservative scoring decisions. Terms such as "probable substance abuser" or "needs a comprehensive assessment" may be used to identify an individual's use [24]. This is done to avoid the mistake of claiming that there is no substance use problem when in fact there is one. A screening tool's full value is appreciated when it is used to determine whether a more complete assessment is necessary and to decide upon the treatment needs of the individual [25].

Among the most popular available self-report screening scales are the CAGE (Cut down, Annoyed, Guilty, Eye-opener) and the Michigan Alcoholism Screening Test (MAST), neither of which are listed below. The MAST exists in two versions: the original version consisting of 25 items in weighted question form, and a shorter version containing 13 discriminating questions. The Short Michigan Alcoholism Screening Test (SMAST) has a greater than 90% sensitivity for identifying alcoholism [24–26]. Though both the CAGE and the MAST instruments can help identify alcohol problems, each has shortcomings. The CAGE performs less reliably in women and adolescents than in men, and its validity depends on the patient's sensitivity to the emotional impacts of alcohol dependence. The original MAST is long (25 items), concentrates on late-stage alcoholism symptoms, and uses differential weighting of particular items, not validated in subsequent studies, in deriving the score [27].

Adolescent Alcohol Involvement Scales (AAIS) The AAIS is a 14-item self-report scale that looks at the type of alcohol abuse and how often it occurs. Questions on the AAIS address topics such as the last drinking

episode, reasons for the initial drinking behavior, the situation in which the drinking occurred, short- and long-term effects of drinking, the adolescent's perception about drinking, and the ways in which others perceive his/her drinking. The severity of the adolescent's alcohol abuse is determined by the overall score, which can range anywhere between 0 and 79. The major scales include non-user/normal, misuser, and abuser/dependent. The test scores are related to a substance abuse diagnosis as well as ratings from other sources. These other sources include independent clinical assessments and the adolescent's parents, as well as the consistency for each individual – ranging from 0.55 in a clinical sample to 0.76 in a general sample. The norms for both of these samples are available in the 13–19-year-old range [28].

Adolescent Drinking Index (ADI) The ADI is a 24-item self-administered test that examines adolescent drinking. It does so by measuring psychological, physical, and social symptoms as well as loss of control. This test is written at a fifth-grade reading level. The results of this test provide a single score as well as two subscale scores. The subscale scores include self-medicating drinking and rebellious drinking. These two scales are intended as research scales. The reliability of the ADI is good. Results are shown to be consistent and accurate (coefficient alpha 0.93–0.95) in measuring the severity of adolescent drinking problems. Studies show a moderate correlation with alcohol consumption as well as significant differences between groups with different levels of alcohol problem severity. In addition, there was a hit rate of 82% in classification accuracy of the ADI. This means that 82% of the time, when a drinking problem was identified using this scale, the test was accurate in classifying the drinking as a problem and the test accurately determined the level of severity of the drinking problem [29].

Adolescent Drug Involvement Scale (ADIS) Moberg and Hahn modified the AAIS (described above) to address drug use problem severity. The ADIS is a 13-item questionnaire written at an eighth-grade reading level. This scale correlates (0.72) with drug use frequency and (0.75) with independent rating by clinical staff. When matched up with the frequency of drug use and the ratings that clinical staff gave, the scale correlates with their findings, therefore providing evidence of the validity of this test [27].

Personal Experience Screening Questionnaire (PESQ) The PESQ is a brief, 40-item screening instrument that consists of a scale that measures the severity of the drinking problem (coefficient alpha 0.91–0.95), drug use history, select psychosocial problems, and response distortion tendencies ("faking good" and "faking bad"). Norms for normal juvenile offender and drug-abusing populations are available. The test is estimated to have an accuracy rate of 87% in predicting the need for further drug abuse assessment [30].

Interviews for Adolescents Based on a Well-known Adult Tool, the Addiction Severity Index (ASI) [31]

Adolescent Drug Abuse Diagnosis (ADAD) The ADAD is a 150-item structured interview that looks at the following content areas: medical status, drug and alcohol use, legal status, family background and problems, school/employment, social activities and peer relations, and psychological status. The interviewer uses a 10-point scale to rate the patient's need for additional treatment in each content area. These severity ratings translate to a problem severity dimension (no problem, slight, moderate, considerable, and extreme problem). The drug use section includes a detailed drug use list and how often the use occurs, and a brief set of items that looks at specific areas of drug involvement (e.g., polydrug use, attempts at abstinence, withdrawal symptoms, use in school). Psychometric studies on the ADAD, using a broad sample of clinic-referred adolescents, provide favorable evidence for its reliability and validity. A shorter form (83 items) of the ADAD intended for treatment outcome evaluation is also available [32–34].

Teen Severity Index (T-ASI) Another adolescent version of the ASI was adapted by Kaminer *et al.* [31]. The T-ASI consists of seven content areas: chemical use, school status, employment-support status, family relationships, legal status, peer-social relationships, and psychiatric status. A medical status section was not included because it was thought to be less relevant to adolescent drug abusers. Patient and interviewer severity ratings are rated on a five-point scale for each of the content areas. Preliminary data indicate adequate inter-rater agreement and initial validity data [35].

"Paper-and-Pencil" Questionnaires

Personal Experience Inventory (PEI) The PEI is a 276-item, multi-scale questionnaire that measures chemical involvement problem severity (10 scales), psychosocial risk (or protective) factors (12 scales), and the tendency for subjects to distort responses (five scales). Supplemental problem screens measure eating disorders, suicide potential, physical/sexual abuse, and parental history of drug abuse. The scoring

program provides a computerized report that includes narratives and standardized scores for each scale, as well as other clinical information. Extensive normative and psychometric data (including test-retest reliability and convergent and predictive validity) are available [36,37].

CONCLUSION

Psychosocial assessment is fundamental to beginning the treatment process. It is a critical element of treatment, for without comprehensive assessment, appropriate patient–treatment matching is not possible. Just as it would be inappropriate to treat diabetes with chemotherapy intended for cancer patients, it is similarly unsuitable to provide a drug-involved adolescent with treatment intended for an adult male alcoholic. Wise, effective use of scarce treatment resources necessitates careful assessment of patients prior to treatment planning. Comprehensive assessment improves the overall cost-effectiveness of providing treatment.

Assessment is also important in the coordination of services. Focused initial and subsequent comprehensive information ensures that the most appropriate services for individuals are delivered at the community level. Aggregated information also assists state and local decision-makers in determining priorities, setting standards, and developing resources according to the areas of greatest need.

Substance use disorders inevitably extend to affect other areas of an individual's life. This is particularly true for adolescents, who are at a critical developmental stage emotionally, intellectually, socially, and physically. Assessing the individual problems of substance-abusing adolescents underlies the development and implementation of effective treatment, positive outcomes, and reduced recidivism. These efforts invariably also address fundamental and broader community and societal problems, which in turn contribute to adolescents' substance use disorders, thus potentially disrupting this lethal cycle.

References

1. Babbit N. *Adolescent Drug and Alcohol Abuse: How to Spot It, Stop It, and Get Help For Your Family*. Sebastopol, CA: O'Reilly & Associates, Inc., 2000.
2. Catalano RF, Hawkins JD, Wells EA, Miller J, Brewer D. Evaluation of the effectiveness of adolescent drug abuse treatment, assessment of risks for relapse, and promising approaches for relapse prevention. *Int J Addict* 1991;**25**:1085–1140.
3. Dembo R. Problems among youths entering the juvenile justice system, their service needs and innovative approaches to address them. *Subst Use Misuse* 1996;**31**:81–94.

4. Dembo R, Williams L, Schmeidler J, Wish ED, Getreu A, Berry E. Juvenile crime and drug abuse: A prospective study of high risk youth. *J Addict Dis* 1991;**11**:5–31.

5. Brook JS, Brook DW, De laRosa M, Whiteman M, Johnson E, Montoya I. Adolescent illegal drug use: The impact of personality, family, and environmental factors. *J Behav Med* 2001;**24**:183–199.

6. Beschner GM, Friedman AS (eds). *Youth Drug Abuse: Problems, Issues, and Treatment*. Lexington, MA: DC Health, 1979.

7. Dishion TJ, McCord J, Poulin F. When interventions harm: Peer groups and problem behavior. *Am Psychol* 1999;**54**:755–764.

8. National Center on Addiction and Substance Abuse at Columbia University. *Adolescent Substance Use: America's #1 Health Problem*. Available from: http://www.casacolumbia.org/upload/2011/20110629 adolescentsubstanceuse.pdf; June 2011.

9. Latimer WW, Winters KC, Stinchfield RD. Screening for drug abuse among adolescents in clinical and correctional settings using the Problem-Oriented Screening Instrument for Teenagers. *Am J Drug Alcohol Abuse* 1997;**23**:79–98.

10. Henggeler SW. The development of effective drug abuse services for youth. In: Egerston JA, Fox DM, Leshner AI (eds), *Treating Drug Abusers Effectively*. New York, NY: Blackwell Publishers, 1997.

11. Lewis RA, Piercy FP, Sprenkle DH, Trepper TS. Family-based interventions for helping drug-abusing adolescents. *J Adolesc Res* 1990;**50**:82–95.

12. Santisteban DA, Szapocznik J, Perez-Vidal A. Kurtines WM, Murray EJ, LaPerriere A. Efficacy of intervention for engaging youth and families into treatment and some variables that may contribute to differential effectiveness. *J Fam Psychol* 1996;**10**:35–44.

13. Bukstein OG, Tarter RE. Substance use disorders. In: Coffey CE, Brumback RA (eds), *Textbook of Pediatric Neuropsychiatry*. Washington, DC: American Psychiatric Press, 1998; pp. 595–616.

14. Liddle HA. Adolescent substance abuse derails development. *American Association for Marriage and Family Therapy: Clinical Update* 2001;**3**(3), April.

15. Martin CS, Winters KC. Diagnosis and assessment of alcohol use disorders among adolescents. *Alcohol Health Res W* 1998;**22**:95–105.

16. Jessor R. Risk behavior in adolescence: A psychosocial framework for understanding and action. *J Adolescent Health* 1991;**12**:597–605.

17. DiIulio JJ, Grossman JB. *Youth Crime and Substance Abuse: Act-Now Strategies for Saving At-Risk Children*. Philadelphia, PA: Public/Private Ventures, 1997.

18. Farrow JA, Smith WR, Hurst M. *Adolescent Drug and Alcohol Assessment Instruments in Current Use: A Critical Comparison*. Olympia, WA: Washington State, Division of Alcohol and Substance Abuse, 1993.

19. Department of Mental Health and Substance Abuse, Prochaska JO, DiClemente CC. Substance Abuse. Guam: DMHSA, 2011. Available from: http://dmhsa.guam. gov/services/substance_abuse/.

20. Winters, KC, Stinchfield RD, Henly GA. Further validation of new scales measuring adolescent alcohol and other drug abuse. *J Stud Alcohol* 1993;**54**:534–541.

21. Bazemore G, Nissen L. Mobilizing social support and building relationships: Broadening correctional and rehabilitative agendas. *Corrections Management Quarterly* 2000;**4**(4):12–21.

22. Perrin S, Last CG. Dealing with comorbidity. In: Eisen AR, Kearney CA, Schaefer CE (eds), *Clinical Handbook of Anxiety Disorders in Children and Adolescents*. Northvale, NJ: Jason Aronson, Inc., 1995; pp. 412–435.

23. Dakof GA, Tejeda M, Liddle HA. Predictors of engagement in adolescent drug abuse treatment. *J Am Acad Child Adolesc Psychiatry* 2001;**40**:274–281.

24. Seltzer ML. The Michigan Alcoholism Screening Test: The quest for a new diagnostic instrument. *Am J Psychiatry* 1971;**127**:89–94.

25. Seltzer ML, Vinokur A, Van Rooijen LJ. A Self-Administered Short Michigan Alcohol Screening Test (SMAST). *Stud Alcohol* 1975;**36**:117–126.

26. Mayfield D, McLeod G, Hall P. The CAGE questionnaire: Validation of a new alcoholism instrument. *Am J Psychiatry* 1974;**131**:1121–1123.

27. Moberg, DP, Hahn L. The adolescent drug involvement scale. *J Adolesc Clin Dependency* 1991;**2**:75–88.

28. Moberg DP. Identifying adolescents with alcohol problems: A field test of the Adolescent Alcohol Involvement Scale. *J Stud Alcohol* 1983;**44**:701–721.

29. Harrell AV, Wirtz, PW. *Adolescent Drinking Index Professional Manual*. Odessa, FL: Psychological Assessment Resources, 1989.

30. Winters KC. Development of an adolescent alcohol and other drug abuse screening scale: Personal Experience Screening Questionnaire. *Addict Behav* 1992;**17**:479–490.

31. Kaminer Y, Bukstein O, Tarter RE. The Teen-Addiction Severity Index: Rationale and reliability. *Int J Addict* 1991;**26**:219–226.

32. Williams RJ, Chang SY. A comprehensive and comparative review of adolescent substance abuse treatment outcome. *Clin Psychol Sci-Pract* 2000;**7**:138–166.

33. Weinberg NZ, Rahdert E, Colliver JD, Glantz MD. Adolescent substance abuse: A review of the past 10 years. *J Am Acad Child Adolesc Psychiatry* 1998;**37**:252–297.

34. Friedman AS, Utada A. A method for diagnosing and planning the treatment of adolescent drug abusers: The Adolescent Drug Abuse Diagnosis (ADAD) Instrument. *J Drug Educ* 1989;**19**:285–312.

35. Kaminer Y, Wagner E, Plummer B, Seifer R. Validation of the Teen Addiction Severity Index (T-ASI). *Am J Addiction* 1993;**2**:250–254.

36. Henley GA, Winters KC. Development of psychosocial scales for the assessment of adolescents involved with alcohol and drugs. *Int J Addictions* 1989;**24**:973–1001.

37. Winters KC. Treating adolescents with substance abuse disorders: An overview of practice issues and treatment outcome. *Subst Abuse* 1999;**20**:203–225.

8

The Neurobiology of Adolescent Addiction

Michael Boucher,[1] and Preetpal Sandhu[2]

[1]*David Geffen School of Medicine, University of California at Los Angeles, Los Angeles, CA, USA*
[2]*David Geffen School of Medicine at UCLA, Los Angeles, CA, USA*

The neurobiology of adolescent addiction involves a complex interaction of different parts of the brain as well as different neurotransmitter systems. And while many details remain unclear at this point, we are learning more and more about the process of addiction and its relation to risk-tasking behavior in adolescents. Our goal in writing this chapter is to elucidate the mechanisms and hypotheses that currently explain a majority of what is known regarding neurodevelopmental changes in adolescence and their impact on addiction. It is important to note that a great deal of the conclusions drawn from the experimental research at this point rely heavily on correlation and that causation has not been proven in the majority of cases. As our knowledge of the human brain and its development continues to grow, we are hopeful that we will have an even larger body of evidence supporting these conclusions.

This chapter focuses on the neurobiology of adolescent substance abuse and addiction. We explore the relationship between risk-taking behavior, substance use and abuse, and adolescent developmental neurobiology. The chapter is divided into four sections. First, we describe normal adolescent brain development. Next, we propose a psychological and biological model of adolescent addiction and risk-taking behavior. Then, we summarize the latest research on the neurobiology of adolescents at risk for substance abuse. Finally, we discuss the neurotoxic effects of substance abuse on the adolescent brain.

ADOLESCENT BRAIN DEVELOPMENT

Most brain growth occurs during the first 10 years of life, but the adolescent brain continues to mature via axonal growth, myelination, and synaptic pruning [1]. Myelination is the glial cell deposition of myelin around axons, insulating the neural connections, resulting in faster and more efficient neural circuitry. Synaptic pruning refers to the removal of excess, unhelpful connections (synapses) between neurons. The child's brain has trillions of synapses between neurons. As the child's brain responds to the environment and learns new skills and behaviors, certain connections are used, retained, and strengthened, and those connections that are not used are eliminated via synaptic pruning. This results in the development and use of dedicated connections and neural circuits, improving efficiency and reducing metabolic demand. It is important to recognize that this is a longitudinal process and that any distinct milestones tend to be variable from one individual to another.

Changes in Gray Matter and White Matter

Two major trends occur during this developmental process: the decline of gray matter and the growth of white matter. We divide the brain into gray matter and white matter based on early pathology studies that recognized that the brain has two distinct layers of color: gray and white. The gray layer, or gray matter, is composed mainly of neural cell bodies, where the cell's nucleus and genetic material is stored. Gray matter volume peaks at age 13 and then begins to decline in volume and thickness, beginning first in the striatum and sensorimotor cortices, progressing to the frontal poles, and ending with the dorsolateral prefrontal cortex [1].

The cerebral cortex is the gray matter on the outer surface of the brain, and we measure the thickness of the cortex over the course of time and in certain diseases and conditions. During adolescence, the brain undergoes marked cortical thinning, most strongly in the parietal lobe, the medial and superior frontal regions, the cingulum, and the occipital lobe. It is believed that decreases in volume and thickness come from selective synaptic pruning, reduction in glial cells, and decreased intracortical myelination [1].

White matter is composed mainly of myelinated axonal tract and is defined by the relatively white appearance of its myelin sheath, and by the absence of neural cell bodies. In contrast to gray matter's volume reduction, the white matter volume increases during adolescence, most strongly in the fronto-parietal regions [1]. To study white matter, researchers are now using a new neuroimaging technique called diffusion tensor imaging (DTI), which uses the diffusion properties of water molecules to explore white matter anatomy in finer detail. Two variables used to describe the white matter quality and architecture are fractional anisotropy (FA) and mean diffusivity (MD). High FA values mean greater myelination and fiber organization, whereas low MD values mean greater white matter density. DTI studies of normal adolescent brains show age-related increases in FA and decreases in MD. The most prominent FA changes during adolescence occur in the superior longitudinal fasciculus, superior corona radiata, thalamic radiations, and posterior limb of the internal capsule. Fiber tracts of the fronto-temporal pathways mature relatively later [2].

There is a temporal relationship between gray matter volume reduction and white matter growth and development. Temporally, the dorsal parietal and prefrontal brain regions experience concomitant gray matter volume reductions and white matter growth and DTI-demonstrate strengthening, though the biological underpinnings of this developmental cross-talk have not yet been well described [1].

Gender and the Brain

As male and female bodies differentiate significantly during adolescence, the male and female brains begin to show differences as well. Male children and adolescents have larger overall brain volumes and proportionally larger amygdala and globus pallidus volumes. Female children and adolescents have larger caudate nuclei and cingulate gyrus volumes. Girls' gray matter volumes typically peak 1–2 years earlier than boys', whereas male adolescents have larger gray matter volume reductions and white matter volume increases. While both genders have the most prominent white matter growth in the frontal lobes, boys have larger white matter volumes around the lateral ventricles and caudate nuclei [1]. Finally, white matter growth in boys is marked by an increase in axonal diameter, with testosterone as a possible etiological factor, whereas white matter growth in girls is driven by an increase in myelin content, with luteinizing hormone associated with greater white matter content [3]. The functional significance of these differences is not known and caution is urged before ascribing explanatory power to these preliminary findings.

THE NEUROPSYCHOLOGY AND NEUROBIOLOGY OF ADOLESCENT RISK-TAKING BEHAVIOR

The preceding section briefly described the neuroanatomical development of the adolescent brain. These changes most likely underlie the primary cognitive and psychological maturations seen in the adolescent development of executive function, which includes tasks such as complex decision-making, self-monitoring, impulse control, and delay of gratification. A popular hypothesis regarding the neuroanatomical correlate of executive function lies in the functional and anatomical relationship between the prefrontal cortex (PFC) and the ventral striatum (VS). In many adolescents, poor executive function is associated with increased risk-taking behavior, and can be theoretically viewed neurobiologically as an unequal relationship between the prefrontal cortex and the ventral striatum.

It has been well demonstrated that adolescents engage in more risk-taking behaviors than their younger and older counterparts, including more experimental substance use [4]. Adolescents are described as impulsive and greater risk-takers, and while these two terms are often conflated, it is very important to distinguish impulsivity from risk-taking across cognitive and neuranatomical domains. One hypothesis that is gaining popularity states that impulsivity is thought to arise from poor "top-down" cognitive control from the prefrontal cortex, and that risk-taking is related to sensation-seeking behavior driven by the ventral striatum.

Impulsivity in adolescence can be seen as a form of poor cognitive control. Cognitive control is defined as the ability to resist temptation in favor of long-term goals, or the ability to delay immediate gratification. Operationalized, it is "the ability to accomplish goal-directed behavior in the face of salient, competing inputs and actions" [5]. Developmental studies demonstrate that cognitive control shows linear improvement from infancy to adulthood, correlating with the pattern of myelination of the prefrontal cortex [6]. Clinically, we observe this behavioral control in the go/no-go task, the Simon task, and the task-switching paradigms, when we are asked to suppress the pre-programmed response to achieve the correct alternative response. For example, imagine the following:

A child, adolescent, and adult are all trained to clap their hands when the light turns blue. Thirty times the light turns blue, and thirty times they clap. Then, we change the rules, and ask them to tap their feet when the light turns blue. The impulse is to clap, and it is hardest for the child and easiest for the adult to control that impulse and adapt to the new rule.

The first 10 times the light turns blue, the child claps by impulse six times, the adolescent four times, and the adult two.

Cognitive control increases linearly with age, but when rewards are linked to behavior, this linear development gets skewed. When we receive an appealing award for completing a task demanding cognitive control, our performance improves. However, when we must suppress an impulse that is linked to an appealing cue, our performance suffers [5]. This idea should fit well with our basic understanding of human nature. When we are rewarded for good behavior, we are more likely to perform that behavior. This is the basis of positive reinforcement. However, for the person on a diet, it is harder to resist an appealing appetizer than the bland sandwich, even though both have the same number of calories. This relates to our basic understanding of addiction: initially, the behavior – drug use – is linked to a positive reinforcement, the euphoria or "high" we experience from the drug, and we quickly learn to like using drugs. However, when we try to stop using the drug, we are trying to choose the behavior – abstinence – that has little to no immediate positive reward associated with it. Thus, in choosing abstinence, we are choosing against the behavior, drug use, that has the appealing reward. This choice is hard, and the more times we use the drug, the harder it becomes to choose abstinence, because our brain is strengthening the link between the behavior and the reward. To compound matters further, after continued drug use, our brain adjusts its response and begins to depend on the drug to feel "normal." We begin to crave the drug, and now choosing abstinence not only has no positive reinforcement, but also negative reinforcement: the craving to feel "normal." At this point, we have reached physiological addiction, and in order to get the euphoria from the drug, we must use an increasing quantity and potency each time. Finally, now that we are addicted and we get less euphoria for each unit of drug use, we experience less reward.

It is a rather simple concept that appealing behaviors are easy to choose and hard to ignore. However, this concept will be explored in detail because, as it turns out, adolescents are much more sensitive than children or adults to these motivational incentives. The teenager is highly responsive to positive reinforcement, but is also highly driven towards appealing-though-dangerous enticements.

In many behavioral studies, adolescents are more sensitive than adults to the promise of financial rewards for accurate performance. In other words, their performance improves more than adults because they are more motivated by the financial reward [7]. This also holds true for social rewards as simple as a happy face. However, this heightened response to rewards can lead to risker decisions. In gambling studies, adolescents will make riskier decisions than adults or children, but only when they know they will be given immediate feedback on their gamble [8]. Knowledge of this immediate feedback elicits an emotional response, and this emotional activation promotes riskier gambles. In the delayed feedback group, the participant is given 30 playing cards, all face down in a grid. He is asked to choose how many playing cards to flip over, and for each red card he will receive $10, but for each black card he will lose $5. He picks his cards all at once and awaits the results. In the immediate gratification group, the participant selects cards one at a time, flipping each card over and finding out if she won or lost money, then being told how many red cards were left. In the delayed group, adolescents and adults did not significantly differ in their gambling risk, but in the immediate gratification group, adolescents were significantly riskier gamblers than adults [8].

Social incentives, ranging from a happy face to peer group acceptance, also influence cognitive control most strongly in adolescents. From epidemiological studies, we know that teenagers are much more likely to try drugs or alcohol if their peers are using substances [9]. On a simulated driving test, adolescents are riskier and more dangerous drivers when peers are in the car than when they are alone, and this risk decreases with age [10].

These findings suggest that risk-taking behavior is the result of the interplay between cognitive control and sensitivity to rewards. While cognitive control increases in a linear fashion with age, sensitivity to rewards appears to peak in adolescence, with teenagers more influenced by rewards than their younger and older counterparts. While toddlers and children are very impulsive, they are also fairly risk-averse, displaying lower sensation-seeking and reward sensitivity. At the other end, adults have reached their maximum level of cognitive control, and they are better able to suppress their motivational, sensation-seeking drives. Adolescents fall right in the middle, but unlike Goldilocks, their motivational drive is too hot and their cognitive control is too cold.

Functional Neuroanatomy and the Neuroimaging Correlates of Cognitive Control and Reward Sensitivity

Galvan *et al.* [11] propose a neurobiological model of adolescent risk-taking behavior that implicates the prefrontal cortex as the location of cognitive control, and the ventral striatum as coordinator of reward sensitivity.

Goal-directed behavior is driven by the interaction between the prefrontal cortex and the ventral striatum, and risky behavior occurs when there is an imbalance in the circuit between the prefrontal cortex and the ventral striatum, henceforth known as the frontostriatal circuit. First, let us define our terms.

The prefrontal cortex (PFC) is located in the anterior part of the frontal lobes of the brain, and the PFC is the primary neuroanatomical location of cognitive control. The development of the PFC is linear, as evidenced by DTI studies of myelination, and the human brain does not complete myelination of the PFC until at least 25 years of age [12]. Clinically, we see impulse control develop linearly, and functional magnetic resonance imaging (fMRI) studies correlate PFC activation with impulse control.

The ventral striatum and the dorsal striatum make up the neostriatum, which is part of the basal ganglia, along with the substantia nigra, globus pallidus, and the subthalamic nucleus. The neostriatum is divided by its anatomical and neurochemical boundaries into the dorsal striatum, made up of the caudate and putamen, and the ventral striatum, consisting of the nucleus accumbens and the olfactory tubercle. The ventral striatum is strongly innervated by dopaminergic fibers from the ventral tegmental area (VTA), a key anatomical player in the mesolimbic dopamine system and highly implicated in all addictive and motivational behaviors [13]. The ventral striatum (henceforth VS) is implicated in motivational drives and sensation-seeking behavior, and appears to be most active during adolescence, as our review of the research will indicate.

Thus, Galvan's model hypothesizes the following:

1. Substance abuse during adolescence can be thought of as a form of risk-taking behavior.
2. Risk-taking behavior is psychologically modeled by the interaction between cognitive control and motivational drives. Risky behavior occurs when the motivational drive is "stronger" than the cognitive control.
3. Risk-taking behavior peaks during adolescence, with children's behavior being "too timid" and adults' too "in control".
4. Neuroanatomically, cognitive control is found in the PFC, and the motivational drive is driven by the VS.
5. During adolescence, the VS is hyperactive compared to its child and adult states, overwhelming the still immature PFC, and ultimately correlating with the adolescent's peak in risk-taking behavior.

Evidence for the first three points has been presented in the preceding sections. The last two points concern the

neurobiology of risk-taking behavior, and evidence for those contentions is reviewed below:

1. Risk-taking behavior is a form of goal-directed behavior, and the frontostriatal circuit is necessary for learning goal-directed behavior.
   - Using lesion studies and single-unit neuronal recordings, we have discovered that when monkeys and humans learn goal-directed behaviors, the VS is activated early on to learn and remember the association between behavior and reward. The PFC later is engaged in maintaining and optimizing behavioral patterns to receive the reward [14].
2. The neuroanatomy of the frontostriatal circuit changes during adolescence.
   - As highlighted earlier, the frontal-temporal white matter circuitry undergoes significant growth in myelination and axon strength during adolescence. DTI and fMRI studies show that the frontostriatal circuit is strengthened via myelination and axonal size during adolescence, and that the strength of the circuit's connection is temporally related to people's ability to display cognitive control [1]. Dopamine receptor density in the striatum peaks early in adolescence, while in the PFC, dopamine receptor density peaks later in young adulthood [12]. It is unclear exactly how dopamine receptor density changes affect behavior, but it is thought to be functionally related to sensation-seeking behavior.
3. Ventral striatal activation is sensitive to reward, and most sensitive during adolescence.
   - Galvan has linked the behavioral studies of reward sensitivity to VS activation, showing that the VS activation was sensitive to the amount of financial reward, and this response was strongest in adolescent brains, showing either signal increases or longer activation [15]. VS activity is positively linked to a self-reported likelihood to engage in risky behavior[11]. Previous imaging studies with adults have also linked the VS activity with risky choices [16].
   - Van Leijenhorst et al. [17] studied gambling, and showed increased VS activation during high-risk gambles, and increased PFC activation during low-risk gambles.
4. Prefrontal cortex activation is related to cognitive control and impulsivity. There is a significant body of evidence documenting PFC activation during impulse control tasks, and as people age the recruitment of PFC is stronger, and impulse control better. Ratings of impulsivity are inversely correlated with brain volume in the PFC [18], and disorders of

impulsivity like attention-deficit/hyperactivity disorder demonstrate decreased activation in prefrontal regions compared with controls [19].

- The PFC, and the science of brain localization in general, gained widespread attention following the curious case of Phineas Gage. On 13 September 1848, 25-year-old Phineas Gage was working as a railroad foreman in Vermont, preparing to blast away rock to clear land for the developing railway. Gage added the blasting powder into a burrowed hole in the rock, and used a large iron rod to compress the charge. By tragic accident, the fuse lit early, the powder exploded, and the large iron rod flew from the hole, entered the left side of his face, through his left eye, and out the top his head. Amazingly, Gage survived, but eventually those around him noticed a distinct change in personality [20], as described eloquently by his doctor, John Martyn Harlow [21]:

The equilibrium or balance, so to speak, between his intellectual faculties and animal propensities, seems to have been destroyed. He is fitful, irreverent, indulging at times in the grossest profanity (which was not previously his custom), manifesting but little deference for his fellows, impatient of restraint or advice when it conflicts with his desires, at times pertinaciously obstinate, yet capricious and vacillating, devising many plans of future operations, which are no sooner arranged than they are abandoned in turn for others appearing more feasible. A child in his intellectual capacity and manifestations, he has the animal passions of a strong man. Previous to his injury, although untrained in the schools, he possessed a well-balanced mind, and was looked upon by those who knew him as a shrewd, smart businessman, very energetic and persistent in executing all his plans of operation. In this regard his mind was radically changed, so decidedly that his friends and acquaintances said he was "no longer Gage."

- From this tragedy, neurologists began to speculate about the function of the part of Gage's brain that was injured. Gage donated his brain to science, and modern researchers have confirmed what Harlow originally posited, namely that Gage suffered severe damage to his left frontal lobe, but all other brain areas were spared. Clinically, as Harlow described, Gage's personality changed drastically: he became impulsive and seemingly governed by his desires. His story serves as a famous and useful reminder of the power of the frontal lobe, and the PFC in particular, in controlling our impulses and restraining our desires.

5. The frontostriatal circuit responds to reward-based cognitive control.

- We previously discussed that rewards improved cognitive control, most strongly in adolescence. Geier *et al*. [22] present evidence for the neural substrate of this enhanced cognitive control, using fMRI during the anti-saccade task. The anti-saccade task is a common experimental tool to study flexible control over behavior. As explained by Douglas *et al*. [see ref. 23], "In this task, participants must suppress the reflexive urge to look at a visual target that appears suddenly in the peripheral visual field and must instead look away from the target in the opposite direction. A crucial step involved in performing this task is the top-down inhibition of a reflexive, automatic saccade." In the study, monetary reward resulted in improved performance, most strongly in adolescents. Anatomically, adolescents showed exaggerated activity in the VS, as expected, and increased activity in the precentral sulcus within the PFC – involved in controlling eye movements – providing visual evidence for the reward-related upregulation in cognitive control.

- Additional evidence highlights the neural correlates of diminished cognitive control when faced with appealing alternatives. Somerville *et al*. [24] tested the go/no-go task with neutral and appealing cues (happy faces). When faced with neutral cues, children, adolescents, and adults all show gradual improvement with practice. The prefrontal cortex activation was associated with accuracy and showed linear changes with age of participant. However, when forced to choose against the appealing cue, adolescents didn't show the steady improvement expected by their neutral performance, and this reduced cognitive control was paralleled by increases in VS activation.

In summary, we postulate that adolescent substance abuse can be seen as an example of risky behavior. Adolescents have consistently been demonstrated to engage in more risky behavior than either children or adults. Neuropsychological research suggests that this risky behavior is the result of highly active motivational drives exerting exaggerated influence over cognitive control. Neurobiologically, it can be inferred that in the adolescent brain, which has a hyperactive VS actively seeking out rewards, and an immature, poorly myelinated PFC, a struggle to control impulsivity will inevitably ensue.

The Role of Neurotransmitters in Risk-Taking Behavior: Serotonin and Dopamine Receptor Systems

Neurotransmitters are amino acids, peptides, and mono-amines that transmit signals from a neuron to a target cell across a synapse. Several neurotransmitter systems exhibit change and development in the adolescent brain. This section focuses on the roles of dopamine and serotonin. The details are nuanced, confusing, and still being discovered, but the take-home message (based on current research) is straightforward: Dopamine is a driving force in all addictive and risk-taking behaviors, and it acts directly on the frontostriatal circuit. Serotonin (5-hydroxytryptamine, or 5-HT) acts as a brake on dopamine, and works to curb impulsive, sensation-seeking, and addictive behavior. First, we will describe the development of the dopamine and serotonin neuro-transmitter systems. Then we will look at their role in risk-taking behavior and addiction.

Dopamine is a catecholamine neurotransmitter pro-duced in the ventral tegmental area (VTA), the hypo-thalamus, and the substantia nigra, along with other brain areas. There are four major pathways through which dopamine exerts its effects: the mesocortical pathway, connecting the VTA with the PFC; the mes-olimbic pathway, connecting the VTA to the nucleus accumbens, amygdala, and hippocampus; the nigrostria-tal pathway, connecting the substantia nigra with the basal ganglia and dorsal striatum; and the tuberoinfun-dibular pathway, connecting the hypothalamus with the pituitary gland. Given the wide distribution of dopa-mine, it is not surprising to learn that it has many effects on the brain. In this chapter we are most interested in the mesolimbic and mesocortical pathways, connecting the VTA with the PFC and the nucleus accumbens. Notably, another major psychiatric illness is also modeled as a disease of dopamine dysregulation. Schizophrenia is defined by positive symptoms (hallucinations, delu-sions, and bizarre behavior) and negative symptoms (blunted affect, poverty of speech, anhedonia, asociality, and avolition). The dopamine hypothesis for schizophre-nia [25] posits that the positive symptoms are driven by excessive activation of D2 receptors in the mesolimbic pathway. Typical antipsychotic medications block D2 receptors and work primarily to lessen the positive symptoms of schizophrenia; many of these medications' side effects are through inadvertent blockade of dopa-mine receptors in the nigrostriatal and tuberoinfundib-ular pathways.

When a person is exposed to novel situations, risky behaviors, or intoxicating substances, the VTA releases dopamine into the nucleus accumbens (NAc). The NAc is activated, evaluates the exposure's appeal, and sends projections to the PFC, amygdala, and other brain areas to influence the person's behavior and memory regard-ing the exposure. In a simplified interpretation, the more dopamine that is released into the NAc, the more it likes the exposure, and the more likely it is we will want that exposure again. Food, sex, and drugs all are associated with dopamine release in the NAc. Certain drugs, like cocaine, cause strong releases of dopamine into the NAc, inducing significant desire as well as neuroplastic changes to the downstream circuits that are thought to be hallmarks of the development of addiction [12].

The dopamine receptor profile changes dramatically in the brain's anatomical reward circuitry – the PFC and the NAc. The density of D1 and D2 receptors peaks in the striatum early in adolescence, followed by loss of these receptors by young adulthood. In the PFC, the D1 and D2 receptor density does not peak until late adoles-cence. Dopamine (DA) fiber density increases in the PFC of adolescent rats and NAc of gerbils, and DA inputs to the primate PFC peak in adolescence [26]. It must be noted that the significance of these findings is not yet clear.

Serotonin is produced in the raphe nucleus and proj-ects to the PFC, NAc, hippocampus, and limbic system [27]. NAc serotonin turnover is four times lower in adolescent rats than in younger or older rats [28]. In men, serotonin receptor binding decreases the most during adolescence [29]. There is some evidence that serotonin input to the NAc is underdeveloped compared to dopamine input to the NAc during adolescence [12]. In functional studies, serotonin is found to be important to control and shape dopamine-related learning. In control rats, conditioned behavior (as driven by dopa-mine) extinguishes after prolonged absence of the cue. However, when rats were exposed to a chemical (MDMA) that is toxic to serotonin projection, they continue to perform the conditioned behavior for more than a week in the absence of the behavioral cue [30]. In other words, without serotonin, there was no brake on the dopamine-driven learned behavior. Similarly, other studies have shown higher serotonin activity correlated with less aggression and impulsivity [31].

AT-RISK ADOLESCENTS: AT-RISK FOR DISINHIBITION

Risk-taking behavior is a hallmark of adolescence, and while it is common for teenagers to experiment with illicit substances, most adolescents do not develop drug addictions, or substance use disorders (SUD). Identifying the at-risk adolescent is a primary goal of public policy, and understanding the neurological markers for at-risk adolescents will provide further insight into the disease of addiction.

One of the most studied neurological risk markers for SUD is the P300 event-related potential (ERP). ERPs are electroencephalogram (EEG) voltage changes in response to events or stimuli from sensory, motor, or cognitive input. The P300 ERP is named for the positive voltage deflection read by electrodes over the parietal lobe, with a latency (delay between stimulus and response) of 300–600 ms. The more attention the patient gives to the stimulus, the stronger the P300 ERP will be recorded. Initially, research found that the P300 ERP was diminished in children of alcoholics, and that a reduced P300 was a predictor of later alcohol abuse [32]. Further research suggested that a reduced P300 ERP was more strongly correlated with conduct disorder and overall trait disinhibition [33], as defined by impulsivity and externalizing behavior, though it must be noted that even this research is viewed as controversial. So, while P300 may not be a specific predictor of SUD, it may serve as a useful and interesting physiological marker of disinhibition, one of the main risk factors for SUD.

In high-risk children (from families with significant alcohol dependence), fMRI studies suggest poor frontal functioning even before drug use began, and this impaired frontal function can predict later substance use [34].

Serotonin and Dopamine

Endogenous serotonin (5-HT) levels have been studied as a risk factor for substance use, given previous research suggesting that serotonin dampens the impact of dopamine in our reward-seeking behavior. Because it is difficult to measure the levels of 5-HT in the brain, researchers have used peripheral markers, including platelet 5-HT, whole blood 5-HT concentration, or platelet MAO (monoamine oxidase) activity. In children of alcoholics, lower whole-blood 5-HT was correlated with more externalizing behavior [35]. Higher platelet 5-HT concentrations were associated with greater impulsivity [36], and certain 5-HT transporter polymorphisms [37] and transporter gene combinations [38] appear to increase the risk for SUD. However, like the P300 ERP, 5-HT dysfunction is more strongly correlated with disinhibition than with SUD [12].

Dopamine receptors have shown some genetic variability linked with SUD development. In children of addicts, the A1 allele of the D2 receptor (DRD2) was linked to higher rates of SUD [39]. The A1 allele is thought to result in reduced dopamine binding and lower D2 receptor expression [40]. However, the A1 allele has also been linked to antisocial behavior and negative affect [12], and to date no studies have controlled for these covariables. It is possible, and indeed probable, that the A1 DRD2 allele is a non-specific risk factor for disinhibition in general.

The Hypothalamic–Pituitary–Adrenal Axis

The hypothalamic–pituitary–adrenal (HPA) axis has a central role in much of our emotional life, and it is not surprising that it is an important player in the neurobiology of substance abuse. In response to stress, HPA axis activation results in the release of cortisol, which has been shown to enhance dopamine release from the VTA into the ventral striatum, like addictive drugs [41]. High-risk children of addicts have a blunted cortisol response to stress, and also have higher levels of impulsivity and externalizing behavior [42]. The level of cortisol response was negatively related to levels of externalizing behavior, and this relationship was stronger in adolescent girls than boys [43]. Thus, externalizing behavior, SUD, and a hypoactive HPA axis are all linked together. However, this finding is not consistent with other studies, which have identified a link between a hyperactive HPA axis, elevated cortisol response, internalizing disorders like depression and anxiety, and SUD [44]. Therefore, both HPA hyperactivity and hypoactivity pose a risk for SUD, most likely mediated by the hypoactive response to stress in the externalizing disorders (antisocial, conduct) and the hyperactive response to stress in the internalizing (anxious, depressed). Taken together, these findings indicate the complicated nature of substance use disorders, and the multiple pathways that can lead to substance abuse.

THE NEUROTOXIC IMPACT OF ALCOHOL AND MARIJUANA

Next, we move on to a discussion about the biological impact of illicit substances on the adolescent brain. Because research on the neurotoxic effects of drugs on the adolescent brain is ethically challenging, we have focused our discussion on the available literature surrounding abuse of alcohol and marijuana, the two drugs most commonly abused by adolescents.

Alcohol

Alcohol is the most abused drug in adolescence, and it is the most studied, with the majority of research done with animals, for obvious ethical reasons. Adolescents appear to be less sensitive than adults to alcohol's behavioral effects, at least in rats. Spear [45] has shown that adolescent rats are less affected than adult rats by the social, motor, sedation, acute withdrawal, and "hangover effects" of ethanol. However, alcohol may be more toxic to the adolescent brain. Adolescent rat brains exposed to ethanol show less neural growth in the hippocampus, and those adolescent rats have worse hippocampal-dependent memory problems [46]. In human imaging studies, alcohol-abusing adolescents were compared with healthy peers and were found to have smaller frontal and hippocampal volumes, altered white matter microstructure, and poorer memory. The hippocampus was smaller in patients who began drinking earlier and who used for longer. Alcohol-using adolescents show altered anisotropy in the corpus callosum, and in adolescent binge drinkers, the frontal, cerebellar, temporal, and parietal regions all showed altered anisotropy. Heavy drinking is associated with diminished frontal cortex activation during spatial working memory tasks, as well as neuropsychological tests of attention, memory retrieval, and visuospatial functioning [5,47]. In longer-term follow-up studies, Squeglia identified gender differences. Girls who drank more often had a greater loss in visuospatial functioning. Alcohol-abusing girls had smaller PFC volumes than controls, while their male counterparts had larger PFC volumes than controls. Girls may be more sensitive than boys to the neurotoxic effects of alcohol: alcohol-abusing girls had a decreased frontal response to spatial working memory and reduced gray matter in comparison to alcohol-abusing boys [1,48].

Marijuana

In studies using fMRI, adolescent marijuana users have less efficient activation in working memory, verbal learning, and cognitive control tasks. Studies consistently show use of alternate brain networks in marijuana-using adolescents [1]. Smokers have larger cerebellar volumes, and female smokers have larger prefrontal cortex volumes than female non-smokers, with both findings suggestive of impaired synaptic pruning [49]. White matter integrity is worse in fronto-parietal and fronto-temporal circuits [50], and as a corollary, adolescent marijuana smokers are at greater risk for depression, and have worse performance on psychomotor speed, complex attention, verbal memory, planning and sequencing ability, even after a month-long abstinence [51].

CONCLUSION

The study of adolescent brain development and the changes that predispose it to risk-taking behaviors such as substance abuse is a fast-changing landscape. Ultimately, a theoretical construct that will likely withstand the test of time will include an "accelerator" currently thought to be located in the ventral striatum and a "brake" currently thought to be a part of the prefrontal cortex. The overall balance and development of these two opposing forces will likely govern the behavioral phenotypes observed in adolescents as they transition into young adulthood. Current thoughts on this subject include the idea that our somewhat arbitrary cut-off definitions for adolescence may not accurately represent neurodevelopmental changes related to risk-taking behavior. In fact, when actuarial data are taken into consideration (as is most frequently done by car-rental and insurance companies) the time period to stability in impulse-control/modulation most likely occurs in the mid-20s. Interestingly, this is when car insurance rates begin to decline for most drivers and when young adults are actually allowed to rent cars. As we begin to understand more about our brains and the manner in which they develop, we will continue to improve our understanding of modulating risk-taking behavior.

References

1. Bava S, Tapert SF. Adolescent brain development and the risk for alcohol and other drug problems. *Neuropsychol Rev* 2010;**20**:398–413.
2. Tamnes CK. Brain maturation in adolescence and young adulthood: regional age-related changes in cortical thickness and white matter volume and microstructure. *Cereb Cortex* 2009;**20**:534–548.
3. Perrin JS, Hervé P-Y, Leonard G, *et al.*Growth of white matter in the adolescent brain role of testosterone and androgen receptor. *J Neurosci* 2008;**28**:9519–9524.
4. Eaton LK, Kinchen S, Ross J, Hawkins J, Harris WA, Lowry R. Youth risk behavior surveillance – United States, 2005, surveillance summaries. *Morbidity and Mortality Weekly Report* 2006;**55**:1–108.
5. Casey BJ, Jones RM. Neurobiology of the adolescent brain and behavior: implications for substance use disorders. *J Am Acad Child Adolesc Psych* 2010;**49**:1189–1201.
6. Davidson MC, Amso D, Anderson LC, Diamond A. Development of cognitive control and executive functions from 4–13 years: evidence from manipulations of memory, inhibition, and task-switching. *Neuropsychologia* 2006;**44**:2037–2078.
7. Hardin MG, Mandell D, Mueller SC, Dahl RE, Ernst M. Inhibitory control in anxious and healthy adolescents is modulated by incentive and incidental affective stimuli. *J Child Psychol Psych* 2009;**50**:1550–1558.
8. Figner B, Mackinlay RJ, Wilkening F, Weber EU. Affective and deliberative processes in risky choice: age differences in risk taking in the Columbia Card Task. *J Exp Psychol Learn* 2009;**35**:709–730.
9. Chassin L. Adolescent substance use. In: Lerner R, Steinberg L (eds), *Handbook of Adolescent Psychology*, 2nd edn. New York: John Wiley & Sons, Ltd, 2004; pp. 655–696.

10. Gardner M, Steinberg L. Peer influence on risk taking, risk preference, and risky decision making in adolescence and adulthood: an experimental study. *Dev Psychol* 2005; **41**:625–635.

11. Galvan A, Hare TA, Davidson M, Spicer J, Glover G, Casey BJ. The role of ventral frontostriatal circuitry in reward-based learning in humans. *J Neurosci* 2005; **25**:8650–8656.

12. Schepsis TS, Adinoff B, Rao U. Neurobiological processes in adolescent addictive disorders. *Am J Addiction* 2008; **17**:6–23.

13. Martin JJ. *Neuroanatomy: Text and Atlas*. New York: McGraw-Hill, 2003.

14. Pasupathy A, Miller EK. Different time courses of learning-related activity in the prefrontal cortex and striatum. *Nature* 2005;**433**:873–876.

15. Galvan A, Hare T, Voss H, Glover G, Casey BJ. Risk-taking and the adolescent brain: who is at risk? *Dev Sci* 2007;**10**:F8–F14.

16. Gill TM, Castaneda PJ, Janak PH. Dissociable roles of the medial prefrontal cortex and the nucleus accumbens core in goal-directed actions for differential reward magnitude. *Cereb Cortex* 2010;**20**:2884–2899.

17. VanLeijenhorst L, Moor BG, Op de Macks ZA, Rombouts SA, Westenberg PM, Crone EA. Adolescent risky decision-making: neurocognitive development of reward and control regions. *Neuroimage* 2010;**51**:345–355.

18. Boes AD, Bechara A, Tranel D, Anderson SW, Richman L, Nopoulous P. Right ventromedial prefrontal cortex: a neuroanatomical correlate of impulse control in boys. *Soc Cogn Affect Neurosc* 2009;**4**:1–9.

19. Vaidya CJ, Austin G, Kirkorian G. Selective effects of methylphenidate in attention deficit hyperactivity disorder: a functional magnetic resonance imaging study. *Proc Natl Acad Sci USA* 1998;**95**:14494–14499.

20. Macmillan M. A wonderful journey through skull and brains: the travels of Mr. Gage's tamping iron. *Brain Cognition* 1986;**5**:67–107.

21. Harlow JM. Recovery from the passage of an iron bar through the head. *Publications of the Massachusetts Medical Society* 1868;**2**:327–347.

22. Geier CF, Terwilliger R, Teslovich T, Velanova K, Luna B. Immaturities in reward processing and its influence on inhibitory control in adolescence. *Cereb Cortex* 2010; **20**:1613–1629.

23. Munoz D, Everling S. Look away: the anti-saccade task and the voluntary control of eye movement. *Nat Rev Neurosci* 2004;**5**:218–228.

24. Somerville LH, Hare TA, Casey BJ. Frontostriatal maturation predicts cognitive control failure to appetitive cues in adolescents. *J Cogn Neurosci* 2011;**23**:2123–2134.

25. Diaz J. *How Drugs Influence Behavior*. Englewood Cliffs: Prentice Hall, 1996.

26. Weickert CS, Webster MJ, Gondipalli P. Postnatal alterations in dopaminergic markers in human prefrontal cortex. *Neuroscience* 2007;**144**:1109–1119.

27. Kalivas P. Neurotransmitter regulation of dopamine neurons in the ventral tegmental area. *Brain Res Rev* 1993;**18**:75–113.

28. Teicher M, Anderson S. Limbic serotonin turnover plunges during puberty. Poster presented at the Meeting of the Society for Neuroscience, Miami Beach, FL, 1999.

29. Dillon K, Gross-Isseroff R, Israeli M, Biegon A. Autoradiographic analysis of serotonin 5-HT1A receptor binding in the human brain postmortem: effects of age and alcohol. *Brain Res* 1991;**554**:56–64.

30. Taylor J, Jentsch J. Repeated intermittent administration of psychomotor stimulant drugs alters acquisition of Pavlovian approach behavior in rats: differential effects of cocaine, d-amphetamine and 3,4-methylenedioxymethamphetamine ("ecstasy"). *Biol Psychiatry* 2001;**50**: 137–143.

31. Hollander E, Rosen J. Impulsivity. *J Psychopharmacol* 2000;**14**:S39–S44.

32. Begleiter H, Porjesz B, Bihari B, Kissin B. Event-related brain potentials in boys at risk for alcoholism. *Science* 1984;**225**:81–96.

33. Iacono WG, Carlson SR, Malone SM, McGue M. P3 event-related potential amplitude and the risk for disinhibitory disorders in adolescent boys. *Arch Gen Psychiatry* 2002; **59**:750–757.

34. Schweinsburg AD, Paulus MP, Barlett VC. An FMRI study of response inhibition in youths with a family history of alcoholism. *Ann NY Acad Sci* 2004;**1021**: 391–394.

35. Twitchell G, Hannah G, Cook E, Fitzgerald H, Little K, Zucker R. Overt behavior problems and serotonergic function in middle childhood among male and female offspring of alcoholic fathers. *Alcohol Clin Exp Res* 1998;**22**:1340–1348.

36. Askenazy F, Caci H, Myque M, Darcourt G, Lecrubier Y. Relationship between impulsivity and platelet serotonin content in adolescents. *Psychiatry Res* 2000;**94**:19–28.

37. Twitchell G, Hanna G, Cook E, Stoltenberg S, Fitzgerald HE, Zucker R. Serotonin transporter promoter polymorphism genotype is associated with behavioral disinhibition and negative affect in children of alcoholics. *Alcohol Clin Exp Res* 2001;**25**:953–959.

38. Nilsson K, Sjoberg R, Damberg M. Role of the serotonin transporter gene and family function in adolescent alcohol consumption. *Alcohol Clin Exp Res* 2005;**29**: 564–570.

39. Connor BT, Noble EP, Berman SM. DRD2 genotypes and substance use in adolescent children of alcoholics. *Drug Alcohol Depend* 2005;**79**:379–387.

40. Thompson J, Thomas N, Singleton A. D2 dopamine receptor gene (DRD2) TaqI polymorphism: reduced dopamine D2 receptor binding in the human striatum associated with the A1 allele. *Pharmacogenetics* 1997;**7**:479–484.

41. Barrot M, Piazza P. The dopaminergic hyperresponsiveness of the shell of the nucleus accumbens is hormone-dependent. *Eur J Neurosci* 2000;**12**:973–939.

42. Moss H, Vanyukov M, Martin C. Salivary cortisol responses and the risk for substance abuse in prepubertal boys. *Biol Psychiatry* 1995;**38**:547–555.

43. Dawes M, Dorn L, Moss H. Hormonal and behavioral homeostasis in boys at risk for substance abuse. *Drug Alcohol Depend* 1999;**55**:165–176.

44. Rao U, Hammen C, Poland RE. Relationship among depression, cigarette smoking and HPA activity in adolescents. Poster presented at the Annual Meeting of the International Society for Research in Child and Adolescent Psychopathology, 2003, Sydney, Australia.

45. Spear L. Anxiogenic effects during withdrawal from acute ethanol in adolescent and adult rats. *Pharmacol Biochem Behav* 2003;**75**:411–418.

46. Witt E. Research on alcohol and adolescent brain development: opportunities and future directions. *Alcohol* 2010;**44**:119–124.

47. DeBellis M, Clark D, Beers S. Hippocampal volume in adolescent-onset alcohol use disorders. *Am J Psychiatry* 2000;**157**:737–744.

48. Squeglia L, Jacobus J, Tapert S. The influence of substance use on adolescent brain development. *Clin EEG Neurosci* 2009;**40**:31–38.

49. Medina K, Nagel B, Tapert S. Abnormal cerebellar morphometry in abstinent adolescent marijuana users. *Psychiatry Res* 2010;**182**:152–159.

50. Bava S, Frank L, McQueeny T, Schweinsburg B, Schweinsburg A, Tapert S. Altered white matter microstructure in adolescent substance abuse. *Psychiatry Res* 2009;**173**:228–237.

51. Medina K, Hanson K, Schweinsburg A, Cohen-Zion M, Nagel B, Tapert S. Neuropsychological functioning in adolescent marijuana users: subtle deficits detectable after a month of abstinence. *J Int Neuropsychol Soc* 2007;**13**:807–820.

9

Psychiatric Comorbidities in Adolescent Substance Use Disorders

Todd Zorick

UCLA Department of Psychiatry; VA West Los Angeles Medical Center, Los Angeles, CA, USA

INTRODUCTION

Adolescent substance use, abuse, and dependence represent a spectrum of maladaptive behavioral disorders with considerable importance both from a societal standpoint, and from the point of view of healthcare practitioners [1,2]. Substance use disorders are highly maladaptive behaviors in adolescents (and other age groups), and result in considerable harm to afflicted individuals, families, and societies [3]. From a health utilization point of view, a study performed in a managed care setting showed that adolescents with substance use disorders both utilized more medical services and were more costly to treat than a matched control group with similar medical problems [4]. Strikingly, adolescents with substance use disorders were found to require continued high levels of expensive treatment services even after discharge from hospital, unlike the non-substance using group, which had decreased healthcare costs after treatment [4]. From a neurobiological point of view, adolescence is characterized by the early maturation of limbic reward areas (which is thought to provide the "drive" to engage in exploratory behavior), with delayed maturation of frontal lobe structures, which are implicated in providing a "brake" to potentially harmful behavioral choices (reviewed in ref. [5]). Therefore, adolescent risk-taking and impulsivity are facilitated by neurobiological changes specific to adolescents, which later in development are normally ameliorated during the transition to early adulthood [5].

However, by and large, most individuals who experiment with drugs and alcohol as adolescents do not go on to suffer from either abuse or dependence syndromes, and it has been hypothesized that adolescent impulsivity in normal development can help establish boundaries for appropriate adult behavior [5,6]. Healthy adolescence is characterized by high levels of impulsivity and risk-taking behavior, and frequently is accompanied by "sampling" of alcohol, nicotine, and illicit drugs [7]. In fact, some data have demonstrated that community-normative adolescent experimentation with alcohol and illicit substances is associated with decreased anxiety, improved psychological health, and better social skills than adolescent peers who never have experimented with alcohol or drugs (e.g. ref. [8]). Therefore, clinicians treating adolescents and counseling families of adolescents who may be using drugs and alcohol should have a sensitivity to the boundaries of normal adolescent behavior, which may be community specific [8]. Conversely, however, most individuals with substance use disorders have histories of early adolescent experimentation with drugs and alcohol, which likely has primed these individuals to develop maladaptive behavioral addictions that eventually cause serious psychosocial dysfunction [1]. Given this, clinicians involved in the care of adolescent substance users can have an important role in the future life trajectory of these individuals, since early interventions to reduce maladaptive behavioral usage patterns of alcohol and other substances can prevent some of the ravages that may result from future addictions [9].

SUBSTANCE ABUSE AND DEPENDENCE SYNDROMES IN ADOLESCENTS

Given these considerations – that substance use disorders in adolescence are harmful, but that abuse and dependence syndromes should be differentiated from community-normative, age-appropriate experimentation – clinicians have several tools available to help

Clinical Handbook of Adolescent Addiction, First Edition. Richard Rosner.
© 2013 John Wiley & Sons, Ltd. Published 2013 by John Wiley & Sons, Ltd.

differentiate the level of potential risk in a given adolescent presenting for treatment. The *Diagnostic and Statistical Manual of Mental Disorders, Fourth Edition, Text Revision* (DSM-IV-TR) criteria for substance abuse and dependence can be assessed during evaluation, in order to clarify whether it appears that problematic drug or alcohol abuse leads to "clinically significant impairment or distress . . . within a 12-month period" [10]. Criteria for DSM-IV-TR substance abuse and dependence are clear and straightforward for clinical diagnostic purposes. However, clinicians treating adolescents with problematic substance use are faced with a conundrum: on a population basis, meeting DSM criteria for abuse and dependence of drugs and alcohol is relatively uncommon among adolescents, with estimates for the proportion of US adolescents meeting criteria for either substance abuse or dependence ranging from 5 to 11% [11,12]; in fact, these clinical syndromes do not reach their population peaks in incidence until age 20 (for abuse syndromes) or age 22 (for dependence syndromes) [13]. By contrast, experimentation with alcohol and illicit drugs is extremely common among US adolescents: in 2009, in a survey of US 12th-graders, 44% reported having drunk alcohol within the last 30 days, around 20% had smoked cigarettes during the last 30 days, and more than 50% reported having tried at least one illegal drug during their lifetime [3]. Therefore, many clinicians will be treating adolescents with concomitant alcohol and illicit drug use who may not meet strict DSM-IV-TR criteria for abuse or dependence syndromes, making clinical decision-making with regard to treatment options more challenging.

PSYCHIATRIC COMORBIDITIES IN ADOLESCENT SUBSTANCE USE DISORDERS

While the evaluation of the severity of substance use in an adolescent presenting for mental health treatment can be problematic in many cases, an understanding of the epidemiology and likely comorbidities of adolescent substance use disorders and mental illness can assist clinicians in the identification of those patients who may be more likely to have or develop a substance use disorder. A considerable body of research has been established using community samples and case reports, which demonstrates the striking commonality of behavioral, mood, anxiety, and substance use disorders among adolescents (reviewed in ref. [12]). However, until recently, there was no comprehensive, statistically valid data sample to be able to accurately estimate either the prevalence, demographic covariates, or psychiatric comorbidity of adolescent mental illness and substance abuse in the US population [14]. In order to address this need, the National Institute of Mental Health (NIMH) established the National Comorbidity Survey Adolescent Supplement (NCS-A), which provided for a nationally representative sample of face-to-face survey interviews of more than 10 000 US adolescents aged 13 to 18 [12,14]. In this comprehensive survey, the lifetime risk for adolescent drug or alcohol use disorder (either DSM-IV abuse or dependence) was 11%, somewhat higher than earlier estimates, with a higher risk for males, and older adolescents [12]. The median age of onset of substance use disorders was age 15, which was much older than the median age of onset for mood and anxiety disorders in this sample, demonstrating that later adolescence (especially age 17 and older) is the riskiest time for developing a substance use disorder [12]. Interestingly, differences in ethnicity, parental divorce, and socioeconomic status did not contribute significantly to the risk of development of substance use disorders among adolescents, so that substance use disorders seem to cut across class and ethnic divides nationwide [12]. With regard to psychiatric comorbidity with substance use disorders, the presence of a substance use disorder increased the proportion of adolescents who suffered from more than one class of disorder, showing that comorbidity with either behavioral (e.g., attention-deficit/hyperactivity disorder (ADHD)), mood, or anxiety disorders is very common with substance use disorders among US adolescents [12]. These data reinforce and extend many previous studies conducted in regional sample populations demonstrating that substance use disorders among adolescents are highly comorbid with behavioral, mood, and anxiety disorders (e.g., ref. [11]).

Utilizing data from a representative sample of some 4000 adolescents in east Texas as part of the Teen Health 2000 (TH2K) survey, Roberts and colleagues [11] found an approximately 5.3% incidence of substance use disorder in this population, again somewhat lower than the estimate for the NCS-A survey [12]. However, in other respects the TH2K data compared favorably with the NCS-A data, showing that substance use disorders were much more common in later adolescents, and that propensity to develop substance use disorders among adolescents cuts across demographic profiles [11,12]. The TH2K data demonstrated that adolescent substance use disorders were highly comorbid with anxiety, attentional, behavioral, and mood disorders, in that 17% of adolescents with substance use disorders met DSM-IV criteria for at least one other Axis I psychiatric condition (aside from substance use) during the last year [11]. Intriguingly, the overall median number of comorbid psychiatric diagnoses in this population was ~2, indicating that those adolescents with comorbid psychiatric conditions were very likely to have several additional psychiatric diagnoses [11]. Psychiatric comorbidity in adolescent substance use disorder was associated with more impairment as measured by the Child Global Assessment Scale, indicating that comorbid psychiatric conditions were associated with worse psychosocial functioning than for pure substance use disorder cases [11]. Increased severity of addiction was associated with an increased risk of psychiatric comorbidity, in that adolescents with substance dependence had a higher mean number of comorbid psychiatric conditions than adolescents with substance abuse diagnoses [11]. In order to estimate the relative association of a given psychiatric diagnosis with the development of substance use disorder, odds ratios (ORs) were calculated for each of the categories of mental illness (ADHD/attentional, anxiety disorders, behavioral disorders, and mood disorders) [11]. It was found that not all psychiatric diagnoses were equally likely to be comorbid with substance use disorders among adolescents: conduct/oppositional disorders and mood disorders had highly elevated odds ratios for developing any substance use disorder (14 and 5.1, respectively), whereas anxiety disorders seemed only to confer risk to develop alcohol dependence (2.8 odds ratio), and not other substance use disorders [11]. By contrast, comorbid ADHD/attentional psychiatric diagnoses by themselves did not seem to result in a relative risk to develop substance use disorders in this adolescent population [11]. The relationship between ADHD diagnosis, behavioral disorders (conduct and oppositional disorders), and liability to develop substance use disorders among adolescents is an extremely complicated and contentious topic that will be addressed subsequently in the chapter, but these data are consistent with prior reports showing that adolescent behavioral disorders tend to be highly associated with propensity to develop substance use disorders, more so than "pure" ADHD in the absence of conduct/oppositional disorder (cf. ref. [14]).

These results also parallel results from data collected in other populations. In a German study of 151 adolescent inpatients with substance use disorders, 41.5% had comorbid conduct disorders, 22.5% had comorbid anxiety disorders, 19.2% had comorbid mood disorders, and 9% were found to have somatoform disorders [15]. In previous epidemiological studies, the rate of comorbidity for other Axis I clinical disorders in adolescents with substance use disorder was 32% [16]. Therefore, multiple lines of evidence collected from different adolescent populations suggest that anxiety disorders, mood disorders, and, especially, behavioral disorders are particularly common comorbid psychiatric diagnoses among adolescents with substance use disorders.

DISRUPTIVE BEHAVIORAL DISORDERS AND SUBSTANCE USE DISORDERS IN ADOLESCENTS

Oppositional defiant disorder (ODD) and conduct disorder are classified by the DSM-IV-TR as disparate, persistent patterns of maladaptive disruptive behaviors that, by definition, result in impaired social or educational functioning in children and adolescents [10]. ODD is defined as a pattern of oppositional, negativistic behavior that far exceeds what is normal, which may include temper tantrums, argumentation with adults, defiance, deliberate annoyance of others, blaming others for one's own misbehaviors, frequent anger, excessive interpersonal sensitivity, and/or vindictiveness [10]. These behaviors, while significant, do not involve "serious violations" of societal norms or of the rights of others (i.e., they do not meet criteria for conduct disorder) [1,10]. Children with ODD seem to be highly susceptible to develop problems with depression as adults, even with the resolution of behavioral problems in adolescence [17]. In a national sample, ODD was found to have a lifetime prevalence of about 10% in the United States [18]. The presence of childhood ODD (even without progression to conduct disorder) was found to convey a high likelihood of later psychopathology as adults, with 68% having impulse control disorders, 62% having anxiety disorders, 47% having substance use disorders, and roughly 46% having mood disorders [18]. Therefore, children with ODD have a greatly increased risk of future psychopathology, including substance use disorders, not to mention their frequent current comorbidity with ADHD [17].

Conduct disorder, by contrast, is seen as a more severe pattern of maladaptive disruptive behaviors, which is distinguished from ODD by virtue of displaying interpersonal aggression and violation of the rights of others (e.g., bullying, frequent fighting) [1]. Symptoms of conduct disorder may also include aggression toward people or animals, destruction of property, frequent lying or theft, and/or serious violations of rules set by authority figures [10]. Adolescents and children with ODD are at increased risk to develop conduct disorder, and both conditions are associated with an elevated risk for ADHD [1]. Interestingly, 90% of adolescents with conduct disorder have been found to meet premorbid criteria for ODD, demonstrating the strong relationship between externalizing disruptive behavior disorders of childhood and later in adolescence [19]. However, only 40–50% of children with ODD will typically go on to develop conduct disorder [17].

Conduct disorder is thought to be present in roughly 7–10% of adolescents in communities worldwide, and is much more common in males (anywhere from 3 to 10 times more prevalent) [1,20,21]. Risk factors for developing conduct disorder include low IQ and poor school performance, harsh and/or erratic parental discipline, chaotic family environments, childhood abuse, parental and peer sociopathy, poverty, and high crime neighborhoods [21].

Conduct disorder in children and adolescents confers a greatly increased risk for future criminality and antisocial personality disorder (reviewed in ref. [23]). In a 40-year follow-up of a cohort of British youths, adolescent conduct disorder was found to lead to a higher rate of school dropout, and the subjects experienced high levels of adversity as adults, including elevated indices of problems with relationships, money, and mental health, compared to non-behaviorally disordered youths [20]. Therefore, adolescent conduct disorder, by and large, leads to poor outcomes in psychosocial functions during adult life [20].

Since the diagnosis of conduct disorder is dependent more upon violation of societal laws than symptomatology (making it somewhat unusual among psychiatric diagnoses), this has led to criticism of the validity of the construct as different from severe ADHD (e.g., ref. [23]). In order to address these criticisms, recent neuroimaging studies have sought to clarify the neurobiology of conduct disorder as an independent entity. ADHD, substance use disorder, and conduct disorder are highly comorbid with one another, but there appears to be a distinct, though overlapping neurobiological substrate to conduct disorder itself [24–26]. In order to assess disorder-specific differences in brain activation during different cognitive tasks, a study was conducted using event-related functional magnetic resonance imaging (fMRI) with three subject groups: adolescents with only conduct disorder, adolescents with only ADHD, and healthy control adolescents [25]. Distinct (though overlapping) patterns of brain activation in different cognitive tasks were found for ADHD and conduct disorder, which provides support for the idea that there is an independent neurobiological basis for conduct disorder [25]. Interestingly, this study found that adolescents with pure conduct disorder showed decreased activation in the right orbitofrontal cortex in response to a reward task, compared to the ADHD-only and healthy control subjects [25]. These findings corroborate earlier reports of reduced orbitofrontal cortex gray matter volume in adolescents with conduct disorder [24]. Given that the orbitofrontal cortex has been hypothesized to signal cognitive representations of the relative reward potential of a given behavior, orbitofrontal cortex dysfunction (especially right-sided) would theoretically impair the ability of individuals with conduct disorder to appropriately weigh the benefits and drawbacks of a given action, thereby resulting in maladaptive behaviors

[25]. In a study looking at neural responses to rewarding tasks, a group of adolescents with comorbid conduct disorder and substance use disorder showed reduced activation in other reward-specific brain areas, which was thought to reflect deficient reward circuitry [26]. Therefore, conduct disorder can be linked to specific neurobiological deficits that have been hypothesized to contribute to behaviors that violate community norms, which are distinct from those typically seen in ADHD.

Most strikingly, conduct disorder is highly comorbid with substance use disorders among adolescents and in later adulthood, especially in the presence of ADHD [11,17]. The interaction between ADHD, conduct disorder, and substance use disorder will be discussed further in the next section; however, the data unambiguously demonstrate that adolescent conduct disorder makes the likelihood of current substance use disorder and later psychopathology much greater. As discussed in the section above, the presence of conduct disorder greatly increases the likelihood that a given adolescent will develop a substance use disorder, much more so than other comorbid anxiety, attentional, or mood disorders [11]. In a study of British youths with conduct disorder, conduct disorder itself did contribute to an increased risk for substance use disorder, independent of the additive risks of associating with substance-using friends (which also increased risks [27]). Additionally, adolescent conduct disorder is associated with poor adult psychosocial functioning (reviewed in ref. [20]). Conduct disorder is therefore perhaps the most important psychiatric comorbid diagnosis to consider among adolescents with substance use disorders or mental health problems, given its poor general prognosis and strong link to later psychopathology, including mood disorders, antisocial behavior, and substance use disorders.

ATTENTION DEFICIT DISORDERS AND SUBSTANCE USE DISORDERS IN ADOLESCENCE

Attention deficit disorders, including ADHD and attention deficit disorder (ADD), are common childhood conditions that affect approximately 6–8% of children in the United States and worldwide (reviewed in ref. [28]). While inattention is primarily diagnosed in children, many of its symptoms continue to be experienced by adolescents and adults even when formal criteria for ADHD are no longer met [28]. In order to diagnose ADHD/ADD, DSM-IV-TR stipulates that symptoms of the disorder must have been present by age 7, and as a result of the symptoms, the behavioral dysfunction must be present in at least two separate settings, either interfering with functioning at home, at school, or in social extracurricular activities [10]. Additionally, symptoms must be present for at least 6 months "to a degree that is maladaptive and inconsistent with the developmental level" [10]. Inattentive symptoms may include failure to pay attention to details in schoolwork, difficulty sustaining attention in play or tasks, not seeming to listen when spoken to, not following through on chores or duties, difficulty in organization, avoidance of tasks that require sustained effort, frequently losing necessary items, easily distractible, and forgetfulness [10]. Hyperactive-impulsive symptoms include fidgeting while sitting, inability to remain seated, inappropriate running/climbing, difficulty remaining quiet, behaviorally "driven," impulsive verbal outbursts, difficulty in waiting, and problems with frequent intrusions and interruptions into the activity of others [10]. There is no known cause of ADHD, although based upon genetic studies it has been linked to familial genetic predisposition, as it is highly heritable, with up to 60–90% of the risk for ADHD being attributed to genetic factors [29]. Similar to other complex neurobehavioral disorders, the inheritance risk for ADHD is not thought to be due to changes in one or a few genes; rather, it is more likely due to a complex interaction between many genes each with only a small effect on the predisposition [29]. ADHD is frequently found in families with other childhood disorders, especially autism spectrum disorders, and recently evidence of a shared genetic liability to both autism and ADHD has been found [30]. Similar to autism, ADHD predominantly affects boys, with a prevalence ratio of at least 4:1 [29].

Attention-deficit/hyperactivity disorder has been found to associate with specific patterns of abnormal brain function in adolescents, which correlate with the degree of pathology and attentional problems [1]. Children with ADHD have deficits in sustained attention during cognitive testing, structural abnormalities in fronto-striatal-parietal brain networks responsible for maintaining attention, and evidence of abnormal glucose metabolism in these same areas [25]. Sustained attentional deficits seen on cognitive testing in ADHD have also been found to correlate with decreased activation in fronto-striatal-parietal network areas via event-related fMRI, including the ventrolateral prefrontal cortices [25]. Summarizing the results of studies of clinical observations, cognitive testing, and neuroimaging, the construct of ADHD can be seen as a coherent diagnostic formulation: it is associated with deficient brain networks that are normally responsible for maintaining attention.

The diagnosis of childhood and adolescent ADHD has also been found to correlate with a strong propensity to develop both current and future mental illness [28]. ADHD was found to be a risk factor for adolescents with major depression to switch into mania [31]. The lifetime risks for the development of various comorbid psychiatric illnesses include: antisocial personality disorder, ~5–10%; major depression, ~25–35%; bipolar disorder, 10–15%; anxiety disorders, 30–50%; and up to 40–50% lifetime risk for substance use disorders [28]. Therefore, beyond the diagnosis and implications of ADHD itself, there is a considerable increased future psychiatric burden often associated with ADHD.

There has been a long-recognized association between ADHD, externalizing behavioral disorders, and the propensity to develop substance use disorders, both in adolescence and adulthood (reviewed in ref. [32]). It has been estimated based upon community samples that 20–40% of children with ADHD have comorbid ODD [29], and that up to 30–50% of ADHD cases will go on to develop conduct disorder [22]. It is also important to point out that the best available evidence indicates that stimulant treatment of children and adolescents with ADHD does not increase the risk of future substance use disorder; rather, most likely it reduces the risk [33]. Clinicians can therefore be reasonably assured that treatment for the condition will not somehow "cause" their adolescent patients to be addicted, as has been claimed.

The presence of comorbid conduct disorder in adolescents with ADHD is a particularly ominous sign, which associates with a worsening of the severity of the behavioral dysfunction, a higher likelihood of developing a substance use disorder, and an increased future rate of adult psychopathology [1,21]. In a longitudinal study of 30 boys with ADHD and conduct disorder followed over 10 years, as adults more than 60% of these individuals continued to meet criteria for ADHD, conduct disorder, and antisocial personality disorder [17]. Additionally, this group was highly afflicted by mood disorders, with approximately 25% developing a major depressive episode, and nearly 40% eventually meeting criteria for bipolar disorder [17]. Additionally, among these youths with both ADHD and conduct disorder, substance use disorders were nearly ubiquitous: more than 70% of these individuals were tobacco smokers and met criteria for a substance use disorder at 10-year follow-up [17].

Given the statistical association between conduct disorder, substance use disorders, and premorbid ADHD, much work has been devoted to understand the relationship between the three dysfunctional behavioral syndromes (discussed in ref. [14]). As discussed previously in this chapter, from an epidemiological standpoint, pure ADHD itself (in the absence of conduct disorder) does not seem to predispose to the development of a substance use disorder [11]. In fact, the best evidence is for a "mediational" model between ADHD, conduct disorder, and substance use disorder [14]. A large sample of children and adolescents in New York state with ADHD (with and without comorbid conduct disorder) was followed in a longitudinal study for more than 20 years to assess whether they developed a substance use disorder, either in adolescence or adulthood [14]. After controlling for possible confounding factors (premorbid substance use disorder, demographic variables, and presence of conduct disorder), the authors found that ADHD did not, by itself, associate with a future propensity for substance use disorder [14]. Rather, the presence of comorbid conduct disorder mediated the strong relationship between ADHD and substance use disorder in this cohort [14]. Therefore, the presence of ADHD and conduct disorder together is associated with a greater severity of ADHD diagnosis [32], highly elevated propensity to both substance use disorder and current and future psychopathology [17], and worsened future psychosocial dysfunction [20]. Taken together, the presence of comorbid conduct disorder with ADHD is a particularly ominous clinical comorbidity that should deserve particular consideration by clinicians treating adolescents, both because of the inherent likely worsening of the clinical disorders, and the high likelihood of concurrent substance use disorder. By contrast, "pure" ADHD, without any evidence of ODD or conduct disorder, does not seem to independently predict an elevated propensity toward developing substance use disorders [14].

SUBSTANCE USE DISORDERS AND COMORBID MOOD DISORDERS IN ADOLESCENTS

In epidemiological studies of adolescents, mood disorders have been found to associate with an increased risk for the development of a substance use disorder [11]. In terms of comorbidity with substance use disorders, the presence of any mood disorder has been shown to produce an increased relative risk for substance use disorder (OR 5.1 [11]).

While mood disorders are known to be common in adult populations, until recently estimates of the rate of mood disorders among US adolescents were made using community samples by extrapolation (discussed in ref. [34]). However, thanks to data from the NCS-A, a statistically valid estimate for the risk of mood disorders among US adolescents is available [12]. The lifetime prevalence for any mood disorder among US adolescents was estimated at 14.3%, making mood disorders relatively common conditions in this population [12]. Of those, 11.7% suffer from either dysthymia or major depression, and 2.7% suffer from either bipolar I or II [12]. The median age of onset of mood disorders was 13 years, indicating that the burden of mood disorder in US

youths often starts at the very beginning of adolescence, somewhat earlier than the median age of onset of substance use disorders (15 years [12]). More than 40% of adolescents with an Axis I diagnosis will also have additional Axis I diagnoses, including substance use disorders, which indicates that there is a high rate of comorbidity for other diagnosable mental illnesses in adolescents with mood disorders [12]. Therefore, mood disorders are common among adolescents, and they are frequently comorbid with both substance use disorders and other comorbid psychiatric conditions.

BIPOLAR DISORDER AND SUBSTANCE USE DISORDERS IN ADOLESCENTS

Bipolar disorder has long been recognized as having a strong association with the propensity to develop a comorbid substance use disorder [1]. Given that the average age of onset of a diagnosis of bipolar disorder is 24 years of age, bipolar disorder has traditionally been regarded as relatively rare in children and adolescents as compared to adults [1]. However, as discussed above, more accurate population incidence data indicate that bipolar disorder is not uncommon in adolescence [12]. Despite controversy about the diagnosis in youth, childhood and adolescent bipolar disorder is persistent across the lifespan, and very frequently continues as adult bipolar disorder [35]. Bipolar disorder, especially in childhood or adolescence, is often a devastating diagnosis from the point of view of ongoing lifetime psychosocial dysfunction, including poor psychosocial functioning, and is associated with a very high risk for suicidal behavior [1]. Indeed, more than 90% of adolescents with bipolar disorder were classified as having "severe impairment" in terms of psychosocial function, a rate higher than that for other primary psychiatric diagnoses among adolescents [12]. Therefore, adolescent bipolar illness is fairly common, and is associated with elevated morbidity in terms of poor psychosocial functioning.

While a complete understanding of the etiology, genetics, and pathophysiology of bipolar disorder is beyond the scope of this chapter, it is important to summarize a few key issues with regard to bipolar disorder in adolescents. The criteria for a (hypo)manic episode in children and adolescents is the same as for adults: abnormally expansive or irritable mood for at least 1 week (4 days in hypomania), which "causes marked impairment,", with symptoms including grandiosity, decreased need for sleep, pressured speech, racing thoughts, distractibility, agitation, and engagement in risky behavior [10]. However, adolescents with new-onset bipolar often have a history of ADHD [1,17], may not have a classic history of cycling between mania and depression, often exhibit severe irritability rather than grandiosity *per se*, and often present with psychotic features [1]. Bipolar disorder is highly heritable, as adolescents with bipolar will often have afflicted family members, and it seems to have a complex polygenic inheritance pattern, similar to most other mental illnesses [1].

Bipolar disorder in adolescents has been found to have a high rate of comorbidity with other Axis I clinical disorders, including anxiety disorders, ADHD, conduct disorder, and substance use disorders (discussed in ref. [36]). Interestingly, the risk for substance use disorders in adolescent bipolar disorder seems to be largely independent of comorbid conduct disorder, unlike the case for ADHD/substance use disorders [14,37]. In fact, it has been shown that the associated risk for comorbid substance use disorders is greater in adolescent-onset bipolar disorder (39% frequency) than in childhood-onset bipolar disorder (only 8%) [37]. In a larger, controlled study to assess specifically the risks of adolescent bipolar disorder and substance use disorder while controlling for potential confounding variables, Wilens *et al.* [36] studied a group of 105 adolescents with bipolar disorder (34 with substance use disorders, and 71 without), compared to a matched group of healthy control adolescents. Independent of age, demographics, or comorbid psychiatric conditions (including conduct disorder), adolescent bipolar disorder alone conferred an elevated risk for any substance use disorder (OR 8.7), compared to healthy controls [36]. Adolescent bipolar illness is therefore associated with severe deficits in psychosocial functioning and psychiatric comorbidities. Additionally, adolescent bipolar disorder by itself clearly and demonstratively increases the risk for development of a comorbid substance use disorder, and clinicians treating these patients should be aware of this risk, which is unlike the case for ADHD (see sections above for a more complete discussion).

DEPRESSION AND ADOLESCENT SUBSTANCE USE DISORDERS

Data from the NCS-A demonstrate that depression is distressingly common among US adolescents, with the risk for developing either dysthymia or major depressive disorder estimated to be 11.7% [12]. Clinical depression is an extremely common psychiatric condition across the lifespan, but a complete discussion of the epidemiology, etiology, and pathophysiology of even adolescent depressive syndromes is beyond the scope of this chapter. However, we will briefly present an understanding of clinical syndromes of depression primarily as they relate to adolescent substance use disorders, and the reader is referred to comprehensive texts for more information (e.g., ref. [1]).

The diagnosis of major depressive disorder in children and adolescents differs somewhat from that of adults, with several of the criteria being modified to better account for the symptoms likely to be experienced in youths [1]. DSM-IV-TR criteria for major depression stipulate that mood symptoms must be present for at least 2 weeks, and that these symptoms "must produce social or academic impairment" [1,12]. Depressive symptoms in adolescents may include depressed or irritable mood states, anhedonia, failure to make weight gains (due to poor appetite), sleep alterations, agitation or lethargy, fatigue, guilty feelings, poor concentration, and in severe cases, thoughts of death or suicidal ideation [10]. Among adolescents, commonly seen symptoms of depression include social isolation, poor family relationships, rejection sensitivity, school difficulties, and deficits in grooming [1]. Adolescent depression, like other psychiatric disorders, has a polygenetic predisposition with a considerable environmental influence, as having parents with depression greatly increases the risk for adolescent depression [1].

Interestingly, the diagnosis of major depression in childhood and adolescence is associated with an elevated risk for future manic switching, with a future incidence anywhere from 20% to 50%, depending upon the time-frame and population studied [31]. As discussed in a previous section, the presence of comorbid ADHD increases the risk of a subsequent switch to mania in adolescents with major depression [31]. These data are consistent with epidemiological studies of adult mood disorders, which show that a risk factor for subsequent manic switching is early-onset depressive episodes [1].

Substance use disorders in adolescents have long been associated with an elevated risk for comorbid major depression [1,38]. In a study of 100 Australian adolescents and young adults (aged 12–22) with substance use disorders, 27% met current criteria for major depressive disorder, with the lifetime rate for any mood or anxiety disorder being 68% [16]. However, given that in adolescents major depression is more common than substance use disorders, a causal relationship between substance use disorders and depression has been difficult to establish, and statistical associations in clinical populations have not produced consistent results [38]. To address the issue of causality, Marmorstein and colleagues [38] used data from 1200 youths who were followed from ages 17 to 24 as part of the Minnesota Twin Family Study. These data indicated that depression at age 17 modestly (but statistically insignificantly) predicted substance use disorders in the same age group [38]. However, depression among 20- to 24-year-olds was predicted by substance use disorder at age 17, indicating that the presence of substance use disorder in adolescents may result in later depressive symptoms [38]. The presence of comorbid conduct disorder was found to greatly increase the rate of problematic alcohol use in depressed adolescents, demonstrating that certain psychiatric comorbidities are associated with increased risk for adolescent substance use disorders [39].

In addition to the frequent comorbidity of depression in substance use disorders, depression may impair the ability of adolescents to benefit from treatment. Comorbid depressive symptoms in adolescents with substance use disorders have been found to associate with poor response to treatment after hospitalization [40]. Taken together with evidence showing that comorbid psychiatric diagnoses tend to associate with worse psychosocial functioning among adolescents with substance use disorders, depression in substance-abusing adolescents is a common comorbid psychiatric condition that will require clinical consideration during treatment.

CO-OCCURRING ANXIETY AND SUBSTANCE USE DISORDERS IN ADOLESCENTS

Anxiety disorders are perhaps the most common form of recognizable mental disorder, and they are exceedingly common in children and adolescents [1]. In fact, data from the NCS-A have shown that the overall risk for developing an anxiety disorder in adolescence is 31.9%, with specific phobia (19.1%) being most common among them [12]. However, the incidences of social phobia (9.1%), separation anxiety disorder (7.6%), and post-traumatic stress disorder (PTSD, 5%) are also very high among US adolescents [12]. Therefore, childhood and adolescence is particularly afflicted with the burdens of anxiety disorders, and these are frequently encountered in clinical populations [1].

Here, we will briefly summarize the clinical and biological understanding of adolescent anxiety disorders as they pertain to comorbid substance use disorders. According to the DSM-IV-TR, separation anxiety disorder can only be diagnosed in childhood and adolescence [1,10]. Across the lifespan, social phobia has been found to be more prevalent in adolescence than in childhood and adulthood [1,10]. Symptoms commonly seen in anxiety disorders in adolescence differ slightly from those in adulthood, in that somatic symptoms are more prominent, and dysfunction due to symptoms often involves difficulties in peer relationships [1]. Childhood-specific anxiety conditions tend to result in chronic adult anxiety disorders like agoraphobia, indicating the lifetime pervasiveness of the underlying propensity to anxiety [1]. Risk factors for adolescent anxiety disorders include: female gender, low socioeconomic status, overprotective parenting style, childhood adversity (including trauma and abuse), and a family history of anxiety disorders [41].

Based upon data from laboratory experiments, animal models, and clinical populations, vulnerability to child and adolescent anxiety disorders is thought to reflect hyperactive fear response circuitry involving the amygdalae [42]. Evidence of increases in the right ventrolateral prefrontal cortex activity were found in response to angry facial cues in adolescents with generalized anxiety disorder, which was hypothesized to represent a compensatory mechanism in reaction to an amygdalar anxiety signal [43]. This evidence was subsequently supported by the demonstration that both effective psychotherapy and medication treatment for adolescent generalized anxiety disorder produced increased activation in the right ventrolateral prefrontal cortex, showing the cortical adaptation that may underlie successful treatment [44]. Therefore, anxiety disorders can be seen as resulting from specific neurobiological abnormalities in fear circuitry, which show evidence of improved modulation concomitant with clinically effective treatments.

Of note, the development of a primary anxiety disorder in childhood or adolescence presaged the future diagnosis of adult bipolar in 14–16% of subjects in a longitudinal cohort study, a rate much higher than for control youths ($\sim$3%); this finding was shown to be independent of comorbid depressive symptoms [45]. Factors that predict bipolar switching in anxiety-disordered youths include comorbid conduct disorder, and family histories of depression and alcoholism [45]. Therefore, similar to ADHD and major depression, anxiety disorders in youths have an elevated risk for later manic switching.

Because anxiety disorders in adolescence are highly prevalent, they are frequently comorbid with substance use disorders [11]. Indeed, in longitudinal studies, the presence of adolescent anxiety disorders increased the relative risk for comorbid alcohol dependence (OR 2.8) [11]. In an Australian sample of adolescent substance users, comorbid PTSD was found to be present in 27% of inpatients studied, indicating that the psychological sequelae of traumatic life events are common among adolescents with severe substance use disorders [16]. In community sample studies of adolescents with anxiety disorders, anywhere from 9% to 12% were found to have comorbid substance use disorders, a lower relative comorbid proportion than that seen for major depression and other mood disorders [46]. However, for adolescents with both an anxiety disorder and major depression, the rate of comorbid substance use disorder increased to $\sim$20%, again indicating that multiple psychiatric comorbid diagnoses produce an increased risk for developing a comorbid substance use disorder [46].

In a comprehensive study of a community sample of adolescents with anxiety disorders, Wu and colleagues found that the relative risk for comorbid substance use disorders was influenced by gender [47]. For adolescent girls (but not boys), anxiety disorders, agoraphobia, separation anxiety disorder, and obsessive-compulsive disorder were associated with frequent/heavy drinking behavior and illicit drug use, whereas among boys, anxiety disorders did not significantly contribute to risky behavior [47]. Therefore, female adolescents with anxiety disorder may be particularly vulnerable to developing substance use disorders, a pattern that has been seen in other adolescent subject populations [46]. Anxiety disorders in general are also more frequent in female adolescents than in males [41]. Taken together, the case for adolescent anxiety disorders being frequently comorbid with substance use disorders is likely to be especially true among females.

CONCLUSIONS: ADOLESCENT SUBSTANCE USE DISORDERS AND COMORBID PSYCHIATRIC CONDITIONS

Misuse of alcohol and illicit substances is highly prevalent in adolescent populations worldwide, including North America. Recent research highlights that substance use disorders among adolescents are likely to be more common than previously thought, indicating the large scale of the problem facing families, communities, and clinical services. Substance use disorders in adolescents exist in a continuum of use patterns with varying levels of community-normative alcohol and drug experimentation at one end of the spectrum, making the clinical assessment of adolescents with substance misuse often problematic. Aside from careful assessment for DSM-IV criteria for substance use disorders, clinicians should also assess adolescent patients for potential psychiatric comorbid conditions that may impact the clinical risk of ongoing or future substance misuse. While incidence data may vary in different populations, a large proportion (up to 40%) of adolescents with substance use disorders will have comorbid psychiatric illnesses. The presence of comorbid psychiatric illness with substance use disorders in adolescents is associated with worse psychosocial functioning, poorer response to treatment, and more severe substance use disorder pathology. Additionally, adolescents with comorbid psychiatric illness and substance use disorder are likely to have multiple additional axis I comorbidities, which tends to further compound the overall clinical severity.

Among comorbid psychiatric conditions, the presence of conduct disorder has been shown to produce the highest relative risk for the development of substance use disorders in adolescence. The presence of ADHD with comorbid conduct disorder is an extremely poor prognostic sign among adolescents, which results in poor psychosocial functioning, extremely high rates of substance use disorders, and elevated risks for adult psychiatric illness, including depression and bipolar disorder. By contrast, the best available data support the view that ADHD itself, without disruptive behavioral manifestations, does not result in an elevated risk for adolescent substance use disorders. ODD has been shown to both associate with later substance use disorder, and to frequently presage conduct disorder, indicating the strong tendency for externalizing disruptive disorders to increase the risk for adolescent substance use disorders. Mood disorders are common in adolescence, and are frequently comorbid with substance use disorders. Among mood disorders, bipolar disorder in adolescence in particular greatly increases the risk for substance use disorder, an effect that is independent of other diagnoses and behavioral problems. Given the elevated prevalence of major depression and dysthymia in adolescence, comorbidity with substance use disorders is frequently seen, though the relative associative risk is lower than for disruptive disorders and bipolar disorder. Adolescent substance use disorder has been shown to confer a risk for the subsequent development of depressive symptoms in early adulthood. Anxiety disorders in adolescence are extremely common, particularly among females, and have been associated with an increased risk for substance use disorders in females compared to males.

While much has been elucidated with regards to the epidemiology and pathophysiology of comorbid substance use disorders and psychiatric illness in adolescents, many issues continue to stand out bereft of research-based clinical guidance. Adequate studies on evidence-based treatment modalities for adolescents with comorbid substance use disorders and psychiatric illness are sorely lacking, possibly confounded by the difficulties of performing studies in this population. Additionally, many adolescent psychiatric diagnoses (including ADHD, conduct disorder, major depression, and anxiety disorders) are associated with a high rate of manic switch in later adolescence and early adulthood. The clinical significance of this phenomenon is poorly understood: should clinicians treat adolescents with risk factors for manic conversion differently than those without, for example? Taken together, significant questions remain about the understanding, treatment, and prognosis of adolescents with comorbid substance use disorder and psychiatric illness that future research should be directed to help clarify.

To conclude, clinicians treating adolescents should screen carefully for both substance use disorders and psychiatric illness, as they will frequently interact to affect the relative clinical course. Among the large proportion of adolescents using alcohol and illicit drugs, the presence of the comorbid psychiatric illnesses listed above may raise the relative risk of clinical severity, psychosocial dysfunction, and likelihood of development of substance use disorders.

References

1. Sadock B, Sadock V (eds). *Kaplan and Sadock's Concise Textbook of Child and Adolescent Psychiatry*, 10th edn. LWW: Philadelphia, PA: Lippincott Williams & Wilkins, 2008.

2. French MT, Zavala SK, McCollister KE, *et al.*Cost-effectiveness analysis of four interventions for adolescents with a substance use disorder. *J Subst Abuse Treat* 2008;**34**:272–281.

3. Johnston LD, O'Malley PM, Bachman JG, *et al.* Monitoring the future: national results on adolescent drug use: Overview of key findings, 2009. NIH Publication No. 10-7583. Bethesda, MD: National Institute on Drug Abuse, 2010.

4. Parthasarathy S, Weisner C. Health care services use by adolescents with intakes into an outpatient alcohol and drug treatment program. *Am J Addictions* 2006;**15**: 113–121.

5. Schepis TS, Adinoff B, Rao U. Neurobiological processes in adolescent addictive disorders. *Am J Addictions* 2008;**17**:6–23.

6. Gullo MJ, Dawe S. Impulsivity and adolescent substance use: rashly dismissed as "all-bad"? *Neurosci Biobehav Rev* 2008;**32**:1507–1518.

7. Casey BJ, Jones RM. Neurobiology of the adolescent brain and behavior: implications for substance use disorders. *J Am Acad Child Adolesc Psychiatry* 2010;**49**:1189–1201.

8. Szapocznik J, Prado G, Burlew AK, *et al.*Drug abuse in African American and Hispanic adolescents: culture, development, and behavior. *Ann Rev Clin Psychol* 2007;**3**:77–105.

9. McClain DB, Wolchik SA, Winslow E, *et al.* Developmental cascade effects of the New Beginnings Program on adolescent adaptation outcomes. *Dev Psychopathol* 2010;**22**:771–784.

10. American Psychiatric Association. *Diagnostic and Statistical Manual for Mental Disorders, Fourth Edition, Text Revision (DSM-IV-TR)*. Washington, DC: APA, 2000.

11. Roberts RE, Roberts CR, Xing Y. Comorbidity of substance use disorders and other psychiatric disorders among adolescents: evidence from an epidemiologic survey. *Drug Alcohol Depend* 2007;**88**(Suppl 1):S4–S13.

12. Merikangas KR, He JP, Burstein M, *et al.* Lifetime prevalence of mental disorders in U.S. adolescents: results from the National Comorbidity Survey Replication–Adolescent Supplement (NCS-A). *J Am Acad Child Adolesc Psychiatry* 2010;**49**:980–989.

13. Compton WM, Thomas YF, Stinson FS, *et al.* Prevalence, correlates, disability, and comorbidity of DSM-IV drug abuse and dependence in the United States: results from the national epidemiologic survey on alcohol and related conditions. *Arch Gen Psychiatry* 2007;**64**:566–576.

14. Brook DW, Brook JS, Zhang C, *et al.* Association between attention-deficit/hyperactivity disorder in adolescence and substance use disorders in adulthood. *Arch Pediatr Adolesc Med* 2010;**164**:930–934.

15. Langenbach T, Spönlein A, Overfeld E, *et al.* Axis I comorbidity in adolescent inpatients referred for treatment of substance use disorders. *Child Adolesc Psych Ment Hlth* 2010;**28**:25.

16. Lubman DI, Allen NB, Rogers N, *et al.* The impact of co-occurring mood and anxiety disorders among substance-abusing youth. *J Affect Disorders* 2007;**103**:105–112.

17. Biederman J, Petty CR, Dolan C, *et al.* The long-term longitudinal course of oppositional defiant disorder and conduct disorder in ADHD boys: findings from a controlled 10-year prospective longitudinal follow-up study. *Psychol Med* 2008;**38**:1027–1036.

18. Nock MK, Kazdin AE, Hiripi E, *et al.* Lifetime prevalence, correlates, and persistence of oppositional defiant disorder: results from the National Comorbidity Survey Replication. *J Child Psychol Psych* 2007;**48**:703–713.

19. Wilson JJ, Levin FR. Attention-deficit/hyperactivity disorder and early-onset substance use disorders. *J Child Adolesc Psychopharmacol* 2005;**15**:751–763.

20. Colman I, Murray J, Abbott RA, *et al.* Outcomes of conduct problems in adolescence: 40 year follow-up of national cohort. *Brit Med J* 2009;**338**:a2981.

21. Murray J, Farrington DP. Risk factors for conduct disorder and delinquency: key findings from longitudinal studies. *Can J Psychiatry* 2010;**55**:633–642.

22. Mannuzza S, Klein RG, Moulton JL3rd. Lifetime criminality among boys with attention deficit hyperactivity disorder: a prospective follow-up study into adulthood using official arrest records. *Psychiatry Res* 2008;**160**:237–246.

23. Banaschewski T, Hollis C, Oosterlaan J, *et al.* Towards an understanding of unique and shared pathways in the psychopathophysiology of ADHD. *Dev Sci* 2005;**8**:132–140.

24. Huebner T, Vloet TD, Marx I, *et al.* Morphometric brain abnormalities in boys with conduct disorder. *J Am Acad Child Adolesc Psychiatry* 2008;**47**:540–547.

25. Rubia K, Smith AB, Halari R, *et al.* Disorder-specific dissociation of orbitofrontal dysfunction in boys with pure conduct disorder during reward and ventrolateral prefrontal dysfunction in boys with pure ADHD during sustained attention. *Am J Psychiatry* 2009;**166**:83–94.

26. Crowley TJ, Dalwani MS, Mikulich-Gilbertson SK, *et al.* Risky decisions and their consequences: neural processing by boys with Antisocial Substance Disorder. *PLoS One* 2010;**5**:e12835.

27. Glaser B, Shelton KH, van denBree MB. The moderating role of close friends in the relationship between conduct problems and adolescent substance use. *J Adolesc Health* 2010;**47**:35–42.

28. Wilens TE. ADHD: prevalence, diagnosis, and issues of comorbidity. *CNS Spectr* 2007;**12**(Suppl. 6):1–5.

29. Stergiakouli E, Thapar A. Fitting the pieces together: current research on the genetic basis of attention-deficit/hyperactivity disorder (ADHD). *J Neuropsychiatr Dis Treat* 2010;**6**:551–560.

30. Lichtenstein P, Carlström E, Råstam M, *et al.* The genetics of autism spectrum disorders and related neuropsychiatric disorders in childhood. *Am J Psychiatry* 2010;**167**:1357–1363.

31. Biederman J, Petty CR, Byrne D, *et al.* Risk for switch from unipolar to bipolar disorder in youth with ADHD: a long term prospective controlled study. *J Affect Disorders* 2009;**119**:16–21.

32. Flory K, Lynam DR. The relation between attention deficit hyperactivity disorder and substance abuse: what role does conduct disorder play? *Clin Child Family Psychol Rev* 2003;**6**:1–16.

33. Wilens TE, Adamson J, Monuteaux MC, *et al.* Effect of prior stimulant treatment for attention-deficit/hyperactivity disorder on subsequent risk for cigarette smoking and alcohol and drug use disorders in adolescents. *Arch Pediatr Adolesc Med* 2008;**162**:916–921.

34. Kessler RC, Avenevoli S, Costello EJ, *et al.* Design and field procedures in the US National Comorbidity Survey Replication Adolescent Supplement (NCS-A). *Int J Meth Psych Res* 2009;**18**:69–83.

35. Geller B, Tillman R, Bolhofner K, *et al.* Child bipolar I disorder: prospective continuity with adult bipolar I disorder; characteristics of second and third episodes; predictors of 8-year outcome. *Arch Gen Psychiatry* 2008;**65**:1125–1133.

36. Wilens TE, Biederman J, Adamson JJ, *et al.* Further evidence of an association between adolescent bipolar disorder with smoking and substance use disorders: a controlled study. *Drug Alcohol Depend* 2008;**95**:188–198.

37. Wilens TE, Biederman J, Millstein RB, *et al.* Risk for substance use disorders in youths with child- and adolescent-onset bipolar disorder. *J Am Acad Child Adolesc Psychiatry* 1999;**38**:680–685.

38. Marmorstein NR, Iacono WG, Malone SM. Longitudinal associations between depression and substance dependence from adolescence through early adulthood. *Drug Alcohol Depend* 2010;**107**:154–160.

39. Marmorstein NR. Longitudinal associations between depressive symptoms and alcohol problems: The influence of comorbid delinquent behavior. *Addict Behav* 2010;**35**:564–571.

40. Dobkin PL, Chabot L, Maliantovitch K, *et al.* Predictors of outcome in drug treatment of adolescent inpatients. *Psychol Rep* 1998;**83**:175–186.

41. Beesdo K, Knappe S, Pine DS. Anxiety and anxiety disorders in children and adolescents: developmental issues and implications for DSM-V. *Psychiatr Clin N Am* 2009;**32**:483–524.

42. McClure EB, Monk CS, Nelson EE, *et al.* Abnormal attention modulation of fear circuit function in pediatric generalized anxiety disorder. *Arch Gen Psychiatry* 2007;**64**:97–106.

43. Monk CS, Nelson EE, McClure EB, *et al.* Ventrolateral prefrontal cortex activation and attentional bias in response to angry faces in adolescents with generalized anxiety disorder. *Am J Psychiatry* 2006;**163**:1091–1097.

44. Maslowsky J, Mogg K, Bradley BP, *et al.* A preliminary investigation of neural correlates of treatment in adolescents with generalized anxiety disorder. *J Child Adolesc Psychopharmacol* 2010;**20**:105–111.

45. Goldstein BI, Levitt AJ. Prevalence and correlates of bipolar I disorder among adults with primary youth-onset anxiety disorders. *J Affect Disorders* 2007;**103**:187–195.

46. O'Neil KA, Conner BT, Kendall PC. Internalizing disorders and substance use disorders in youth: comorbidity, risk, temporal order, and implications for intervention. *Clin Psychol Rev* 2011;**31**:104–112.

47. Wu P, Goodwin RD, Fuller C, *et al.* The relationship between anxiety disorders and substance use among adolescents in the community: specificity and gender differences. *J Youth Adolesc* 2010;**39**:177–188.

10

Toxicology of Substances of Abuse

Eleanor Vo,[1] and Dean De Crisce[2]

[1] Psychiatric Screening Center, Department of Psychiatry; Capital Health Regional
Medical Center, Trenton, NJ, USA
[2] New York University School of Medicine, Brooklyn, NY, USA

Basic knowledge of the toxicology and detection of substances of abuse is helpful in the evaluation of, and monitoring for, addictive disorders in youth. "Drug testing" is common and frequently used by both clinicians and parents. Such testing is utilized for clinical evaluation, monitoring compliance, intervention, prevention, and control of school and workplace safety.

There is a high prevalence of alcohol and illicit substance use among US teens. The 2008 Monitoring the Future National Survey demonstrated that 37% of 12th-graders, 27% of 10th-graders, and 14% of 8th-graders had at some point used illicit substances [1]. A 2007 Survey reported that 72.7% of surveyed students had used alcohol or other illicit substances on at least one occasion [2]. Some students experiment with substances of abuse in, arguably, a developmentally appropriate manner. However, some do progress to develop clinical stigmata of abuse or dependence.

Drug testing serves a role in clinical treatment, jurisprudence, athletics, and scholastic and workplace monitoring, justified by the high societal costs of substance of abuse. A 2011 US Department of Justice National Drug Intelligence Center report noted that substance misuse results in an economic impact on US society of approximately $193 billion dollars annually, as per their 2007 data [3]. Of that number, $68 billion resulted from loss of productivity, along with additional costs secondary to crime, premature death, property loss and health-related costs. For comparison, a 2008 study estimated that diabetes costs the United States more than $174 billion each year, and heart disease costs an estimated $316 billion dollars [3].

Substances of abuse play a costly role in employment, health, and criminal systems. Bureau of Labor Statistics 1998 data from the Census of Fatal Occupational Injuries estimated that 10–20% of employees who died while working had post-mortem toxicology findings indicating alcohol or other drug use [4]. The cost of illicit substances to the health and criminal systems was estimated by the Office of National Drug Control Policy (ONDCP) in 2002 to be $180.9 billion, representing a 5% increase in the prior decade [5]. Crime costs associated with substances of abuse, alone, have been estimated at $61 billion dollars annually [3]. It has been proposed that greater use of drug screening procedures might result in reduced losses and resources resulting from substance use and misuse.

Drug testing is commonly and sensationally used in professional sports to monitor athletes, and it was increasingly used in school-based athletics. The US Supreme Court ruled in 1995 that drug testing was appropriate to reduce drug use in school sports programs [6]. This program was extended in many school systems [7–10]. In 2003 the US Supreme Court ruled that drug testing could be expanded to all school programs [11]. Many of those expansions have been reduced, or discontinued altogether, as a result of funding considerations. In 2009, Florida schools stopped testing due to funding issues and a negative cost to benefit ratio, leaving only three states with drug testing options in schools, including New Jersey, Illinois, and Texas [12].

Drug screening is also routinely used for compliance monitoring in drug diversion programs, treatment programs, and for individuals in community supervisory programs such as parole and probation. A Canadian study showed that in contrast with monitoring outcomes for adult chemical dependency outpatients, adolescents had improved outcomes when utilizing drug testing in an outpatient program [13].

Primary prevention for substance abuse in youth occurs in middle high schools; drug testing functions as

Clinical Handbook of Adolescent Addiction, First Edition. Richard Rosner.
© 2013 John Wiley & Sons, Ltd. Published 2013 by John Wiley & Sons, Ltd.

secondary prevention when utilized by parents, drug courts, drug programs, school systems, and mental health providers. A key advantage of monitoring for substance use by these systems is that it provides for early intervention and potential reduction in later, poorer outcomes. Drug use in adolescence is associated with higher rates of use in adulthood [1]. In addition, adolescent substance abuse is related to comparatively poorer physical and mental health, and delinquent behaviors [14].

There are various recommendations with regard to ethical considerations in drug testing, involving informed consent and limitations on use. The US Preventive Services Task Force (USPSTF) supports drug testing in a clinical setting when there is a reasonable suspicion of substance abuse and recommends informed consent be obtained when completing those tests [15]. The American Academy of Pediatrics (AAP) recommends limiting drug testing to situations in which it is useful to aid in diagnosis and formatting treatment plans, but advises against its use as a screening tool; informed consent is recommended [16,17].

HISTORY OF DRUG TESTING

Mandates for a "drug-free workplace" arose from federal guidelines regarding federal employees. The Federal Regulation Executive Order 12564 (1986) signed in law by President Ronald Reagan noted:

> The federal government, as the largest employer in the Nation, can and should show the way towards achieving drug-free workplaces through a program designed to offer drug users a helping hand and, at the same time, demonstrating to drug users and potential drug users that drugs will not be tolerated in the Federal workplace; The profits from illegal drugs provide the single greatest source of income for organized crime, fuel violent street crime, and otherwise contribute to the breakdown of our society; The use of illegal drugs, on or off duty, by Federal employees is inconsistent not only with the law-abiding behavior expected of all citizens, but also with the special trust placed in such employees as servants of the public; Federal employees who use illegal drugs, on or off duty, tend to be less productive, less reliable, and prone to greater absenteeism than their fellow employees who do not use illegal drugs [18].

Executive Order 12564 led to the creation of the Drug-Free Workplace Act of 1988, establishing federal drug-testing programs, education and training programs, and employee assistance programs. Technical guidelines were established for federal workplace drug-testing programs and certification of laboratories engaged in drug testing for federal agencies [19]. Initially involving primarily the Department of Transportation, the guidelines have been revised and expanded to address the collection and testing of urine specimens, the requirements for certification of test facilities, and the role of and standards for collectors and Medical Review Officers for testing of individuals in safety sensitive positions [20].

Drug-testing guidelines and processes are regulated by the Substance Abuse and Mental Health Services Administration (SAMHSA) in conjunction with the National Institute on Drug Abuse (NIDA) and the Department of Health and Human Services (DHHS), setting the standards for most drug-testing methods in use in the United States today [21].

TESTING STANDARDS

The Substance Abuse and Mental Health Administration devised the standard urine screening panel used by the Department of Transportation, commonly referred to as the NIDA-5, SAMHSA-5 or DOT-5 panels [21]. Other expanded tests are available such as the NIDA-9, and a urine drug screen that tests for 12 potential substances of abuse.

The NIDA-5 panel, frequently the standard panel available in hospitals, laboratories, and home kits, screens for the marijuana metabolite (delta-9-tetrahydrocannabinol-9-carboxylic acid), cocaine metabolite (benzyolecgonine), phencyclidine, amphetamines (D-amphetamine, D-methamphetamine), and opiates (heroin, morphine, and codeine) [21].

Expanded panels might include additional substances of abuse such as ethanol (alcohol), propoxyphene (Darvocet, Darvon), hydrocodone (Lortab, Vicodin), oxycodone, barbiturates, methaqualone (Quaalude), anabolic steroids, benzodiazepines (e.g., Valium), MDMA (ecstasy) and therapeutic pharmaceuticals such as tricyclic antidepressants, and methadone [22]. The NIDA-9 routine panel includes the NIDA-5 with the addition of barbiturates, benzodiazepines, methadone and propoxyphene [22].

Standards for drug testing might involve either therapeutic or regulatory purposes. Both seek to confirm the presence of the potential abused substance; however, therapeutic purposes might require lower testing thresholds for purposes of monitoring and substance identification [23].

SAMPLE SOURCES

Samples utilized as substrates for drug testing may be obtained from urine, blood, serum, saliva, hair, and sweat. Although the present standard remains urine for most substances, other samples and methods might be chosen in consideration of such variables as substance metabolism, population, monitoring period, ease of sample acquisition, application of results, and expense. Detection times for samples vary based on sample characteristics, as well as substance metabolism and interference.

Substances ingested, inhaled, injected, and smoked "pass through" the circulatory system to later undergo hepatic metabolism, tissue sequestration or urinary elimination. Products of metabolism are generally eliminated through the urinary system, with a smaller portion eliminated through respiration and sweat mechanisms [24]. Typically serum drug testing provides the shortest time-frame for detection, whereas hair samples provide for much longer detection times [24]. Therefore, certain substances of abuse that are present in the blood only for brief periods may be better detected in urine, which contains metabolites with longer half-lives [25]. Likewise, long-term compliance monitoring might be better using testing of hair or sweat samples. All methods have advantages and disadvantages.

Urine

Urine is the most common sample source for drug testing, and considered to be the "gold standard" for most substances of abuse; it is relatively non-invasive and readily obtainable. An additional advantage is that it allows detection of some parent compounds along with more enduring metabolites [26]. The metabolites have a longer half-life compared to the parent compound, with most being found in the urine for 1 to 5 days depending on the drug [26,27]. The NIDA-5 or NIDA-9 panels are the typical screening panels for urine samples; results may be available in a matter of hours.

Disadvantages of utilizing urine as a testing substrate include such considerations as the inability to detect substances used immediately before collection (inadequate time for metabolism), the ease with which the sample can be adulterated or substituted, and limitations of urine detection of alcohol. Alcohol (ethanol) in its parent form can be detected in urine for only approximately 8 hours, leaving serum detection of alcohol levels a more useful instrument (discussion of the use of ethyl glucuronide as an alcohol use biomarker is discussed later in this chapter) [28].

Adulterants for urine sampling are readily available online and in stores; a search of online retailers produces multiple products advertised to assist in evading positive urine results [29]. Although the mechanism of action of these adulterants is discussed in a later section, one example is pyridinium chlorochromate (PCC), an active ingredient of "Urine Luck," originally marketed as a urine "detoxifier" [30]. Early publications reported efficacy only in evading detection of cannabis and opiates. Now it is marketed as a way to obscure detection of nicotine in urine samples. PCC is easily identified in urine samples [30].

Urine toxicology screening, despite potential disadvantages, is still the most frequent and standard method for determining the presence of substances of abuse. It is routinely used in emergency, clinical, and monitoring settings because of the ease of collection, relative low cost, and rapid results, which aid in diagnostic formulation, treatment planning, and legal outcomes.

Blood/Serum

A more invasive but still common sample source for drug testing is blood/serum. Although useful in deterring adulteration or substitution, serum samples are limited by the time window available for substance detection. As a result of the parent compound "passing through" the circulatory tree prior to hepatic metabolism and renal elimination, serum generally has the disadvantage of detecting only parent substances and not metabolites [26,27]. Therefore serum sample detection times are much shorter than for urine samples. Serum detection times for substances of abuse are generally between 12 and 24 hours [26].

Additional disadvantages associated with blood testing are the difficulties in obtaining access in drug abusers, minor risks associated with blood draws, and invalidation of hemolysed samples.

Serum is typically used to measure serum alcohol levels. On occasion the NIDA-5 and NIDA-9 panels are used to screen for fentanyl, ketamine, and oxycodone. Results may be available in hours to days (detection times for specific substances are identified below) [22].

Hair

Hair is the only sample source that provides a cumulative measure of drug use and a long time-frame for detection. Hair sampling offers a non-invasive and easily obtained testing method that is difficult to adulterate. Hair testing can detect the parent drug and its metabolites. Metabolite testing allows for differentiation between environmental exposure and ingested substances. Ease in retesting is an additional benefit, as results are expected to be replicated over brief time periods. Frequency of use is expected to yield correspondingly higher concentrations of the substance in the hair [22].

Hair analysis is a testing method used primarily in forensics and research; however, recent options do include workplace testing or treatment purposes. It is a growing adjunct to other standard methods of drug screening. Hair testing is routinely used for NIDA-5 screening, and results are available in 1 to 4 days [22].

Hair samples are taken from the scalp line, and the first 3 cm of hair is analyzed to detect use over a period of 60 to 90 days, the longest drug detection period available [24]. Scalp hair growth is about 0.3 mm/day for the average person. It takes approximately 4 to 10 days from the time of drug use for the hair to grow above the scalp, therefore preventing hair testing as a method for detection of acute usage and intoxication.

Substances of abuse and their metabolites are keratinized within growing hair strands, related to the melanin content of the hair. Therefore hair with higher melanin content, and thus darker pigmentation, contains higher concentrations of incorporated substances [26]. A minimum of approximately 1 cm of hair is required for analysis, detecting substances used in the prior 30 days [31]. As in other sample sources, initial screening is performed, followed by confirmatory testing [31]. It is more labor intensive than other sample testing methods, and costs substantially more [32].

Samples may be taken from various scalp sites and, less desirably, from body hair. There has been concern about the reliability of alternative hair sampling sites, such as body, beard, and pubic areas, in providing results similar in accuracy to scalp hair. Fatty acid ethyl esters (FAEEs) are utilized in the keratinizing process of hair growth, and were originally thought to be key for detecting alcohol consumption. Hartwig et al. demonstrated that FAEE effects were similar for all body sites in alcohol users [33]. However, body hair growth is more variable, and substantially slower than scalp hair, leading to difficulty in interpreting time of use for suspected users. According to one laboratory, body hair yields results that give an indication of substance use over a period of 1 year, because of the differential rate of hair growth [31]. Using non-scalp hair presents additional challenges related to collection and invasiveness.

Environmental contaminants and chemical treatments can affect the validity of hair testing. For example, bleaching, dyeing, perming, straightening, and UV light exposure may decrease drug concentrations. Chemical processing causes changes to hair structure, growth, and porosity. Exposure to environmental pollutants, and confounders such as environmental marijuana smoke, has been proposed to affect test results [34]. As such, there are a number of retail products available as shampoos that are marketed to obscure hair testing results. One product advertised as "Ultra Clean," however, did not reduce drug levels significantly when tested on 14 post-mortem hair samples from known substance abusers [35].

Although hair drug testing has not been approved for use by the Department of Transportation for employment purposes, it has been used by other governmental agencies and has been upheld in arbitrations by various court rulings and appeals [36,37]. Guidelines published by the Society of Hair Testing provide collection procedures, testing standards, and thresholds for detection [38].

Recent developments in the field of hair analysis include a novel rapid cocaine screen, requiring only a small hair sample of 2.5 mg taken from either scalp or pubic hair, providing results in 5 minutes. The method of analysis used in this technique, matrix-assisted laser desorption/ionization-mass spectrometry (MALDI-MS), has shown significant promise. Vogliardi et al. demonstrated 100% specificity and sensitivity for detection of cocaine by MALDI-MS, referenced to gas chromatography-mass spectrometry (GC-MS), even when analyzing samples with low concentrations of cocaine [39].

Saliva

Like hair testing, the use of saliva or oral fluids is a rapidly growing technique. It is a sensitive technique that is non-invasive, readily obtainable, and allows direct observation to prevent adulteration [40]. Oral fluid refers to saliva excreted by the three main salivary glands: parotid, sublingual, and submaxillary [41]. Samples are collected by either swab or an absorbent foam pad, which is then diluted to approximately 1 mL volume [41]. The solution is then subject to analysis, primarily for the parent compounds of the NIDA-5 panel. Immunoassay screening is followed by confirmatory testing, as in most other drug testing methods. Preliminary screening results are provided in minutes.

Oral fluid samples are affected by fluid pH, drug concentration, membrane characteristics, protein binding, and lipophilicity of the substance [40]. Drugs that have a higher protein-bound fraction are represented in lower concentrations in oral fluid, as the latter contains only the unbound drug [42]. Lipophilic substances likewise are present in greater concentration as a result of the increased membrane permeability [42]. Oral fluid testing is more sensitive for those substances having a higher pH, such as cocaine and amphetamine, which are more easily detected in the acidic oral environment [43].

Direct observation during the collection of oral fluid allows for easy validation. Although oral fluid is not readily adulterated, assisted methods of collection, referred to as "stimulated," can affect result outcomes. Oral fluid is obtained by either stimulated or non-stimulated methods. The non-stimulated method is most accurate and involves draining, swabbing, and absorbent pad collection methods. Stimulated methods involve mechanical or chemical manipulation, involving instructing the subject to move their mouth, tongue, lips, and cheek to increase saliva production. Other mechanical methods may include chewing wax or rubber bands, which can alter oral fluid production. Chemical stimulation might involve the use of citric acid candy, chewing gum, or other agents designed to increase oral fluid production. This may lead to drug concentration and pH changes in the oral fluid [41,42] and has been shown to substantially decrease concentrations of codeine, methamphetamine, and cocaine [41].

There is an abundance of retail products available on the internet advertising the ability to reliably provide for negative oral drug testing. Various mouthwashes and tablets are available such as Supreme Klean Saliva Wash, Ultra Wash Toxin-Cleansing Mouthwash, Detox Mouthwash by Stinger, and Saliva Detox Kit [44,45]. One study of some commercially available adulterants or potential adulterants (Clear Choice, Fizzy Flush, Spit and Clean Mouthwash, and Cool Mint Listerine) had no substantial effect on oral testing results after 30 minutes [41]. A brief rinsing effect may be possible with these agents, including water [41].

Limitations to oral fluid testing include short detection periods, similar to serum testing. Orally ingested and smoked substances may have higher concentrations in oral fluid than in actual serum levels; however, oral samples give evidence of drug use generally only in the last 12 to 24 hours, though reports vary [26,40]. Additionally, it has been reported that contamination of oral samples can occur with cigarette smoking, commonly found amongst adolescent substance abusers [43].

Sweat

Sweat drug testing is a unique non-invasive technique that can be used to detect or confirm suspected drug use, providing a method of monitoring and deterrence. A tamper-proof semi-permeable patch is placed on the skin of the subject and collected at intervals of 1 to 7 days. Perspiration is captured in the patch, and analyzed. The method screens for the NIDA-5 panel and can detect both parent compounds and metabolites [46]. Patches prevent sample substitution or dilution, but allow for normal activities such as bathing and exercising; an overlay is available for those performing strenuous activity or in humid environments [46].

PharmChek, a manufacturer of the sweat patch, reports that positive results give evidence of suspected drug use but cannot be extrapolated to determine the dose of drug taken, nor the time or pattern of use. A positive result indicates usage during the time when the patch was worn, or within 24 to 48 hours before the patch was applied [46]. Drugs and metabolites are excreted through the sweat over a period of time similar to that seen with urine. Differential excretion of substances in the sweat, and small sample volumes may affect testing accuracy [47]. Environmental contamination of patch results may be possible.

Sweat patch testing has been increasingly used in the criminal justice system because of ease of use, resistance to adulteration, and the ability to detect use over prolonged periods of time [48]. The use of the sweat patch was upheld in a 2006 US Court of Appeals Eighth Circuit decision in which Honorable O'Connor remarked:

Today, we join the other courts that have previously determined that sweat patch results are a generally reliable method of determining whether an offender has violated a condition of his or her probation. It is important to note that the Food and Drug Administration cleared the PharmChem sweat patch technology back in 1990. Today, the sweat patch is a widely used method for drug testing that is authorized by the Administrative Office of the United States Courts. [48].

Hair, oral fluid, and sweat drug testing are alternative, useful adjuncts to urine and serum testing methods. Urine is still the specimen of choice when confirming or exploring suspicions of drug or alcohol use [41].

TESTING METHODS

All sample specimens, described above, are methods of body fluid collection subjected to similar biochemical testing. Routine testing methods employ screening by immunoassay, with confirmatory testing by gas chromatography-mass spectrometry for positive results. The tests vary in sensitivity, specificity, accuracy, and cost [49].

Immunoassay

Immunoassays use selective antigen-antibody binding to detect the presence of drugs or their metabolites. Immunoassays are available for commercial purchase and are the initial and often primary source for substance abuse testing. They may be used by "point-of-care" personnel such as physicians, nurses, substance abuse counselors, probation officers, or parents [31,32,50]. Detection of binding, proportional to the concentration of the suspected substance present, is measured with enzymes, radioisotopes, or fluorescent compounds [49].

Immunoassays may not differentiate between specific drugs in a given class. False positives occur as a result of antibody binding to non-target compounds similar in structure to the desired target [50]. Therefore, positive results are reported as "presumptive," with further clarification by confirmatory testing with greater specificity. The quality of commercial products may vary in specificity and thresholds for detection [50]. Commercial products generally have package inserts that describe cross-reactivities. Federal guidelines for qualified laboratories utilize cut-off thresholds for detection of substances of abuse, by both immunoassay and confirmatory methods, established by SAMHSA [51]. These are discussed in more detail below.

Immunoassays provide inexpensive, rapid, and automated results to detect multiple suspected substances in a minimum of sample material. Among the many types of techniques available, the most widely used is the enzyme multiplied immunoassay technique (EMIT). Other forms include enzyme-linked immunosorbent assay (ELISA), radioimmunoassay (RIA), fluorescence polarization immunoassay (FPIA), latex agglutination immunoassay, cloned enzyme donor immunoassay, and immunoturbidimetric assay [22,49].

The EMIT uses enzymatic reaction as the detection mechanism. It is simple, inexpensive and relatively user independent. RIA identifies desired targets with radiolabeled isotopes, and is less prone to dilution or adulteration effects, but is more costly and time consuming. FPIA uses fluorescein-labeled drugs that compete with an unlabeled drug for antibody. Although highly sensitive and specific, the method allows for background interference in serum samples. Latex agglutination immunoassay is a unique technique that pairs a sample with latex beads coated with antibodies. Presence of the target causes agglutination. Samples are incubated at room temperature for 1–8 hours [49,50,52].

Chromatography

Chromatography is a specific technique utilized for confirmatory testing. Inert gas carries urine and other substrates through chromatographic columns. Components are then separated by boiling points and affinity for the column. The compounds are identified by separation and retention time, which are unique and reproducible for each substance. Common methods of chromatography are gas chromatography-mass spectrometry (GC-MS), thin-layer chromatography (TLC), and high-performance liquid chromatography (HPLC).

Gas chromatography-mass spectrometry is the standard for confirmatory drug testing. Compounds are separated by gas chromatography and analyzed by mass spectrometry. This method is highly accurate and able to detect small concentrations of multiple substances in a single sample [49,50,53]. Results identify molecular weights and chemical structures of the compounds, providing definitive identification of the retrieved substance [54], rather than the similarities in structure indicated by immunoassay.

A disadvantage of GC-MS is that it requires a labor-intensive, and thus costly, process, rendering it impractical for initial testing [49]. False positives, although rare, can occur with substances that have the same mass spectrum layout or ionization, affecting retention time [53]. A similar but more recent method, termed tandem mass spectrometry (MS-MS), utilizes dual mass spectrometers to increase test sensitivity [55]. Another limitation of GC-MS is that unlike immunoassays, which can screen for multiple substances simultaneously, a particular GC-MS study is directed toward a specific substance in question. Therefore a substance that is not specified will not be found on GC-MS.

Thin-layer chromatography is generally considered a screening method used to test for a number of agents. This method is not as accurate as GC-MS, and requires up to 4 hours and a minimum concentration to detect the target substance. Samples are applied to a prepared plate, and components are identified by separation using a solvent. Separation of compounds is identified manually as spots on the TLC plate. A significant disadvantage of this technique is the user-dependent results in interpreting colors, peaks, and spots on the plate [56].

High-performance liquid chromatography achieves compound separation on a column using a principle similar to TLC. In this method, however, the solvent is introduced to the column at high pressure through smaller particle-sized column materials, allowing for better separation at a fast rate. The technique is detailed and costly, but offers high specificity. Liquid chromatography with mass spectrometry has the advantage of being able to detect low concentrations of drugs. This method also uses smaller samples, requires less preparation, and provides less interference than GC-MS [56].

TESTING RELIABILITY AND RESULT INTERPRETATION

Interpretation of test results by clinicians, parents, and others requires a basic discussion and understanding of statistical measures. The general consideration of test "reliability" actually involves measures of precision, accuracy, sensitivity, specificity, and predictive value.

Validity refers to "accuracy," and indicates the test's ability to measure what it claims to measure. Reliability refers to "precision," and is defined as a test's ability to provide a consistent, reproducible result. A laboratory test might be reliable, without being valid. That is, consistent results might be reported that do not represent the true target measurement of the test. Reliability is a necessary but insufficient requirement for validity. Therefore a useful test leading to various treatment and forensic outcomes must be both reliable (precise) and valid (accurate).

Of great importance is the understanding that a negative test result does not exclude the use of the substance. It might indicate that the substance was not present at the detection threshold, the test did not assess for the actual substance used (e.g., "designer drugs") or there was interference by faulty collection methods or tampering. Clinical correlation must always be applied when interpreting results.

Precision

Reliability of drug screening and confirmatory methods is provided for by quality assurance methods, and standardization of specimen collection and handling. For greatest reliability, these quality control methods must be assured both in the laboratory and at point-of-care.

Drug testing, which frequently is used for judiciary and forensic purposes, mostly in the adult population but also in adolescents, must reliably and defensively determine specimens that contain drugs of abuse, or their metabolites, and identify specimens that have been tampered.

Testing reliability is monitored by the National Institute of Drug Abuse, the Substance Abuse and Mental Health Services Administration (SAMHSA), and other federal agencies, which provide certification and regulation for laboratories approved for forensic use. Mandatory Guidelines are established by the National Laboratory Certification Program (NLCP), setting comprehensive testing standards, quality assurance, chain of custody procedures, personnel training, and reporting confidentiality [57].

Laboratory quality assurance procedures are inspected from specimen collection through result confirmation and reporting. Mandatory NLCP guidelines require inspection of each certified laboratory at least twice a year to document performance, quarterly proficiency challenges, and an external blind control specimen program [57]. Laboratories may additionally obtain certification from the College of American Pathologists (CAP). SAMHSA maintains a list of all certified laboratories by state, on their website (http://workplace. samhsa.gov). Not all laboratories are certified; however, those approved for use in the federal workplace program require such certification.

Forensic standards and chain of custody procedures are perhaps outside of the scope of this chapter, which is geared to clinicians treating adolescents, unlikely to require such stringent collection methods. Frequently,

screening tests are administered at point-of-care, and are used to guide clinical decision-making. However, it is important to note that collection procedures might affect both precision and test accuracy, and it is not uncommon for substance-abusing adolescents to be involved in various disciplinary processes. Various certification programs are offered to provide training in proper collection techniques.

In brief, urine is collected under direct observation and properly identified. Secure transfer, preventing unauthorized access to the specimen, is assured. Often samples are split into two separate aliquots, allowing retesting and laboratory confirmation if necessary. On-site validity testing is completed, as described below. Samples that require formal laboratory testing, must be delivered in a timely manner, as determined by guidelines for the particular sample and laboratory. Laboratories can be contacted for procedures associated with their specific products.

Test methods themselves are approved for use by the US Food and Drug Administration (FDA) prior to marketing, and undergo extensive tests for reliability, and validity.

Accuracy

Accuracy, the ability to identify true drugs of abuse in samples in which they are actually present, is affected by standards set for sensitivity and specificity. Sensitivity may be defined as the ability of a test to identify all those cases in which the target drug of abuse is present in the sample source (true positives). A test with a very high sensitivity might have such low thresholds for detection that although a negative result provides strong assurance that the sample is drug free, the proportion of false positives increases. Therefore sensitivity must be balanced by specificity.

Specificity represents the ability of the test to rule out those samples that do not have drugs of abuse present (true negatives). A test with very high specificity might utilize such high thresholds for detection, that although a positive result strongly indicates the presence of the drug, the proportion of false negatives increases. That is, a highly specific test will exclude samples that truly have drugs of abuse present, but at lower concentrations than the threshold level of detection. Ideally tests aim for both high sensitivity and specificity.

NIDA and SAMHSA determine cut-off thresholds for reporting of results positive for the presence of substances of abuse. Threshold standards are examined and updated, and represent a compromise between sensitivity and specificity, in an attempt to identify the majority of true substance use in submitted samples while avoiding false positives secondary to passive contact and

Table 10.1 Federal drug-testing cut-off thresholds.

Substance	Screening/immunoassay cut-off [51]	Confirmation/GC-MS cut-off [51]
Amphetamine (amphetamine and methamphetamine)	500 ng/mL	250 ng/mL
Cocaine metabolites (benzoylecgonine)	150 ng/mL	100 ng/mL
Heroin (6-acetylmorphine)	10 ng/mL	10 ng/mL
Marijuana metabolites (delta-9-tetrahydrocannabinol-9-carboxylic acid)	50 ng/mL	15 ng/mL
MDMA, MDA, MDEA (methylenedioxymethamphetamine, also including methylenedioxyamphetamine and methylenedioxyethylamphetamine)	500 ng/mL	250 ng/mL
Opiate metabolites (morphine, for heroin, morphine and codeine use)	2000 ng/mL	2000 ng/mL
Phencyclidine	25 ng/mL	25 ng/mL

other test confounders. Cut-off thresholds tend to higher specificity to eliminate the "passive inhalation" explanation.

Table 10.1 illustrates the most recent federally determined thresholds for the detection of substances of abuse in urine, effective October 2010 [51]. Laboratories might adopt these recommended thresholds, or expand their cut-offs to lower thresholds, or to include additional substances. Of note, detection thresholds developed for adult populations may be inadequate for the child and young adolescent population, as urine is more dilute [49].

In developing accurate methods for drug abuse screening, results are compared with GC-MS, which represents the "gold standard" or best testing method available to identify drugs of abuse in sample sources. As previously described, GC-MS is impractical for use as a routine screening method. The accuracy of the EMIT immunoassay, the most commonly utilized routine screening method, has been reported to range from approximately 87% to 99% [58,59]. Such studies have indicated that EMIT immunoassays can accurately identify drugs of abuse in urine samples, in which their presence was confirmed by GC-MS.

Predictive Value

In addition to reliability (reproducibility) and validity (accuracy), another important distinction in interpreting drug tests is the "predictive value" of a positive result. Positive predictive value refers to the probability that a positive is indeed evidence of the use of a targeted substance. This term appears deceptively similar to accuracy. Whereas accuracy in drug testing indicates that the tests can reliably identify substances of abuse when they are actually present, positive predictive value

looks toward the value of a positive result in predicting actual use. High specificity, such as employed by federal cut-off thresholds, is expected to minimize false positives.

Prevalence of drug use in a specific population statistically affects the predictive power of the test results. That is, given the same test accuracy and specificity, a positive result in a population with low prevalence of substance abuse (e.g., young children) has substantially less predictive value than in a population with high prevalence of substance abuse (e.g., an adult population of recent arrestees) because of the high ratio of false positives to true positives. The same is true with regards to the actual substance; in a population in which MDMA is more prevalent (e.g., "rave club" attendees), a positive result has greater predictive value than in a population in which its use is rare (e.g., Vietnam veterans), as the ratio of false positives to true positives is lower than in the latter population.

Few recent studies of rates of overall false positives in immunoassay drug screens in general samples have been designed with enough statistical power to draw substantial conclusions. This is understandable as such studies would require large numbers of random urines to undergo screening tests followed by GC-MS for a wide variety of substances to exclude cross-reactivities and reagent interference, and to examine for substances that might be present at subthreshold levels. Various specific contributors to false positive and false negative results are examined below.

False positive rates in immunoassays have been reported to be as high as 28.8% for opiates, 25.9% for amphetamines, 7.9% for cocaine, and 7.8% for cannabis [49]. Rates differ dependent upon the particular test and manufacturer. Some potential contributors to false positive results remain unknown. Further, the actual incidence of false positives in the absence of known cross-reactants is unknown.

There are various studies examining routine medication known to cross-react with immunoassay antibodies that lead to positive results in the absence of the actual drug of abuse. Brahm *et al.* demonstrated that upon an examination of routine medication in an urban clinic, 21.5% of formulary medications were reported to be associated with false positive urine drug screens, with amphetamine representing the highest false positive result [60].

Consideration of these factors, and the potential for adverse clinical and judiciary outcomes, indicates that positive results from screening exams should be considered "presumptive" and followed by confirmatory testing prior to result reporting [60].

Factors Affecting Reliability and Validity

False positive immunoassay findings may result from cross-reactivity of medications, reagent interference, test operator errors, equipment contamination, and sample mislabeling. Table 10.2 illustrates routine medications that are known to cross-react with immunoassays [27,49,60–62]. Special care must be taken when interpreting positive results from individuals with significant metabolic derangement, renal disease, and liver disease [49].

False negative immunoassay findings are often the result of tampering to obscure a positive finding; however, they might also occur secondary to improper specimen handling and significantly delayed transport of specimens to a designated laboratory (allowing for target agent degradation). Tampering generally takes the form of specimen substitution or dilution, and adulteration. Physiological characteristics of urine can be used in some cases to determine substantial tampering, referred to as validity testing.

Specimen substitution is a means by which the evaluee purposely offers a "clean" urine sample, or synthetic substitute, from another individual or animal. This may be accomplished in non-observed urine collection by emptying a sample, often kept close to the body in order to maintain temperature, previously brought by the evaluee, into the collection cup. In observed collections, substitution is still possible through catheterization of "clean" urine into the evaluee's bladder prior to the testing [63].

In 2003 SAMHSA first began investigating urine substitutes when a product, "Minuteman," was found at a workplace site subjected to drug testing. The product was a dehydrated drug-free urine sample that could be used as a substitute for an individual urine sample. Since 2003, multiple kits that range in cost from 50 to 100s of dollars are available for purchase. Other products, such as catheterization kits, elaborate devices such as a prosthetic penis, "clean" samples, and synthetic urine (e.g. "Quick Fix Synthetic Urine") containing physiologic pH, specific gravity, and creatinine, are also available [29,63]. Physiologic temperatures might be

Table 10.2 Cross-reactivities associated with immunoassay false positives.

Target agents	Agents associated with false positives [27,49,60,61]
Amphetamine/methamphetamine	Amantadine, brompheniramine, bupropion, chloroquine, chlorpromazine, desipramine, ephedrine, fenfluramine, labetalol, MDMA, methylphenidate, *N*-acetylprocainamide, phentermine, phenylephrine, phenylpropanolamine, promethazine, propranolol, pseudoephedrine, quinacrine, ranitidine, ritodrine, selegiline, trazodone, trimethobenzamide, trimipramine, tyramine, Vick's Inhaler (L-methamphetamine)
Barbiturates	Ibuprofen, naproxen
Benzodiazepines	Oxaprozin, sertraline
Cannabinoids	Dronabinol, efavirenz, esomeprazole, hemp, ibuprofen, lansoprazole, naproxen, omeprazole, pantoprazole, tolmetin
Cocaine	Fluconazole, topical anesthetics containing cocaine
Lysergic acid diethylamide (LSD)	Amitriptyline, chlorpromazine, doxepin, fluoxetine, haloperidol, metaclopramide, risperidone, sertraline, verapamil
Methadone	Chlorpromazine, clomipramine, diphenhydramine, doxylamine, ibuprofen, quetiapine, verapamil
Opiates	Dextromethorphan, diphenhydramine, poppy seeds, quinine, quinolones, rifampin, verapamil
Phencyclidine	Dextromethorphan, diphenhydramine, desmethylvenlafaxine, doxylamine, ibuprofen, imipramine, ketamine, meperidine, tramadol, venlafaxine

easily reached through the use of heating pads and microwaves [29]. This type of tampering, although extreme, might be expected in high stakes testing such as in legal proceedings or athletics, as well as workplace testing for adults, particularly among professionals.

Dilution refers to attempts to dilute a urine specimen to such a degree as to effectively decrease the concentration of drug below cut-off levels. Urine can be diluted externally through the addition of water to the sample, or internally through the use of diuretics or the ingestion of large volumes of water prior to testing.

Adulteration is another method to obscure a positive test result, whereby the evaluee adulterates the urine sample through the use of additives that affect test results. Various substances may be added to the urine sample that purport to degrade or obscure the drug and/or drug metabolites, or alter urine pH to adversely affect the assay or reagent interaction. Adulterants can be additionally ingested by the donor to alter urine pH or aid in renal clearance and elimination. Information on these techniques is widely available to the public online. As is evident below, delta-9-tetrahydro-cannabinol (THC) assays are most sensitive to adulteration [49].

Common substances added to urine samples leading to false negative results include:

- salt;
- baking soda;
- bleach – false negative for THC, lysergic acid diethylamide (LSD), benzodiazepines, codeine and morphine;
- peroxide – false negative for THC, LSD, benzodiazepines, codeine and morphine;
- detergents – false negative for THC, phencyclidine (PCP), benzodiazepines;
- liquid soaps;
- ammonia;
- vinegar – false negative for THC, opiates, and cocaine;
- lemon juice;
- Visine (eyedrops) – false negative for THC; and even
- bathroom cleaning solutions.

Most current drug tests can detect common household adulterants, but may not be able to distinguish the use of Visine (tetrahydrolozine) [29].

Various products might be ingested to adulterate urine samples. These include Golden Seal (false negative for THC), fluconazole (false negative for cocaine), or any of a number of commercially available products such as "Klear," "Whizzies," "Urine Luck," and "Premium Detox 7 Day Kit," which contain glutaraldehyde,

nitrates, or other substances that affect urine test results [29,49,63]. Other attempts to adulterate urine involve ingestion of salicylates, large quantities of vitamin C, vinegar, and acidic fruit juices to acidify the urine and enhance elimination of amphetamines and PCP, thereby decreasing drug detection time [63].

Validity Testing

Validity testing is used to identify specimen substitution, dilution, and adulteration. Physiologic urinary ranges are measured to exclude samples suggestive of tampering. Tampering is generally considered to be evidence of a presumptive positive result. SAMHSA sets guidelines for validity testing [64].

Urine is considered substituted to beyond characteristics associated with normal human urine if the creatinine concentration is less than 5 mg/dL and the specific gravity is outside of the range of 1.001 to 1.020 [64]. Temperature strips are additionally available for most commercial urine screening tests, and values outside of 89.6°F to 100.4°F (32–38°C), within 4 minutes of collection, suggest substitution [49].

A urine sample is considered dilute if the creatinine is less than 20 mg/dL and the specific gravity is less than 1.003, unless the criteria for a substituted specimen are met [64].

Evidence of an adulterated sample is demonstrated with a nitrite concentration less than 500 fg/mL, a pH outside the range 3 to 11, the presence of an exogenous substance, or the presence of an endogenous substance at a higher than physiologic concentration [64]. Results indicating values outside the normal range, or noted precipitants, may indicate the use of such adulterants as salt or Golden Seal.

Additional measures, which might be used by point-of-care providers, as well as laboratory technicians, to ensure sample integrity include observation of expected color and odor to detect some adulterants such as ammonia, bleach, or vinegar.

COMMON SUBSTANCES OF ABUSE

What follows is a brief discussion of common substances of abuse. Full treatment of each of these specific substances is outside the scope of this chapter. Table 10.3 illustrates detection periods for common drugs of abuse, based on sample type.

Detection times are often given as ranges, as clearance times for individuals may vary based on age, drug concentration consumed, body mass index, gender, and renal and hepatic function. Higher ranges are more likely in chronic users with higher body mass

Table 10.3 Comparison ranges of detection times between various sample sources [27,31,43,49,62].

Drug	Serum detection time	Oral detection time	Urine detection time	Hair detection time
Alcohol	7–24 h			
Amphetamine	46 h	20–50 h	1–9 days	Up to 90 days
Barbiturates:				
short–acting	2–4 h	50 h	1–6 days	
long–acting			7–21 days	
Benzodiazipines:				
short–acting	2–7 h		72 h	
long–acting		5–50 h	2–30 days	
Benzoylecgonine (cocaine metabolite)	48 h	12–24 h	48–72 h	
Buprenorphine		5 days	4–8 days	
Cannabis (single dose)	5 h	2–34 h	9–78 h	
Cannabis (chronic use)	2–14 days		Up to 95 days	Up to 90 days
Cocaine (single dose)	6–12 h	5–12 h	14–59 h	Up to 90 days
Cocaine (chronic use)	48 h	8–48 h	5–9 days	Up to 90 days
Codeine		7–21 h	24–48 h	Up to 90 days
Gamma–hydroxybutyric acid (GHB)	5–8 h	5 h	12 h	
Heroin	20 h	2–24 h	7–54 h	Up to 90 days
Hydrocodone		7–21 h	11–36 h	
Hydromorphone (single dose)		6 h	6–24 h	
Ketamine			3 days	
Lysergic acid diethylamide (LSD)	N/A	N/A	36–96 h	
MDMA (ecstasy)	24 h	24 h	1–3 days	Up to 90 days
Methamphetamine	24–48 h	6–76 h	1–6 days	Up to 90 days
Methadone		24 h	24–96 h	
Nicotine (continine, >28 g)	4–6 h	4 days	4 days	
Phencyclidine (PCP)	1–3 days	N/A	8–30 days	Up to 90 days

indices, older age, and impaired metabolic function [27,31,43,49].

Alcohol

Alcohol is the most widely used intoxicant in the world [49] and the most accessible of all abused substances for adolescents. According to the US Monitoring the Future survey of 2010, alcohol was easily accessible to 60% of 8th-graders, 80% of 10th-graders and 90% of 12th-graders [65]. In 2010, 14%, 29%, and 41% of 8th-, 10th-, and 12th-graders, respectively, had used alcohol in the prior 30 days. Additionally, 12th-graders did not perceive binge drinking as a significant concern [65].

Alcohol is a centrally acting depressant, leading to, in extreme cases, coma or respiratory failure. It serves as a disinhibitor and intoxicant. Within 30–60 minutes of ingestion, ethanol is absorbed through the gastrointestinal tract and primarily metabolized in the liver at an average rate of 0.015–0.020 g/dL/h, increasing to up to 0.030 g/dL/h in certain users [66,67]. Metabolism and absorption are affected by food intake, chronicity of use, age, gender, ethnicity, genetics, and other factors. A small proportion of unchanged alcohol is excreted in the urine, sweat, and breath. Various stereotypic toxic effects of heavy alcohol use may be measured, providing the basis for the use of biomarkers in complementary assessment of problematic alcohol use [68].

Blood alcohol level (BAL), or blood alcohol concentration (BAC), is the accepted measure of alcohol exposure and intoxication. Alcohol can be detected in the blood only for a brief period of approximately 8–12 hours [28].

Detection of alcohol use may also be assessed through the use of Evidence Breath Test Devices (EBT), which measure breath alcohol content (BrAC) and indirectly estimate BAC with accurate correlation [67]. They are commercially available as handheld devices and utilize semiconductor oxide sensor or fuel cell sensor technologies. The devices are reliable and may be used in the measurement of BrAC for evidential purposes [67].

Difficulties with breathalyzers include inability for later test confirmation, potential calibration issues, and errors in estimating BAC from the BrAC. Forensic users require basic training with the device, and repeat testing, following a blank test, is advised 15 to 30 minutes after the initial test. False positives or inaccurately elevated results have been reported in diabetics (acetone in breath), individuals with obstructive lung diseases, or the use of other volatile substances such as breath spray containing isopropyl alcohol. A 15-minute period of observation is recommended prior to testing, at least in part to ensure against inaccurate readings due to residual alcohol in the mouth [67].

Alcohol use can be assessed in select urine drug screens that assay for the presence of the alcohol metabolite ethyl glucuronide (EtG), referred to as a biomarker, which can be identified in urine for up to 72 hours after alcohol ingestion. According to a SAMHSA Advisory, as a new technology, ethyl glucuronide tests lack sufficient proven specificity for use as primary evidence that an individual has engaged in alcohol use [68]. Standard thresholds for EtG detection have not yet been established, and the predictive value of a positive test result is in question. Furthermore, test result variation in the presence of diseases, gender, ethnicity, and other variables is unclear. Potential false positives of this highly sensitive test may occur with incidental exposure to alcohol found in medications, hygiene products, and food, as well as urine alcohols resulting from fermentation in diabetics.

Additional biomarkers useful in assessing for problematic alcohol use include gamma-glutamyltransferase (GGT), alanine aminotransferase (ALT), aspartate aminotransferase (AST), mean corpuscular volume (MCV), and others. When associated with actual alcohol use, these biomarkers indicate chronic alcohol consumption, and therefore are not useful in determining acute usage. They are, rather, useful clinical tools to aid in treatment intervention. A new and promising alcohol marker, phosphatidyl ethanol (PEth), might allow serum-based detection of alcohol use for up to 3 weeks [68].

Amphetamines and Ephedra Derivatives

Amphetamines were developed in the late 1880s as a derivative of plant-based ephedra, followed by the development of methylphenidate in 1919, and methamphetamine in 1920. Amphetamines were not generally used until the 1930s when stimulant and decongestant properties were identified [69]. Amphetamine and methamphetamine have high potential for abuse.

Ephedra, from the Chinese herb ma-huang (*Ephedra sinica*), yields 1–3% ephedrine. This compound is often marketed as a legal stimulant and used in weight loss products. Due to widespread availability and marketing as "natural" or "herbal," ephedra is often mistakenly thought of by consumers as entirely safe for use. In 2006 the FDA banned ephedra-containing dietary supplements due to association with severe cardiovascular side effects and deaths [70]. Derivatives such as ephedrine and pseudoephedrine continue to be used in decongestant medication. Ma huang remains commercially available in energy-promoting, weight loss, and thermogenic supplements.

Amphetamine and methamphetamine are Schedule II drugs available as Adderall (amphetamine) and Desoxyn (methamphetamine). Commercial use has included indications as antidepressants, weight loss agents, stimulants, decongestants, and as treatment for attention-deficit/hyperactivity disorder and narcolepsy. Amphetamine and methamphetamine are available in pill form and as crystalline powders, manufactured by illegal laboratories, on the illicit market.

Methamphetamine is known crystal, glass, ice, tina, tweek, and meth. Amphetamine is known as crank and speed. They are chemically related centrally acting stimulants providing euphoria, increased energy, and appetite suppression [62]. Routes of administration include oral ingestion, nasal inhalation, smoking, and intravenous administration.

Methamphetamine in its crystallized form grew in popularity in the 1980s due to wide availability and low cost. In 1990 the use in 12th-graders was approximately 1.3%, increasing in 1998 to approximately 3%. Prevalence of methamphetamine use in 2010, was 1.2% for 8th-graders, 1.6% for 10th-graders and 1% for 12th-graders, representing a dramatic decline (greater than 70%) from its use in 1999 [65].

Therapeutic doses of amphetamine range from 5 to 60 mg daily, with common abused doses of 100 to 1000 mg/day, and up to 5000 mg/day in chronic users [62]. The average half-life for amphetamine detection in urine is 7 to 34 hours.

Variability in urine pH affects elimination rates. In the presence of neutral urinary pH, 30% of amphetamine is excreted unchanged in the urine. As urine is acidified toward a pH of 5, the proportion excreted unchanged increases to 75% [27]. Acidic pH aids in rapid urinary elimination of the drug. Amphetamines can be detected in the blood for up to 46 hours at a cut-off level of 4 ng/mL, oral fluid analysis allows detection for up to 50 hours with a cut-off level of 10 ng/mL [27].

Therapeutic doses of methamphetamine range from 2.5 to 10 mg daily, with abused doses similar to those for amphetamine. The mean elimination half-life of methamphetamine (10 h) is similar or slightly shorter than that of amphetamine (12 h). As peak blood methamphetamine concentrations occur moments after injection, minutes after smoking, and approximately 3 hours after oral dosing, detection times are dependent upon the route of administration [62]. Up to 54% of an oral dose is excreted in urine as methamphetamine and 23% as the metabolite amphetamine, dependent upon urinary pH. Following intravenous use, 45% is excreted as methamphetamine and 7% as amphetamine [62].

Smoked methamphetamine can be detected in the blood for 4 to 48 hours. The metabolite amphetamine is only detectable in blood samples for 4 hours (cut-off 1 ng/mL), whereas methamphetamine may be detected for up to 48 hours (cut-off 4 ng/mL) [27].

Oral detection of methamphetamine depends on chronicity of use. Following a single dose, methamphetamines can be detected orally for approximately 24 hours; however, following more heavy use (three to four times), the substance can be detected in oral samples for up to 72 hours. Interestingly, the oral fluid concentration has been found to be two to four times higher than plasma levels. A unique, processed, smokable form of methamphetamine called 'ice' can be detected in the urine for up to 60 hours [27].

To summarize, a positive urine screening generally indicates use within 24 to 72 hours, but may indicate usage greater than 1 week prior, following chronic use. Common sources of false positive results are summarized in Table 10.2, and include trazodone, bupropion, desoxyephedrine-based nasal inhalers, and ephedrine-based cold medication (the latter two may result in false positive results on GC-MS, requiring additional testing to provide discrimination) [27,49,60,61].

As previously discussed, amphetamines have been reported to have false positive results of up to 25.9% on immunoassays, with one study finding that amphetamines represented the highest rate of false positives associated with cross-reactivities [49,59]. It should be noted that the "club drug" ecstasy (MDMA) requires high concentrations in the urine to lead to positive results on amphetamine immunoassays [49].

Benzodiazepines

Benzodiazepines are a Schedule IV sedative drug class commonly prescribed for anxiety, sleep, and seizure disorders. Common forms include diazepine, clonazepam, alprazolam, and lorazepam. These medications are sold on the illicit market as the result of drug diversion and theft, and are used for their sedative qualities as well as their ability to potentiate other substances of abuse, such as alcohol or opiates.

With increasing use of prescription medication in adults and teens, benzodiazepine abuse has increased; these drugs are easily obtained from legitimate users as well as on the street. Benzodiazepine abuse declined in the late 1970s to early 1990s; however, in the early 2000s use doubled and has continued to rise. As of 2010, 2.8% of 8th-graders, 5.1% of 10th-graders, and 5.6% of 12th-graders have abused these substances [65].

The pharmacokinetics of benzodiazepines vary, according to the lipophilicity and half-life of the individual drugs. Screening tests do not discriminate between single or chronic use, nor do they distinguish between individual drugs. Serum testing can identify lipophilic agents such as diazepam within minutes, and its metabolites (oxazepam and temazepam conjugates) in the urine within 36 hours. Agents, including metabolites, with long half-lives can be identified in the urine for up to 30 days after use [49,62].

False positives in urine immunoassays for benzodiazepines have been reported to be associated with sertraline and oxaprozin use [27,49,60,61].

Cocaine

Cocaine is derived from the leaves of the coca plant, used by Native Americans for thousands of years in Peru and Bolivia as a mild stimulant. Albert Neimann, a German chemist, isolated cocaine hydrochloride (methylbenzoylecgonine) from the plant in the mid-1800s. Cocaine has since had a colorful history, and books have been written touting its virtues as an anesthetic, appetite suppressant, stimulant, analgesic, "addiction cure," and antidepressant, including "On Coca" by Sigmund Freud [71,72].

By the early 1900s, cocaine was used in many products in Europe and the United States for medicinal purposes (anesthetics, tonics, and psychoactive compounds) as well as in wines, elixirs and soft drinks such as Coca-Cola. However, adverse reactions as the result of its use had already been documented. In 1903 Coca-Cola removed cocaine as an ingredient in its popular soft drink, and by 1914, the Harrison Narcotic Act banned cocaine from all the over-the-counter medications along with its use in food and beverages [71].

Cocaine is a Schedule II drug, used as a 4% solution of hydrochloride salt, by otolaryngologists and emergency room physicians as a topical anesthetic and vasoconstrictive agent. The National Survey on Drug Use and Health in 2006 reported that cocaine was the second most commonly used illicit substance following marijuana [73]. It is available on the illicit market as powder, or as small, smokable rocks in the case of the cocaine base ("crack" cocaine). Cocaine is referred to as blow, snow, coke, or toot, and the cocaine base is referred to as rock or crack. It can be ingested orally, nasally, through smoking, or intravenously.

Cocaine was generally used as an inhaled or injected substance until the mid-1980s, when cocaine base (first as "freebase," then as "crack") spread throughout the United States as an epidemic. Use progressively increased until the sensational death of Leonard Bias, a top draft pick in the 1986 National Basketball League, after his purported initial use of cocaine. The sensation led to the passage of the 1986 Federal Anti Drug Abuse Act, providing for more stringent penalties and educational programs. Cocaine use decreased until the early 1990s and then remained stable throughout the 1990s.

The Monitoring the Future Survey of 2008 found that 1.8% of 8th-graders, 3.0% of 10th-graders and 4.4% of 12th-graders had used cocaine [1]. The most recent Survey in 2010 showed that use in the prior 12 months for all three groups was below 4%. Over 30% of 12th-graders reported access to cocaine in 2010 [65].

Cocaine is commonly abused in doses of 10 to 120 mg. The half-life of cocaine is very short, 1 hour or less; the inactive metabolite, benzoylecgonine, has a half-life about 6 hours. Cocaethylene, formed during the metabolism of cocaine, in the presence of concurrent alcohol use, is an active and potent metabolite [62].

The major metabolite of cocaine, benzoylecgonine (BE), can be detected in the urine for up to 3 to 4 days after a single dose [27,62]. However, intravenous cocaine users may show detectable levels of BE in the urine for only 1 to 2 days [27]. Chronic use of cocaine can result in detection in urine for up to 10 days [62]. When cocaine is used for nasal surgery either as an anesthetic or vasoconstrictor, BE is detectable in the urine for up to 24 hours, clearing within 72 hours [74].

Detection of cocaine in the blood ranges from 5 to 12 hours, varying with doses from 20 to 100 mg. In chronic users, BE can be detected in the blood for up to 8 days (cut-off of 25 ng/mL) [27].

Oral fluid detection of the parent compound, cocaine, after a single dose is between 5 and 12 hours; however, the major metabolite can be detected orally for up to 24 hours (cut-off 1 ng/mL). Chronic cocaine users can submit positive oral tests for up to 10 days (cut-off of 0.5 ng/mL) [27].

Hair sampling tests for the presence of cocaine, using the MALDI-MS technique for cocaine, can identify 10–100 ng/mL of the substance and its metabolites in as little as 1 mg of hair [39].

Cocaine has few cross-reactions leading to false positives on immunoassays. Reports have noted fluconazole to be associated with false positive results [61]. The predictive value of a positive immunoassay ranges from 92% to 97.8% [49]. Non-cocaine topical anesthetics such as procaine, lidocaine, and benzocaine are amides not detected as cocaine.

Inhalants

Inhalant abuse refers to the use of commonly obtained commercial volatile substances to achieve intoxication. Substances used are generally aromatic hydrocarbons (adhesives), aliphatic hydrocarbons (aerosols or fuels), alkyl halides (solvents or paints), and nitrites. Use of inhalants is a worldwide problem particularly affecting adolescents in developing countries because of their ready accessibility and very low cost. Commonly used inhalants include all toluene-containing substances, whiteout correction fluid, various cleaning products, paint thinner, whipped cream gas dispensers, amyl nitrate "poppers," freon-based computer keyboard dusters, glue, and many other daily use products that are virtually ubiquitous [75,76].

The US Monitoring the Future survey in 2010 found approximately 8% of 8th-graders, 6% of 10th-graders, and 4% of 12th-graders had used inhalants in the prior 12 months [65]. The prevalence of inhalant abuse appears to decline with age [76].

Toluene, the most widely abused inhalant, is rapidly absorbed following inhalation and is detectable in blood within 10 seconds of inhalation exposure. It is highly lipophilic; the initial half-life ranges approximately from 3 to 6 hours. Up to 20% is excreted unchanged in the lungs, and the remainder as inactive metabolites in urine.

Inhalants are not routinely included in serum or urine drug screens, however, they may be specifically requested if suspicion is high. Urinary o-cresol and hippuric acid concentrations correlate with blood toluene concentrations [62,76]. Results are not immediately available and therefore clinical correlation is recommended for immediate treatment, including perhaps arterial blood gas testing.

Lysergic Acid Diethylamide (LSD)

LSD was synthesized by Albert Hoffman in 1938 while exploring ergot derivatives for various pharmaceutical uses. Ergotamine-producing rye mold is suspected to have produced cases of psychosis in the Middle Ages because of its psychoactive properties. It was first marketed by Sandoz Laboratories in 1947 as a psychiatric medication.

Like cocaine and opiates, LSD has had profound cultural and sociological effects. Considered to be the herald of the 1960s "flower power revolution," LSD use was promoted by Harvard psychologist Timothy Leary,

Aldous Huxley, and others, and stood as the essential base from which many 1960s era musical bands such as the Doors, Grateful Dead, and Pink Floyd grew. It has been, and continues to be, studied for psychiatric, military, and medical purposes as an agent of chemical warfare, psychotherapy, "consciousness expansion," end-of-life care, addiction treatment, and other uses related to its unique psychedelic properties [77] Attitudes toward LSD in the lay and professional community range from an almost fanatical promotion as a pseudo-religious sacrament to its consideration as a dangerous street drug, similar to stances towards psilocybin, mescaline, ibogaine, salvia, ayahuasca, fly agaric, morning glory, jimsonweed, deadly nightshade, and more modern substances such as ketamine and MDMA.

LSD is a Schedule I drug, referred to as blaze, tabs, blotter, microdot, trips, and window panes on the illicit market. It is generally orally ingested.

US-based studies demonstrate slight increases in prevalence of use amongst adolescents and children between 1991 and 1996. Use has since decreased in 8th-, 10th-, and 12th-graders to approximately 3% or less [65].

LSD is ingested in small doses of 50 to 200 μg, and has a half-life of only 2.5 to 5 hours. Metabolites are inactive, and 1% of LSD is excreted in the urine unchanged [27].

LSD and other hallucinogens are not routinely included in urine or serum immunoassays, but can be separately requested. LSD can be detected in urine for 24 hours, with longer detection times of 2 to 5 days related to higher ingested doses [27,62]. The metabolite 2-oxo-3-hydroxy-LSD can be detected in higher concentrations in the urine, with detection times of up to 96 hours [27]. In subjects receiving 200–400 μg of LSD, concentrations in urine ranged from 1 to 55 ng/mL [62].

Table 10.2 includes routine medications that cross-react with urine immunoassays leading to potential false positive results [27,49,60,61].

Marijuana

Marijuana, the common term for the leaves and flowers of the *Cannabis sativa* plant, is the most prevalent illicit substance among adolescents (and in general, worldwide), and is the source for all derived cannabinoids. Marijuana has the least perceived risk and the lowest risk of disapproval of all the substances that adolescents are exposed to [65].

Delta-9-tetrahydrocannabinol (THC) is the primary active agent in cannabis, and produces mild sedative, disinhibitory, and euphoric effects, although long-term use has been associated with increased risk of anxiety, depressive, and psychotic disorders [78]. In its native form as a plant, resin, powder, and oil, cannabis is a Schedule I drug, generally smoked or orally ingested. The scheduling has been challenged on repeated occasions by medical marijuana advocates, and routine medicinal derivatives have been marketed with Schedule II (Canada) and III designations. Various US states have, additionally, reclassified scheduling to allow the legalization of medical marijuana use. This is a contemporary and controversial issue.

THC has been used in medications such as Marinol (dronabinol), Cesamet (nabilone – Canada) and Sativex (THC and cannabidiol – Canada) for anorexia, nausea, pain relief, and spasticity. Therapeutic uses of marijuana have been documented as an antiemetic [79–81], appetite stimulant for cachectic patients [82], anticonvulsant [83,84], and for movement disorders [85], pain control [86–89], and glaucoma [90,91].

Cannabis, widely available on the illicit market, is referred to as weed, herb, pot, grass, ganja, sinse, bud, and reefer, among other terms, and its use spans all age groups and socioeconomic strata. The US National Survey on Drug Use and Health in 2006 found that 44% of males and 35% of females had used marijuana at least once [73]. This high percentage is likely applicable to children and adolescents, as THC is the most frequently detected drug in adolescents.

Marijuana's peak use occurred in the late 1970s, followed by a brief decline, and subsequent increase in the early 1990s. The Monitoring the Future 2008 survey reported that 11% of 8th-graders, 24% of 10th-graders, and 32% of 12th-graders had exposure to marijuana use [1,2]. The 2010 survey demonstrated significant increases in use, with 1.2% of 8th-graders, 3.3% of 10th-graders, and 6.1% of 12th-graders reporting daily use. Up to 80% of 2010 US high school students reported that marijuana was readily accessible to them [65].

Synthetic cannabinoids have been synthesized since the mid-1990s and on sale since 2000. There are approximately 470 synthetic cannabinoids, only five of which have been regulated, despite a 2010 temporary emergency ban of the Drug Enforcement Agency, which was enacted in March 2011. The five synthetics included in the scheduling and temporary ban that came into effect on 1 March 2011 include, JWH-018, JWH-073, JWH-200, CP-47,497, and cannabicyclohexanol [92].

Many other synthetic cannabinoids have eluded regulation, and are available at convenience stores, novelty shops, and online [93–95]. These synthetic forms, marketed as herbal incense and organic spice blends, are available as commercial products such Pep Spice X, Pep Pourri Twisted, Genie, Spice Diamond, K1 Fire Blend, Ex-SES Platinum, and K2 Premium Blend [96]. The continuous manufacture of synthetic cannabinoids and other designer drugs for sale in the public market, over the last 20 years, illustrates the savvy nature of these amateur, and sometimes professional chemists in evading bans and regulations.

Common abuse of THC involves variable intake doses, generally 5 to 30 mg, which the user self-regulates through smoking, or oral ingestion. Smoking results in absorption of THC to peak levels within approximately 10 to 20 minutes, whereas oral ingestion results in peak levels after 1 to 3 hours. Levels do not correspond directly to intoxicating effects or impairment. THC is highly lipophilic and sequestered in tissues. Elimination half-life is estimated at 3 to 4 days, with plasma concentrations in occasional users falling below detection thresholds within 8 to 12 hours [27,62].

THC is extensively metabolized to the active metabolite 11-hydroxy-THC initially, and then to the inactive metabolite 11-nor-9-carboxy-THC (THC-COOH). Very little THC is excreted unchanged. Thirty percent of metabolites are eliminated in the urine, and the remainder through feces. THC metabolism is affected by cytochrome P450 induction and inhibition [62].

Cannabis use can be detected in routine urine immunoassays through identification of THC-COOH, appearing in urine 4 hours after use. Periods of detection generally in the ranges of 10 to 75 hours or 3 to 13 days have been noted for occasional and chronic smokers, respectively. Positive urine immunoassays generally provide evidence for recent use in the prior 1 to 3 days; however, times vary based on route and chronicity of use. Oral ingestion leads to prolonged urinary detection times of up to 6 days (cut-off 20 ng/mL). Heavy chronic use leads to prolonged urinary detection of up to 3 months following last use, as the result of tissue sequestration [27,31,43,49,62].

THC, subject to rapid metabolism, can only be detected in plasma for 5 hours using a very low cut-off threshold of 1 ng/mL [27]. Serum measurement of THC is an impractical method of cannabis use detection.

Synthetic cannabinoids are not detected in routine urine immunoassays. Properties of these substances, including chemical structure, absorption, distribution, metabolism, and excretion, have not yet been determined for each unique form, which makes their unique detection challenging. However, up to 12 specific compounds can be identified in urine (HPLC-MS-MS), blood (HPLC-MS-MS), and submitted herbal product samples (GC-MS) [97].

Substances associated with false positive results on urine immunoassay are illustrated in Table 10.2, including common non-steroidal anti-inflammatory agents, proton pump inhibitors, and efavirenz [27,49,60,61]. Hemp products may contain low concentrations of THC, and their use may result in positive urine cannabinoid test findings [62]. The predictive value of a positive cannabis urine immunoassay is 92 to 100% [49].

Opioids

Opioids are a class of natural or synthetic derivatives of the opium poppy. They have analgesic, sedative, and euphoria-producing properties. Derivatives of the opium poppy have been used for thousands of years in China, India, and the Near East. Opium has been used in Western medicine since the 1500s, appearing in various tonics and elixirs throughout the 1700s and 1800s including as treatment for pain and psychiatric disorders [98].

Morphine, the active agent of the opium poppy, was first isolated in 1803 by German pharmacist Frederick Sertürner, and later commercially manufactured by Merck laboratories in 1827. In 1895 Bayer produced heroin (diacetylmorphine) for medicinal use. In response to rising misuse of opium and available derivatives, and rooted in US indirect involvement in the "opium wars" between China and Britain, the US Harrison Act of 1914 was passed, which strictly regulated non-clinical use. The history of the opium poppy in recent times has involved significant sociological, political, military, and financial upheavals [98].

Modern medical use of opioids includes products available for treatment of pain, cough, diarrhea, and replacement therapy for opioid addiction. Scheduling for these medications includes heroin (Schedule I), morphine (Schedule II), acetaminophen (paracetamol) and codeine (Schedule III), propoxyphene (Schedule IV), and diphenoylate and atropine (Schedule V) [99].

Opioids are abused in almost every available natural, semi-synthetic, and synthetic form available. Historically, this abuse refers primarily to the natural opiates morphine and codeine, and the semi-synthetic opioid heroin. However, in recent years the availability of additional semi-synthetic and synthetic forms has drastically increased, and abuse of those medications has far surpassed classical opiates in adolescent groups. Semi-synthetic forms include hydromorphone, hydrocodone, oxycodone, and buprenorphine; synthetic forms include fentanyl, methadone, and tramadol [100].

Heroin and many other opioids are abused by intravenous injection, oral ingestion, or by smoking. Most semi-synthetic or synthetic forms, as prescribed medications, are available as tablets, but also as transdermal patches or suppositories. Heroin is referred to as dope, smack, junk, tar, white, and other names. Available tablets containing, for example, codeine, oxycodone, or hydromorphone are referred to in the illicit market as loads, M, roxy, monkey, TNT, cody, and other terms.

The 2010 Monitoring the Future survey reported use of heroin in the prior 12 months as approximately 1% for 8th-, 10th-, and 12th-graders. However, oxycontin use was reported at between 2 and 5% in those same groups over the prior year, with vicodin at between 3 and 8% [65].

Heroin and codeine are metabolized to morphine; however, each has a unique metabolite allowing specific identification in the urine. Norcodeine is a specific product of codeine metabolism, and 6-acetylmorphine is unique to the heroin metabolic pathway. Morphine is metabolized to nor-morphine and the active metabolite morphine-6-glucuronide [101]. Heroin is used intravenously or inhaled at doses ranging from 10 mg to up to 2 g by chronic users. The half-life of heroin (diacetylmorphine) is 2 to 7 minutes, followed by the half-lives of 6-acetylmorphine at 6 to 25 minutes, morphine at 2 to 7 hours, and morphine-6-glucuronide at 2.5 to 6.5 hours [27,62,101].

Heroin is rarely detected in the urine; the metabolite 6-acetylmorphine is generally detectable for only 2–8 hours following use. However, morphine metabolites (resulting from heroin, codeine, or morphine use) are detectable in urine for 2 to 4 days, with the longer periods associated with chronic use [27,62]. As previously described, 6-acetylmorphine is indicative of heroin use; norcodeine is indicative of codeine use.

Contrary to expectation, urine drug screens generally identify only heroin, opium, morphine, and codeine use. Most other semi-synthetic and synthetic forms, such as oxycodone, hydrocodone, and tramadol, are not detected on routine urine panels, and do not confirm as morphine on GC-MS. They require expanded panels and specific assays to identify their unique metabolites [101]. Methadone, a synthetic used in opiate replacement therapy, is likewise not generally included on routine panels. It does not cross-react with heroin or morphine on urine immunoassays, and must be included as a separate panel item.

Heroin, morphine, and their metabolites can be identified in plasma. Detection times vary depending on the route of administration, rate of elimination, and specific substance used. Intranasal heroin use can lead to detection of morphine for up to 12 hours. Intravenous heroin use can lead to detection of morphine and its metabolites for up to 1 to 5 days in heavy chronic users. Oral fluid testing identifies 6-acetylmorphine from 30 minutes to 8 hours, morphine for 12 to 24 hours, and codeine for up 21 hours [27].

Cross-reactivities for urine opiate immunoassays are listed in Table 10.2. Common medications associated with false positives include dextromethorphan, diphenhydramine, quinolone antibiotics, and verapamil. Quetiapine, ibuprofen, and chlorpromazine have been reported to be associated with false positives on methadone urine immunoassays [27,49,60,61]. A predictive value of a positive urine immunoassay is quite low, at 71% [49].

Poppy seed ingestion can additionally lead to positive results for opiate use on both urine immunoassays and GC-MS, depending on the cut-off threshold used. Ingestion of cookies, rolls, cakes, or bagels containing as little as one teaspoon of poppy seed filling, have been demonstrated to cause positive urine drug screen results for heroin and morphine for up to 60 hours. This result is an essential "true positive," as poppy seeds contain low concentrations of morphine and codeine, and therefore cannot be discriminated on GC-MS. It is commonly referred to as a "false positive" when utilized to indicate illicit use [49,102,103].

Phencyclidine (PCP) and Ketamine

Phencyclidine (PCP) is a dissociative anesthetic marketed by Parke-Davis in 1956 under the name Sernyl for its anesthetic qualities. It was later reserved for veterinary use only, after reports of postoperative agitation, delirium, and psychosis emerged in 1965. Ketamine was developed in 1962 by Parke-Davis as an alternative to phencyclidine [104,105], and has been explored as a psychotherapy agent and as a treatment for addiction.

PCP is a Schedule II drug (veterinary use) and continues to be used in illicit markets, along with other derivatives and structurally related analogs, generally created in "underground" laboratories. MK801, dexoxadrol, 2-MDP, tiletamine, and N-ethyl-1-phenylcyclohexylamine are examples of such analogs. It is unclear if these analogs are available presently on the illicit market, are marketed as other "club drugs" (see below). Ketamine, a Schedule III pediatric and veterinary anesthetic, along with other uses, is a structural analog of PCP. It is presently more popular than PCP in the adolescent population and is obtained by theft or diversion from legitimate laboratories. The effects of these substances include euphoria, perceptual distortion, depersonalization, and analgesia [104,105].

PCP is typically ingested by smoking, either by mixing the crystalline substance in tobacco and other herbal materials, or by dipping a smokable material in its liquid form. Injectable, intranasal, and transdermal uses are also reported. It is referred to as dust, sherm, boat, water, and fry. Ketamine can be smoked or used intranasally, intramuscularly, or intravenously. It is referred to as special K, jet, bump, or K [62,106].

Popular in the 1970s, use of PCP has since significantly declined among youths. In 2010 it had been used by approximately 1% of 12th-graders in the prior year, representing a decline by over 50% since 1996.

Ketamine had been used by 1.6% of 12th-graders in the prior year, declining from its peak use in 2000 [65]. As mentioned, ketamine has been marketed as ecstasy or other club drugs, and has been reportedly added to marijuana, heroin, and cocaine without user knowledge [62,106].

PCP is used in doses of 3 to over 10 mg, titrated by the user. It is highly lipophilic and sequestered in tissues. Blood levels of PCP peak 1 to 4 hours after use; half-life ranges from 7 to 46 hours, with an average of 21 hours. It is extensively metabolized to inactive metabolites. Common abused doses of ketamine range from 25 to 300 mg. The half-life is 2 to 3 hours. It is metabolized to the active metabolites norketamine and dehydronorketamine [62].

PCP is routinely included in urine immunoassays. It can be identified in the urine for up to 7 to 8 days following use. Within 10 days, 97% of a heavy dose is excreted. However, due to sequestration, heavy users have reported positive urine tests for up to 30 days. Serum testing is impractical, as the detection time is 5 to 15 minutes in blood [27,31,43,49,62]. Acidification of the urine is reportedly used to hasten elimination of the weakly basic PCP. Urine PCP concentrations may be followed over time for clinical correlation with psychiatric symptoms. Ketamine is not routinely included in urine immunoassay panels; however, it can be detected in urine for approximately 3 days [62].

Medications known to cross-react with PCP antibodies on urine immunoassays are listed in Table 10.2. Common medications include dextromethorphan, venlafaxine, ibuprofen, meperidine (pethidine), and diphenhydramine [49,61]. Discrimination is possible by GC-MS.

"Club Drugs"/Designer Drugs

The term "club drugs" generally refers to a wide variety of intoxicants used by adolescents and college-aged adults in bars and "rave" clubs throughout the 1990s until the present. The substances are chemically unrelated, including both traditional and designer drugs such as ecstasy (MDMA), LSD, GHB (gamma-hydroxybuturate), poppers (amyl nitrate), DXM (dextromethorphan), synthetic cannabinoids, ketamine, and Rohypnol (flunitrazepam). Viagra (sildenafil) has also been used as a club drug, or in conjunction with others, although it is not considered to be an intoxicant. Ketamine and LSD have been discussed in other sections of this chapter.

Rohypnol and GHB have gained particular infamy as drugs used in sexual assaults ("date rape drugs"), although they are abused themselves for their sedative, amnestic, dissociative, and euphoria-producing properties. MDMA has been examined extensively as a

psychotherapeutic and "empathogenic" agent [107]. Ketamine is a dissociative anesthetic. All of these drugs have a relatively low incidence of use in the general population. Dextromethorphan, the common antitussive, is abused at high doses, providing a dissociative effect similar to ketamine.

According to results of the 2010 Monitoring the Future survey, 0.6% of 8th-graders and 1.4% of 12th-graders reported use of GHB in the past year, representing a 50% decrease in the prior 5 to 10 years. Likewise Rohypnol use, reported at similar rates, has declined in preference. MDMA, however, declined in incidence after its peak use in 2000 to 2001, but has risen among younger users, associated with decreased perceived risk and disapproval. In 2010, 2.4% of 8th-graders, 4.7% of 10th-graders, and 4.5% of 12th-graders had used MDMA at least once in the prior year, with lifetime use at 3.3, 6.4, and 7.3%, respectively [1,2,64].

Methylenedioxymethamphetamine (MDMA)

MDMA is a derivative of methamphetamine that has both stimulant and hallucinogenic properties. Initially MDMA was designed as an appetite suppressant and adjunct to psychotherapy, later diverted to recreational use until its ban in the mid-1980s. The acute effects of MDMA include extroversion, mood elation, and perceptual distortion [107,108].

MDMA, a Schedule I drug, is termed ectasy, XTC, X, E, rolls, and Molly on the illicit market. It is available in colorful engraved tablets (butterflies, doves, and other markings similar to Valentine's Day candies) and powders for use. MDMA has had significant sociological effects among adolescents and young adults as the basis for the "rave scene" and electronic dance music ("jungle," "acid," "psychedelic trance," and other styles) arising since the mid-1980s. The phenomenon has been associated with musicians such as the Chemical Brothers, Astral Projection, and Aphex Twin. The rave scene has promoted messages of "peace and love," differing in its cultural effects from LSD only in the extent of political activism and influence.

Common doses of MDMA in tablets can range between 10 and 150 mg. Doses ingested range between 50 mg and 700 mg, with an average dose of 120 mg. Street purity is surprisingly low and tablets often contain various other drugs and adulterants. MDMA is rapidly absorbed, with a half-life of 7 to 8 hours, and produces various metabolites including methylenedioxyamphetamine (MDA), a club drug in its own right. Peak concentrations of MDMA and MDA are reached at approximately 2 and 4 hours, respectively [62,108].

MDMA is not routinely included in urine immunoassays. It is detectable in urine for 1 to 3 days [27].

Methylenedioxyethylamphetamine (MDEA), chemically related to MDMA and often found as a component of club drugs, can be detected in urine for 1.5 to 2.5 days [108].

MDMA can be detected in plasma through identification of both the parent compound and the metabolite, MDA, for approximately 24 hours (cut-off 20 ng/mL) [27]. Common sources for false positives are unknown.

Gamma-Hydroxybutyric Acid (GHB)

Gamma-hydroxybutyric acid (GHB) was researched in the 1960s as a GABA analog, and sold in nutritional food stores in the early 1990s as a body-building supplement secondary to its ability to elevate levels of growth hormone [109]. It was restricted and classified as a Schedule I drug in 2000, although Xyrem (sodium oxybate) is available as a Schedule III drug in the United States for treatment of narcolepsy and cataplexy. Sodium oxybate continues to be used as an anesthetic adjunct and treatment for substance withdrawal and addiction in Europe [62,99]. GHB has been used recreationally in both the United States and Europe for its sedative, euphoria-producing, empathogenic, and aphrodisiac properties.

Following the 2000 ban, various precursors (such as GBL) were readily available as "solvents" and kits, to evade regulation and allow users to produce GHB. Many of these precursors are listed as controlled substance analogs, and sales are monitored. There are multiple analogs available that have avoided regulation, and at least one, beta-phenyl-gamma-aminobutyric acid (phenibut) is available as a commercial supplement from legitimate nutritional stores advertised as a natural relaxant and sleep aid [110,111].

GHB is available on the illicit market as a powder or liquid, and is orally ingested or used intravenously. It is referred to as GBH, Georgia home boy, G, scoop, liquid X, and various other terms that may refer to GHB precursors and analogs. GHB was reported in 2010 to have been used at least once in the prior year by 1.6% of US 12th-graders in the Monitoring the Future 2010 survey [65].

Xyrem (sodium oxybate) is utilized in doses of 6 to 9 mg daily. Common abused doses of GHB are typically 1 to 5 g, with up to 100 g used per day [62]. GHB peak plasma levels are reached within 15 to 20 minutes, and the drug is rapidly eliminated. Serum detection is possible within 5 to 8 hours after use, rendering blood testing a relatively impractical method of detection [27,62].

GHB is not included in routine urine immunoassays; however, urine tests designed to identify GHB are useful for only 5 to 12 hours. The longest period of detection is provided by sweat patch testing within 24 hours [27,62]. Common sources for false positives are unknown.

Flunitrazepam (Rohypnol)

Flunitrazepam is a Schedule IV benzodiazepine, not approved for use in the United States, but produced in Europe and Mexico for treatment of sleep and anxiety disorders. It is manufactured in 1 to 2 mg tablets, and available on the illicit US market through illicit importation [112], being referred to as R2, roofies, roach, and rope. The incidence of flunitrazepam use among youths is similarly low, or less, than that for GHB [65]. Methods of abuse include oral ingestion and smoking.

Flunitrazepam is a potent benzodiazepine used at low dosages. Urine immunoassays for benzodiazepines are not specific for flunitrazepam, and may result in false negatives [113]. The metabolite 7-aminoflunitrazepam can be detected in urine by GC-MS for 14 to 28 days. In one study, oral fluid detection did not exceed 6 hours after ingestion of 1 mg [27].

Anabolic Steroids

Anabolic steroids (AAS) are a class of synthetic androgenic and anabolic compounds related to, and derived from, testosterone. AAS are Schedule III medications used to treat endocrinological disorders, age-related bone loss, cachexia, and anemias. Preparations such as Equipoise, Anadrol, Winstrol, Primobolan, and available precursers have permeated professional sports as performance-enhancing drugs used along with non-steroidal medication such as erythropoietin, growth hormone, diuretics, and stimulants [114]. In 1990 the US Anabolic Steroid Act classified anabolic steroids as controlled substances; it was amended in 2004, adding precursors and "prohormones" to the controlled classification [115].

Anabolic steroids are available for purchase on the internet, and through illicit importation from laboratories and distributors outside the United States [116]. In the illicit market, AAS are referred to as juice and roids, and are administered via oral ingestion, topical gels, transdermal routes, and intramuscular injection. Although not intoxicants, they are viewed as potential substances of abuse.

Adolescents and young adults are particularly vulnerable to athletic performance pressures, which can be perceived to be alleviated by the use of AAS. The prevalence of anabolic steroid use is illustrated by the mandatory school testing programs that have been enacted in the last 10 years [6–12]. Perhaps as a result of those measures, use has declined by 50% in the last 8 years as noted by the Monitoring the Future Survey of 2010. In that study, 1.1%, 1.6%, and 2% of 8th-, 10th- and 12th-graders reported ever having used anabolic steroids [65].

Anabolic steroids undergo extensive metabolism and are excreted in urine. Metabolites produced are often indistinguishable from endogenous sources; ratios of testosterone and the naturally occuring isomer epitestosterone are compared in the urine to detect abuse [117].

Methenolone (Primobolan), a common target for testing, is generally detectable by GC-MS as the glucuronide-conjugated metabolite in the urine for only 5 days following use. Sulfated conjugated metabolites are detectable by GC-MS for up to 9 days, with more sensitive techniques increasing the window of detection to up to 14 days [118].

Detection periods for other anabolic steroids depend primarily on the half-lives, elimination rates, and route of administration of the various drugs. Commercial laboratories offer urine testing for multiple steroids of abuse by LC-MS-MS and GC-MS. Detection times range from days to 18 months for oil-based decanoate preaprations [117].

CONCLUSIONS

This chapter has reviewed major substances of abuse, and their detection. Methods of testing and source samples have been discussed. Substance abuse toxicology is a rapidly growing field, and testing of abused substances is common in schools, clinics, substance abuse treatment programs, and legal, domestic, and employment settings. Testing contributes to treatment planning, but can also be used in high-stakes settings.

Testing is not without its pitfalls and drawbacks. Cross-reactivities on screening exams are poorly quantified, identified incidentally in clear cases of the absence of substance abuse. More specific tests can be costly and impractical for regular use. Many of the methods are proprietary.

Clinicians and others using these tests are advised to educate themselves regarding the limitations of, and substances included in, the panels they choose, and to consult with the manufacturer if questions arise. Clinical correlation is always advised, as testing methods are unable to detect all designed substances of abuse.

References

1. Johnston L, O'Malley P, Bachman J, *et al. Monitoring the Future National Survey Results on Drug Use, 1975–2007: Volume I, secondary school students.* NIH Publication No. 08-6418A. Bethesda, MD: National Institute on Drug Abuse, 2008.
2. Johnston L, O'Malley P, Bachman J, Schulenberg J. *Monitoring the Future National Survey Results on Adolescent Drug Use. Overview of key findings, 2006.* NIH Publication No. 07-6202. Bethesda, MD: National Institute on Drug Abuse, 2007.
3. National Drug Intelligence Center. *The Economic Impact of Illicit Drug Use on American Society.* Washington, DC: US Department of Justice, 2011.
4. Weber W, Cox, C. Analysis of toxicology reports: Work-Related Fatal Injuries in 1998. *Compensation and Working Conditions* 2001; Spring: 27–29.
5. Dasgupta A. The effects of adulterants and selected ingested compounds on drug-of-abuse testing in urine. *Am J Clin Pathol* 2007;**128**:491–503.
6. *Vernonia School District 47 vs Acton*, 15S CT 2386 (1995).
7. Florida to begin drug test for prep athletes. *USA Today* 2007; 19 June.
8. Sterling E. UIL adopts rules for athlete drug testing. *Raymondville Chronicle/Willacy County News* 2008; 16 January. Available from: http://www.raymondvillechroniclenews.com/news/2008/0116/news/024.html.
9. Temkin B. Teen athletes face drug test: for 1st time, state requires random testing. *Chicago Tribune* 2008; 14 January.
10. Smith P. Feature: Number of schools embracing random drug testing on the rise – So is opposition. StoptheDrugWar.org, 2008. Available from: http://stopthedrugwar.org/print/14756.
11. *Board of Ed. of Independent School Dist. No. 92 of Pottawatomie City vs Earls*, (01-332) 536 U.S. 822, 242 F.3d 1264 (2002).
12. Larimer S. Steroid testing of Florida schools' athletes ends over money. *TCPalm* 2009. Available from: http://www.tcpalm.com/news/2009/feb/16/fla-school-steroid-testing-ends-over-money/.
13. Vakili S, Currie S, El-Guebaly N. Evaluating the utility of drug testing in an outpatient addiction program. *Addictive Disorders and Their Treatment* 2009;**8**:22–32.
14. Sobada Z, Bukoswki W. *Handbook of Drug Abuse Prevention: Theory, Science and Practice.* New York: Kluwer Academic/Plenum Publishers, 2003.
15. U.S., Preventative Services Task Force. Screening for drug abuse. In: DiGiuseppe C, Atkins D, Woolf SH (eds), *Guide to Clinical Preventive Services.* Baltimore: Williams & Wilkins, 1996; pp. 588–594.
16. Anon. Testing for drugs of abuse in children and adolescents. *Pediatrics* 1996;**98**:305–330.
17. Knights J, Mears C. Testing for drugs of abuse in children: addendum – Testing in schools and at home. *Pediatrics* 2007;**119**:627–630.
18. Executive Order 12564 of Sept. 15, 1986, appear at 51 FR 32889, 3 CFR, 1986 Comp., p. 224.
19. Section 503 of Public Law 100-71, 5 U.S.C. Section 7301 (1988).
20. *Federal Register* 2010; 30 April **75** (83): 22809–22810. Retrieved from: http://www.gpo.gov/fdsys/pkg/FR-2010-04-30/html/2010-10118.htm.
21. *Federal Register* 2008; 25 November **73** (228): 71857–71907. Retrieved from: http://www.gpo.gov/fdsys/pkg/FR-2008-11-25/html/E8-26726.htm.
22. Quest Diagnostics Inc. Standard urine testing for drug and alcohol abuse. c. 2000–12. Retrieved from: http://www.questdiagnostics.com/home/companies/employer/drug-screening/drug-test-types/lab-based/urine-testing.html.
23. Pesce A, West C. Drugs-of-abuse testing and therapeutic-drug monitoring. *Medical Laboratory Observer* 2011; March:42–46. Available from: www.mlo-online.com.

24. Pragst F, Balikova M. State of the art in hair analysis for detection of drug and alcohol. *Clin Chim Acta* 2006;**370**:17–49.

25. Dolan K, Rouen D, Kimber J. An overview of the use of urine, hair, sweat, and saliva to detect drug use. *Drug Alcohol Rev* 2004;**23**:213–217.

26. Warner E, Sharma N. Laboratory diagnosis. In: Ries R, Fiellin D, Miller S, Saitz R (eds), *Principles of Addiction Medicine*. Philadelphia: Lippincott Williams & Wilkins, 2009; pp. 295–303.

27. Verstraete A. Detection times of drugs of abuse in blood, urine, and oral fluid. *Ther Drug Monit* 2004;**26**:200–205.

28. Jaffee W, Trucco E, Levy S, *et. al.*Is this urine really negative? A systematic review of tampering methods in urine drug screening and testing. *J Subst Abuse Treat* 2007;**33**:33–42.

29. Dasgupta A. The effects of adulterants and selected ingested compounds on drug-of-abuse testing in urine. *Am J Clin Pathol* 2007;**128**:491–503.

30. Wu A, Bristol B, Sexton K, *et al.*Adulteration of urine by "Urine Luck." *Clin Chem* 1999;**45**:1051–1057.

31. HairConfirm. Forensic drug of abuse testing; Frequently asked questions. Craig Medical Distribution Inc., c. 1997–2011. Available from: http://www.craigmedical.com/Hair_Drug-Test_FAQ.htm.

32. Hair drug test kit follicle. Medimpex United Inc. c. 2000–11. Available from: http://www.meditests.com/hairdrugtest.html.

33. Hartwig S, Auwarter V, Pragst F. Fatty acid ethyl esters in scalp, pubic, axillary, beard and body hair as markers of alcohol misuse. *Int Leg Med* 2003;**38**:163–167.

34. Kidwell D, Blank L. Environmental exposure: The stumbling block of hair testing. In: Kintz P (ed.), *Drug Testing in Hair*. Boca Raton, FL: CRC Press, 1996; pp. 17–68.

35. Rohrich J, Zornthlein S, Porsch L, *et al.*Effects of the shampoo Ultra Clean on drug concentrations. *Int J Legal Med* 2000;**113**:102–106.

36. *Gregory Hicks et al. vs City of New York et al.,* Index No. 119154 (1999).

37. *In the Matter of Patrick Forte*, New York Appeal Board No. 477610 (2000).

38. Society of Hair Testing. Recommendations for hair testing in forensic cases. SOHT, 2003. Available from: http://www.soht.org/pdf/Consensus_on_Hair_Analysis.pdf.

39. Vogliardi S, Favretto D, Frison G, et al. Validation of a fast screening method for the detection of cocaine in hair by MALDI-MS. *Anal Bioanal Chem* 2010;**396**:2435–2440.

40. Cone E, Jenkins A. Saliva drug analysis. In: Wong S (ed.), *Handbook of Analytical Therapeutic Drug Monitoring and Toxicology*. London: CRC Press, 1997; pp. 303–333.

41. Drummer OH. Drug testing in oral fluid. *Clin Biochem Rev* 2006;**27**:147–159.

42. Crouch D. Oral fluid collection: the neglected variable in oral fluid testing. *Forensic Sci Int* 2005;**150**:165–173.

43. Cone E, Huestis M. Interpretation of oral fluid tests for drugs of abuse. *Ann NY Acad Sci* 2007;**1098**:51–103.

44. Passing All Drug Test.com. Beat saliva drug test. Passingalldrugtest.com, c. 2006–11. Available from: http://www.passingalldrugtest.com/drug-testing-information/beat-saliva-drug-test.html.

45. AlwaysTestClean.com. Pass a saliva swab drug test. Available from: http://www.alwaystestclean.com/saliva_drug_test.htm.

46. PharmChem Inc. PharmChek drugs of abuse patch; Technical questions and answers. 2007. Retrieved from: http://www.pharmchem.com/pharmchem/files/download_files/Patch_Technical_Q_and_A.pdf

47. Kidwell D, Holland J, Athanaseli S. Testing for drugs of abuse in salvia and sweat. *J Chromatogr B Biomed Sci Appl* 1998;**713**:111–135.

48. *United States vs Meyer*, 485 F. Supp.2d 1001, 1001 (N.D. Iowa 2006). Available from: http://www.ca8.uscourts.gov/opndir/07/04/062961P.pdf.

49. Moeller KE, Lee KC, Kissack JC. Urine drug screening: Practical guide for clinicians. *Mayo Clin Proc* 2008;**83**:66–76.

50. Mitchell JM. Immunoassays as an initial test in drug testing. Center for Forensic Sciences RTI International, 2008. Available from: http://nac.samhsa.gov(DTAB (Presentations(Aug08(JohnMitchellDTAB0808_508.pdf.

51. US Department of Health and Human Services. Mandatory guidelines and proposed revisions to mandatory guidelines for federal workplace drug testing programs: Notices. *Federal Register* 2008; November 25 (73 FR 71858), Section 3.4, effective October 2010. Available from: http://workplace.samhsa.gov/Dtesting.html.

52. Meegan J, Brigetti K, Horstmann D. Use of enzyme immunoassays and the latex agglutination test to measure the temporal appearance of immunoglobin G and M antibodies after natural infection or immunization with rubella virus. *J Clin Microbiol* 1983;**18**:745–748.

53. Wu A. Mechanism of interferences for gas chromatography/mass spectrometry analysis of urine for drugs of abuse. *Ann Clin Lab Sci* 1995;**25**:319–329.

54. NIST Standard Reference Database Number 69. In: Linstrom PJ, Mallard WG (eds), *NIST Chemistry WebBook*. National Gaithersburg, MD: Institute of Standards and Technology. Available from: http://webbook.nist.gov.

55. Strathmann FG, Hoofnagle AN. Current and future applications of mass spectrometry to the clinical laboratory. *Am J Clin Path* 2011;**136**:609–616.

56. Pesce A, West C. Drugs-of-abuse testing and therapeutic-drug monitoring. *Medical Laboratory Observer*. NP Communications, 2011. Available from: http://www.mlo-online.com/features/201103/current_buzz.aspx.

57. Autry JD. Testimony on Federal workplace drug-testing by Acting Director Center for Substance Abuse Prevention Substance Abuse and Mental Health Services Administration, U.S. Department of Health and Human Services Before the House Committee on Commerce, Subcommittee on Oversight and Investigations July 23, 1998. Department of Health and Human Services. Available from: http://www.hhs.gov/asl/testify/t980723f.html.

58. Wilson JF, Smith BL, Toseland PA, *et al.* External quality assessment of techniques for the detection of drugs of abuse in urine. *Ann Clin Biochem* 1994;**31**:335–342.

59. Gibb RP, Cockerham H, Goldfogel GA, Lawson GM, Raisys VA. Substance abuse testing of urine by GC/MS in scanning mode evaluated by proficiency studies, TLC/GC, and EMIT. *J Forensic Sci* 1993;**38**:124–133.

60. Brahm NC, Yeager LL, Fox MD, Farmer KC, Palmer TA. Commonly prescribed medications and potential false-positive urine drug screens. *Am Soc Health-Sys Pharm* 2010;**67**:1344–1350.

61. Colbert D. Drug abuse screening with immunoassays: Unexpected crossreactivities and other pitfalls. *Br J Biomed Sci* 1994;**51**:136–146.

62. Couper FJ, Logan BK. Drugs and human performance. National Highway Traffic Safety Administration Fact Sheets, Publication HS 809 725. Washington, DC: Department of Transportation, 2004. Available from:

http://.ntl.bts.gov/lib/26000/26000/26092/164-Drugsand HumanPerf.pdf.

63. Berge K, Bush D. The subversion of urine drug testing. *Minnesota Medicine* 2010; 45–47. Available from: http://www.minnesotamedicine.com/tabid/3533/Default.aspx.

64. Department of Health and Human Services, Substance Abuse and Mental Health Services Administration, Center for Substance Abuse Prevention, National Laboratory Certification Program (NLCP). Notice to HHS certified and applicant laboratories subject: Guidance for reporting specimen validity test results. NLCP Program Document #35. DHHS, 1998. Retrieved from: http://workplace.samhsa.gov/DrugTesting/pdf/Program%2035%20-%20Guidance%20for%20Reporting%20Specimen%20Validity%20Test%20Results%20-%20September%2028,%201998.pdf.

65. Johnston J, O'Malley P, Bachman J, Schulenberg J. *Monitoring the Future: National Results and Adolescent Drug Use, Overview of Key Findings 2010.* Ann Arbor, MI: Institute for Social Research, University of Michigan, 2011. Available from: http://www.monitoringthefuture.org/pubs/monographs/mtf-overview2010.pdf.

66. Montgomery MR, Reasor MJ. Retrograde extrapolation of blood alcohol data: An applied approach. *J Toxicol Environ Health* 1992;**36**:281–292.

67. Glinn M, Adatsi F, Curtis P. Comparison of the analytical capabilities of the BAC Datamaster and Datamaster DMT; Forensic breath testing devices. *J Forensic Sci* 2011;**56**:1632–1638.

68. Center for Substance Abuse Treatment. The role of biomarkers in the treatment of alcohol use disorders. Substance Abuse Treatment Advisory 5(4). DHHS Publication No. (SMA) 06-4223. DHHS, 2006. Available from: http://kap.samhsa.gov/products/manuals/advisory/text/0609_biomarkers.htm.

69. Rasmussen N. *On Speed: The Many Lives of Amphetamine.* New York: New York University Press, 2008; pp. 87–113.

70. Haller C, Benowitz N. Adverse cardiovascular and central nervous system events associated with dietary supplements containing ephedra alkaloids. *N Engl J Med* 2000;**343**:1833–1838.

71. Rawson R. *Treatment Improvement Protocol 33; Treatment for Stimulant Use Disorders.* DHHS Publication No. (SMA) 09-4209. Rockville, MD: Substance Abuse and Mental Health Services Administration, 1999.

72. Byck R. *Cocaine Papers by Sigmund Freud.* New York: Stonehill, 1974.

73. Office of Applied Studies. *Results from the 2006 National Survery on Drug Use and Health: National Findings.* Rockville, MD: Substance Abuse and Mental Health Services Adminstration, 2007.

74. Reichman O, Otto R. Effects of intranasal cocaine on the urine drug screen for benzoylecgonine. *Otolaryngol Head Neck Surgery* 1992;**106**:223–225.

75. Joseph DE. Inhalants. In: Joseph D (ed.), *Drugs of Abuse.* Washington, DC: United States Drug Enforcement Administration, 2005; pp. 58–60. Available from: http://www.justice.gov/dea/pubs/abuse/doa-p.pdf.

76. Jauch EC, Cadena RS, Kuo JD. Inhalants. In: Ramachandran TS (ed.), *Medscape Reference* [online], 2010. Available from: http://emedicine.medscape.com/article/1174630-overview.

77. Nichols D. LSD: Cultural revolution and medical advances. *Chem World* 2006;**3**(1). Available from: http://www.rsc.org/chemistryworld/Issues/2006/January/LSD.asp

78. Moore TH, Zammit S, Lingford-Hughes A, *et al.* Cannabis use and risk of psychotic or affective mental health outcomes: A systematic review. *Lancet* 2007;**370**:319–328.

79. Jordan K, Schmol H, Aapro M. Comparative activity of antiemetic drugs. *Crit Rev Oncol Hematol* 2007;**61**:162–175.

80. Slatkin N. Cannabinoids in the treatment of chemotherapy-induced nausea and vomiting: Beyond prevention of acute emesis. *J Support Oncol* 2007;**5**(5 Suppl. 3):1–9.

81. Parker L, Burton P, Sorge R, *et al.* Effect of low doses of delta9-tetrahydrocannabinol and cannabidiol on the extenction of cocaine-induced and amphetamine-induced conditioned place preference learning in rats. *Pharmacol Biochem Behav* 1991;**40**:695–700.

82. WhitField R, Bechtel L, Statich G. The impact of ethanol and Marinol/marijuana usage on HIV+/AIDS patients undergoing azidothymidine, azidothymidine/dideoxycytidine, or dideoxyinosine therapy. *Alcohol Clin Exp Res* 1997;**21**:122–127.

83. Davis J, Ramsey H. Antiepileptic action of marijuana-active substances. *Feder Proc* 1949;**8**:284–285.

84. Cortesi M, Fusar-Poli P. Potential therapeutical effects of cannabidiol in children with pharmacoresistant epilepsy. *Med Hypothesis* 2007;**68**:920–921.

85. Bisogno T, DiMarzo V. Short- and long-term plasticity of the endocannabinoid system in neuropsychiatric and neurological disorders. *Pharmacol Res* 2007;**56**:428–442.

86. Noyes RJ, Brunks S, Avery D, *et al.* The analgesic properties of delta-9-tetrahydrocannabinol and codeine. *Clin Pharmacol Ther* 1975;**18**:84–89.

87. Herzberg U, Eliav E, Bennett G, *et al.* The analgesic effects of R(+)-WIN 55,212-2 mesylate, a high affinity cannabinoid agonist, in a rat model of neuropathic pain. *Neurosci Lett* 1997;**221**:157–160.

88. Mao J, Price D, Lu J, *et al.* Two distinctive antinociceptive systems in rats with pathological pain. *Neurosci Lett* 2000;**280**:13–16.

89. Kawaski Y, Kohno T, Ji R. Different effects of opioid and cannabinoid receptor agonists on C-fiber-induced extracellular signal-regulated kinase activation in dorsal horn neurons in normal and spinal nerve-ligated rats. *J Pharmacol Exp Ther* 2006;**316**:601–607.

90. Noyes RJ, Baram D. Cannabis analgesia. *Compr Psychiatry* 1974;**15**:531–535.

91. Pacher P, Bakai S, Kunos G. The endocannabinoid system as an emerging target of pharmacotherapy. *Pharmacol Rev* 2006;**58**:389–462.

92. Drug Enforcement Agency. (2010) DEA moves to emergency control synthetic marijuana. DEA Public Affairs News Release: Number: 202-307-7977. Washington, DC: DEA, 2010. Available from: http://www.justice.gov/dea/pubs/pressrel/pr112410p.html.

93. K2 Herb Blends. K2 Herb Store, c. 2012. Available from: www.k2herbstore.com.

94. Wicked X Herbal Potpourri. Herbal Magics, c. 2008–10. Available from: www.herbalmagics.com/.

95. Wang L. John W. Huffman. Organic chemist invented a compound in 1995 that is now at the center of a controversy brewing over synthetic marijuana. *Chem Eng News* 2010;**88**:43. Available from: http://pubs.acs.org/doi/abs/10.1021/cen-v088n026.p043.

96. Heltsley R, Shelby M, Crouch D, *et al.* Detection of synthetic cannabinoids in US athletes suspected of spice

use. *ToxTalk, Society of Forensic Toxicology Inc* 2011;**35**:13–15.

97. NMS Labs. K2 Spice and other synthetic cannabinoids testing. NMS Labs, c. 2010. Available from: http://www.nmslab.com/services-forensic-K2-testing.

98. PBS Frontline. Opium throughout history. PBS and WGBH/Frontline, 1998. Available from: http://www.pbs.org/wgbh/pages/frontline/shows/heroin/etc/history.html.

99. Drug Lookup. Epocrates Online. Reference [website]. Epocrates, Inc., c. 2012. Available from: https://online.epocrates.com.

100. Trescot AM, Datta S, Lee M, Hansen H. Opioid pharmacology. *Pain Phys* 2008;**11**:S133–153.

101. Smith H. Opioid metabolism. *Mayo Clin Proc* 2009;**84**:613–624.

102. Moeller MR, Hammer K, Engel O. Poppy seed consumption and toxicological analysis of blood and urine samples. *Forensic Sci Int* 2004;**143**:183–186.

103. Meadway C, George S, Braithwaite R. Opiate concentrations following the ingestion of poppy seed products – evidence for 'the poppy seed defense'. *Forensic Sci Int* 1998;**96**:29–38.

104. Beagle JQ. Synthesis and effects of PCP analogues. Erowid archives, c. 1995-2010. Available from: http://www.erowid.org/archive/rhodium/chemistry/pcp/pcp_index.html.

105. Davies BM, Beech HR. The effect of 1-arylcyclohexylamine (Sernyl) on twelve normal volunteers. *Brit J Psych* 1960;**106**:912–924.

106. DanceSafe.org. Ketamine. c. 2012. Available from: http://dancesafe.org/drug-information/ketamine.

107. Sessa B, Nutt DJ. MDMA, politics and medical research: Have we thrown the baby out with the bathwater? *J Psychopharmacol* 2007;**21**:787–791.

108. Glennon R. The pharmacology of classical halucinogens and related designer drugs. In: Ries R, Fiellin D, Miller S, Saitz R (eds), *Principles of Addiction Medicine*, 4th edn. Philadelphia: Lippincott Williams & Wilkins, 2009; pp. 215–230.

109. Volpi R, Chiodera P, Caffarra P, Scaglioni A, Saccani A, Coiro V. Different control mechanisms of growth hormone (GH) secretion between γ-amino- and γ-hydroxy-butyric acid: neuroendocrine evidence in Parkinson's disease. *Psychoneuroendocrinology* 1997;**22**:531–538.

110. National Drug Intelligence Center. Informational bulletin: GHB analogs. NDIC, 2002. Available from: http://www.justice.gov/ndic/pubs1/1621/index.htm#Tests.

111. The Vitamin Shoppe Inc. Other supplements [website]. c. 2012. Available from: http://www.vitaminshoppe.com/store/en/browse/sku_detail.jsp?id=M3-1005&sourceType=cs&source=FG&ci_src=14110944&ci_sku=M3-1005.

112. University of Maryland, Center for Substance Abuse Research. Flunitrazepam (Rohypnol). Available from: http://www.cesar.umd.edu/cesar/drugs/rohypnol.pdf

113. Wang PH, Liu C, Tsay WI, Li JH, Liu RH, Wu TG. Improved screen and confirmation test of 7-aminoflunitrazepam in urine specimens for monitoring flunitrazepam (Rohypnol) exposure. *J Anal Toxicol* 2002;**26**:411–418.

114. Hoffman JR, Ratamess NA. Medical issues associated with anabolic steroid use: Are they exaggerated? *J Sport Sci Med* 2006;**5**:182–193.

115. Rannazzisi JT.'Anabolic Steroid Control Act of 2004.' Office of Diversion Control Drug Enforcement Administration before the House Committee on the Judiciary Subcommittee on Crime, Terrorism and Homeland Security March 16, 2004. Available from: http://www.justice.gov/dea/pubs/cngrtest/ct031604.html.

116. SteroidPortal.com. Available at: http://www.steroidportal.com/.

117. Redwood Toxicology Laboratory. Steroid/sports drug testing. Available from: http://www.redwoodtoxicology.com/services/steroid_testing_faq.html.

118. Baumann S. Longterm detection of anabolic steroid metabolites in urine. Agilent Technologies, 2010. Available from: http://www.chem.agilent.com/Library/applications/5990-5748EN.pdf.

Section Three

Risk and Prevention

Edited by Avram H. Mack

11

Prevention of Adolescent Psychoactive Substance Use

Maria E. McGee and Avram H. Mack

Georgetown University School of Medicine, Washington, DC, USA

INTRODUCTION

The prevention of psychoactive substance use among adolescents continues to be one of the highest international public health priorities [1]. Various prevention approaches have evolved in recent years in an attempt to delay the onset of substance use or reduce and/or prevent "high risk" or harmful substance use. The early initiation of substance use predicts later misuse, abuse, and dependence. Prevention approaches are less expensive and more efficacious than treatment approaches [2]. Thus, if we can prevent substance misuse/abuse, we can prevent substance dependence. The earlier prevention strategies can be initiated, the better.

Psychoactive substance use disorders are forms of neurodevelopmental disorders that typically begin during adolescence. These disorders are influenced by a complexity of genetic, environmental, and phenotypic liabilities. Adolescents are at a heightened psychosocial vulnerability to a variety of risk-taking and health-compromising behaviors including experimentation with substances. Rates of risk-taking behavior peak in middle to late adolescence [3–6]. In general, prevention efforts should always focus on their specific audience with sensitivity to developmental stages and appropriate timing. These often revolve around theories of both risk and protective factors inherent in use at particular developmental stages. Prevention efforts for adolescents require an understanding of the adolescents' developmental level and because of this there is a renewed interest in prevention strategies in child and adolescent psychiatry [7].

This chapter reviews the manner in which prevention leaders have been able to fit their message to the developmental needs of adolescents. These efforts require a focus on normal child/adolescent development and pathological risk factors discussed in the other six chapters in this section.

PROTECTIVE FACTORS

Adolescents might have some factors protecting them from the risk of psychoactive substance use. These factors have a moderating or buffering effect; that is, they possess characteristics that reduce the impact of risk factors on outcomes [8]. They are associated with a positive adjustment during adolescence and are facilitators of healthy prosocial behaviors. These protective factors might counteract the negative influences of a few risk factors. The more protective factors are promoted and risk factors are reduced, the more likely risk-taking and health-compromising behaviors and their associated sequelae might be prevented. Child and adolescent psychiatrists need to understand and integrate these factors into preventive strategies.

Psychoactive substance use problems usually arise from a combination of individual, familial, and community related influences. Therefore, potential protective factors can be divided into: (i) individual factors, (ii) connectedness to family factors, and (iii) connectedness to community factors [2,9]. These are described in the following paragraphs.

Individual Protective Factors

An adolescent's phenotypic profile plays a vital role in the prevention of psychoactive substance use and the promotion of healthy behaviors. Individual protective factors are those such as religiosity (of both the adolescent and parent(s)), perceived risk of use, a positive sense of self, disapproval and avoidance of peers who use substances, affiliation with prosocial peers, a focus on academic performance, academic competence, healthy social skills, healthy coping styles (including empathy and problem-solving skills), a strong internal locus of control, and the use of psychopharmacotherapy when indicated for attention-deficit/hyperactivity disorder (ADHD) and other possible childhood psychiatric disturbances. These may operate as significant buffering agents for the prevention of adolescent substance use [8,10,11–13].

Religiosity refers to one's behavioral and attitudinal religious devotion regardless of the content of the beliefs [2,14]. Research has demonstrated a strong inverse correlation between religiosity and substance use. This suggests that religiosity might operate as a protective factor against substance use [15]. Also, religious parents tend to rear religious children and those parents share their behavioral values with their children. Likewise, they are more likely to support and monitor their children; they tend to be more actively engaged in authoritative parenting (rather than authoritarian parenting); and, they are more likely to set a strong and clear example of healthier lifestyles [10].

Self-regulation refers to the ability to alter one's responses; that is, an adolescent's affect, behavior, and cognition are consistent with an adolescent's ideals, values, morals, and social expectations supportive of the pursuit of his/her long-term best interests. Self-regulated behaviors include the ability to: 1) delay gratification, 2) rapidly transition between different tasks, 3) focus attention, and 4) control one's emotions and behaviors. Adolescence is a critical period for the formation of the brain mechanisms related to self-regulation. Impaired self-regulation (that is, self-dysregulation) is associated with the initiation and maintenance of a variety of risk-taking and health-compromising behaviors including the experimentation and use of substances. Research has demonstrated an inverse correlation between self-regulation and substance use. Thus, when self-regulatory skills fail to emerge or are impaired during adolescence the likelihood of serious substance use-related harm is increased.

Connectedness to Family Protective Factors

An adolescent's family plays a vital role in the prevention of psychoactive substance use and the promotion of healthy behaviors. They can help to reinforce individual protective factors against substance use. Protective factors related to connectedness to family include healthy family relationships, cohesion within the family, positive parental guidance in the avoidance of substance use, increased parental presence and the display of a strong example at home, increased parental supervision and monitoring of adolescent's activities with peers, clear and consistent rules of conduct and boundary setting that are followed within the family structure, constructive parental involvement in the lives of their children, and, most importantly, a strong and stable attachment to parent(s) [2,9,12].

Authoritative parenting, as opposed to rigid authoritarian parenting, is a key protective factor. Despite the fact that adolescence is a time when youths are in the process of asserting their autonomy from the adults in their lives, parents continue to have a positive influence on their children's behaviors. This includes decision-making related to substance use [11,16] and judicious parental monitoring. Parental monitoring refers to the degree to which parents supervise their children's activities and their whereabouts [16,17]. It involves ensuring age-appropriate adult supervision of activities outside and inside the home, enforcing household rules, establishing curfews, and knowing their child's friends. These alone do not explain lower levels of substance use among adolescents; however, they are a strong predictor of an adolescent's personal norms regarding substance abuse and his/her decision-making skills to avoid their use [16]. Adolescents with a strong sense of attachment to their parents and a cohesive family might be more inclined to seek out their parents' help if they encounter a significant problem related to substance use. In essence, cohesive and loving families provide support for youths and a context in which to learn, enact, and be reinforced for prosocial coping behaviors [10].

Connectedness to Community Protective Factors

An adolescent's community can provide a vital culturally based role in the prevention of psychoactive substance use and the promotion of healthy behaviors. This connectedness refers to the interrelated welfare of an individual with one's community. It can help to reinforce individual and connectedness to family protective factors against substance use. Connectedness to community protective factors include success in school performance, strong bonds with institutions (such as school and religious organizations), adoption of conventional norms about substance use, anti-substance use policies at school and community, the availability and continuity of healthy community-based social support and ties, strong neighborhood attachment, and affiliation with prosocial peers [2].

Significant school protective factors can be divided into: (i) positive academic achievement, (ii) high academic aspirations, and (iii) supportive teachers. Teachers can be a tremendous source of support for adolescents, especially when familial support is lacking or nonexistent. Teachers can provide a non-judgmental point of view, help adolescents feel connected to school as a social body, provide prosocial examples, and buffer negative peer interactions [10].

Significant peer protective factors include having friends that are not engaged in violent behaviors or psychoactive substance use as well as peer disapproval of its use. The perception that substances are not "normative" among peers and in the general school environment is an important protective factor against their use [11,18].

Developmental Processes and Outcomes

Developmental processes and outcomes of younger adolescents are different from those of older ones. These factors are distinct depending on a youth's developmental stage. The potential impact of particular risk and protective factors changes with a youth's developmental stage. For younger adolescents family and community factors are more salient, whereas for older adolescents peer and school influences are more important. Familial influences (such as healthy parent-child bonds) are important in childhood and early adolescence but recede in relative importance as older adolescents spend more unsupervised time with their peers [19]. Social connectedness (that is, one's connection with one's family, friends, and school) plays an increasingly vital role among older adolescents in reducing the risk of substance use [9]. Therefore, prevention strategies for adolescents need to attend to these distinct developmental needs.

TYPES OF PREVENTION STRATEGIES

While prevention strategies are traditionally organized in a continuum of primary, secondary, and tertiary strategies, the need for an increased emphasis on creating programs that match the risk-needs of specific targeted groups of individuals requires a more specific classification scheme. These strategies need to change the balance between risk and protective factors so that protective factors outweigh risk factors. They also need to take into consideration the normal course of human development. The United States Institute of Medicine (US IOM) adopted a prevention continuum based on Gordon's classification scheme that goes beyond traditional primary, secondary, and tertiary strategies [20]. Its focus is the target population. This approach encompasses a three-tiered preventive intervention classification system based on the targeted population:

1. the general population, a universal approach;
2. those "at risk," a selective approach; and,

3. those who exhibit early stages of use or related problem behaviors, an indicated approach.

These categories represent the population groups toward whom the interventions are directed and are thought to be most optimal. It also makes assumptions concerning the targeted group's risk for substance use. The following paragraphs analyze each of these tiers.

Universal Prevention Strategies

Universal strategies are a form of primary prevention. Their purpose is to delay the onset of substance use or reduce and/or prevent new cases of psychoactive substance use and misuse in the general population at any social level – national, state, city, neighborhood, school district, or local school. This generalized approach is implemented regardless of individual risk factors. Its intent is to reach a broad audience in which all individuals, without prior screening for substance abuse risk, are provided with information and skills necessary to prevent or delay the onset of substance use. This targeted group encompasses individuals from "low" to "high risk" for substance use, misuse, abuse, and dependence. Since it is so broad, it is typically less intensive [21,22]. It involves the dissemination of comprehensive health education and decision-making skills related to prevention to all children regardless of risks [22]. This broad focus includes areas related to social marketing, regulatory control, and law enforcement initiatives as well as a range of psychosocial programs aimed at preventing or delaying the use of substances [21].

There are two categories of universal prevention strategies based on either a consumption model or a sociocultural model. When creating a universal prevention strategy, one must be aware of the link between the consumption and sociocultural models in an attempt to understand the contributing factors of substance use among adolescents.

The first category emphasizes a consumption model aimed at societal control of the availability of psychoactive substances. It includes social change initiatives such as increasing the age at which legal substances can be legally purchased, increasing the price of these substances through taxation or with price controls, limiting sale hours, stronger enforcement of underage purchase laws, and state-mandated "zero tolerance" legislation for driving under the influence of alcohol.

The second category focuses on a sociocultural model that emphasizes education and enhancement of individuals' competencies through information, values' clarification, and skill-building techniques. These are delivered in various ways such as school-based programs and curricula for all children within a school district, media campaigns, and community interventions aimed at strengthening families to prevent drug use, such as the Iowa Strengthening Families Program [23], Guiding Good Choices (GGC, formerly known as Preparing for the Drug-Free Years Program) [24], Families and Schools Together (FAST) [25], Project ALERT [26], and the Adolescent Transition Program [27]. These types of prevention programs can encompass community-wide efforts through media campaigns that target schools, recreational activities, and/or physicians' offices. In general, schools appear to be the primary mode of program delivery. The school is a common sense place for prevention efforts because it is the environment in which large numbers of youths are available for long periods of time and it is the setting in which problems relating to parental substance abuse/dependence or other familial risk factors will be most consistently discernible [21,28].

The goal of universal prevention is to deter the onset of substance use and misuse by providing all individuals with the information and skills necessary to prevent the problem. All members of the targeted population share the same general risk for substance use and misuse, although the risk may vary greatly among individuals or subgroups. The entire population is assessed as "at risk" for substance use and misuse and capable of benefiting from prevention programs. Targeting risk and protective factors in a substance use prevention program can have benefits for a broad range of adolescent risk behaviors [6,29].

The advantages of universal prevention include a broad political appeal, the avoidance of labeling or stigmatizing children and their families as "high risk," and the ground work for more targeted programs [22]. However, perhaps a more prudent prevention strategy would be to identify "high risk" youths and those with substance use problems rather than to treat everyone as if one size fits all [30].

Educational Programs

Historically, primary prevention efforts have focused heavily on school-based education programs and mass media campaigns. Programs targeted at students and parents have a significantly increased knowledge base regarding psychoactive substance use. However, it has been difficult to effectuate change in attitudes toward substances, and changes in behaviors have been modest or difficult to demonstrate.

National programs for teaching children to refuse or abstain from psychoactive substances have only been partially successful. Because of the ubiquitous presence of substances in the culture, coming to personal terms with substance abuse/dependence represents a complex developmental task for some adolescents. A "Just Say No" approach might be important for those at "low risk" for developing a substance abuse problem. However, "Just Say No" has been criticized by some for reducing a multifaceted matter into a catch phrase. In addition, adolescents need to be educated on what the reasons are for saying "No" in the first place [31].

Twelve-Step and other Self-Help Programs

Self-help programs such as Alateen (for teenagers whose lives have been affected by someone else's alcohol use problem), Alanon (for family members and significant others of people with substance use disorders), Alcoholics Anonymous, Narcotics Anonymous, Cocaine Anonymous, Adult Children of Alcoholics, and Mothers Against Drunk Driving (MADD) provide support and dissemination of educational materials. Some groups provide important lobbying power. These organizations can also help disseminate information and, indirectly through twelve-step work, aid at early case finding and intervention.

Mass Media Campaigns

Mass media prevention campaigns often use popular peer role models as well as messages delivered by prominent sports figures, celebrities, or parental role models (such as Nancy Reagan, Rosalynn Carter, Betty Ford, and Tipper Gore). Public service announcement campaigns are used in an attempt to increase knowledge and awareness of the public health problem, alter perceptions of community norms, change attitudes, challenge myths, and promote increased communication between parents and children.

Social Policy and Legal Efforts

Given that the availability of addictive substances leads to greater use among adolescents and given that alcohol and tobacco are widely available, cheap, and legal, their impact on adolescent behavior is powerful. Limiting availability of alcohol and tobacco through increased taxation, decreasing outlet availability, decreasing hours of sale, and age restriction policies are ways to reduce overall consumption. After the legal drinking age was raised to 21 throughout the United States, studies have indicated that this approach decreased teenage motor vehicle collisions and deaths. Unfortunately, too little effort has been put into enforcing this limit on college campuses, where binge drinking has become endemic. Some colleges have attempted to address the issue of alcohol use of their students by enforcing "dry" campuses instead of "wet" campuses. Limiting tobacco advertising and use in public places has been another effective measure in an effort to achieve the US Surgeon General's goal of a "smokeless" society.

Selective Prevention Strategies

Selective strategies are also a form of primary prevention. Like universal prevention, their purpose is to delay the onset of substance use or reduce and/or prevent new cases of psychoactive substance use and misuse. Unlike universal prevention, they do not focus on the general population, but target "high risk" individuals or families as possible members of "high risk" subgroups (such as adolescents with parents and/or siblings dependent on substances; families who live in high crime, high alcohol outlet density, high illicit drug use, and/or extremely impoverished neighborhoods; associates of peers who abuse substances; young offenders; youths involved with gangs; victims of physical and/or sexual abuse; youths in foster homes; homeless youths; youths displaying behavioral problems; school dropouts; school truants; or academically failing students) regardless of the degree of risk of any individual within the subgroup. No single individual in the subgroup may be at personal risk for substance abuse, while another person in the same subgroup may be abusing substances. These individuals are targeted not because of specific individual needs assessments or diagnoses, but because the subgroup as a whole is at heightened risk. Thus, the targeted individuals are deemed to be "at risk" for substance abuse/dependence solely due to their membership in a particular population subgroup. The risk groups may be distinguished by demographic characteristics (such as age, gender, family history, or economic status), biological genetic risk factors, or psychosocial environmental risk factors known to be associated with substance abuse [32].

Examples of selective family interventions are the Strengthening Families Program [33] for psychoactive substance-abusing families, and other culturally modified versions for certain "high risk" African American, Latin American, Native American, Asian, and Pacific Islander families. The determination of "high risk" by ethnicity might be a shallow designation. The common bond in almost all of these groups is extreme poverty, high unemployment, poor educational opportunities, and highly marginalized individuals. Caution must be used to avoid any type of stereotyping, and studies of intervention strategies should include all socioeconomic groups as "at risk" [34].

Determining "High Risk" Groups

Efforts to target programs for those at "high risk" for heart disease, obesity, hypertension, and cholesterol have been paralleled by programs to help the "high risk" group of children of alcoholics adopt alternative alcohol-free lifestyles. Given the impact of genetic risks, it is important to target those in this "high risk" group (although all genetic factors may create varying degrees of risk). Familial alcoholics often have earlier onset of problem drinking, more severe social consequences, less consistently stable family involvement, poor academic and social performance, more antisocial behavior, and poorer prognosis in treatment. There is evidence that genetic risks can be addressed through preventive strategies [35].

Violent Youths

One "high risk" group involves adolescents who display violent behaviors. Various hospital emergency rooms (ERs) have initiated efforts to identify and mollify (if not prevent) psychoactive substance use among adolescents presenting for emergent treatment around violence. In one study, among adolescents identified in the ER with self-reported alcohol use and aggression, a brief intervention resulted in a decrease in the prevalence of self-reported aggression and alcohol consequences [36].

High School and College Students

Despite continued efforts to reduce alcohol abuse/dependence among adolescents, including college students, problems continue. Binge drinking among high school and college students is rampant. College freshmen are often away from home for the first time and might think that psychoactive substance experimentation is stylish and a symbol of friendship. Some colleges have taken a lead in developing programs to help students in recovery by providing a campus free of alcohol (that is, a "dry" instead of a "wet" campus) and other substances, counseling, and peer mentoring. Yet, access to substances is often readily available.

Indicated Prevention Strategies

Indicated strategies are a form of secondary prevention. They seek to limit harm in the early stages of a psychoactive substance use disorder through considering the developmental stage of an adolescent. The goal is to identify "high risk" individuals who are exhibiting early signs of substance use (such as students who have initiated binge drinking) and to prevent the onset of substance abuse/problematic use in these individuals who do not meet the *Diagnostic and Statistical Manual of Mental Disorders, Fourth Edition, Text Revision* (*DSM-IV-TR*) criteria for substance abuse or dependence [37] and target them with special programs. These targeted individuals exhibit substance abuse-like behavior at a subclinical level and other related problem behaviors associated with substance abuse [32]. Thus, unlike universal or selective prevention strategies, the goal of indicated strategies is not to prevent substance use or its initiation, but rather to prevent the development of substance abuse/dependence, diminish frequency of substance use, and prevent problematic patterns of substance use. It also addresses risk factors associated with the individual including conduct disorders, poor academic performance, school truancy, depression, suicidal behavior, and interpersonal social problems such as alienation from parents, school, and positive peer groups. Less emphasis is placed on assessing or addressing environmental influences such as community values. Individuals are often referred to indicated prevention programs by their parents, teachers, school counselors, school nurses, youth workers, friends, or the courts.

Examples of indicated family interventions include: structured family therapy [38] and Functional Family Therapy (FFT) [39], systems behavioral family therapy [40], multi-dimensional family therapy [41], multi-target ecological treatment [42], and multi-systemic family therapy [43,44].

CONCLUSIONS

The prevention of psychoactive substance use among adolescents is an important public health priority because use often begins during adolescence, and the early initiation of use is associated with greater risk for later serious health and behavior problems. No single approach has been identified as effective for preventing substance use among adolescents. In fact, different factors in separate programs appear to be effective in certain communities with certain age groups. A multi-pronged approach to prevention is often necessary [45]. Research has suggested that although universal programs can be effective in reducing and preventing substance use, selective and indicated programs are more effective and have a greater cost-benefit ratios [46,47].

The American Medical Association's (AMA's) Guidelines for Adolescent Preventive (GAP) Services [48] recommend both primary and secondary prevention strategies to reduce adolescent substance use. These guidelines also recommend that physicians routinely determine their patients' risk factors including a family history of alcoholism and other substance use disorders,

and conduct screenings for all schoolchildren. Preventive efforts should start during prenatal visits and continue with developmentally appropriate information as the child and family mature [47].

References

1. The National Center on Addiction and Substance Abuse at Columbia University. Adolescent Substance Use: America's #1 Public Health Problem. June 2011. Available at: http://www.casacolumbia.org/templates/NewsRoom.aspx?articleid=631&zoneid=51. Accessed 15 December 2011.
2. Beyers JM, Toumbourou JW, Catalano RF, Arthur MW, Hawkins JD. A cross-national comparison of risk and protective factors for adolescent substance use: the United States and Australia. *J Adolesc Health* 2004;**35**:3–16.
3. Stronski SM, Ireland M, Michaud P, Narring F, Resnick MD. Protective correlates of stages in adolescent substance use: a Swiss National Study. *J Adolesc Health* 2000;**26**:420–427.
4. Crone EA, Bullens L, van derPlas EA, Kijkuit EJ, Zelazo PD. Developmental changes and individual differences in risk and perspective taking in adolescence. *Dev Psychopathol* 2008;**20**:1213–1229.
5. Haegerich TM, Tolan PH. Core competencies and the prevention of adolescent substance use. *New Dir Child Adolesc Dev* 2008;**122**:47–60.
6. Bailey JA. Addressing common risk and protective factors can prevent a wide range of adolescent risk behaviors. *J Adolesc Health* 2009;**45**:107–108.
7. Beardslee WR, Chien PL, Bell CC. Prevention of mental disorders, substance abuse, and problem behaviors: a developmental perspective. *Psychiatr Serv* 2011;**62**:247–254.
8. Wills TA, Ainette MG. Good self-control as a buffering agent for adolescent substance use: an investigation in early adolescence with time-varying covariates. *Psychol Addict Behav* 2008;**22**:459–471.
9. Anteghini M, Fonseca H, Ireland M, Blum RW. Health risk behaviors and associated risk and protective factors among Brazilian adolescents in Santos, Brazil. *J Adolesc Health* 2001;**28**:295–302.
10. Kliewer W, Murrelle L. Risk and protective factors for adolescent substance use: findings from a study in selected Central American countries. *J Adolesc Health* 2007;**40**:448–455.
11. Kulig JW, American Academy of Pediatrics Committee on Substance Abuse. Tobacco, alcohol, and other drugs: the role of the pediatrician in prevention, identification, and management of substance abuse. *Pediatrics* 2005;**115**:816–821.
12. Brown EC, Catalano RF, Fleming CB, Haggerty KP, Abbott RD. Adolescent substance use outcomes in the Raising Healthy Children project: a two-part latent growth curve analysis. *J Consult Clin Psychol* 2005;**73**:699–710.
13. Herman-Stahl MA, Krebs CP, Kroutil LA, Heller DC. Risk and protective factors for nonmedical use of prescription stimulants and methamphetamine among adolescents. *Addict Behav* 2007;**32**:1003–1015.
14. Amey CH, Albrecht SL, Miller MK. Racial differences in adolescent drug use: the impact of religion. *Subst Use Misuse* 1996;**31**:1311–1332.
15. Marsiglia FF, Kulis S, Nieri T, Parsai M. God forbid! Substance use among religious and non-religious youth. *Am J Orthopsychiatry* 2005;**75**:585–598.

16. Parsai M, Kulis S, Marsiglia FF. Parental monitoring, religious involvement and drug use among Latino and non-Latino youth in the southwestern United States. *Br J Soc Work* 2010;**40**:100–114.

17. Bahr SJ, Maughan SL, Marcos A, Li B. Family, religiosity, and the risk of adolescent drug use. *J Marriage Fam* 1998;**60**:979–993.

18. Suís JC, Parera N. Protective factors against drug use among young adolescents. *J Adolesc Health* 2004;**34**:135.

19. Cleveland MJ, Feinberg ME, Bontempo DE, Greenberg MT. The role of risk and protective factors in substance use across adolescence. *J Adolesc Health* 2008;**43**:157–164.

20. Gordon R. An operational classification of disease prevention. In: Steinberg JA, Silverman MM (eds), *Preventing Mental Disorders*. Rockville, MD: U.S. Department of Health and Human Services, 1987.

21. Lubman DI, Hides L, Yücel M, Toumbourou JW. Intervening early to reduce developmentally harmful substance use among youth populations. *Med J Aust* 2007;**187**(7 Suppl.):S22–25.

22. Zavela KJ. Developing effective school-based drug abuse prevention programs. *Am J Health Behav* 2002;**26**:252–265.

23. Molgaard V, Kumpfer KL. *The Iowa Strengthening the Families Program for Families with Pre- and Early Teens.* Ames, IA: Iowa State University, 1995.

24. Hawkins JD, Catalano RF, Miller JY. Risk and protective factors for alcohol and other drug problems in adolescence and early adulthood: Implications for substance abuse prevention. *Psychol Bull* 1992;**112**:64–105.

25. McDonald L. Families and schools together (FAST). In: Talley R, Walz G (eds), *Safe Schools, Safe Students*. Washington, DC: NECP, NAPSO, APA, ERIC, 1996; pp. 59–63.

26. Ghosh-Dastidar B, Longshore DL, Ellickson PL, McCaffrey DF. Modifying pro-drug risk factors in adolescents: Results from Project ALERT. *Health Educ Behav* 2004;**31**:318–334.

27. Dishion TJ, Kavanagh K. *Intervening with Adolescent Problem Behavior: A Family-Centered Approach*. New York: Guilford Press, 2003.

28. Emshoff JG, Price AW. Prevention and intervention strategies with children of alcoholics. *Pediatrics* 1999;**103**:1112–1121.

29. Ellickson PL, McCaffrey DF, Klein DJ. Long-term effects of drug prevention on risky sexual behavior among young adults. *J Adolesc Health* 2009;**45**:111–117.

30. Black DR. Peer helping/involvement: an efficacious way to meet the challenge of reducing alcohol, tobacco, and other drug use among youth? *J Sch Health* 1998;**68**:87–93.

31. Government Accounting Office. DARE Long-Term Evaluations and Federal Efforts to Identify Effective Programs. GAO, 2003. Available at: http://www.gao.gov/products/GAO-03-172R. Accessed 15 December 2011.

32. Institute of Medicine. New directions in definitions. In: Mrazek PJ, Haggerty RJ (eds), *Reducing Risks for Mental Disorders: 96 Frontiers for Preventive Intervention Research*. Washington, DC: National Academy Press, 1994.

33. Kumpfer KL, Pinyuchon M, Teixeira de Melo A, Whiteside HO. Cultural adaptation process for Iinternational dissemination of the strengthening families program. *Eval Health Prof.* 2008;**31**(2):226–39.

34. Fang L, Schinke SP, Cole KC. Preventing substance use among early Asian-American adolescent girls: initial evaluation of a web-based, mother-daughter program. *J Adolesc Health* 2010;**47**:529–532.

35. Brody GH, Chen YF, Beach SR, Philibert RA, Kogan SM. Participation in a family-centered prevention program decreases genetic risk for adolescents' risky behaviors. *Pediatrics* 2009;**124**:911–917.

36. Walton MA, Chermack ST, Shope JT, *et al.* Effects of a brief intervention for reducing violence and alcohol misuse among adolescents: a randomized controlled trial. *JAMA* 2010;**304**:527–535.

37. American Psychiatric Association. Diagnostic and statistical manual of mental disorders (4th ed., text rev.). Washington, DC: American Psychiatric Press, 2000.

38. Szapocznik J, Perez-Vidal A, Brickman AL, *et al.* Engaging adolescent drug abusers and their families in treatment: a strategic structural systems approach. *J Consult Clin Psychol* 1988;**56**:552–557.

39. Alexander JF, Parsons V. *Functional Family Therapy*. Monterey, CA: Brooks/Cole, 1982.

40. Rowe CL. Family therapy for drug abuse: review and updates 2003–2010. J Marital Fam Ther. 2012 Jan;**38**(1):59–81.

41. Liddle HA, Dakof GA. Family-based treatment for adolescent drug use: state of the science. *NIDA Res Monogr* 1995;**156**:218–254.

42. Chamberlain P, Rosicky JG. The effectiveness of family therapy in the treatment of adolescents with conduct disorders and delinquency. *J Marital Fam Ther* 1995;**21**:441–459.

43. Henggeler SW, Borduin CM. *Family Therapy and Beyond: A Multisystemic Approach to Treating the Behavior Problems of Children and Adolescents*. Pacific Grove, CA: Brooks/Cole, 1990.

44. Henggeler SW, Melton GB, Smith LA. Family preservation using multisystemic therapy: an effective alternative to incarcerating serious juvenile offenders. *J Consult Clin Psychol* 1992;**60**:953–961.

45. Johnson EM, Amatetti S, Funkhouser JE, Johnson S. Theories and models supporting prevention approaches to alcohol problems among youth. *Public Health Rep* 1988;**103**:578–586.

46. Shamblen SR, Derzon JH. A preliminary study of the population-adjusted effectiveness of substance abuse prevention programming: towards making IOM program types comparable. *J Prim Prev* 2009;**30**:89–107.

47. Emshoff JG, Price AW. Prevention and intervention strategies with children of alcoholics. *Pediatrics.* 1999;**103**(5 Pt 2):1112–21.

48. Elster AB, Kuznets NJ (eds). *American Medical Association's Guidelines for Adolescent Preventive Services (GAPS): Recommendations and Rationale*. Baltimore: Williams & Wilkins, 1994.

12

Developmental Risks for Substance Use in Adolescence: Age as Risk Factor

Manuel Lopez-Leon[1] and Jesse A. Raley[2]

[1] New York University School of Medicine; New York University
Child Study Center, New York, NY, USA
[2] Adult, Child & Adolescent, and Forensic Psychiatrist, Columbia, SC, USA

INTRODUCTION

The use, abuse, prevention, and treatment of substance use disorders in children and adolescents is of grave concern; not the least since its prevalence is rising, the age of first usage is falling, and the morbidity and mortality of youths with any substance use is increasing. Substance abuse can interfere with natural growth and normal interaction and development, including relationships with peers, performance in school, attitudes toward law and authority, and acute and chronic organic effects. The question of when use becomes abuse and dependency in adolescents is controversial. There is a continuum between hazardous, harmful use and abuse – and it appears that such a dimensional model will be codified by the forthcoming *Diagnostic and Statistical Manual of Mental Disorders, Fifth Edition* (DSM-5). It is more difficult to diagnose dependence in adolescents because of the reduced likelihood of signs and symptoms of withdrawal that frequently occur later in addiction. Adolescents are less likely to report withdrawal symptoms, have shorter periods of addiction, and may recover more rapidly from withdrawal symptoms. Early identification of patterns of drug use that interfere with relationships, school performance, and ability to provide good self-care are important in addition to physiological symptoms of tolerance and withdrawal.

Consideration of the factors that create risk that adolescents will use a substance of abuse must first address that these are individuals who are undergoing a peculiar phase of their lives where their own peer, social, family, biological, and educational domains are themselves risk factors for the initiation or the maintenance of substance misuse. While the other chapters in this book's section on "Risk" will deal with specific problems that are risk factors (e.g., the presence of fetal alcohol syndrome or of maltreatment), this chapter will review the normal adolescent's experience and the attendant risk for misuse, whether "experimental," occasional, uncontrollable, or otherwise.

It is clear that exposure to substances is not uncommon among adolescents. Data from the "Monitoring the Future" study reported that lifetime use of any illicit drug had risen to 48% in 2010 after having remained at 47% for 2007, 2008, and 2009 [1]. In 2010 daily use of cannabis significantly rose for 8th-, 10th-, and 12th-graders. In 2009, 10.0% of youths aged 12 to 17 were current illicit drug users: 7.3% used cannabis, 3.1% engaged in non-medical use of prescription-type psychotherapeutics, 1.0% used inhalants, 0.9% used hallucinogens, and 0.3% used cocaine, according to the National Surveys on Drug Use and Health (NSDUH) 2009. Through the adolescent years from 12 to 17, the rates of current illicit drug use in 2009 increased from 3.6% at ages 12 or 13, to 9.0% at ages 14 or 15, to 16.7% at ages 16 or 17. The types of drugs used in the past month varied by age group, and it is important to note that while cannabis use continued to rise in 2010, overall use of illicit drugs other than cannabis declined in 2010. Among 12- or 13-year-olds, 1.6% used prescription-type drugs non-medically, 1.4% used inhalants, and 0.8% used cannabis. Among 14- or 15-year-olds, cannabis was the most commonly used drug (6.3%), followed by prescription-type drugs used non-medically (3.3%); inhalants and hallucinogens tied for third rank (0.8%).

Clinical Handbook of Adolescent Addiction, First Edition. Richard Rosner.
© 2013 John Wiley & Sons, Ltd. Published 2013 by John Wiley & Sons, Ltd.

Cannabis also was the most commonly used drug among 16- or 17-year-olds (14.0%); followed by prescription-type drugs used non-medically (4.3%), hallucinogens (1.6%), inhalants (0.8%), and cocaine (0.6%).

Substances other than heroin, alcohol, and cocaine are of increasing importance. It is notable that abuse of "prescription medications" is a new and significant, albeit poorly documented concern. Among teens in the United States, prescription medications have been replacing alcohol as the second most common category of abused substances, and if this trend continues they will also soon replace cannabis as the most common substance of abuse through all age brackets [2]. In 2005, for the first time the number of new abusers (aged 12 and older) of prescription drugs was on a par with that for new abusers of cannabis. In 2005, the estimated number of 12–17-year-olds who started using prescription drugs in the 12 months prior to the survey was 850 000, compared with 1 139 000 cannabis initiates [3]. In 2003 the estimates were 913 000 for prescription medications, compared to 1 219 000 cannabis initiates [4–6]. In 2005, 2.1 million teens abused prescription drugs. Teens aged 12 to 17 have the second-highest annual rates of prescription drug abuse after young adults (18–25). Prescription drugs are the most commonly abused drugs among 12–13-year-olds. Teens (12–17) in western and southeastern US states are more likely to abuse prescription pain relievers. The most recent research on deaths in the United States due to poisoning over a 5-year period (1999–2004) shows that nearly all poison deaths in the country are attributed to drugs, and most drug poisonings result from the abuse of prescription and illegal drugs [7,8]. Pain relievers, like Vicodin and OxyContin, are the prescription drugs most commonly abused by teens [5]. Nearly half of teens who have abused prescription painkillers also report the use of two or more other drugs, most commonly alcohol and cannabis. Nearly 40% of teens report having friends who abuse prescription pain relievers and nearly 30% report having friends who abuse prescription stimulants. Over half of teens say they abuse prescription painkillers because the medications aren't illegal; one in three believes there is less shame attached to using prescription drugs than illicit drugs; and one in five said parents "don't care as much if you get caught" abusing prescription drugs. Among 12th-graders, past-year abuse of OxyContin increased 30% between 2002 through 2007 [8]. Past year abuse of Vicodin is particularly high among 8th-, 10th-, and 12th-graders, with nearly 1 in 10 high school seniors reporting taking it in the past year without a prescription.

As discussed in this text (see Chapter 14), the greatest risk for substance use of any form in adolescence is the effect of peers, which may be followed by

psychiatric conditions, genetic components, and other social forces. But for each individual adolescent other non-diagnostic forces include thrill-seeking or sensation-seeking behavior, insufficient impulse control, insufficient abstract reasoning or planning, and omnipotent feelings. Adolescents often engage in periods of anger or rejection of "authority." Furthermore, the maintenance of use may be more tolerable because of a lack of effects on the adolescent's social or biological world. Psychological resilience of adolescents may protect them from consequences while failing to impede use.

ADOLESCENT SUBSTANCE MISUSE: "EXPERIMENTAL" AND OTHER FORMS

Given that any exposure to some substances can have lasting deleterious effects, it is important to consider the factors that lead to occasional, experimental or sub-diagnostic use among adolescents – even experimental use is dangerous and should not be ignored. Such factors include peer or family influences (discussed in next chapter), as well as curiosity, judgment, impulse control, sensation-seeking or thrill-seeking behavior, or challenges to authority. Substance use – even experimentation – need not necessarily be normalized in terms of it being seen as acceptable, but clearly occasional misuse among adolescents is common. It does not always lead to discernible pathology, although adolescents are obviously poor observers of whether or not substances harm them. Some studies have used lack of functional impairment as the sole defining criteria for experimentation [9].

Adolescents' perception and self-report on whether substance use constitutes experimentation or problem use has also been explored. Unfortunately, adolescents who define themselves as experimenting users vary widely among the parameters of amount, frequency, and duration [10,11]. This significantly limits the utility of solely relying on self-report to define whether an adolescent's substance use constitutes experimentation.

DEVELOPMENTAL CONTRIBUTIONS TO RISK-TAKING BEHAVIOR

Biological, social, and psychological development persists throughout the adolescent period. Adolescence has traditionally been regarded as a time of dramatic transitions. As part of the process of developing into a young adult, adolescents undergo a series of changes in their attitudes and behaviors [12]. The last region of the brain to develop via myelination and synaptic pruning is the prefrontal cortex. During late adolescence, this area reaches maturation and is associated with substantial white matter volume increases. This plays a critical part in the higher cognitive functions relevant to judgment such as risk estimation, risk choices, the ability to evaluate short- versus long-term consequences, and, therefore, executive decision-making functions. As this region normally matures, adolescents are able to better reason, develop self-control, and make increasingly more mature judgments. This might explain why exposure to psychoactive substances at this time might affect propensity for future addiction. Brain structure and function changes across adolescence may underlie the differences that are observed in risk-taking behavior [13]. This developmental period produces several phenotypic behaviors that may impact both misuse and advanced forms of use:

- *Inexperience and risky behaviors:* Risk-taking behavior may or may not include substance experimentation, but does include several dangerous activities. The described neurodevelopmental reasons why adolescents are more likely to engage in risky behavior should lead clinicians to assess for risk-taking behaviors in their adolescent patients. Information from this assessment may guide the clinician's substance history and overall evaluation.
- *Rebelliousness:* In their search for identity and independence, adolescents often demonstrate a desire to resist authority and experiment the opposite of whatever is conventional. They are faced with either becoming submissive and accepting of the norms imposed on them, or attempting to become independent by rejecting them [14]. Not only does rebellion among adolescents occur, but there is also an identified neurobiological basis for this behavior. Studies show that the prefrontal cortex regulates risk-taking behavior, and that this part of the brain is relatively underdeveloped in the adolescent brain [15–17]. Adolescents who have hypoactive prefrontal cortices – particularly anterior cingulate cortex, orbitofrontal cortex, and medial prefrontal cortex – tend to engage in more risk-taking behavior than the typical adolescent [18].
- *Sensation-seeking:* Interest in sensations may come from boredom or from some reaction to one's psychological environment. This may account for interest in hallucinogens as adolescents are enthralled with the capacities around abstract thought. Biological mechanisms might make substances more appealing: Teenagers experimenting with alcohol may experience less sedation or more stimulation; both scenarios suggest that an inherited differential response to alcohol may make alcohol more reinforcing for adolescents with a genetic predisposition to alcoholism. Alcohol addiction is more likely to occur in adolescents who drink to feel the alcohol's effects rather than those who drink to fit in or experiment with alcohol.
- *Identity formation:* Adolescence is a period in which youths develop sexual maturity and establish their identity as individuals in society [19]. Most often it can be a period of strength and resilience [20]. During this period, youths often spend more time with peers and are more influenced by their peers than by their parents. Also, during this period, youths are at a heightened psychosocial vulnerability to a variety of risk-taking behaviors including experimentation with psychoactive substances. Rates of risk-taking behavior peak in middle or late adolescence [13,21,22]. Difficulties in behavioral and emotional control are major causes of morbidity and mortality in adolescence [20,23].

ATTITUDES REGARDING USE OF ILLICIT SUBSTANCES

One measure of the above components of adolescent misuse is adolescent assessment of the risk of various substances. NIDA's Monitoring the Future study addressed this issue for various substances. Awareness of attitudes regarding addictive substances is critical for practicing clinicians. The national trends are important because they may pique the clinician's vigilance for use among a clinical population. And, assessing the attitude of individual patients is also important, especially as one checks their attitudes against the national trends for that age group.

Historically, overall substance use trends have followed cannabis use. Since 2006, 8th-, 10th-, and 12th-graders' views of dangerousness and disapproval of cannabis use have both trended downward [1]. In 2010, 51.6% of 12th-graders, 59.2% of 10th-graders, and 73.5% of 8th-graders reported that they "disapprove" or "strongly disapprove" of trying cannabis "once or twice." Correspondingly, in 2010 rates of use "in the last 30 days" were 21.4%, 16.7%, and 8.0%, respectively. This reiterates that attitudes relating to substance use reflect individuals' likelihood to experiment with the substance.

While cannabis use may mirror trends for overall substance use, alcohol disapproval is much lower. Only 30.7% of 12th-graders report they "disapprove" or "strongly disapprove" of trying one to two drinks. Other illicit substances such as cocaine, crack, heroin, MDMA ("ecstasy"), LSD, amphetamine, and steroids have higher rates of disapproval. Interestingly, overall disapproval for 12th-, 10th-, and 8th-graders using LSD and ecstasy "once or twice" is steadily trending downward over the past 5 years. LSD use has been steady and low since the 1990s but ecstasy use has been inconsistent and increased in 2010.

THEORIES OF ADOLESCENT PSYCHOACTIVE SUBSTANCE USE

Given the importance of understanding, treating, and preventing all forms of substance use among adolescents, it is also valuable to appreciate theories of how this use progresses.

The Gateway Hypothesis: the Risk of "Experimental" Use

Kandel's Gateway Hypothesis was developed in the 1970s; it posited a progressive causal chain sequence of psychoactive substance use that begins with experimentation with legalized psychoactive substances (i.e., alcohol and/or tobacco), followed by cannabis use, and then continues with other illegal psychoactive substances, for example, cocaine, heroin, amphetamines, and LSD [24–26]. Cannabis use is considered a crucial step on the path to other "harder" illicit substances and thus opens a floodgate that can spiral the adolescent downward into more potent drugs. It assumes that psychoactive substances are arranged in a hierarchical status with some psychoactive substances being worse than others. The "gateway drugs" are considered "softer" psychoactive substances, that is, alcohol, tobacco, and cannabis. They are the "stepping stones" to "harder" psychoactive substance use. As mentioned earlier, these are the three psychoactive substances most commonly used by adolescents in the United States. This hypothesis assumes that the "gateway drugs" increase the proportion of users going onto more potent substances [25,27–30]. It also assumes that "gateway drugs" sensitize maturing reward pathways to the effects of more potent substances [31].

Some of the explanations used in the literature to support the Gateway Hypothesis are as follows:

- *Biochemical level:* At a biochemical level, the nexus between cannabis use and other illicit psychoactive substance use results from changes in brain chemistry due to the increasing use of cannabis. This biochemical change might lead to increases in an individual's responsiveness to other illicit substances. This might create a psychological or physiological need for further and stronger experiences of the same type [32,33].
- *Individual learning level:* At an individual learning level, the nexus between cannabis use and other illicit psychoactive substance use results from an individualized learning process in which an adolescent first experiments with cannabis and learns that it has gratifying euphoric effects and low rates of adverse side effects. This explanation assumes that experimentation with cannabis might reduce the perceived risks in the use of other illicit substances with gratification overpowering any adverse side effects. This gratification, in turn, undermines the strong negative publicity directed against all illicit drug use. A cannabis user might become emboldened to take the next step to the use of other illicit and more potent psychoactive substances. These experiences subsequently can form the grounds for further experimentation with other illicit substances [32–34].
- *Societal level:* At a societal level, the nexus between cannabis use and other illicit psychoactive substance use results from the differential association of cannabis users and non-users within the drug culture, that is, the cannabis user and buyer often must associate with hard drug users and drug dealers whom they would not otherwise have met. Regular cannabis users often need to remain in contact with the drug culture in order to obtain cannabis. Cannabis dealers might also sell other "harder" psychoactive substances. This nexus of cannabis users with the drug culture can provide multiple opportunities for regular cannabis users both to learn about other illicit psychoactive substances and to obtain them [28,33,34].
- *Cognitive impairment level:* At a cognitive impairment level, the nexus between cannabis use and other illicit psychoactive substance use results from an intoxicated cannabis user becoming more likely to be lured toward experimentation with other illicit psychoactive substances secondary to cognitive impairment [34] (see also Chapter 17).

Prevention programs based on Kandel's hypothesis are directed toward preventing the use of specific "gateway drugs," which in turn might help reduce the initiation of more potent ones [32,35]. This implies that if smoking of nicotine-containing products were restricted there would be less use of cannabis. This also implies that if cannabis were legalized there would be greater use of more potent psychoactive substances [27]. In many countries drug policy and legislation have been significantly influenced by this hypothesis [33].

There are frequent exceptions to the gateway sequence model. For example, not all nicotine smokers or alcohol consumers go onto use cannabis, and not all cannabis users first smoked nicotine or consumed alcohol [27]. Some cannabis users never move on to "harder" psychoactive substance use [34]. Thus, "softer" psychoactive substance use does not necessarily lead to "harder" psychoactive substance use [36]. Also, "gateway sequence" violations have been found to be more common in studies of disadvantaged or deviant groups [30]. Perhaps some individuals are more willing to try any psychoactive substance, and the "gateway drugs" are merely the ones that are most commonly available at an earlier age than the "harder" ones and therefore are used first.

Besides the gateway sequence model, other variables can affect the course of psychoactive substance use, and these are described in greater detail in this section. Some of these are important in the context of the Gateway Hypothesis:

- *Substance availability:* As discussed in the next chapter, simply the accessibility of a psychoactive substance might explain why some substances are used over others. Accessibility refers to a substance's availability, affordability, and acceptance within a culture. Even current drug legislation and sentencing protocols influence accessibility; for example, cocaine appears to be less frowned upon than crack when in reality they are the same [33,35]. Thus, "gateway sequence" violations might reflect a greater and earlier prominence of "non-gateway" drugs in the user's drug history [35].
- *Birth cohort:* Some illicit substance use is significantly more common among more recent birth cohorts. Present generation adolescents have a much broader range of exposure and accessibility to drugs and, therefore, a much wider gateway. Many drugs that exist today did not exist in previous generations. Even the potency of specific substances varies with the different birth cohorts. This broader exposure significantly complicates the hypothesis. For example, today in the United States there is a broader array of "gateway drugs" such as ecstasy [37] and oxycodone [38].
- *Comorbid psychiatric illnesses/dual diagnoses:* As discussed later in this section, both internalizing and externalizing disorders pose immense risk for substance use among adolescents. There is a high frequency of comorbid mental disorders in individuals with a high intake of psychoactive substances [39]. These samples commonly display much earlier initiation into significantly more potent first substance use [40–42]. Thus, comorbid psychiatric illnesses appear to be important for both the order of initiation of illicit drug use and particularly for the development of dependent use once initiation begins.
- *Non-diagnostic personal characteristics:* As discussed above, some studies have shown that personal characteristics might be responsible for "gateway sequence" violations such as impulsivity and risk-taking behaviors. Violations reflecting precocious entry into psychoactive substance use were found to be associated with elevated risks for later dependence. This would be consistent with the possibility

that "gateway sequence" violations reflect a broader underlying vulnerability to drug problems [35]. The longstanding causal debate has revolved around the precise identification of the problem. Does the fact that cigarette smokers are more likely to go on to use cannabis result from unobserved heterogeneity? That is, do people with a greater susceptibility to smoke cigarettes also have a greater susceptibility to consume cannabis, or is it the result of a treatment effect, namely exposure to cigarettes (the treatment) induces cannabis use (the outcome)? The vast number of empirical papers on the Gateway Hypothesis have not resolved the identification problem [27].

The Reverse Gateway Hypothesis

The Reverse Gateway Hypothesis posits that for some nicotine smokers, cannabis use precedes nicotine [43,44]. Thus, it assumes that cannabis use predicts later nicotine initiation and/or nicotine dependence in those who had not used nicotine before. Thus, cannabis might be a "gateway drug" to nicotine. Some of the explanations used in the literature to support this hypothesis include:

- *Reducing the sedative effects and enhancing the rewarding effects:* For some cannabis-oriented youths, nicotine might reduce the sedative effects of cannabis and both increase and prolong its rewarding effects [45]. Thus, nicotine might enhance the physiological, behavioral, and rewarding effects of tetrahydrocannabinol [46].
- *Reinforcing effects of cannabis:* For some cannabis-oriented youths, their cannabis use appears to support and reinforce their nicotine use [47]. Some studies demonstrate that significant cannabis use during adolescence predicts initiation of nicotine use in non-nicotine-smoking adolescents and that young adult cannabis use predicted a transition to later nicotine dependence [44,48]. Moreover, in Australia a "reverse gateway" has been described for cannabis where its use has been linked to increased risk of subsequent initiation to nicotine use and dependence [35,44]. However, this study could not rule out the fact that cannabis is commonly mixed with nicotine in joints to enhance burning and stretch supplies.

CONCLUSIONS

Subthreshold use of addictive substances occurs not uncommonly during adolescence. While "experimentation" may be difficult to define, it is understood that many people experiment with addictive substances for the first time during adolescence, and some people will continue to use these substances into adulthood. There are risk factors associated with experimentation including availability, attitudes, and family dynamics. The clinician's job is to assess for both experimentation and the risk of experimentation as well as to continually assess for the risk of experimentation transitioning to substance abuse or dependence.

References

1. Johnston LD, O'Malley PM, Bachman JG, Schulenberg JE. *Monitoring the Future national results on adolescent drug use: Overview of key findings, 2010*. Ann Arbor: Institute for Social Research, The University of Michigan, 2011.
2. Office of National Drug Control Policy. Teens and Prescription Drugs, an analysis of recent trends on the emerging drug threat. Washington, DC: Office of National Drug Control Policy. Executive Office of the President, 2007.
3. Substance Abuse and Mental Health Services Administration. *Results from the 2005 National Survey on Drug Use and Health: National Findings*. Office of Applied Studies, NSDUH Series H-30, DHHS Publication No. SMA 06-4194. Rockville, MD: SAMHSA, 2006.
4. Substance Abuse and Mental Health Services Administration, Office of Applied, Studies. *Drug Abuse Warning Network, 2005: national estimates of drug-related emergency department visits*. DAWN Series D-29, DHHS Publication No. (SMA) 07-4256. Rockville, MD: SAMHSA, 2007.
5. Substance Abuse and Mental Health Services Administration. *Results from the 2004 National Survey on Drug Use and Health: National Findings*. Office of Applied Studies, NSDUH Series H-28, DHHS Publication No. SMA 05-4062. Rockville, MD: SAMHSA, 2005.
6. Substance Abuse and Mental Health Services Administration. *Results from the 2006 National Survey on Drug Use and Health: National Findings*. Office of Applied Studies, NSDUH Series H-32, DHHS Publication No. SMA 07-4293. Rockville, MD: SAMHSA, 2007.
7. Paulozzi LJ, Annest J. Unintentional poisoning deaths –United States, 1999–2004. *MMWR* 2007;**56**:93–96.
8. Wu LT, Pilowsky DJ, Patkar AA. Non-prescribed use of pain relievers among adolescents in the United States. *Drug Alcohol Depend* 2008;**94**:1–11.
9. Lee SS, Humphreys KL, Flory K, Liu R, Glass K. Prospective association of childhood attention-deficit/hyperactivity disorder (ADHD) and substance use and abuse/dependence: A meta analytic review. *Clin Psychol Rev* 2011;**31**:328–341.
10. Andrews JA, Duncan SC. Examining the reciprocal relationship between academic motivation and substance use: Effects of family relationships, self-esteem, and general deviance. *J Behav Med* 1997;**20**:523–549.
11. Thurman PJ, Green VA. American Indian adolescent inhalant use. *Am Indian Alsk Native Ment Health Res* 1997;**8**:24–40.
12. Erickson E. *Identity and the Life Cycle*. New York: International Universities Press, 1959.
13. Crone EA, Bullens L, Van Der Plas EAA, Kijkuit EJ, Zelazo PD. Developmental changes and individual differences in risk and perspective taking in adolescence. *Dev Psychopathol* 2008;**20**:1213–1229.
14. Anthony EJ. Between yes and no: The potentially neutral area where the adolescent and his therapist can meet. *Adolesc Psychiat* 1976;**3**:323–344.
15. Casey BJ, Giedd JN, Thomas KM. Structural and functional brain development and its relation to cognitive development. *Biol Psychol* 2000;**54**:241–257.
16. Gogtay N, Giedd JN, Lusk L, *et al.* Dynamic mapping of human cortical development during childhood through early adulthood. *Proc Natl Acad Sci USA* 2004;**25**:8174–8179.
17. Spear LP. Modeling adolescent development and alcohol use in animals. *Alcohol Res Health* 2000;**54**:241–257.
18. Shad MU, Bidesi AS, Chen L, Thomas BP, Ernst M, Rao U. Neurobiology of decision-making in adolescents. *Behav Brain Res* 2011;**217**:67–76.
19. Rodrigues MC, de Assis Viegas CA, Gomes EL, deGodoy Morais JPM, de Oliveira Zakir JC. Prevalence of smoking and its association with the use of other drugs among students in the Federal District of Brasília, Brazil. *J Bras Pneumol* 2009;**35**:986–991.
20. Dahl RE. Adolescent brain development: vulnerabilities and opportunities. *Ann NY Acad Sci* 2004;**1021**:1–22.
21. Bailey J. Addressing common risk and protective factors can prevent a wide range of adolescent risk behaviors. *J Adolesc Health* 2009;**45**:107–108.
22. Stronski SM, Ireland M, Michaud P, Narring F, Resnick MD. Protective correlates of stages in adolescent substance use: A Swiss national study. *J Adolesc Health* 2000;**26**:420–427.
23. Anteghini M, Fonseca H, Ireland M, Blum RW. Health risk behaviors and associated risk and protective factors among Brazilian adolescents in Santos, Brazil. *J Adolesc Health* 2001;**28**:295–302.
24. Kandel DB. States in adolescent involvement in drug use. *Science* 1975;**190**:912–914.
25. Kandel DB, Faust R. Sequence and stages in patterns of adolescent drug use. *Arch Gen Psychiat* 1975;**32**:923–932.
26. Hamburg BA, Kraemer HC, Jahnke W. A hierarchy of drug use in adolescence: behavioral and attitudinal correlates of substantial drug use. *Am J Psychiat* 1975;**132**:1155–1163.
27. Beenstock M, Rahav G. Testing Gateway Theory: do cigarette prices affect illicit drug use? *J Health Econ* 2002;**21**:679–698.
28. Fergusson DM, Boden JM, Horwood LJ. Cannabis use and other illicit drug use: Testing the cannabis Gateway Hypothesis. *Addiction* 2006;**101**:556–569.
29. Yamaguchi K, Kandel DB. Patterns of drug use from adolescence to young adulthood: III. Predictors of progression. *Am J Publ Hlth* 1984;**74**:673–681.
30. Wells JE, McGee MA. Violations of the usual sequence of drug initiation: prevalence and associations with the development of dependence in the New Zealand Mental Health Survey. *J Stud Alcohol Drugs* 2008;**69**:789–795.
31. McQuown SC, Belluzzi JD, Leslie FM. Low dose nicotine treatment during early adolescence increases subsequent cocaine reward. *Neurotoxicol Teratol* 2007;**29**:66–73.
32. Fergusson DM, Boden JM, Horwood LJ. The developmental antecedents of illicit drug use: Evidence from a 25-year longitudinal study. *Drug Alcohol Depend* 2008;**96**:165–177.
33. Bretteville-Jensen AL, Sutton M. The income-generating behaviour of injecting drug-users in Oslo. *Addiction* 1996;**91**:63–79.

34. Choo T, Roh S, Robinson M. Assessing the "gateway hypothesis" among middle and high school students in Tennessee. *J Drug Issues* 2008;0022-0426/08/02: 467–492.

35. Degenhardt L. Evaluating the drug use "gateway" theory using cross-national data: Consistency and associations of the order of initiation of drug use among participants in the WHO World Mental Health Surveys. *Drug Alcohol Depend* 2010;**108**:84–97.

36. Peele S, Brodsky A. Gateway to nowhere: how alcohol came to be scapegoated for drug abuse. *Addiction Res* 1997;**5**:419–426.

37. Reid LW, Elifson KW, Sterk CE. Ecstasy and gateway drugs: initializing the use of ecstasy and other drugs. *Ann Epidemiol* 2007;**17**:74–80.

38. Grau L, Dasgupta N, Harvey A, *et al*. Illicit use of opioids: is OxyContin a 'gateway drug'? *Am J Addictions* 2007;**16**:166–173.

39. Langås AM, Malt UF, Opjordsmoen S. Comorbid mental disorders in substance users from a single catchment area – a clinical study. *BMC Psychiat* 2011;**11**:25.

40. Golub A, Johnson BD. The shifting importance of alcohol and marijuana as gateway substances among serious drug abusers. *J Stud Alcohol* 1994;**55**:607–614.

41. Golub A, Johnson BD. The misuse of the 'Gateway Theory' in US policy on drug abuse control: a secondary analysis of the muddled deduction. *Int J Drug Policy* 2002;**13**:5–19.

42. Mackesy-Amiti ME, Fendrich M, Goldstein PJ. Sequence of drug use among serious drug users: typical vs atypical progression. *Drug Alcohol Depend* 1997; **45**:185–196.

43. Humfleet GL, Haas AL. Is marijuana use becoming a 'gateway' to nicotine dependence? *Addiction* 2004; **99**:5–6.

44. Patton G, Coffey C, Carlin J, Sawyer SM, Lynskey M. Reverse gateways? Frequent cannabis use as a predictor of tobacco initiation and nicotine dependence. *Addiction* 2005;**100**:1518–1525.

45. Tullis LM, Frost-Pineda K, Dupont R, Gold MS. Marijuana and tobacco: A connection. *J Addictive Dis* 2003;**22**: 51–62.

46. Valjent E, Mitchell JM, Besson MJ, Caboche J, Maldonado R. Behavioural and biochemical evidence for interactions between D9-tetrahydrocannabinol and nicotine. *Br J Pharmacol* 2002;**135**:564–578.

47. Highet G. The role of cannabis in supporting young people's cigarette smoking: a qualitative exploration. *Health Educ Res* 2004;**19**:635–643.

48. Viveros MP, Marco EM, File SE. Nicotine and cannabinoids: parallels, contrasts and interactions. *Neurosci Biobehav Rev* 2006;**30**:1161–1181.

13

Genetic Risk Factors for Substance Use During Adolescence

Hallie A. Lightdale

Georgetown University Counseling and Psychological Services; Georgetown University School of Medicine, Washington, DC, USA

INTRODUCTION

The past 20 years have seen elucidation of many "biological" aspects of substance use and substance dependence, especially findings on neuronal circuits and abnormal neuroanatomy. Genetic understanding is another perspective – an important and powerful one – that has also developed in this period. Family studies have demonstrated familial transmission of a propensity not just to a particular substance of abuse, but also perhaps a vulnerability to addiction in general. Individuals with alcohol dependence are not only more likely to have relatives in their families who are also dependent on alcohol, but they are more likely to have relatives with dependence on other substances, such as cocaine, opioids, and tobacco. For example, the risk of alcohol dependence in relatives of proband alcohol-dependent patients compared with controls is about two-fold [1]. While it could be argued that familial patterns of addiction are affected by a variety of social and environmental factors, twin studies have demonstrated that considerable variability in risk for developing addiction is due to genetics.

What is meant, then, by "genetics?" We may refer to "genetic factors" as the qualities transmitted through genes and chromosomes, and those components may be differentiated from the impact of the family as a social unit affecting the individual's use (see Chapter 14), or the genetic influences upon the production of various psychiatric disorders (discussed in Chapters 15 and 16) or upon the development of various medical or neurological conditions. While all of these factors may have genetic components, they have not been analyzed in terms of their risk for substance use. This chapter generalizes among substances only when warranted. And, as elsewhere in this text, one must remember that this discussion relates to adolescents (including many college students) rather than to adults. We also exclude discussion of the normal neurological development that is affected by genes – here we discuss genetic variations that have been specifically linked to substance use. This chapter begins with a short review of human genetics as it relates to adolescent substance use, followed by a review of candidate genes and then a discussion of the gene × environment paradigm.

There are limitations to applying current genetics as it relates to adolescent substance use – one is that the data specific to this age group are few. Secondly, most of the information described below is regarding substance *dependence* diagnoses – which are rare among adolescent substance users. Third, the determinative role of genetic factors in an individual's use is far from conclusive: genetic factors contribute only some risk for use in this population, and genetic factors are likely intertwined with other behaviors, personality styles, and mental disorders that produce, among others, antisocial or impulsive actions. For example, among unaffected monozygotic twins reared in a non-abusing household, the risk of alcohol misuse was no greater than among controls, suggesting that environment, as a part of gene × environment interaction, matters [2]. Another limitation is that the natural history of use differs by each substance, and so generalizability is questionable, especially in non-dependent use situations. It is necessary to consider adolescent development. Crowley and others have intensely researched whether or not there is a generalized risk that comes during adolescence – they have not linked this generalized "use" risk with specific loci, but there is evidence of generalized risk associated with developmental level [3,4]. As a result of these issues, the study of the genetics of substance use among adolescents is concurrently complex, unresolved, and *vital* to prevention and treatment.

GENETIC METHODS AND THE LITERATURE

A full review of genetic methods and the genetics of behavioral phenotypes is beyond the scope of this chapter (see Lynskey *et al.* [5] for a review). What are some of the ways in which we learn from genetics? Genes that influence heritable traits may be identified. Linkage studies point to chromosomal locations. Association studies and other methods of analysis that make up linkage disequilibrium relationships, point to specific genes. Indeed, that alcoholism occurs in families was established nearly 60 years ago by Jellinek and Jolliffee. In alcohol dependence, genetic influences are greater in early- rather than late-onset dependence [6]. Although genetic influences in alcoholism and other drug abuse by both males and females have become fairly well established through twin, adoption, and split sibling studies, the mode of transmission is not clear nor is the answer to the question: what is being transmitted? Some studies have suggested that tolerance to alcohol is the transmitted trait. In establishing the genetic bases of cocaine abuse and cannabis abuse, other studies have proposed that it is a general vulnerability to a particular substance that is transmitted, such that the affected proband might become addicted after only one exposure [1]. Other studies have focused on abnormalities in dopamine receptor subtypes in the nucleus accumbens; the ventral striatum; NMDA (*N*-methyl-D-aspartate) glutamate receptors; alcohol dehydrogenase enzyme (ADH2*2 as protective), the synthesis of neuropeptide Y (Pro7 allele), and others that are described in this chapter.

In terms of specific genetic methods, rapid technological advances have made feasible the identification of specific gene variants that influence risks for substance-use disorders, and linkage and association (including genome-wide association studies) have identified promising candidate genes implicated in the development of substance-use disorders [5]. Here we review some current commonly employed methods.

1. *Adoption, twin, and extended-family study* designs have been used for some time, and they have established a heritable component to liability to nicotine, alcohol, and illicit drug dependence in adults. However, this must be understood in the context that shared environmental influences are relatively stronger in youth samples and at earlier stages of substance involvement (e.g., use) [5].

2. *Genome-wide linkage studies* are used to identify risk genes without knowing the mechanism they affect. Genome-wide linkage studies are the traditional method for identifying loci – they are family-based studies that require the investigation of markers that map throughout the entire genome, allowing the identification of chromosomal regions where markers are co-inherited with the phenotype of interest. What would a successful genome-wide linkage study provide? It would demonstrate the loci on a chromosome, but would not identify genes. However, a genome-wide association study could provide gene identification. Genome-wide linkage scans have been completed for alcohol dependence, conduct disorder, and opioid dependence.

3. *Genome-wide association studies (GWAS)* use different strategies. GWAS have been performed throughout a range of psychiatric diagnoses; and although the genetic mechanisms are still unknown, associations are elicited through the process [7]. Genome-wide association studies may feature a newer method in which very closely spaced markers are studied in an effort to discern those that vary in frequency. The intention is to genotype a sufficient number of markers so that there is at least one with *linkage disequilibrium*, which is indicative of an association. To date, use of GWAS analyses have produced information for one specific substance-dependent trait: the genotyping of those with nicotine dependence [8]. One large study on Nicotine Dependence using a two-stage design analyzed pooled DNA, leading to 30 000 single nucleotide polymorphisms (SNPs) that were assessed in both cases and controls. This process identified genes possibly associated with nicotine dependence (including neurexin 1, *NRXN1* or *VPS13A*). It is not yet known, however, whether or not these were in fact "false positives." Another method that utilizes GWAS has been the application of pooling strategies: DNA pooling provides an easier way to do a GWAS analysis, but no findings have been made to this point.

ABNORMAL GENETIC FACTORS AFFECTING USE OF SPECIFIC SUBSTANCES

The main research in this area is regarding substance dependence defined as "genetically influenced" [9] in a complex manner. It is not simply mendelian inheritance, which is to say that no one gene translates into substance dependence; probably many different genes are implicated. And environmental cues and other phenotypic components of personality and temperament, such as self-efficacy, do have an effect in determining use or dependence, or even the presence of the substance in the individual's life (that availability or presence of the substance impacts use compels us to consider this as a gene × environment interaction). There is much overlap in the genetic influences associated with abuse/dependence across drug classes, and shared genetic influences contribute to the commonly observed associations between substance use disorders and externalizing and, to a lesser extent, internalizing psychopathology [5].

It is also important to maintain the awareness that each drug is different and may have a different pattern of use and effects of genes. McGue and colleagues found that a significant genetic influence existed on the use and abuse of nicotine but not on the use and abuse of other substances (however, their study did not include alcohol). This finding supports the concept that experimentation may lead to continued drug use based on genetic factors [10]. Nicotine, being often the first drug used by adolescents, is the drug with which most adolescents experiment (although the most recent studies suggest cannabis has moved close to nicotine in this regard). Whether a nicotine-experienced adolescent continues to smoke may be influenced by the effects he or she obtains from nicotine, which may be genetically influenced. A study by Biederman *et al.* [11] found different effects based on substance of abuse.

Alcohol Dependence

Twin, family, and adoption studies all have demonstrated the heritability of alcohol dependence. The disorder is heritable around 50–60%, meaning more than half of the risk is genetic [12]. Kendler found the rate of alcohol dependence to be the same in monozygotic and dizygotic twins over a near-50-year sample, yet concordance was higher in monozygotic cases [13]. The rate was relatively stable over time.

Linkage Studies for Alcohol Dependence

There are promising leads for identifying alcohol dependence susceptibility loci. These are measured in terms of logarithm of odds (LOD) scores. Both the Collaborative Studies on Genetics of Alcoholism (COGA) study [14] and the NIAAA study [15] found loci influencing risk close to the alcohol dehydrogenase (ADH) gene cluster on the long arm of chromosome 4. Some have studied other concepts, such as the "response to alcohol," which, in one study by Wilhelmsen *et al.* [16], was shown to be lower in a chromosomal area – in that study a low response was a risk factor for the development of alcohol dependence. Furthermore, linkages for behavioral

entities other than the diagnosis of alcohol dependence have been examined, such as for consumption severity, and withdrawal (chromosomes 6, 15, 16, 4 and 12 respectively).

Other Substances of Abuse

In studying abuse and genetics beyond simply alcohol, the work of Ming Tsuang has been seminal, highlighted by his 1998 work, which used a Vietnam-era twin registry and found evidence of heritable risk for use of substances. In this study "use" was defined as use of a substance at least once weekly. The study showed that there was a familial basis for all of the substances through "significant pairwise concordance rates." And, a difference was seen in monozygotic versus dizygotic twin users for cannabis, stimulant, and cocaine abuse and dependence and for all drugs overall. Nicotine dependence was shown to have heritability of more than 60%; for opioid dependence the heritability was 0.43, and for stimulants it was 0.44. Other studies have identified linkages for other substances: nicotine dependence and its related traits as discussed above [17,18], cocaine dependence [19] and opioids [20]. Uhl *et al.* [21] showed that there is convergence among many of these studies that show dependence traits.

Cocaine Dependence

Earlier reviews by Kendler and Prescott [22] used twin study data showing "unexpectedly high" heritability for cocaine abuse and dependence (0.79 and 0.65); for males, heritability was 0.79 for dependence [23]. One recent analysis demonstrated the findings of a linkage scan that was performed on a sample of families where two siblings had conduct disorder. This report included data that suggested linkage on chromosome 10. The study further reviewed distinctions between European-American and African-American cases, with a LOD of 4.66 on chromosome 12 for "heavy use" among European-Americans and 3.65 on chromosome 18 for "moderate cocaine and opioid use" among European0-Americans. A genome-wide LOD score of 3.65 on chromosome 9 was seen in the African-American cases for the existence of cocaine-induced paranoia [19].

Opioid Dependence

Another study by Gelernter [24] regarding opioid use included a genome-wide linkage scan into heavy use clusters. In this report the best linkages were found for the traits. Glatt *et al.* [20] reported the initial results of a linkage scan for opioid dependence in a sample of Han subjects in China, showing the highest statistical significance to be a region on chromosome 17q.

GENETICALLY CHARACTERIZED PSYCHIATRIC DISORDERS OR CONDITIONS THAT AFFECT RISK OF USE

These include internalizing and externalizing disorders as well as "non-psychiatric" disorders (see other chapters in this section). Attention-deficit/hyperactivity disorder (ADHD) is a neurodevelopmental disorder that has some genetic component. Biederman and colleagues [25] studied ADHD as a familial risk of substance use: ADHD in the proband was consistently associated with a significant risk for ADHD in relatives. Drug dependence in probands increased the risk for drug dependence in relatives irrespective of ADHD status, whereas alcohol dependence in relatives was predicted only by ADHD probands with comorbid alcohol dependence. In addition, ADHD in the proband predicted drug dependence in relatives, and drug dependence in comparison probands increased the risk for ADHD in relatives. Both alcohol dependence and drug dependence bred true in families without evidence for a common risk between these disorders.

Overall, patterns of familial risk analysis suggest that the association between ADHD and drug dependence is most consistent with the hypothesis of variable expressivity of a common risk between these disorders, whereas the association between ADHD and alcohol dependence is most consistent with the hypothesis of independent transmission of these disorders. Findings also suggest specificity for the transmission of alcohol and drug dependence. Separating drug use from alcohol use is necessary in the approach to substance use disorders and the treatment of ADHD. Equal concern should be given in cases of conduct disorder and, perhaps to a lesser extent, in cases of oppositional defiant disorder.

Sub-diagnostic temperament deviations, which probably have a genetic basis, also are associated with an increased risk for psychopathology and substance abuse (see other chapters in this section). For example, children with a "difficult temperament" more commonly manifest externalizing and internalizing behavior problems by middle childhood and in adolescence, compared with children whose temperament is normative. Increased behavioral activity level is noted in both youths at high risk for substance abuse and those having a substance use disorder. Other temperamental trait deviations found in high-risk youths include reduced attention-span persistence [26], increased impulsivity [27], and such negative affect states as irritability [28]

and emotional reactivity [29]. Tarter *et al.* [30] developed a difficult temperament index to classify adolescent alcoholics. Those adolescents with a difficult temperament displayed a high conditional probability to develop psychiatric disorders such as conduct disorder, ADHD, anxiety disorders, and mood disorders.

CANDIDATE GENES FOR SUBSTANCE USE RISK IN ADOLESCENTS

This section reviews some of the specific enzymes or other gene products that are involved in substance use in which variations have been identified.

Alcohol Dependence Candidate Gene Studies

Alcohol-Metabolizing Enzymes

The risk of alcohol dependence in some populations is influenced by genetic polymorphisms at certain loci that encode alcohol dehydrogenase (ADH) and aldehyde dehydrogenase (ALD), the enzymes that metabolize alcohol in the liver. There are variants of ADH: especially well studied are *ADH1B* and *ADH1C*. Several genome-wide linkage scans have highlighted a region of chromosome 4q that contains a cluster for the ADH gene. Variants of these genes have been studied. In a case-control sample, Luo *et al.* [31] highlighted 16 markers within the ADH gene cluster that were identified and genotyped, with four markers within *ALDH2*. Edenberg *et al.* [32] similarly genotyped single nucleotide polymorphisms (SNPs) across the ADH gene cluster on chromosome 4q in a set of families with high risk for alcohol from the COGA study. This group also found information suggestive of an association with Alcohol Dependence for both *ADH1A* and *ADH1B*.

GABRA2

This refers to gamma-aminobutyric acid (GABA) A receptor alpha-2 subunit, a variant of the gene for the GABA-A receptor, for which several lines of evidence have shown an association with alcohol dependence in adults. The COGA study [33] showed evidence of the significance of chromosome 4p. This was the result of the convergence of two findings – one was that beta waves on the electroencephalogram were associated with a pertinent factor and that there was a finding of linkage disequilibrium to a GABA-A receptor gene cluster in this same chromosome region, which later showed association with *GABRA2*, one of four GABA-A genes in this region [34]. Several groups of investigators in case-control samples have replicated this finding. Alcohol dependence is associated with a haplotype at

GABRA2 in multiple populations [35]. The association has been demonstrated in both Plains Indians and Finn populations [36]. Nonetheless, the mechanism of risk of *GABRA2* remains uncertain.

CHRM2

There is also interest in the muscarinic acetylcholine receptor M2 (encoded by the genetic locus *CHRM2*, for cholinergic receptor, muscarinic 2) as a risk factor for alcohol dependence [37]. *CHRM2* is located in a region that has been identified as linked to alcohol dependence. SNPs from this area have been reported to be significantly associated with major depressive disorder. Luo *et al.* [38] later related this locus to personality measures, but no association with a specific mechanism for alcohol use risk has so far been found.

Opioid Receptors in Alcohol Use

Given the discovery that naltrexone can be helpful in alcohol dependence, there is interest in the genetic basis of the mu opioid receptor. Initial studies examining the association of the mu receptor (OPRM1) with substance dependence focused on the A118G polymorphism, which encodes a Asn40Asp amino acid substitution and which has been shown to be functional. Zhang *et al.* [39] reviewed 13 SNPs in this region: significant differences were found between cases and controls for those mapping into both types of use. The relationship to alcohol dependence was replicated in Russian subjects.

Candidate Genes for Other Substances of Abuse

Dopa Decarboxylase (DDC)

Dopa decarboxylase is of course an enzyme of major importance for the synthesis of monoamines. The gene encoding this protein is *DDC*, which was studied by Ma [40] with regard to nicotine dependence. Ma and colleagues used family-based association tests to show association between some *DDC* haplotypes and various traits of smoking behavior. These findings were added to in the study by Yu *et al.* [41], which reported an association of alleles and haplotypes at *DDC*.

DRD2/ANKK1/TTC12

These are another group of proteins in which there has been interest. There has been a long-running controversy about the significance of *DRD2* (dopamine receptor D2), but still no clear consensus. Gelernter *et al.* [42] showed a linkage peak (LOD 1.97) for nicotine dependence in

the European-American part of the sample at the region of chromosome 11 that includes the *NCAM1-TTC12-ANKK1-DRD2* gene cluster. One explanation for the inconsistency is that the data reflect an effect that is actually mediated through variation at a nearby locus.

Nicotine Dependence

In an array-based candidate gene study, Saccone *et al.* [43] found 3713 candidate SNPs from 348 candidate genes that might be related to nicotine dependence (ND). And the strongest results from this range were concentrated in an area of genetic import to nicotine dependence, especially cholinergic receptor genes such as *CHRNB3* (a locus also seen as important in GWAS studies [8]) and *GABRA4*. In terms of nicotine dependence and related traits specifically, Li *et al.* [44] found that putative linkages in numerous genome-wide linkage scans for use and related phenotypes had been identified on at least 12 chromosomes, and others have found other sites as well [18]. Further, Gelernter *et al.* [42] showed a linkage for chromosome 5 markers in African American men with a positive score on the Fagerstrom Test for Nicotine Dependence. In a 2011 article Li *et al.* [45] described a study on Han Chinese adolescents that found a single SNP (rs2298122) in the *CALY* gene that was positively associated with nicotine cigarette initiation, although only in females. Supportive evidence for this association was subsequently observed in an independent sample of Caucasian adolescents [45].

GENE × ENVIRONMENT INTERACTIONS THAT AFFECT RISK OF USE

The gene × environment paradigm reflects a renewed focus on the potential interactions between genetic and environmental stimuli, and this is of great importance when considering adolescent use. It focuses on the situations in which environmental effects on a phenotype differ depending upon the genotype. This effect may be an important factor in modulating risk for psychiatric phenotypes. It is possible that different genes react to different neurobiological substrates, that the environmental cues develop and change which makes this unique. Environmental cues may matter more or less at different ages, so this is both complex and important.

The magnitude can be large enough to be detected reliably. Couvault *et al.* [46] found that an interaction between a *5-HTTLPR* polymorphism and negative life events moderated alcohol and drug use in college students. In findings that are consistent with earlier results showing that this allele increases the risk for depression under conditions of increased stress, those homozygous for the short allele who experienced multiple negative life events reported more frequent and heavy drinking and greater non-prescription drug misuse. Kaufman *et al.* [47] also examined genetic and environmental predictors of early alcohol use, but in this study the subjects were adolescents and predictors of early alcohol use included maltreatment, family loading for substance dependence, and presence of *5-HTTPR* genotype. Maltreated children and matched controls participated the rate of alcohol use in the maltreated children was more than seven times the rate in controls. And the maltreated children also initiated drinking on average more than 2 years before controls. Consistent with the report by Covault, early alcohol use was predicted by maltreatment. *5-HTTLPR* had a gene × environment interaction, with increased risk associated with the short allele. Another important finding was made by the Mannheim Study of Children at Risk, which has followed the long-term effects of maltreatment and endocrine effects, in particular corticotropin-releasing hormone (CRH) and adrenocorticotropic hormone (ACTH). This study's function is to assess real events and their relationship to real psychopathology. In this case, the psychopathology reviewed is heavy alcohol use. In this study, among 15-year-olds homozygous for the C' allele of a haplotype tagging SNP (rs1876831) of *CRHR1*, the number of negative life events during the past 3 years was significantly related to increasing rates of lifetime heavy use and levels of use per occasion. These events are different from those types of early childhood maltreatment that have featured in the studies by Nemeroff and others, where there is an assumption that a fundamental change in the CRH/ACTH loop is made. However, it is conceivable that this study has uncovered a genetic haplotype that similarly creates abnormal physiology in that neuroendocrine function [48].

Gene × environment interactions have been of great interest in relation to adult subjects, but for adolescent use more and more a predominance of social risk factors is observed. Some studies have demonstrated that in those with alleles identified as high risk, social-based interventions can overcome the genetic risk. This supports the concept that no individual is destined to be addicted or to be a substance user. For example, in terms of adolescent tobacco use, experimentation is common in adolescence, but use is highly affected by environmental features [49]. Similarly, while the risk of some adolescent smoking leading to young adult smoking include an odds ratio of 16 [50], further research has demonstrated the effects of peers, employment, education, and parental influences on the transition to young adult smoking. Greater physical activity is associated with lessened progression to significant use [51], and this has been found to be protective even among those who have the alleles seen as risk factors for smoking [52] (see also Chapter 14).

CONCLUSION

It is exciting to be able to summarize the many genetic methods that have been helpful in elucidating the risks of substance use imparted by genetics. All the more so, because the effects in adolescents are both important and also complex, and this chapter's limitation is that so many of the studies did not necessarily include adolescents. It is in this age range where several forces coalesce, and we look forward to learning more about this phase in particular.

References

1. Nurnberger JI Jr, Wiegland R, Buholz K, *et al.* A family study of alcohol dependence: coaggregation of multiple disorders in relatives of alcohol dependent probands. *Arch Gen Psychiatry* 2004;**61**:1246–1256.
2. Jacob T, Waterman B, Heath A, *et al.* Genetic and environmental effects on offspring alcoholism: new insights using 17. *J Pediatr Psychol* 2004;**29**:299–308.
3. Young SE, Rhee SH, Stallings MC, *et al.* Genetic and environmental vulnerabilities underlying adolescent substance use and problem use: general or specific? *Behav Genet* 2006;**36**:603–615.
4. Palmer RHC, Young SE, Hopfer CJ, *et al.* Developmental epidemiology of drug use and abuse in adolescence and young adulthood: Evidence of generalized risk. *Drug Alcohol Depend* 2009;**102**:78–87.
5. Lynskey MT, Agrawal A, Heath A. Genetically informative research on adolescent substance use: methods, findings, and challenges. *J Am Acad Child Adolesc Psychiatry* 2010;**49**:1202–1214.
6. Liu I-C, Blacker DL, Zu R, *et al.* Genetic and environmental contributions to the development of alcohol dependence in male twins. *Arch Gen Psychiatry* 2004;**61**:897–903.
7. Psychiatric GWAS Consortium Coordinating, Committee. Genome-wide association studies: history, rationale, and prospects for psychiatric disorders. *Am J Psychiatry* 2009;**166**:540–556.
8. Bierut LJ, Cubells JF, Iacono WG, *et al.* Genetic research and smoking behavior. *JAMA* 2007;**297**:809.
9. Gelernter J, Kranzler HR. Genetics of alcohol dependence. *Hum Genet* 2009;**126**:91–99.
10. Derringer J, Krueger RF, McGue Matt, Iacono WG. Genetic and environmental contributions to the diversity of substances used in adolescent twins: a longitudinal study of age and sex effects. *Addiction* 2008;**103**:1744–1751.
11. Biederman J, Monuteaux MC, Mick E, *et al.* Is cigarette smoking a gateway to alcohol and illicit drug use disorders? A study of youths with and without attention deficit hyperactivity disorder. *Biol Psychiatry* 2006;**59**:258–264.
12. Prescott CA, Kendler KS. Genetic and environmental contributions to alcohol abuse and dependence in a population-based sample of male twins. *Am J Psychiatry* 1999;**56**:34–40.

13. Kendler KS, Prescott CA, Neale MC, *et al.* Temperance board registration for alcohol abuse in a national sample of Swedish male twins, born 1902 to 1949. *Arch Gen Psychiatry 1997;* **54**:178–184.

14. Foroud T, Edenberg HJ, Goate A, *et al.* Alcoholism susceptibility loci: confirmation studies in a replicate sample and further mapping. *Alcohol Clin Exp Res* 2000;**24**:933–945.

15. Long JC, Knowler WC, Hanson RL, *et al.* Evidence for genetic linkage to alcohol dependence on chromosomes 4 and 11 from an autosome-wide scan in an American Indian population. *Am J Med Genet* 1998; **81**:216–221.

16. Wilhelmsen KC, Schuckit M, Smith TL, *et al.* The search for genes related to a low-level response to alcohol determined by alcohol challenges. *Alcohol Clin Exp Res* 2003;**27**:1041–1047.

17. Bierut LJ, Rice JP, Goate A, *et al.* A genomic scan for habitual smoking in families of alcoholics: common and specific genetic factors in substance dependence. *Am J Med Genet A* 2004;**124**:19–27.

18. Li MD, Payne TJ, Ma JZ, *et al.* A genomewide search finds major susceptibility loci for nicotine dependence on chromosome 10 in African Americans. *Am J Hum Genet* 2006;**79**:745–751.

19. Gelernter J, Panhuysen C, Weiss R, *et al.* Genomewide linkage scan for cocaine dependence and related traits: significant linkages for a cocaine-related trait and for cocaine-induced paranoia. *Am J Med Genet B Neuropsychiatr Genet* 2005;**136**:45–52.

20. Glatt SJ, Su JA, Zhu SC, *et al.* Genome-wide linkage analysis of heroin dependence in Han Chinese: results from wave one of a multi-stage study. *Am J Med Genet B Neuropsychiatr Genet* 2006;**141**:648–652.

21. Uhl GR. Molecular genetics of substance abuse vulnerability: remarkable recent convergence of genome scan results. *Ann NY Acad Sci* 2004;**1025**:1–13.

22. Kendler KS, Prescott CA. Cocaine use, abuse and dependence in a population-based sample of female twins. *Br J Psychiatry* 1998;**173**:345–350.

23. Kendler KS, Karkowski LM, Neale MC, *et al.* Illicit psychoactive substance use, heavy use, abuse, and dependence in a US population-based sample of male twins. *Arch Gen Psychiatry* 2000;**57**:261–269.

24. Gelernter J, Panhuysen C, Wilcox M, *et al.* Genomewide linkage scan for opioid dependence. *Am J Hum Genet* 2006;**78**:759–769.

25. Biederman J, Petty CR, Wilens TE, *et al.* Familial risk analyses of attention deficit hyperactivity disorder and substance use disorders. *Am J Psychiatry* 2008;**165**: 107–115.

26. Schaeffer KW, Parsons OA, Yohman JR. Neuropsychological differences between male familial and nonfamilial alcoholics and nonalcoholics. *Alcohol Clin Exp Res* 1984;**8**:347–351.

27. Shedler J, Block J. Adolescent drug use and psychological health. A longitudinal inquiry. *Am Psychol* 1990;**45**:612–630.

28. Brook JS, Whiteman M, Gordon AS, Brook DW. The role of older brothers in younger brothers' drug use viewed in the context of parent and peer influences. *J Genet Psychol* 1990;**151**:59–75.

29. Blackson TC. Temperament: a salient correlate of risk factors for alcohol and drug abuse. *Drug Alcohol Depend* 1994;**36**:205–214.

30. Tarter R, Kirisci L, Hegedus A, *et al.* Heterogeneity of adolescent alcoholism. *Ann NY Acad Sci* 1994;**708**:172–180.

31. Luo X, Kranzler HR, Zuo L, *et al.* Diplotype trend regression (DTR) analysis of the ADH gene. *Am J Hum Genet* 2006;78:943–987.

32. Edenberg HJ, Xuei X, Chen HJ, *et al.* Association of alcohol dehydrogenase genes with alcohol dependence: a comprehensive analysis. *Hum Mol Genet* 2006;**15**: 1539–1549.

33. Porjesz B, Almasy L, Edenberg HJ, *et al.* Linkage disequilibrium between the beta frequency of the human EEG and a GABAA receptor gene locus. *Proc Natl Acad Sci USA* 2002;**99**:3729–3733.

34. Edenberg HJ, Dick DM, Xuei X, *et al.* Variations in GABRA2, encoding the alpha 2 subunit of the GABA (A) receptor, are associated with alcohol dependence and with brain oscillations. *Am J Hum Genet* 2004;**74**:705–714.

35. Fehr C, Sander T, Tadic A, *et al.* Confirmation of association of the GABRA2 gene with alcohol dependence by subtype-specific analysis. *Psychiatr Genet* 2006;**16**:9–17.

36. Enoch MA, Schwartz L, Albaugh B, *et al.* Dimensional anxiety mediates linkage of GABRA2 haplotypes with alcoholism. *Am J Med Genet B Neuropsychiatr Genet* 2006;**141**:599–607.

37. Luo X, Kranzler HR, Zuo L, *et al.* CHRM2 gene predisposes to alcohol dependence, drug dependence, and affective disorders: results from an extended case-control structured association study. *Hum Mol Genet* 2005;**14**:2421–2434.

38. Luo X, Kranzler HR, Zuo L, *et al.* CHRM2 variation predisposes to personality traits of agreeableness and conscientiousness. *Hum Mol Genet* 2007;**16**:1557–1568.

39. Zhang H, Luo X, Kranzler HR, *et al.* Association between two opioid receptor gene (OPRM1) haplotype blocks and drug or alcohol dependence. *Hum Mol Genet* 2006;**15**:807–819.

40. Ma JZ, Beuten J, Payne TJ, *et al.* Haplotype analysis indicates an association between the DOPA decarboxylase (DDC) gene and nicotine dependence. *Hum Mol Genet* 2005;**14**:1691–1698.

41. Yu Y, Panhuysen C, Kranzler HR, *et al.* Intronic variants in the DOPA decarboxylase (DDC) gene are associated with smoking behavior in European-Americans and African-Americans. *Hum Mol Genet* 2006;**15**:2192–2199.

42. Gelernter J, Panhuysen C, Weiss R, *et al.* Genomewide linkage scan for nicotine dependence: identification of a novel chromosome 5 risk locus. *Biol Psychiatry* 2007;**61**:119–126.

43. Saccone SF, Hinrichs AL, Saccone NL, *et al.* Cholinergic nicotinic receptor genes implicated in a nicotine dependence association study targeting 348 candidate genes with 3713 SNPs. *Hum Mol Genet* 2007;**16**:36–49.

44. Li MD, Ma JZ, Beuten J. Progress in searching for susceptibility loci and genes for smoking-related behaviour. *Clin Genet* 2004;**66**:382–392.

45. Li D, London SJ, Liu J, *et al.* Association of the calcyon neuron-specific vesicular protein gene (CALY) with adolescent smoking initiation in China and California. *Am J Epidemiol* 2011;**173**:1039–1048.

46. Covault J, Tennen H, Herman AI, *et al.* Interactive effects of the serotonin transporter 5-HTTLPR polymorphism and stressful life events on college student drinking and drug use. *Biol Psychiatry* 2007;**61**:609–616.

47. Kaufman J, Yang BZ, Douglas-Palumberi H, *et al.* Genetic and environmental predictors of early alcohol use. *Biol Psychiatry* 2007;**61**:1228–1234.

48. Blomeyer D, Treutlein J, Esser G, *et al.* Interaction between CRHR1 gene and stressful life events predicts adolescent heavy alcohol use. *Biol Psychiatry* 2008;**63**:146–151.

49. Brook JS, Saar NS, Zhang C, Brook DW. Familial and non-familial smoking: Effects on smoking and nicotine dependence. *Drug Alc Depend* 2009;**101**:62–68.

50. Chasin L, Presson CC, Rose JS, Sherman SJ. The natural history of cigarette smoking from adolescence to adult. *Health Psychol* 1996;**15**:478–484.

51. Rodriguez D, Audrain-McGovern J. Team sport participation and smoking: analysis with general growth mixture modeling. *J Pediatr Psychol* 2004;**29**:299–308.

52. Audrain-McGovern J, Rodriguez D, Wileyto EP, Schmitz KH, Shields PG. Effect of team sport participation on genetic predisposition to adolescent smoking progression. *Arch Gen Psychiatry* 2006;**63**:433–441.

14

Familial and Other Social Risk Factors in Adolescent Substance Use

Michael Brendler

Georgetown University School of Medicine, Washington DC, USA

This chapter reports on factors for which the evidence of risk of substance use is strongest. The deleterious effects of substance abuse and addiction for adults are widely documented, as consequences can manifest in any or all of the following areas: emotional health, physical health, cognition, productivity, finances, and social relationships. For adolescents these consequences may be intensified in concert with the multitude of normal developmental processes, which can be affected by these toxic molecules acting biologically or by the social, attachment, or psychological havoc they wreak. This chapter will highlight two disparate but related categories of social influence upon substance use in adolescents: familial and non-familial. Both of these domains function as systems oriented to supporting adolescent maturation into adulthood; yet, in US culture there is a patterned shift in how teens relate to their families and extrafamilial social systems. Adolescents tend to spend less time with their families and more time with their peers; their opinions and behaviors are shaped more by peers or other external forces. Conflict between adolescents and parents tends to increase and deference toward parents decreases [1].

It is in this context that several types of social influences on adolescent substance use have been identified, even varying by different substances of abuse; this chapter reviews several such factors, but centers around the position that family and peer influences are the most significant relational factors predicting or protecting against substance use among adolescents. Such a position dovetails with the concepts raised by Volkow's perspective of systems risks for adolescent substance use [2]. As an example, in terms of tobacco, experimentation is common in adolescence, and use is highly affected by environmental features [3]. For example, early adolescent smoking has been associated with young adult smoking at a rate of 16 to 1 [4]. Research has demonstrated that there are clear effects of peers, employment, education, and parental influences on the transition from teenage substance abuse to young adult substance abuse. That this social/systems perspective of adolescent substance use differs from that among adults highlights the distinction that is this unique window of human development and vulnerability.

INTERACTION OF ADOLESCENT SOCIAL DEVELOPMENT AND SUBSTANCE ABUSE

Historically, adolescence has been viewed psychologically and developmentally as a time of "storm and stress" [5]. In Western culture, experimentation, individuation, risk-taking, acting out, conflict with parents, and mood fluctuations have all been considered a normal part of adolescent development [6]. Accordingly, this chapter will examine social and developmental issues of adolescence through a Western lens and with the understanding that much of the research reflects large group trends that poorly account for individual differences. As in other chapters in this text, we do not assume that data about one substance of abuse generalizes to others nor that risks for use are equivalent to risks for the development of dependence.

In considering the developmental issues related to adolescence, it is important to focus on those issues most impacted by social and familial factors. Studies of US teens have shown that early adolescence is associated with increased parent–child conflict compared to pre-adolescence [7]. Furthermore, it appears that the

Clinical Handbook of Adolescent Addiction, First Edition. Richard Rosner.
© 2013 John Wiley & Sons, Ltd. Published 2013 by John Wiley & Sons, Ltd.

intensity of this conflict increases toward mid-adolescence before tapering off in late adolescence [7]. In addition to increased conflict, there also appears to be a trend where teens and parents experience less emotional closeness and spend less time together, and the potential influence of peers and social forces becomes more salient. It is only in late adolescence that identity formation, as described by Erikson, becomes consolidated.

THE EXAMPLE OF EARLY ALCOHOL INITIATION AND LATER DEPENDENCE

Early alcohol use has consistently been found to be a risk factor for later alcohol dependence. For example Grant and Dawson [8] found that retrospective reports of alcohol initiation prior to the age of 15 were associated with four times greater risk for later alcohol dependence than peers who did not initiate until 20 years of age or older. While the strength of the association between early adolescent initiation of alcohol consumption and later alcohol dependence has been repeatedly established, the mechanisms underlying this relationship are still not well understood. Several models have been proposed to explain this phenomenon. Dewit *et al.* [9] proposed a developmental model, which suggests that early drinking affects the trajectory of social networks and brain development, placing these teens at higher risk for dependency. According to this model, early drinkers are exposed to community and peer groups who have more permissive views on drinking, provide increased exposure to settings where alcohol is available, and may even reinforce drinking as a means of coping with emotional distress.

PEER FACTORS

While there is a clear link in the literature between parental emotional support and decreased risk of substance abuse in adolescence, the same is not true of peer support. Numerous studies have shown that peer support does not serve as a deterrent for teen substance abuse [10,11]. In fact, peer support has been found to have an inverse relationship to teen substance abuse [12]. Unlike parent emotional support there appears to be a complex relationship to teenage substance abuse. Parental support is consistently positively related to protective factors and negatively related to risk factors. In contrast, peer support is positively correlated with good self-control (a factor that predicts less substance abuse), but is not protective with most risk factors, and for some risk factors is positively correlated. In other words, peer support is beneficial in some ways, but does not serve as a protective factor against early substance abuse in the same way that parental support does. In fact, in some cases, peer support may actually provide a pathway for early substance abuse initiation [12]. One of the

theories explaining this dynamic suggests that parents and peer groups may hold different value systems. As discussed earlier, adolescent development is often marked by attempts to develop a sense of self as separate or different from parents. Peer groups provide a natural and needed social context for support in developing emerging identities, placing peers in a powerfully influential position with respect to teen decisions. Adolescents have consistently been found to be more impulsive, have poorer judgment, and are more invested in peer approval than adults. To this end, peers may positively reinforce impulsive behavior, risk-taking, and their attitudes toward illicit substances may range from tolerant to encouraging.

Peer Attitudes

The effects of peer influence on adolescent substance abuse go well beyond emotional support. The attitudes and experiences with illicit substances have bidirectional effects upon teen decision-making. Adolescents who associate with other teens who use drugs are more likely to try drugs themselves [13]. In contrast, teens whose peer group does not use drugs, rarely use drugs themselves [14]. Both effects are thought to be related to the effects of peer modeling. There is also evidence that modeling is not the only non-adult-child relational factor related to risk or prevention of substance abuse. Brook *et al.* [15] found that both modeling and strong sibling attachment promoted low younger sibling drug abuse.

Other Peer Factors

It is important to consider the role of other components of relationships with peers that may be risk factors for use or disordered substance use among adolescents. One is the engagement in inappropriate sexual activity among peers – another behavior associated with risk – which may be explained by an underlying interest in thrill-seeking behavior. Interaction with deviant peers also predicts substance abuse problems, particularly if that deviation extends to severe antisocial behavior, conduct disorder, and even gang involvement. Finally, the lack of engagement in substance-free activities should be counted as another risk factor for use among adolescents.

FAMILY FACTORS

The evidence highlighting the link between family factors and adolescent substance abuse is well established [16]. Currently, the question is less about whether or not families influence teenage substance abuse, but rather what are the significant family variables and how do those variables interact with genetic factors.

Family History of Substance Abuse

A family history of substance abuse has been found to be the strongest predictor of early initiation of substance abuse [17]. Having a first-degree relative who is an alcoholic is also related to offspring becoming substance abusers [16]. While a family history of substance abuse has been linked to both earlier onset and higher rates of adolescent substance abuse, there is some question about the degree of influence of parenting practices versus the role of genetics. Due to this complexity, there remains a great deal of uncertainty about the specific parenting behavioral pathways that influence adolescent substance abuse. One parenting pathway that has been proposed is that modeling (behavioral imitation) is a causal factor in adolescent substance abuse. Wills et al. [18] suggest that this explanation is insufficient given the modest correlation between parent and teen substance use.

Recent studies have examined the influence of parental substance abuse more closely as a complex predictor for adolescent substance abuse. For example, parent substance abuse is correlated with negative life events, lower levels of parental support, and higher levels of parent–child conflict – both risk factors for adolescent substance abuse [19]. This suggests that parent substance abuse in and of itself may not be the driving factor in leaving teens at greater risk for early initiation of substance abuse. Instead, parental substance abuse may lead to a variety of other problematic behaviors, which in turn have more direct effects on lowering the threshold for early-onset substance abuse.

Sibling Substance Abuse

While most research has focused on the role of parents in terms of family influence of teenage substance abuse, sibling patterns of abuse can be powerfully influential. Siblings can provide a context through which teens are introduced to and may learn about drugs. For example, a high percentage of chemical-dependent teenagers have siblings who are also substance abusers [20]. Moreover, teens who have substance-abusing siblings are more likely to engage in substance abuse at a younger age, and teens whose siblings do not abuse drugs are more likely to abstain as well [21]. Younger siblings often observe and model the behavior of their older siblings. If older siblings have permissive attitudes or are substance abusers themselves, younger siblings may mimic these attitudes and behaviors.

Familial Relationships and Communication

Wills et al. [19] developed an empirically supported model delineating factors related to early-onset substance abuse. They found that teenage expression of good self-control (i.e., no substance abuse) is influenced by a number of family factors. Specifically, adolescent perceptions of both emotional and functional support from parents were predictive of good self-control and were protective factors against early substance abuse. Adolescents who believe that they can be open with their parents and talk frequently also are less likely to engage in early substance abuse. Teenagers who abuse drugs have been found to view communication with their parents as problematic. Specifically, substance-abusing teens describe the communication with their parents as closed and unclear [22] and view their patterns of communication as rigid [23]. Conversely, older siblings may have an inhibitory effect on early substance abuse if their attitudes and behaviors support drug avoidance.

Family bonding has also been found to be related to early initiation of adolescent substance abuse. Lack of closeness between parents and their children has been shown to be a risk factor for early onset of drinking and drug abuse [24,25]. While a lack of closeness is a risk factor, emotional and instrumental support from parents and extended family (or community) buffers against early substance abuse. Having a well-established external support system that encourages a child's own coping is a buffering factor against adolescent substance abuse [26]. Children whose parents have high expectations of them also have lower levels of adolescent substance abuse [27].

Family Structure and Composition

The arrangement and composition of family members has been studied as a predictor of (or protector against) adolescent substance use. One study found that the presence in the home of a father, even if a substance user, provides greater protection against the development of an adolescent addiction than his absence [28]. In other words, adolescents who live only with their mothers are more likely to develop an addiction than adolescents living with both parents. Larger family size has also been shown to increase the risk of adolescent substance experimentation. One study suggests that for adolescent boys, being born to younger parents (i.e., less than 21 years old at the time of the child's birth) increased the risk of developing an addiction by nearly six-fold. Finally, parental influence against using drugs is tempered by whether the adolescent is involved in a peer group that supports experimentation [29].

Parental Monitoring

Parental monitoring is the extent to which parents watch and supervise their children's behavior [30]. Parental monitoring levels have consistently been associated with levels of adolescent substance abuse [31]. Adolescents who perceive their parents to have a high degree of awareness of how they spend their time away from the family (high monitoring) have substantially lower levels of substance abuse than those who see their parents as less aware of their behavior when away from home. While this pattern is well established, what is less clear is why this is the case. To date the literature has not provided much insight into this particular finding. In fact, parental monitoring is generally only measured in subjective and abstract terms. Most measures are self-report and reflect parent and teen perspectives on how aware parents are of their children's behavior. Furthermore, parental monitoring has been shown to be influential regardless of parent attitudes or discipline regarding substance abuse. Given this information, the literature suggests that certain types of parental involvement are very helpful for dissuading kids from substance abuse.

Parental Discipline

The absence of clear rules and consequences in families appears to leave adolescents at higher risk for substance use. In addition, parental habits and attitudes towards alcohol and drug use have consistently related to those of their children [32]. In fact, a permissive attitude toward substance abuse in the family is a stronger predictor of adolescent substance abuse than actual parent substance abuse (although this finding varies according to the type of substance used by parents [33]). For example, parental alcoholism is positively correlated with teenage drinking problems and increases the risk for chemical dependency in general. Beardslee et al. [34], Needle et al. [21], and Gilman et al. [35] report evidence that parental smoking increases the risk for adolescent smoking initiation among a cohort of adolescents enrolled in the New England Family Study. In the Gilman study, current (but not past) parental smoking was associated with an increased risk of smoking initiation during adolescence. In contrast, parental cannabis abuse has not been found to significantly predict substance abuse initiation or abuse in teens [21]. There is some evidence to suggest that parents who use alcohol and drugs as a form of coping may indirectly reinforce similar coping behaviors in their children. Jurich et al. [36] found that adolescents who believe their parents use substances to cope with stress were at greater risk for developing a substance abuse problem themselves. Additionally, they found that fathers who report using alcohol as a means of avoidance tend to have kids who use substances as a means to cope with stress. While these findings are purely correlational and do not represent causal relationships between the substance abuse of parents and that of

their children, they do highlight clear familial patterns associated with higher risk of substance abuse. Parents' behavior and attitudes toward drinking and drugs are clearly related to those of their children. And to the extent that this reflects a parental process for coping with stress, this coping style may also be passed down and become a family pattern in responding to stress.

Parent–Child Conflict

One of the most consistent findings in the literature is that parent–child conflict is a risk factor for early substance abuse. Parent–child conflict across early, middle, and late adolescence all predict greater risk for substance abuse [37]. Patterns of conflict based on destructive arguing and adolescents' perceptions that their interactions with their parents are negative have positive correlations with early substance abuse [38]. Family conflict may also facilitate adolescent disengagement from the family and association with deviant peer groups engaged in high-risk behaviors, including substance abuse. In addition to eroding a central means for emotional support, parent–child conflict may also create additional stress, which may overwhelm adolescent coping, leaving teens at greater risk for substance abuse as a means of compensatory coping.

As a system, the family too may have personality traits that extend throughout the family and affect coping and are risks for substance use. Families with substance use have been found to have personality differences compared with non-using families. Specifically, the subjects with substance use disorders differed on the dimensions of alienation, control, harm avoidance, and the higher-order traits of negative emotionality and constraint. All of these factors reflect attempts to control interpersonal distress between family members either overtly (verbal or physical) or through creating interpersonal distance (alienation or avoidance). Relatives with substance use disorders likewise differed in comparison with non-substance-abusing relatives on the dimensions of control and constraint. Female relatives with histories of substance abuse also had higher scores for stress reactivity and negative emotionality. The identification of persons at high risk on the basis of such personality dimensions may therefore serve as an important source of information for both treatment and prevention efforts [39].

ENVIRONMENTAL EXPERIENCES

Adverse Experiences

A tremendous amount of effort has been given to the study of the relationship between childhood maltreatment and substance use. Over the past decade the Adverse

Childhood Experiences Study (ACES) has documented associations between several forms of maltreatment with earlier age of substance use initiation [40]. The ACES study included 10 forms of adverse experience, although it does not include parental loss of employment and other forms of loss. As one of the 10 adverse experiences defined in the ACES study, it has been recognized that parental separation or divorce is associated with lesser educational achievement, earlier age of entry to the workforce, and earlier substance use initiation.

Work

Youths in the labor force are at high risk of using substances. A 1998 study by the Institute of Medicine [41] found the following:

* High-intensity work (20+ hours per week) is associated with unhealthy behaviors, including substance abuse, insufficient sleep and exercise, and limited time with families.
* The link between intensive work schedules and substance use is found in multiple studies, even after statistical control for background and variables and pre-existing conditions such as parental socioeconomic status, race, family composition, and prior substance use.
* Skill utilization (the use of special skills) at work was associated with decreased cigarette and marijuana use. In females, skill utilization was associated with decreased alcohol use.
* Youths who noted that their jobs did not require their skills, and who perceived their jobs to be unconnected to the future, used more cigarettes as the intensity of their work increased.

The basis for these associations is unknown, but they should be considered in the clinical evaluation of youths who work.

Gender-Specific Adverse Experiences

There are differences in gender-based risks for substance use, which likely reflect both genetic and environmental factors. The distinctions between girls and boys in terms of relationships and extracurricular activities are just some of those differences. Surveying 781 adolescent girls and their mothers, one study found relationships between girls' use of alcohol, prescription drugs, and inhalants with girls' after-school destinations, body images, depression, best friend's substance use, maternal drinking behavior, mother–daughter interactions, and family norms surrounding substance use [42]. The reader is referred to comprehensive reviews for more information [43].

School Factors

Behavioral and Academic Expectations: Lack of clear expectations for both academic performance and in-school behavior from both parents and school is a risk factor for early onset substance abuse. Positive attitudes toward school, attendance, and identifying with the school are protective factors. High academic and behavioral expectations also serve as a buffer against early substance abuse. Goal-setting and orientation to high achievement are also protective factors.

Availability of School-Based Resources: Tutoring, counseling services, and prevention messages impact substance use, and this includes extracurricular activities, especially athletics. Findings from the *2009 National Survey on Drug Use and Health* indicate that adolescents who participate in extracurricular activities are less likely to have used alcohol, cigarettes, and illicit drugs in the past month. In particular adolescents who participated in these activities were half as likely as non-participants to have smoked cigarettes [44]. The choice of engaging in greater physical activity is associated with less risk of progression to significant use [45], and this has been found to be protective even among those who have the alleles seen as risk factors for smoking [46].

Other school characteristics that influence teenage substance abuse behaviors include student commitment and sense of belonging, the academic culture (i.e., the attrition rate, overall school achievement orientation, violence/bullying/deviant behavior), and parental and community involvement.

COMMUNITY AND SOCIAL FACTORS

There are several avenues of impact from community and social forces in the adolescent's life. Certainly community norms favoring alcohol and drug use are one, and this connects with whether or not laws and ordinances on substance use are enforced, or if they are enforced consistently. Below is a brief discussion of those factors.

Media, Marketing, and Entertainment

There has been an immense range of research into the impact of media, marketing, and entertainment upon adolescent substance use. There is evidence that visual media directly influence teenage smoking through observational learning and communication of messages that reinforce smoking. Wellman *et al.* [47] performed a meta-analysis and estimated that high exposure to smoking in the media, including movies, television, videos, and tobacco advertising and promotions, can double the odds of smoking initiation among youths. One interesting avenue of investigation has explored the link between adolescent violence and substance use as stemming from exposure to violent television programming: Brook *et al.* assessed more than 400 African-American and Puerto Rican adolescents during three points in time for their exposure to violent television programs in late adolescence, which predicted exposure to violent television programs in young adulthood, which in turn was related to tobacco/marijuana use, nicotine dependence, and later drug dependence [48].

Availability of Alcohol and Drugs

Increased alcohol availability is associated with increases in drinking prevalence and amount consumed. Availability is also related to the level of use of illegal drugs [49]. The prevalence of specific psychoactive substance use disorders is influenced by regional availability of particular substances and social trends. The 'Monitoring the Future' study revealed that 82.1% of 12th-graders believed marijuana was "fairly easy" or "very easy" to obtain. Permission to use substances has also affected use. In New York City rules on smoking in public places have affected use as local smoke-free restaurant laws may significantly lower youth smoking initiation by impeding the progression from cigarette experimentation to established smoking [50].

Neighborhood Disorganization

Neighborhood characteristics, such as high population density and lack of natural surveillance of public places, high residential mobility, physical deterioration, high concentration of poverty, and high crime, are related to drug abuse, as well as juvenile crime and levels of drug trafficking. Risk factors for alcohol and other drug abuse include community disorganization, lack of community bonding, lack of cultural pride, lack of cultural competence, inadequate youth services, and a lack of opportunities for prosocial behaviors. Research into resilience factors within the community is sparse. There has been some suggestion that neighborhoods supplement the family and individual resilience factors by promoting contexts in which children can be exposed to positive influences [51]. Several factors contributing to resilience in the face of structural and economic disadvantage have been identified, including healthy neighborhood institutions; an abundance of positive role models; opportunities to link children to caring adults; strong social networks; and social cohesion imbued with community willingness to positively intervene. It should be noted that these protective factors are not specific to substance abuse and are presented as conditions that support resilience against general risk factors.

CONCLUSION

The practitioner should gain from consideration of the myriad forces acting upon adolescent substance use. The scientific support for these risk factors is strong, and assessment, care, public policy, and prevention efforts should keep these components in mind in the future.

References

1. Steinberg LD. Transformations in family relations at puberty. *Dev Psychol* 1981;**17**:833–840.
2. Baler RD, Volkow ND. Addiction as a systems failure: focus on adolescence and smoking. *J Am Acad Child Adolesc Psychiatry* 2011;**50**:329–339.
3. Brook JS, Saar NS, Zhang C, Brook DW. Familial and non-familial smoking: Effects on smoking and nicotine dependence. *Drug Alc Depen* 2009;**101**:62–68.
4. Chassin L, Presson CC, Rose JS, Sherman SJ. The natural history of cigarette smoking from adolescence to adult. *Health Psychology* 1996;**15**:478–484.
5. Hall GS. *Adolescence: Its Psychology and its Relation to Physiology, Anthropology, Sociology, Sex, Crime, Religion, and Education* (Vols I & II). Englewood Cliffs, NJ: Prentice-Hall, 1904.
6. Arnett JJ. Adolescent storm and stress, reconsidered. *Am Psychol* 1999;**54**:317–326.
7. Laursen B, Coy KC, Collins WA. Reconsidering changes in parent–child conflict across adolescence: a meta-analysis. *Child Dev* 1998;**69**:817–832.
8. Grant BF, Dawson DA. Age at onset of alcohol use and its association with DSM-IV alcohol abuse and dependence: results from the National Longitudinal Alcohol Epidemiologic Survey. *J Subst Abuse* 1997;**9**:103–110.
9. Dewit DJ, Adlaf EM, Offord DR, Ogborne AC. Age at first alcohol use: a risk factor for the development of alcohol disorders. *Am J Psychiatry* 2000;**157**:745–750.
10. Greenberg MT, Siegel JM, Leitch CJ. The nature and importance of attachment relationships to parents and peers during adolescence. *J Youth Adolescence* 1983;**12**:373–386.
11. Wills TA, Vaughan R. Social support and substance use in early adolescence. *J Behav Med* 1989;**12**:321–339.
12. Wills TA, Resko JA, Ainette MG, Mendoza D. Role of parent support and peer support in adolescent substance use: a test of mediated effects. *Psychol Addict Behav* 2004;**18**:122–134.
13. Huizinga D, Loeber R, Thornberry TP. Urban delinquency and substance abuse (OJJDP Research Summary, NCJ 143454). Washington, DC: Office of Juvenile Justice and Delinquency Prevention, Office of Justice Programs, 1995.
14. Moon DG, Hecht ML, Jackson KM, Spellers RE. Ethnic and gender differences and similarities in adolescent drug use and refusals of drug offers. *Subst Use Misuse* 1999;**34**:1059–1083.
15. Brook JS, Brook DW, Whiteman M. Older sibling correlates of younger sibling drug use in the context of parent–child relations. *Genet Soc Gen Psych Monogr* 1999;**125**:451–468.

16. Jacob T, Johnson S. Family influences on substance abuse. In: Tarter R, Ammernan R, Ott P (eds), *Source Book on Substance Abuse: Etiology, Methodology, and Intervention*. New York: Allyn & Bacon, 1999; pp. 165–175.

17. Costello EJ, Erkanli A, Federman E, Angold A. The development of psychiatric comorbidity with substance abuse in adolescents: effects of timing and sex. *J Clin Child Psychol* 1999;**28**:298–311.

18. Wills TA, Yaeger AM, Sandy JM. Buffering effect of religiosity for adolescent substance use. *Psychol Addict Behav* 2003;**17**:24–31.

19. Wills TA, Cleary S, Filer M, Shinar O, Mariani J, Spera K. Temperament related to early-onset substance use: test of a developmental model. *Prev Sci* 2001;**2**:145–163.

20. Craig SR, Brown BS. Comparison of youthful heroin users and nonusers from one urban community. *Int J Addict* 1975;**10**:53–64.

21. Needle R, McCubbin H, Wilson M, *et al.*Interpersonal influences in adolescent drug use – The role of older siblings, parents, and peers. *Int J Addictions* 1986;**21**:739–766.

22. Rees CD, Wilborn BL. Correlates of drug abuse in adolescents: A comparison of families of drug abusers with families of nondrug users. *J Youth Adolesc* 1983;**12**:55–63.

23. Steier F, Stanton MD, Todd TC. Patterns of turn-taking and alliance formation in family communication. *J Commun* 1982;**32**:148–160.

24. Penning M, Barnes G. Adolescent marijuana use: a review. *Int J Addictions* 1982;**17**:749–791.

25. Brook JS, Brook DW, Gordon AS, Whiteman M, Cohen P. The psychological etiology of adolescent drug use: A family interactional approach. *Genet Soc Gen Psychol Monogr* 1990;**116**:2.

26. Garmezy N. Stress resistant children: the search for protective factors. In: Stevenson J (ed.), *Recent Research in Developmental Psychopathology*. Oxford: Pergamon, 1985; pp. 213–233.

27. Benard, B. *Fostering Resilience in Kids: Protective Factors in Family School and Community*. San Francisco, CA: Western Center for Drug-Free Schools and Communities, 1990.

28. Blackson TC, Butler T, Belsky J, Ammerman RT, Shaw DS, Tarter RE. Individual traits and family contexts predict sons' externalizing behavior and preliminary relative risk ratios for conduct disorder and substance use disorder outcomes. *Drug Alcohol Depend* 1999;**56**:115–131.

29. Ouellette JA, Gerrard M, Gibbons FX, Reis-Bergan M. Parents, peers, and prototypes: antecedents of adolescent alcohol expectancies, alcohol consumption, and alcohol-related life problems in rural youth. *Psychol Addict Behav* 1999;**13**:32–44.

30. Bahr SJ, Maughan SL, Marcos AC, Li B. Family, religion, and the risk of adolescent drug use. *J Marriage Fam* 1998;**60**:979–992.

31. Svensson R. Risk factors for different dimensions of adolescent drug use. *J Child Adolesc Subst Abuse* 2000;**9**:67–90.

32. Cannon SR. *Social Functioning Patterns of Families of Offspring Receiving Treatment for Drug Abuse*. New York: Libra, 1976.

33. Hansen WB, Graham JW, Sobel JL, *et al.* The consistency of peer and parent influences on tobacco, alcohol, and marijuana use among young adolescents. *J Behav Med* 1987;**10**:559–579.

34. Beardslee WR, Son L, Vaillant GE. Exposure to parental alcoholism during childhood and outcome in adulthood: A prospective longitudinal study. *Brit J Psychiat* 1986;**149**: 584–591.

35. Gilman SE, Rende R, Boergers J. Parental smoking and adolescent smoking initiation: an intergenerational perspective on tobacco control. *Pediatrics* 2009;**123**: e274–e281.

36. Jurich AP, Polson CJ, Jurich JA, Bates RA. Family factors in the lives of drug users and abusers. *Adolescence* 1985;**20**:143–159.

37. Brook J, Brook DW, Zhang C, Cohen P. Pathways from adolescent parent–child conflict to substance use disorders in the fourth decade of life. *Am J Addiction* 2009;**18**: 235–242.

38. Wills TA, Sandy JM, Yaeger A, Shinar O. Family risk factors and adolescent substance use: moderation effects for temperament dimensions. *Dev Psychol* 2001;**37**: 283–297.

39. Swendsen JD, Conway KP, Rounsaville BJ, Merikangas KR. Are personality traits familial risk factors for substance use disorders? Results of a controlled family study. *Am J Psychiatry* 2002;**159**:1760–1766.

40. Rothman EF, Edwards EM, Heeren T, Hingson RW. Adverse childhood experiences predict earlier age of drinking onset: results from a representative US sample of current or former drinkers. *Pediatrics* 2008;**122**:e298–304.

41. National Research Council, Institute of Medicine. *Protecting Youth At Work: Health, Safety, and Development of Working Children and Adolescents in the United States*. Washington, DC: National Academy Press, 1998.

42. Schinke SP, Fang L, Cole KC. Substance use among early adolescent girls: risk and protective factors. *J Adolesc Health* 2008;**43**:191–194.

43. Brady KT, Back SE, Greenfield SF. *Women and Addiction: A Comprehensive Handbook*. New York, NY: Guilford Press, 2009.

44. Office of Applied Studies, Substance Abuse and Mental Health Services Administration. *Results from the 2009 National Survey on Drug Use and Health: Volume I. Summary of National Findings*. NSDUH Series H-38A, HHS Publication No. SMA 10-4856. Rockville, MD: SAMHSA, 2010.

45. Rodriguez D, Audrain-McGovern J. Team sport participation and smoking: analysis with general growth mixture modeling. *J Pediatr Psychol* 2004;**29**:299–308.

46. Audrain-McGovern, Rodriguez D, Wileyto EP, Schmitz KH, Shields PG. Effect of team sport participation on genetic predisposition to adolescent smoking progression. *Arch Gen Psychiatry* 2006;**63**:433–441.

47. Wellman R, Sugarman D, DiFranza J, Winickoff J. The extent to which tobacco marketing and tobacco use in films contribute to children's use of tobacco: a meta-analysis. *Arch Pediatr Adolesc Med* 2006;**160**: 1285–1296.

48. Brook DW, Saar NS, Brook JS. Earlier violent television exposure and later drug dependence. *Am J Addict* 2008;**17**: 271–277.

49. Gorsuch RL, Butler MC. Initial drug abuse: a review of predisposing social psychological factors. *Psychol Bull* 1976;**83**:120–137.

50. Siegel M, Albers AB, Cheng DM, *et al.* Local restaurant smoking regulations and the adolescent smoking initiation process: results of a multilevel contextual analysis among Massachusetts youth. *Arch Pediatr Adolesc Med* 2008; **162**:477–483.

51. Wandersman A, Nation M. Urban neighborhoods and mental health: psychological contributions to understanding toxicity, resilience, and interventions. *Am Psychol* 1998;**53**:647–656.

15

Externalizing Disorders

Yasmin Jilla

Department of Psychiatry, Georgetown University Hospital, Washington DC, USA

INTRODUCTION

Research has established that externalizing disorders are commonly comorbid with substance use disorders in adolescents [1–3]. Externalizing disorders are disruptive toward others and include attention-deficit/hyperactivity disorder, oppositional defiant disorder, and conduct disorder. Externalizing disorders have been shown to be a major risk factor for the development of substance use disorders. Many of the risk factors associated with the development of externalizing disorders also predispose to the development of substance use disorders [2].

Attention-deficit/hyperactivity disorder (ADHD) is defined as a syndrome of inattention, hyperactivity, and/or impulsivity with impairment in executive functioning skills before age 7 years old. The impairment of symptoms must occur in two or more settings and lead to impairment in social, academic, or occupational functioning. There are 18 official *Diagnostic and Statistical Manual of Mental Disorders, Fourth Edition* (DSM-IV) symptoms, which can be classified as combined type (both symptoms of inattention and hyperactivity-/impulsivity), predominantly inattentive type, predominantly hyperactive-impulsive type, and not otherwise specified. Inattentive symptoms include failure to give attention to detail, difficulty sustaining attention, not seeming to listen when spoken to directly, having difficulty following through on instructions, having poor organizational skills, being reluctant to engage in tasks that require sustained mental effort, losing things easily, and being easily distracted and forgetful. Hyperactive symptoms include being fidgety, leaving one's seat in situations that require one to be seated, running about or climbing excessively, having difficulty playing or engaging in leisure activities quietly, being "on the go" or "driven by a motor," and talking excessively.

Examples of impulsive symptoms include blurting out answers, having difficulty awaiting turn, and interrupting or intruding on others [4,5]. ADHD is one of the most common childhood psychiatric disorders and affects 3–7% of school-aged youths [6]. Factors associated with a higher prevalence of ADHD are male gender, poor socioeconomic background, and young age.

The category of conduct disorder and oppositional defiant disorder was officially introduced to DSM-III in 1980 [7]. Conduct disorder is defined by a pattern of behavior in which the basic rights of others or major age-appropriate societal norms or rules are violated for at least a 12-month period. Conduct disorder involves aggression to people and animals, destruction of property, deceitfulness or theft, and/or serious violations of rules. The childhood-onset type occurs prior to the age of 10 years [4,5]. Boys are more commonly affected than girls, but as children age, the gap between males and females closes [8]. Poverty and poor socioeconomic background are common in conduct disorder [9]. Oppositional defiant disorder is used to describe children who show persistently disobedient, angry, negative, and provocative opposition to authority by violations of minor rules, temper tantrums, argumentativeness, provocative behavior, and stubbornness for at least a 6-month period with some form of impairment in social, academic, or occupational functioning [4,5].

COMORBIDITY

The Drug Abuse Treatment Outcome Study – Adolescent (DATOS-A) studies found that nearly two-thirds of their adolescent substance-abusing sample had a comorbid diagnosis. Conduct disorder was the most common comorbid diagnosis and ADHD was the second most common [10]. A study of Native American adolescents showed similar results [11].

Clinical Handbook of Adolescent Addiction, First Edition. Richard Rosner.
© 2013 John Wiley & Sons, Ltd. Published 2013 by John Wiley & Sons, Ltd.

Conduct disorder, as well as the association with a deviant peer group, may be partially responsible for the link between childhood ADHD and subsequent substance disorders, but the studies remain inconsistent and inconclusive [12]. The interplay between ADHD and conduct disorder may exert an additive effect on risk. Research suggests that the rate of comorbidity between ADHD and conduct disorder may be between 30% and 45% [13,14].

The most frequent comorbidities for oppositional defiant disorder and conduct disorder are with ADHD, major depression, and substance abuse [15,16]. Many of the risk factors associated with the development of externalizing disorders similarly predispose to the development of substance use disorders. Conduct disorder, in particular, has consistently been shown to be a major predictor of substance use disorders [4]. Rates of conduct disorder range from 50% to 80% in adolescent patients with substance use disorders [17].

EMPIRICAL DATA ON ADHD AND SUBSTANCE USE RISK

Comorbid substance use disorders are often seen in young people with ADHD [18,19]. Early studies have shown conflicting results regarding the association between ADHD and later substance use [12]. In a review of the early literature, it was determined that the relationship between ADHD and substance use may have been overstated and better accounted for by other factors, such as conduct disorder [20]. A recent 10-year follow-up study of monitoring children into young adulthood by Wilens et al. [21] showed that ADHD subjects were 1.47 times more likely to develop substance use disorders compared to controls. ADHD continued to be a significant risk factor for any drug-use disorders and cigarette smoking, but no significant association was found for overall substance use disorders and alcohol use disorders. In this sample, 30% of the children at baseline with ADHD already had conduct disorder, which subsequently increased the risk for substance use disorder by nearly threefold.

Some research suggests that a diagnosis of ADHD increases the initiation and use of particular drugs, specifically cigarette smoking [12]. Charach et al. [22] performed a comparative meta-analysis of 13 studies and examined the link between ADHD and substance use disorders. The meta-analysis showed ADHD was associated with alcohol and drug use disorders in adulthood and nicotine use in adolescence. In a study by Milberger et al. [23], ADHD was a major predictor of early initiation of cigarette smoking into mid-adolescence, after controlling for psychiatric comorbidity. Biederman et al. [24] performed a rigorous 10-year

follow-up study examining the lifetime prevalence of psychopathology in a sample of male youths aged 6 to 17 years, with and without ADHD. The authors found that the lifetime prevalence of nicotine dependence, alcohol dependence, and drug dependence was greater among ADHD youths than control subjects. Lifetime risk of nicotine dependence remained statistically significant even after controlling for baseline psychopathology. ADHD nicotine smokers may begin smoking as an attempt to manage deficits of attention and concentration [25]. It is possible that some ADHD youths who smoke cigarettes may do so in an attempt to self-medicate their ADHD symptoms, since nicotine has been shown to modulate dopaminergic pathways and exert stimulant like effects [23]. It is recommended that smoking prevention and cessation programs be targeted to youths with ADHD not only to decrease the risks of nicotine use but also susceptibility to future illicit drug use via the stage theory and gateway hypothesis. Stage theory postulates that there is a temporal ordering of substance use experimentation in which lower order substances, which are commonly used, precede the use of higher order substances. Hence, usually a legal substance, such as nicotine or alcohol, is followed by marijuana use, usually the first illicit substance used, before progressing to other higher levels of illicit substances. Related to the stage theory is the gateway hypothesis, proposed by Kandel, that postulates that marijuana use facilitates the entry into use of other illicit substances such as cocaine, hallucinogens, opiates, and intravenous drugs. According to Kandel, 26% of adolescents who use illicit drugs progress to the next of the four states, compared with only 4% who have never used marijuana [26]. An overarching goal of prevention is to delay the initiation of the use of gateway substances such as nicotine, alcohol, and marijuana [17].

Risks for specific substance use may vary depending upon the ADHD symptoms present. Burke et al. [27] studied a sample of 177 boys with ADHD between the ages of 7 and 12 years until the age of 18 years and found adolescent hyperactivity/impulsivity symptoms were more associated with alcohol use. Adolescent inattentive symptoms were related to tobacco use and marginally associated with other drug use. Abrantes et al. [28] studied substance use involvement of 191 male and female smokers and found only inattentive symptoms were associated with marijuana and nicotine dependence.

An additional concern regarding the link between ADHD and substance use disorders is associated with prescribed stimulant medications. Stimulant medications are considered the first-line treatment for ADHD. Over the past few decades, stimulant medications have been increasingly prescribed by practitioners for ADHD [29,30]. A majority of reports have found that children with ADHD treated with stimulant medications seem to have a decreased risk of substance use disorders compared with children with ADHD who are not treated with stimulant medications [12]. In 2003, Wilens *et al.* [31] performed a meta-analytic review of six major studies conducted between 1998 and 2002 in order to determine whether or not stimulant treatment affected the development of substance abuse. The meta-analysis comprised 674 medicated individuals (adolescents and young adults) with ADHD and 360 unmedicated subjects, who were followed for at least 4 years. They found that the pooled estimate of the odds ratio indicated a nearly two-fold reduction in the risk for substance use disorders in youths who were treated with stimulants compared with youths who did not receive stimulants for ADHD. An age effect was observed in that studies that followed subjects into adolescence were more likely to find a protective effect for stimulant treatment than were studies that followed individuals into adulthood.

Faraone *et al.* [32] performed a retrospective data study of 206 ADHD adults receiving pharmacotherapy, and no differences were found in the prevalence of cigarette smoking, alcohol or drug abuse, or dependence. A 13-year prospective study by Fischer and Barkley [33] followed 147 children, between the ages of 4 and 12 years, with ADHD and 73 matched control subjects. Results showed no significant increased risk of substance use in adolescents treated with stimulant medications as children. However, in young adulthood, medicated-treated participants were more likely to report cocaine use compared with unmedicated subjects. Once conduct disorder was controlled for, however, cocaine use was no longer significant. Subjects who were treated with stimulants for less than 1 year were more likely to report cocaine or hallucinogen abuse compared to subjects who were treated for more than 1 year. Conduct disorder was found to account for the risk of cocaine use but not hallucinogen abuse.

The mechanism by which ADHD stimulant treatment protects against substance use disorders is unclear. A hypothesis about how ADHD stimulant pharmacotherapy decreases the risk of substance use disorders includes the decreased need for self-medicating of ADHD symptoms with licit and illicit substances. The close monitoring by prescribing practitioners of young people who receive stimulant medications may directly influence substance use risk. Additionally, families who seek medication treatment for their children may be more intact and supportive as well as more invested in their children's educational success. They may be more involved in parenting. It may be that by decreasing ADHD symptoms with pharmacotherapy, the low self-esteem, demoralization, and academic and occupational failure that are often associated with ADHD are decreased, which themselves are associated independently with substance use disorder risk. It may be also that stimulants' pharmacological efficacy in decreasing conduct disorder symptoms may indirectly reduce the risk of substance use [31].

A majority of ADHD individuals use their medications appropriately. However, there is a risk of diversion and misuse with increasing prescriptions. According to the Office of National Drug Control Policy and the National Institute on Drug Abuse, next to marijuana, prescription medications are the most common drugs that teenagers use to get high [34,35]. A survey performed by A Partnership for a Drug-Free America showed that nearly one in five (19%) of teens reported abusing at least once prescription medications not prescribed to them [36]. According to the National Survey on Drug Use and Health, 2% of adolescents aged 12 to 17 years admitted to non-medical use of stimulant medications. Possible reasons why teens may be abusing prescription medications include beyond just getting high. They may believe that since the medication is prescribed by a doctor then it must be safe. Additionally, stimulants may be misused to improve concentration, increase energy, and decrease need for sleep [37,38].

In 2001, Poulin performed a study that found that adolescents' reporting of non-medical use of prescription stimulants correlated with the number of prescription users who reported giving away their medication [39]. Additionally, approximately 30% of adolescents report having a friend who abuses prescription stimulants [35]. Setlik *et al.* [30] performed a study in 2009 in order to better understand the trend of stimulant abuse by ADHD teens. They examined the American Association of Poison Control Center's National Poison Data System for the years 1998 to 2005 for all cases involving teens aged 13 to 19 years for which the reason was intentional abuse or intentional misuse of prescription medications for ADHD. Additionally, they used sales data from IMS Health's National Disease and Therapeutic Index database to compare poison center call trends with probable availability. Over the 8-year period, calls related to adolescent abuse of prescription ADHD medications rose by 76%, and during the same time period prescriptions of these medications for 10–19-year-olds rose by 86%, whereas prescriptions for 3–19-year-olds increased by 80%.

Wilens *et al.* [40] performed a 10-year longitudinal study of youths with ADHD to study the risks and characteristics of youths who misuse or divert their prescribed stimulant ADHD medications. A structured psychiatric interview and self-report questionnaire were used with subjects with ADHD and controls without ADHD. The authors found that 11% of the ADHD group reported selling their medications, and 22% reported misusing their medications. All ADHD subjects diverting their medication had either comorbid conduct disorder or substance use disorder, and 83% of ADHD subjects misusing their medications met criteria for either conduct disorder or substance use disorder. Additionally, the medications that were misused or diverted were immediate-release preparations of stimulants. Hence, careful monitoring and selection of non-stimulant medications (i.e., atomoxetine) and extended-release stimulants should be considered in high-risk groups with ADHD and comorbid conduct disorder and substance use disorders in order to reduce the risks of stimulant misuse and diversion.

EMPIRICAL DATA ON CONDUCT DISORDER/OPPOSITIONAL DEFIANT DISORDER AND SUBSTANCE USE RISK

Several longitudinal studies have shown that early conduct problems or juvenile delinquent behavior increases the risk for later substance use. A study of inner-city London boys showed that convicted men were significantly more likely than unconvicted men to be heavy drinkers as young adults and use other harder drugs compared to unconvicted men [41]. Moffitt et al. [42,43] used a priori classification of juvenile offending groups and found that boys in the life-course-persistent and adolescence-limited offending groups were more likely to show alcohol dependence and marijuana dependence at age 18 years than those in recovery, abstainer, and unclassified groups. Follow-up data for this cohort at age 26 years indicated that life-course-persistent and adolescence-limited offenders were rated by informants as having more alcohol- and drug-related problems. Using data from the Oregon Youth Study, a longitudinal study of 204 at-risk boys in high-crime areas of the Pacific Northwest who were interviewed annually from ages 9 to 10 years to ages 23 to 24 years, Wiesner et al. [44] found that chronic high-level offenders engaged more often in drug use compared to rare and low-level offenders. These findings were consistent with the views that developmental failures associated with higher levels of antisocial behavior and crime were predictive of drug use.

Lynskey and Fergusson [45] studied the relationships between conduct problems and later substance use behaviors in a longitudinal study of 1265 children in New Zealand at birth, 4 months, 1 year, and annual intervals up until the age of 15 years. They gathered information via maternal interviews, child interviews, teacher reports, and official records from hospitals and the police. They studied patterns of alcohol consumption, tobacco smoking, illicit drug use, child behavior, and confounding factors, such as gender, family social position, family living standards, family size, parental discord, parental history of alcohol and drug problems, parental alcohol consumption, parental smoking, parental illicit drug use, and parental attitudes of alcohol use. The results of the study showed that children with tendencies to conduct problems during middle childhood were at a significantly increased risk of tobacco, alcohol, and illicit drug use by the age of 15 years. There was a consistent relationship between the extent of conduct problems during middle childhood and rates of tobacco, alcohol, and illicit drug use. Children who had high conduct problem scores at 8 years of age had elevated levels of alcohol consumption and higher rates of alcohol-related problems (2.3 times more likely), daily cigarette smoking (3.6 times more likely), and illicit drug use (3.0 times more likely) compared to young people with low conduct problem scores. It was found that early conduct problems were a solid predictor of later substance use. This study's findings were consistent with research that suggests that early externalizing behaviors have a highly specific correlation with later developmental outcomes, in particular regarding conduct disorder as an associated risk of later antisocial and norm-violating behaviors.

The second portion of the analysis concerned whether the confounding factors mentioned above could explain the correlation between conduct disorder and substance use. It was found that controlling for confounding factors, such as gender, family socioeconomic circumstances, parental use of illicit drugs, and marital conflict, reduced the observed associations between conduct disorder and substance use; however, even after controlling for such factors, associations remained between early conduct problems and later use of tobacco, alcohol, and illicit drugs. The clinical implications of these conclusions suggest that substance use prevention strategies should be targeted in conduct disorder populations [45]. Such offenders are in greatest need for prevention and intervention efforts in order to avoid the societal costs of their serious adjustment problems in early adulthood.

EXTERNALIZING DISORDERS AND DEVELOPMENTAL OUTCOME

There is a strong interrelation between attention problems and conduct problems, and there are three main perspectives as to how these areas influence developmental outcome [46]. The first perspective suggests that attention problems and conduct problems are part of general externalizing behaviors and, hence, young people with either of these disorders are at an elevated risk of a variety of negative outcomes including substance use, crime, and mental health problems [47,48]. The second perspective views that conduct problems and attention problems each have specific consequences for later development. The dual pathway hypothesis suggested by Fergusson and Horwood [49] posits that conduct problems are related to later crime, substance use, and mental health problems, and attention problems are more linked to educational underachievement. Hence, higher rates of educational problems in conduct individuals are due to attention problems and higher rates of crime, substance use, and mental health problems in inattentive individuals are due to conduct problems. The third perspective in the literature suggests that attention problems and conduct problems combine non-additively to affect later developmental outcomes. It assumes that young people with both conduct problems and attention problems are at higher risk for later adverse outcomes than expected from the additive risk [50–52].

There are two major hypotheses as to how early disruptive behavior may affect later substance use and abuse. The first hypothesis suggests that there are similar temperamental tendencies during childhood into adolescence and young adulthood. Hence, children with a predisposition to antisocial, norm-violating types of behaviors express tendencies in childhood of disruptive behaviors and in adolescence and young adulthood of increased use of tobacco, alcohol, and illicit drugs [53]. Behavioral characteristics might include impulsivity, aggression, high sensation seeking, low levels of harm avoidance, inability to delay gratification, low levels of striving to achieve, lack of religiosity, and psychopathology, particularly conduct disorder [53]. Temperamental precursors such as impulsivity, novelty seeking, and sensation seeking tend to peak in late adolescence [54]. The second hypothesis suggests that social and environmental factors that predispose children to problem behaviors may also lead to them developing substance use problems later in life. Such factors may include disadvantaged socio-demographics, parental substance use and attitudes toward substance use, marital conflict, and individual characteristics [45]. Additional factors that may contribute include stressful life events, lack of support from parents, absence of normative peers, perception of high availability of drugs, social norms that facilitate drug use, and relaxed laws and regulatory policies [53]. Conduct disorder increases the risk of early alcohol and cannabis use and strongly predicts alcohol and cannabis abuse in adulthood, predominantly in males [55].

CONCLUSION

Externalizing disorders have a major role in the development of substance use in adolescents. Though the role of ADHD in the development of substance use

disorders may be variable in research findings, ADHD appears to pose a particular risk leading to nicotine use, which can be a gateway drug toward heavier drug use. Youths treated with stimulant medications appear to have a decreased risk of substance use disorders overall. Research has consistently shown that youths with conduct problems have a significantly increased risk of later illicit drug and alcohol use. Though the link between externalizing disorders and risk for substance use is strong, it is worth mentioning limitations to the empirical data mentioned, mainly that a majority of the studies in youths have been in males. Little is known of the respective risk relationship in males versus females. Temperamental characteristics and environmental factors likely influence later substance use in adolescents. Overall, individuals with externalizing disorders are a high-risk group for future substance use, and specific prevention plans, interventions, and treatments to address these problems should be focused upon this population.

References

1. Biederman J, Munir K, Knee D. Conduct and oppositional disorder in clinically referred children with attention deficit disorder: a controlled family study. *J Am Acad Child Adolesc Psychiatry* 1987;**26**:724–727.
2. Crowley TJ, Riggs PD. Adolescent substance use disorder with conduct disorder and comorbid conditions. *NIDA Res Monogr* 1995;**156**:49–111.
3. Thompson LL, Riggs PD, Mikulich SK, Crowley TJ. Contribution of ADHD symptoms to substance problems and delinquency in conduct-disordered adolescents. *J Abnorm Child Psychol* 1996;**24**:325–347.
4. Martin A, Volkmar FR. *Lewis's Child and Adolescent Psychiatry.* Philadelphia, PA: Lippincott Williams & Wilkins, 2007.
5. American Psychiatric Association. *Diagnostic and Statistical Manual of Mental Disorders, Fourth Edition.* Washington, DC: APA, 1994.
6. American Psychiatric Association. *Diagnostic and Statistical Manual of Mental Disorders, Fourth Edition, Text Revision.* Washington, DC: APA, 2000.
7. American Psychiatric Association. *Diagnostic and Statistical Manual of Mental Disorders, Third Edition.* Washington, DC: APA, 1980.
8. American Academy of Child and Adolescent Psychiatry. *Practice Parameters for the Assessment and Treatment of Children and Adolescents with Conduct Disorder.* Washington, DC: AACAP, 1997.
9. Loeber R, Wung P, Kennan K, *et al.* Developmental pathways in disruptive behavior. *Dev Psychopathol* 1993;**5**:101–132.
10. Grella CE, Hser Y, Joshi V, Rounds-Bryant J. Drug treatment outcomes for adolescents with comorbid mental and substance use disorders. *J Nerv Ment Dis* 2001;**189**:384–392.
11. Novins DK, Duclos CW, Martin C, Jewett CS, Manson SM. Utilization of alcohol, drug, and mental health treatment services among American Indian adolescent

detainees. *J Am Acad Child Adolesc Psychiatry* 1999;**38**:1102–1108.

12. Looby A. Childhood attention deficit hyperactivity disorder and the development of substance use disorders: Valid concerns or exaggeration. *Addict Behav* 2008;**33**:451–463.

13. Barkley RA, Fischer M, Smallish CS. The adolescent outcome of hyperactive children diagnosed by research criteria: An 8-year prospective follow-up study. *J Am Acad Child Adolesc Psychiatry* 1990;**29**:546–557.

14. Gittleman R, Mannuzza S, Shenker R, Bonagura N. Hyperactive boys almost grown up: I. Psychiatric status. *Arch Gen Psychiatry* 1985;**42**:937–947.

15. Angold A, Costello EJ, Erkanli A. Comorbidity. *J Child Psychol Psychiatry* 1999;**40**:57–87.

16. Armstong TD, Costello EJ. Community studies on adolescent substance use, abuse, or dependence and psychiatric comorbidity. *J Consult Clin Psychol* 2002;**70**: 1224–1239.

17. Kaminer Y, Tarter RE. Adolescent substance abuse. In: Galanter M, Kleber HD (eds), *Textbook of Substance Abuse Treatment*, 3rd edn. Arlington: American Psychiatric Publishing, 2004; pp. 505–517.

18. Biederman J, Wilens T, Mick E, Milberger S, Spencer TJ, Faraone SV. Psychoactive substance use disorders in adults with attention deficit hyperactivity disorder (ADHD): Effects of ADHD and psychiatric comorbidity. *Am J Psychiatry* 1995;**152**:1652–1658.

19. Levin FR, Keiber HD. Attention deficit hyperactivity disorder and substance abuse: Relationships and implications for treatment. *Harvard Rev Psychiatry* 1995;**2**:246–258.

20. Lynskey MT, Hall W. Attention deficit hyperactivity disorder and substance abuse: Is there a causal link? *Addiction* 2001;**96**:815–822.

21. Wilens TE, Martelon M, Joshi G. *et al.* Does ADHD predict substance-use disorders? A 10-year follow-up study of young adults with ADHD. *J Am Acad Child Adolesc Psychiatry* 2011;**50**:543–553.

22. Charach A, Yeung E, Climans T, Lille E. Childhood attention-deficit/hyperactivity disorder and future substance use disorders: comparative meta-analyses. *J Am Acad Child Adolesc Psychiatry* 2011;**50**:9–21.

23. Milberger S, Biederman J, Faraone SV, Chen L, Jones J. ADHD is associated with early initiation of cigarette smoking in children and adolescents. *J Am Acad Child Adolesc Psychiatry* 1997;**36**:37–44.

24. Biederman J, Monuteaux MC, Mick E, *et al.* Young adult outcome of attention deficit hyperactivity disorder: A controlled 10-year follow-up study. *Psychol Med* 2006;**36**:167–179.

25. Pomerleau OF, Downey KK, Stelson FW, Pomerleau CS. Cigarette smoking in adult patients diagnosed with attention deficit hyperactivity disorder. *J Subst Abuse* 1995;**7**:373–378.

26. Kandel DB, Yamaguchi K, Chen K. Stages of progression in drug involvement from adolescence into adulthood: Further evidence for the gateway theory. *J Stud Alcohol* 1992;**53**:447–457.

27. Burke JD, Loeber R, Lahey BB. Which aspects of ADHD are associated with tobacco use in early adolescence? *J Child Psychol Psychiatry* 2001;**42**:493–502.

28. Abrantes AM, Strong DR, Ramsey SE, Lewinson PM, Brown RA. Substance use disorder characteristics and externalizing problems among inpatient adolescent smokers. *J Psychoactive Drugs* 2005;**37**:391–399.

29. Safer DJ, Zito JD, Fine EM. Increased methylphenidate usage for attention deficit disorder in the 1990s. *Pediatrics* 1996;**98**:1084–1088.

30. Setlik J, Randall Bond G, Ho M. Adolescent prescription ADHD medication abuse is rising along with prescriptions for these medication. *Pediatrics* 2009;**124**:875–880.

31. Wilens TE, Faraone SV, Biederman J, Gunawardene S. Does stimulant therapy of attention-deficit/hyperactivity disorder beget later substance abuse? A meta-analytic review of the literature. *Pediatrics* 2003;**111**:179–185.

32. Faraone SV, Biederman J, Wilens TE, Adamson J. A naturalistic study of the effects of pharmacotherapy on substance use disorders among ADHD adults. *Psychol Med* 2007;**37**:1743–1752.

33. Fischer M, Barkley RA. Childhood stimulant treatment and risk for later substance abuse. *J Clin Psychiatry* 2003;**64**: 19–23.

34. Johnston LD, Bachman JG, Schulenberg JE. *Monitoring the Future: National Results on Adolescent Drug Use: Overview of Key Findings*. Bethesda, MD: National Institute on Drug Abuse, 2005.

35. Office of National Drug Control Policy, Executive Office of the President. Teens and prescription drugs: an analysis of trends on the emerging drug threat. Washington, DC: Office of National Drug Control Policy, Executive Office of the President, 2008.

36. Partnership for a Drug-Free America. The Partnership Attitude Tracking Study (PATS): teens in grades 7 through 12. Washington, DC: Partnership for a Drug-Free America, 2005.

37. Boyd CJ, McCabe SE, Cranford JA, Young A. Adolescents' motivations to abuse prescription medications. *Pediatrics* 2006;**118**:2472–2480.

38. Teter CJ, McCabe SE, Cranford JA, Boyd CJ, Guthrie SK. Prevalence and motives for illicit use of prescription stimulants in an undergraduate student sample. *J Am Coll Health* 2005;**53**:253–262.

39. Poulin C. Medical and nonmedical stimulant use among adolescents: from sanctioned to unsanctioned use. *Can Med Assoc J* 2001;**165**:1039–1044.

40. Wilens TE, Gignac M, Swezey A, Monuteaux MC, Biederman J. Characteristics of adolescents and young adults with ADHD who divert or misuse their prescribed medications. *J Am Child Adolesc Psychiatry* 2006;**45**: 408–414.

41. Farrington DP. Later adult life outcomes of offenders and nonoffenders. In: Brambring M, Lowesel F, Skowronek H (eds), *Children at Risk: Assessment, Longitudinal Research, and Intervention*. Berlin: Walter deGryter, 1989; pp. 220–244.

42. Moffitt TE, Caspi A, Dickson N, Silva P, Stanton W. Childhood-onset versus adolescent-onset antisocial conduct problems in males: Natural history from ages 3 to 18 years. *Dev Psychopathol* 1996;**8**:399–424.

43. Moffitt TE, Caspi A, Harrington H, Milne BJ. Males on the life-course-persistent and adolescence-limited antisocial pathways: Follow-up at age 26 years. *Dev Psychopathol* 2002;**14**:179–207.

44. Wiesner M, Kim HK, Capaldi DM. Developmental trajectories of offending: validation and prediction to young adult alcohol use, drug use, and depressive symptoms. *Dev Psychopathol* 2005;**17**:251–270.

45. Lynskey MT, Fergusson DM. Childhood conduct problems, attention deficit behaviors, and adolescent alcohol, tobacco, and illicit drug use. *J Abnorm Child Psychol* 1995;**23**:281–302.

46. Fergusson DM, Horwood LJ, Ridder EM. Conduct and attentional problems in childhood and adolescence and later substance use, abuse, and dependence: Results of a 25-year longitudinal study. *Drug Alcohol Depend* 2007;**88S**:S14–S26.

47. Farrington DP, Loeber R, Van Kammen WB. Long-term criminal outcomes of hyperactivity-impulsivity-attention deficit and conduct problems in childhood. In: Robins L, Ruttler M (eds), *Straight and Dubious Pathways from Childhood to Adulthood*. New York: Cambridge University Press, 1990.

48. Loeber R, Stouthamer-Loeber M, White HR. Developmental aspects of delinquency and internalizing problems and their association with persistent juvenile substance use between ages 7 and 18. *J Clin Child Psychol* 1999;**28**:322–332.

49. Fergusson DM, Horwood LJ, Lynskey MT. The stability of disruptive childhood behaviors. *J Abnorm Child Psychol* 1995;**23**:379–396.

50. Flory K, Milich R, Lynam DR, Leukefeld C, Clayton R. Relation between childhood disruptive behavior disorders and substance use and dependence symptoms in young adulthood: individuals with symptoms of attention-deficit-/hyperactivity disorder and conduct disorder are uniquely at risk. *Psychol Addict Behav* 2003;**17**:151–158.

51. Lynam DR. Early identification of chronic offenders: who is the fledgling psychopath? *Psychol Bull* 1996;**120**:209–234.

52. Molina BSG, Smith BH, Pelham Jr WE. Interactive effects of attention deficit hyperactivity disorder and conduct disorder on early adolescent substance use. *Psychol Addict Behav* 1999;**13**:348–358.

53. Bates MD, Labouvie EW. Personality-environment constellations and alcohol use: a process-oriented study of intraindividual change during adolescence. *Psychol Addict Behav* 1995;**9**:23–25.

54. Zuckerman M. *Behavioral Expressions and Biosocial Bases of Sensation Seeking*. New York: Cambridge University Press, 1994.

55. Kramer TL, Han X, Leukfeld C, Booth BM, Edlund C. Childhood conduct problems and other early risk factors in rural adult stimulant users. *J Rural Health* 2009;**25**:50–57.

16

Internalizing Disorders Among Adolescents: A Risk for Subsequent Substance Use

Tiffany G. Townsend and Dionne Smith Coker-Appiah

Georgetown University School of Medicine, Washington, DC, USA

Over the past several decades, attention has been given to the significant health risk posed by adolescent substance misuse. In fact, substance use and abuse has been associated with increased rates of unintentional injury and morbidity among adolescent populations [1]. In addition, the threat to health and well-being increases for those adolescents with co-occurring or comorbid psychiatric conditions [2]. Due to the high rates of comorbidity between substance use disorders (SUDs) and other psychiatric diagnoses, such as conduct disorder and attention deficit disorder [3], the link between SUDs and externalizing disorders among adolescents has been well researched and documented. However, much less attention has been given to the risk of SUDs among adolescents who suffer from internalizing disorders [2,4], although evidence suggests that internalizing disorders and SUDs frequently co-occur among this population [5–9]. For instance, community and clinical study findings indicate that comorbidity rates range from 9% to 47.9% [4]. Adolescents with comorbid internalizing disorders and SUDs generally show poorer treatment outcomes in both areas, including more frequent treatment dropout, and higher relapse rates [2,10–12]. These statistics highlight the need to examine the relationship between SUDs and internalizing disorders among adolescents much more closely.

Internalizing disorders are a class of disorders characterized by inner-directed symptomatology and are among the most common psychiatric disorders that emerge during adolescence [4,13,14]. Among adolescents, internalizing disorders comprise multiple classes including mood disorders (e.g., major depressive disorder, dysthymic disorder, bipolar disorder); anxiety disorders (e.g., avoidant disorder, separation anxiety, phobias, obsessive-compulsive disorder); eating disorders (e.g., anorexia nervosa, bulimia nervosa); and psychotic disorders (e.g., schizophrenia, schizophreniform, schizoaffective disorder, delusional disorder, psychotic disorder NOS) [13]. Although the comorbidity of SUDs and internalizing disorders can have a greater impact on the lives and treatment outcomes of these adolescents (as opposed to their non-comorbid counterparts), substance use issues are often not assessed, addressed, or properly treated in mental health settings [2,15–17]. Similarly, professionals qualified to treat adolescent substance use/abuse may not have the appropriate training to treat co-occurring mental health issues [18]. Given that internalizing disorders increase the risk that an adolescent will develop SUDs, it becomes increasingly important to provide comprehensive psychiatric assessments for adolescents that can test for the presence of more than one Axis I disorder [19] and that can ensure appropriate screening for the presence of SUDs, regardless of the initial psychiatric presentation [5].

This chapter will examine the most common classes of adolescent internalizing disorders (mood disorders, anxiety disorders, eating disorders, and psychotic disorders) and their comorbidity with adolescent SUDs. In the examination of each internalizing disorder, we will discuss prevalence and comorbidity rates, along with illness progression and outcomes. Each section will conclude with a presentation of theories to help explain the predictive relationship between the internalizing disorder and the subsequent development of SUDs among adolescents.

SUDS AND MOOD DISORDERS AMONG ADOLESCENTS

Mood disorders include but are not limited to major depressive, dysthymic, and bipolar disorders, and are characterized by both emotional (e.g., sadness, hopelessness), biological (e.g., appetite and sleep difficulties) and/or cognitive symptoms (difficulty concentrating, thoughts of death) [20]. Depressive disorders, which include major depressive disorder (MDD) and dysthymic disorder, are the most commonly experienced mood disorders among adolescents. According to the 2004 National Survey on Drug Use and Health (NSDUH), the lifetime prevalence of all forms of adolescent depression is 14% [21], compared to a lifetime prevalence of 1% for bipolar disorder among adolescents. In addition, recent surveys indicate that lifetime rates of illicit drug use among adolescents are high. Results from the 2003 Youth Risk Behavior Survey indicate that approximately 40% of adolescents had used or experimented with an illicit substance at least once during their lives [22].

Adolescence is characterized by specific psychosocial challenges and changes in the brain that increase the probability that psychiatric difficulties and substance abuse will emerge during this developmental period in young people who are predisposed to these conditions [23]. Consequently, it is not surprising to see a concomitant increase in the prevalence of depression and substance use among this age group [24], resulting in a strong association between depression, smoking, drinking, and illicit drug use among teens [25]. In fact, depression is second only to externalizing disorders as the most commonly diagnosed comorbid disorder among adolescents with SUDs [26]. Adolescents who have a substance dependency are 5.6 times more likely to have comorbid depression than their counterparts who are not substance dependent [5]. Across several community samples, the prevalence of comorbid depression and SUDs among adolescents has been found to range from 11% to 32% [4]. Findings from studies of clinical samples indicate that these rates are often higher among adolescents in treatment for addictions. For example, Lubman *et al.* [27] found that 27% of adolescents seeking substance abuse treatment met the criteria for current depression, and 46% had experienced a major depressive episode (MDE) in the previous year. It should be noted that these prevalence rates are greatly affected by gender. As internalizing disorders, particularly depression, have been found to occur more frequently among adolescent girls compared to adolescent boys,

who more frequently experience SUDs [6], a similar gender disparity can be seen in the comorbid manifestations of depression and SUDs. Among adolescents referred for substance abuse treatment, 69% of adolescents girls experienced comorbid MDD compared to 37% of adolescent boys [28].

Although the occurrence of bipolar disorder is not as common as depression among adolescent populations, the association between bipolar disorder and SUDs is equally strong [29], if not stronger [30]. Those adolescents who suffer from bipolar disorder are at increased risk for developing SUDs, and this risk may be even greater than the risk faced by adults with bipolar disorder. Specifically, lifetime prevalence rates of alcohol and drug use disorders were found to be greater among those who experienced adolescent-onset bipolar disorder than among those whose bipolar disorder began in adulthood [31]. In addition, Wilens *et al.* [32] found that adolescents with bipolar disorder were 2.8 times more likely than their counterparts without bipolar disorder to experience a substance abuse problem, even after controlling for demographic information and other psychiatric history. It is clear from these findings that SUDs and mood disorders frequently co-occur among adolescents. Unfortunately, those adolescents who suffer from comorbid SUDs and mood disorders often experience negative outcomes and prolonged recovery.

Illness Progression and Outcomes

Adolescents who are concurrently diagnosed with SUDs and a mood disorder may experience a worse prognosis than those adolescents who develop a mood disorder or SUDs separately. For instance, depression in combination with substance use has been shown to increase the risk for adolescent suicide [33], while also increasing the risk for aggressive, high-risk criminal activity when delinquent behaviors are also present [34]. In fact, the widespread use of alcohol and other illicit drugs among adolescents has been identified as an influential factor contributing to the rate of adolescent suicide. Specifically, intoxicating psychoactive substances may increase impulsivity and predispose users to suicide attempts [35]. In addition, co-occurring SUDs and mood disorders may complicate treatment for both illnesses and produce negative outcomes, such as high treatment dropout rates [11], more persistent substance use involvement [3], and an increased risk for substance use relapse [36]. Due to the strong relationship between mood disorders and SUDs, and the increased risk for a negative prognosis for those adolescents who suffer from both, it is important for clinicians to identify the presence of both disorders in order to inform effective treatment.

Theories to Explain the Risk

Many studies seem to indicate that internalizing disorders, such as bipolar disorder and depression, typically precede the onset of SUDs [4,29]. This would suggest that internalizing disorders are a risk factor for later substance use problems. In support of this hypothesis, a youth study conducted by Kaplow and colleagues [37], found that youths with more depressive symptoms at an early age were at an increased risk for developing alcohol problems later in life. In addition, findings from a community sample of adolescents found depression to precede the development of SUDs in 58.1% of the cases [38]. Similarly, among adolescents with comorbid bipolar disorder and SUDs, Wilens *et al.* [39] found that bipolar disorder preceded the onset of SUDs in 55% of the cases in their study; and Goldstein *et al.* [40] found that it preceded SUDs in 60% of their cases. Theories offered to help explain this temporal sequencing purport that adolescents may use substances to self-medicate and cope with the negative affect associated with mood disorders [19,41]. Thus, the treatment of internalizing disorder may help to prevent the subsequent development of SUDs among adolescents [4].

Finally, there is evidence to suggest that the association between SUDs and mood disorder may be due to confounding variables, such as academic problems, discipline problems, and social skills deficits [42], or an underlying factor that may be causing both disorders [4,19]. When examining the underlying factor hypothesis, some studies suggest that the factor may be a health-compromising lifestyle or a disposition toward unconventionality [43]. Another hypothesis focuses on Eysenck and Eysenck's personality model, which identifies three personality dimensions – psychoticism, extraversion, and neuroticism [44]. Neuroticism has been associated with traits frequently seen in internalizing disorders, such as anxiety and depressive symptoms, and this personality trait has been linked to alcohol misuse [45]. Regardless of the mechanism to explain the association, there is a substantial literature to support a strong relationship between mood disorders and SUDs.

SUDS AND ANXIETY DISORDERS AMONG ADOLESCENTS

Anxiety is a natural response to stress and danger, but can become a disorder when it is excessive, uncontrollable and affects daily functioning [46]. The *Diagnostic and Statistical Manual of Mental Disorders, Fourth Edition, Text Revision* (DSM-IV-TR) identifies several anxiety disorders, including generalized anxiety disorder (GAD), social anxiety disorder, specific phobia, panic disorder, obsessive-compulsive disorder (OCD), post-traumatic stress disorder (PTSD), anxiety secondary to medical condition, acute stress disorder (ASD), and substance-induced anxiety disorder [20]. Approximately 2.5–5% of adolescents meet criteria for an anxiety disorder [14,47], and some studies have shown a slight increase in anxiety disorders during adolescence [47,48].

Although occurring less often than comorbid SUDs and depression, co-occurring anxiety and SUDs has a prevalence averaging between 16.2% and 18.2% across studies of adolescents [4]. Lubman *et al.* [27] found the prevalence rates for comorbid anxiety and SUDs to vary as a function of the type of anxiety disorder. Specifically, they found 27% of adolescents in treatment for SUDs had co-occurring PTSD, 10% had co-occurring panic disorder, 2% had social phobia, and 1% had GAD. One of the strongest relationships between SUDs and anxiety tends to occur among adolescents who experience PTSD. This is likely due to adolescents' high risk for trauma exposure [49]. Kilpatrick and colleagues [50] found that adolescents who had a history of witnessed violence were 9.6 times more likely to experience co-occurring SUDs and PSTD than their counterparts without a similar history. Likewise, those with a history of sexual victimization were 6.73 times more likely, and those who experienced physical victimization were 2.84 times more likely to experience comorbid SUDs and PTSD. As with depression, the relationship between anxiety and SUDs tends to vary as a function of gender. Twenty-four percent of adolescent girls who were receiving treatment for SUDs had a comorbid diagnosis of PTSD, compared to 9% of adolescent males [28]. However, the type of substance used/abused may also impact prevalence rates and the gender effects noted above. According to Kilgus and Pumariega [19], those adolescents who abuse cocaine tend to experience comorbid anxiety more often than adolescents who abuse other substances, and this effect seems to be more pronounced among adolescent boys.

Illness Progression and Outcomes

The findings above provide compelling evidence that SUDs and anxiety disorder commonly co-occur among adolescents, particularly those adolescents who are exposed to trauma, violence, and victimization [51–53]. While SUDs and anxiety can be debilitating to adolescents separately, comorbid SUDs and anxiety disorders are associated with a wide range of impairments, including poor school performance, suicidal behavior, communication problems, and somatic complaints [51]. The presence of an anxiety disorder among adolescents with SUDs can contribute to higher craving for substances and may negatively impact treatment outcomes [19]. In addition, Franken *et al.* [54] found that the presence of an anxiety disorder contributed to addiction relapse by interfering with the development of adaptive coping strategies. This suggests that when treating anxiety among adolescents, service providers need to consider and properly address the potential for the subsequent emergence of a substance abuse problem.

Theories to Explain the Risk

As previously mentioned, studies indicate that internalizing disorders, including anxiety, typically precede SUDs [6]. In a study of 1420 youths, those adolescents who experienced anxiety earlier in life were twice as likely to evidence SUDs later [14]. Similarly, Sonntag and colleagues [55] found that social phobia predicted nicotine dependence among a sample of adolescents, although the type of anxiety disorder has been found to moderate the relationship between SUDs and anxiety. For instance, earlier symptoms of GAD predicted later alcohol use among a community sample of adolescents, while separation anxiety did not evidence this same relationship [37].

Similar to depression, hypotheses proposed to help explain this temporal relationship suggest that adolescents may use substances such as alcohol to help cope with and manage their anxiety. This is particularly true among those adolescents who suffer from social anxiety [56], and PTSD [52,53]. Among adolescents who experience social anxiety, substances such as alcohol may help to minimize the anxiety that is experienced during or in anticipation of social situations. In support of this hypothesis, Blumenthal *et al.* [56] found that 13% of the variance in drinking motives among adolescents with social anxiety in their study was accounted for by coping related motives, while other motives for drinking (i.e., increasing positive affect, enhancing social situations, or avoiding peer rejection) did not evidence the same predicative relationship. A similar explanation has been proposed for the association between PTSD and SUDs. Specifically, it is thought that adolescents who have been exposed to traumatic events such as sexual victimization, physical violence, and natural disasters, may use substances to cope with the psychological reactions that result from the traumas they experience [52,57]. Accordingly, studies have found SUDs to follow the onset of trauma in 25–75% of cases, and follow the development of PTSD in 14–59% of cases [51]. In addition, the use of substances to cope with PTSD is much more prevalent among adolescent girls and young women than among adolescent boys and young men [58,59].

SUDS AND EATING DISORDERS AMONG ADOLESCENTS

Eating disorders (ED) are syndromes characterized by severe disturbances in eating behavior and by distress or excessive concern about body shape or weight [20]. The DSM-IV-TR lists three major classes of ED [20]: Anorexia Nervosa (AN) (restricting type and binge-eating/purging type) [60]; Bulimia Nervosa (BN) (purging type and non-purging type); and Eating Disorder, Not Otherwise Specified [20]. In the United States, approximately 10 million females and one million males suffer from an ED [61], and the age of onset typically occurs during mid to late adolescence [20,60,62]. ED and weight control behaviors have been more prevalent in females than males [20,63,64]; while substance abuse has been more prevalent in males [63]. The commonly held perception that individuals with ED are generally upper-middle-class white teenage girls or young women must be challenged as evidence indicates that ethnic minorities [62,65] and males [62,66] also suffer from ED.

The comorbidity of ED and SUD has been well established in the literature [62,63,67–72], and the risk for both is initiated and often increased throughout the mid to late adolescent period [20,62,73–75]. Common substances associated with ED include alcohol, tobacco, marijuana, heroin, cocaine, inhalants, amphetamines, methamphetamines, ecstasy, steroids, hallucinogens, and laxatives [62,63,67]. A report by The National Center on Addiction and Substance Abuse at Columbia University (2003) indicates that approximately 50% of individuals with an ED also abuse or are dependent on alcohol or illicit substances as compared to the 9% of the general population. Further, more than 35% of individuals with a SUD also report some form of an ED, compared with a prevalence of 1–3% in the general population [62]. To show the gravity of the comorbidity problem, the report indicated that "Individuals with eating disorders are up to five times likelier to abuse alcohol or illicit drugs and those who abuse alcohol or illicit drugs are up to 11 times likelier to have eating disorders" [62,p.i].

While the common belief has been that substance use among ED subtypes classified as calorie restrictors (e.g., anorexia nervosa) was less common [68–70,72,76], recent evidence indicates that alcohol and illicit drug use can also be elevated among this subgroup [67,77]. Among those who binge eat, the use of nicotine, alcohol, and illicit drugs is common [62,63,78]. Another study found that approximately 12–18% of individuals suffering from AN abuse alcohol, tobacco, and other drugs, and 30–70% of individuals suffering from BN struggle with substance abuse [71]. Some recent evidence has found that: (i) SUDs are most common among individuals who report lifetime diagnoses of both AN and BN subtypes [72,77]; (ii) those who endorse purging behaviors have higher rates of SUDs as compared to their non-purging counterparts [72,77]; and (iii) those individuals with BN report higher rates of SUDs [68,69,78–80].

Illness Progression and Outcomes

Eating disorders and SUDs are both long-term, treatment-resistant, and life-threatening disorders that are susceptible to relapse and, thus, may require ongoing intensive therapy [62,71]. However, adolescents who suffer from co-occurring EDs with SUDs often experience worse treatment outcomes than those adolescents who suffer from each illness separately. While anxiety may increase the craving for substances [19], food deprivation may increase the reinforcing effect of substances [71], making the combination of EDs and SUDs that much more difficult to treat. In fact, the presence of a comorbid psychiatric illness, including SUDs, has been associated with higher treatment dropout rates, slower responsiveness to treatment, and lower rates of remission for those adolescents who suffer from EDs [71,81]. Again, comprehensive screening, assessment, and treatment may help to improve prognosis when these illnesses co-occur.

Theories to Explain the Risk

The temporal relationship between ED and SUDs has not been clearly established or well understood [62]. Additional research is necessary to determine temporal order. Evidence indicates that the temporal relationship can be bidirectional, in that either disorder can have an initial presentation [62,82]. For example, adolescents with eating disorders can use substances to both assist with weight reduction and as a means to help alleviate the psychological distress associated with having an ED [62]. Likewise, adolescents with SUDs might run the risk of using certain appetite suppressant substances that can play a primary role in the eventual development of an ED [62]. An ED can also develop in cases where individuals are in the process of substance withdrawal, which can often lead to overeating as a compensatory method to replace the loss of stimulation (as a result of substance withdrawal) to certain pleasure centers in the brain [62].

Multiple mechanisms and hypotheses have been proposed to help understand the comorbidity of EDs and SUDs [62,83]. The mechanisms outlined fall into several categories, including psychological/personal, familial, social, and biological. Psychological/personal mechanisms include the addictive personality

hypothesis, the impulsive personality hypothesis, the self-medication hypothesis, and the effects of other co-occurring psychological disorders (e.g., mood, anxiety, personality disorders) and mental health problems (e.g., low self-esteem, stress/coping, child abuse) [62,68]. The familial mechanisms include dysfunctional family interaction patterns (e.g. unhealthy parent–adolescent relationships, low parental monitoring of adolescent behavior), and family histories of ED and SUDs [62,68]. Social mechanisms include peer influences (e.g., unhealthy social norms, peer pressure related to high-risk behaviors) and media influences (e.g., advertising and marketing aimed at dieting, weight loss, and substance use) [62]. Finally, the biological mechanisms include genetic factors, which can predispose individuals to both EDs and SUDs [68]. It is important to note that while these mechanisms and hypotheses seem plausible, the empirical evidence for their existence or confirmation remains inconclusive.

SUDS AND PSYCHOTIC DISORDERS

Psychotic disorders are serious debilitating thought disorders characterized by disturbances in perception and reality testing, and accompanied by delusions and/or hallucinations [20]. Although the onset of psychotic disorders such as schizophrenia and schizoaffective disorders peaks during adolescence the actual prevalence of psychotic disorders among adolescents is low, with community sample estimates ranging from 0.54% to 1% [84].

While not as prevalent among adolescents as some of the other internalizing disorders, there is still a strong association between psychotic disorders and SUDs [85,86]. The lifetime prevalence rate for alcohol abuse in adolescents with schizophrenia has been found to be as high as 53.5%, and for other illicit substances to be 47% [87]. Reimherr and McClellan [85] found that one-third of adolescents with a schizophrenia or a schizoaffective diagnosis also evidenced substance abuse problems, with schizoaffective disorders found to occur more commonly with SUDs among this population. According to Pencer and colleagues [88], adolescents with psychotic symptoms use more illicit substances, particularly cannabis or marijuana, than their adolescent counterparts who do not evidence psychosis, and even more than adults who experience psychotic symptoms. This suggests that substance use is a particularly significant risk for those adolescents diagnosed with psychotic disorders.

A vigorous debate persists over the relationship between cannabis and psychosis. One position is that cannabis can create a lasting psychotic disorder; the other is that those at risk of psychotic disorders or those in a prodromal state are at high risk of substance use [89].

Illness Progression and Outcomes

Unfortunately, the co-occurrence of psychotic disorders and SUDs leads to particularly problematic outcomes, complicating treatment success for both illnesses. Studies have found that the dual diagnosis of schizophrenia and substance use has been linked to an increase in recurrence of symptoms, more violent outbursts, hospitalizations and suicide, an increased susceptibility to victimization, and a decrease in adherence to treatment [90]. Reimherr and McClellan [85] found a similar link to increased hospitalizations for those adolescents dually diagnosed with SUDs and schizophrenia or SUDs and schizoaffective disorder. In addition, they also found a link to poor school performance and low academic achievement.

Theories to Explain the Risk

As with the internalizing disorders discussed above, theories to help explain the development of SUDs among adolescents with psychotic disorders focus on affect regulation or self-medication models. As previously mentioned, these models propose that adolescents use substances to cope with negative affect [23]. Among adolescents suffering from a psychotic disorder, substances can be used to alleviate or numb feelings of alienation, fear, confusion, anxiety, dysphoria, and depression – negative affect frequently reported by adolescents with psychosis [23,87]. In a study of 70 adolescents between the ages of 15 and 20, Pencer and Addington [23] found support for this hypothesis. According to their study findings, negative affect predicted substance use/misuse among adolescents diagnosed with a psychotic disorder, but it failed to predict substance use/misuse among adolescents who did not evidence psychosis.

Another model suggests that there may be underlying personal characteristics that are associated with both illnesses. This model, termed the deviance prone model, purports that psychotic disorders and SUDs frequently co-occur because they are both deviant behaviors, and all deviant behaviors share underlying characteristics that include a difficult temperament, cognitive dysfunction, and a disturbance in psychological self-regulation. According to this model, children begin to develop these deviant characteristics as a result of deficient socialization from the family, which is reinforced later in life through association with deviant

peers [23]. However, the link between deviance and substance use has been established in adolescent populations that do not evidence psychosis [91], so this model may not adequately explain the unique link between psychotic disorders and SUDs.

Finally, there are models that suggest the use of substances may actually contribute to the subsequent development of a psychotic disorder [90,92]. While substance-induced psychosis is typically transient and rarely leads to a more serious psychotic disorder, some studies have shown links to substance use in early adolescence, particularly the use of marijuana and methamphetamines, and the subsequent development of psychotic disorders such as schizophrenia and schizophreniform disorder [92,93]. According to this model, the developing brain during early adolescence may be particularly susceptible to the cumulative neurobiological effects of certain drug exposure, which may lead to the experience of more severe psychosis later in life [90]. Although the direction of the relationship may vary, these models all point to a strong link between psychotic disorders and SUDs, a risk that service providers must consider when treating adolescents with psychotic disorders.

SUMMARY AND CONCLUSIONS

Based on the literature reviewed above, the relationship between SUDs and internalizing disorders among adolescents is strong, particularly among adolescent girls [4,25,26,29,30,50,62,63,85,86]. While several models have been proposed to help explain this strong association, the model that has been cited most often and has received the most empirical support is the affect regulation or self-medication model [19,23,41,56,62,87]. This model suggests that adolescents who are suffering from internalizing disorders use substances to self-medicate in an attempt to regulate or mitigate the negative affect associated with their internalizing illness, ultimately leading to a SUD. Clearly, the risk that adolescents with internalizing disorders may develop a subsequent SUD is high [23,32,37,56,62], which needs to be considered and properly addressed by service providers. The co-occurrence of internalizing disorders and SUDs has definite treatment implications, often complicating illness progression and treatment outcomes for both disorders. This highlights the need to ensure that comprehensive psychiatric assessments for adolescents screen for SUDs, regardless of adolescents' initial psychological presentation, and that adolescents with a dual diagnosis receive a single treatment plan that addresses both SUDs and internalizing disorders as primary concerns [5].

References

1. Brindis C, Park MJ, Ozer EM, Irwin CE Jr. Adolescents' access to health services and clinical preventive health care: crossing the great divide. *Pediatr Ann* 2002;**31**:575–81.

2. Lichtenstein DP, Spirito A, Zimmermann RP. Assessing and treating co-occurring disorders in adolescents: examining typical practice of community-based mental health and substance use treatment providers. *Community Ment Health J* 2009;**46**:252–257.

3. Grella CE, Hser YI, Joshi V, Rounds-Bryant J. Drug treatment outcomes for adolescents with comorbid mental and substance use disorders. *J Nerv Ment Dis* 2001;**189**: 384–392.

4. O'Neil KA, Conner BT, Kendall PC. Internalizing disorders and substance use disorders in youth: Comorbidity, risk, temporal order, and implications for intervention. *Clin Psychol Rev* 2011;**31**:104–112.

5. Bukstein OG, Horner MS. Management of the adolescent with substance use disorders and comorbid psychopathology. *Child Adolesc Psychiatr Clin N Am* 2010;**19**: 609–623.

6. Kessler RC, Nelson CB, McGonagle KA, Edlund MJ, Frank RG, Leaf PJ. The epidemiology of co-occurring addictive and mental disorders: implications for prevention and service utilization. *Am J Orthopsychiatry* 1996;**66**:17–31.

7. DeMilio L. Psychiatric syndromes in adolescent substance abusers. *Am J Psychiatry* 1989;**146**:1212–1214.

8. Clark DB, Bukstein OG. Psychopathology in adolescent alcohol abuse and dependence. *Alcohol Health Res World* 1998;**22**:117–121, 126.

9. Chan YF, Dennis ML, Funk RR. Prevalence and comorbidity of major internalizing and externalizing problems among adolescents and adults presenting to substance abuse treatment. *J Subst Abuse Treat* 2008;**34**:14–24.

10. Winters KC. Treating adolescents with substance use disorders: an overview of practice issues and treatment outcome. *Subst Abuse* 1999;**20**:203–225.

11. Cornelius JR, Maisto SA, Martin CS, *et al.* Major depression associated with earlier alcohol relapse in treated teens with AUD. *Addict Behav* 2004;**29**:1035–1038.

12. Winters KC, Stinchfield RD, Latimer WW, Stone A. Internalizing and externalizing behaviors and their association with the treatment of adolescents with substance use disorder. *J Subst Abuse Treat* 2008;**35**:269–278.

13. Reynolds WM. Introduction to the nature and study of internalizing disorders in children and adolescents. *School Psychol Rev* 1990;**19**:137.

14. Costello EJ, Mustillo S, Erkanli A, Keeler G, Angold A. Prevalence and development of psychiatric disorders in childhood and adolescence. *Arch Gen Psychiatry* 2003;**60**: 837–844.

15. Carey KB, Correia CJ. Severe mental illness and addictions: assessment considerations. *Addict Behav* 1998;**23**: 735–748.

16. Amodeo M. The therapeutic attitudes and behavior of social work clinicians with and without substance abuse training. *Subst Use Misuse* 2000;**35**:1507–1536.

17. Deas-Nesmith D, Campbell S, Brady KT. Substance use disorders in an adolescent inpatient psychiatric population. *J Natl Med Assoc* 1998;**90**:233–238.

18. Grella CE. Contrasting the views of substance misuse and mental health treatment providers on treating the dually diagnosed. *Subst Use Misuse* 2003;**38**:1433–1446.

19. Kilgus MD, Pumariega AJ. Psychopathology in cocaine-abusing adolescents. *Addict Dis Treat* 2009;**8**:138–144.

20. American PsychiatricAssociation. *Diagnostic and Statistical Manual of Mental Disorders: Fourth Edition, Text Revision* (DSM-IV-TR). Washington, DC: American Psychiatric Association, 2000.

21. Substance Abuse and Mental Health Services Administration. Results from the 2004 National Survey on Drug Use and Health: National findings. DHHS Publication No. SMA 05-4062, NSDUH Series H-28. SAMHSA, 2005. Available from: http://www.oas.samhsa.gov/p0000016.htm#2k4.

22. Centers for Disease Control and Prevention. Youth Risk Behavior Surveillance – United States, 2003. CDC, 2004.

23. Pencer A, Addington J. Models of substance use in adolescents with and without psychosis. *J Can Acad Child Adolesc Psychiatry* 2008;**17**:202–209.

24. Kaminer Y, Connor DF, Curry JF. Comorbid adolescent substance use and major depressive disorders: a review. *Psychiatry (Edgmont)* 2007;**4**:32–43.

25. Shaffer D, Fisher P, Dulcan MK, *et al.* The NIMH Diagnostic Interview Schedule for Children Version 2.3 (DISC-2.3): description, acceptability, prevalence rates, and performance in the MECA Study. Methods for the Epidemiology of Child and Adolescent Mental Disorders Study. *J Am Acad Child Adolesc Psychiatry.* 1996;**35**: 865–877.

26. Armstrong TD, Costello EJ. Community studies on adolescent substance use, abuse, or dependence and psychiatric comorbidity. *J Consult Clin Psychol* 2002;**70**:1224–1239.

27. Lubman DI, Allen NB, Rogers N, Cementon E, Bonomo Y. The impact of co-occurring mood and anxiety disorders among substance-abusing youth. *J Affect Disord* 2007;**103**: 105–112.

28. Clark DB, Pollock N, Bukstein OG, Mezzich AC, Bromberger JT, Donovan JE. Gender and comorbid psychopathology in adolescents with alcohol dependence. *J Am Acad Child Adolesc Psychiatry.* 1997;**36**:1195–1203.

29. Goldstein BI, Bukstein OG. Comorbid substance use disorders among youth with bipolar disorder: opportunities for early identification and prevention. *J Clin Psychiatry* 2010;**71**:348–358.

30. Dilsaver SC, Akiskal HS, Akiskal KK, Benazzi F. Dose–response relationship between number of comorbid anxiety disorders in adolescent bipolar/unipolar disorders, and psychosis, suicidality, substance abuse and familiality. *J Affect Disord* 2006;**96**:249–258.

31. Perlis RH, Miyahara S, Marangell LB, *et al.* Long-term implications of early onset in bipolar disorder: data from the first 1000 participants in the systematic treatment enhancement program for bipolar disorder (STEP-BD). *Biol Psychiatry* 2004;**55**:875–881.

32. Wilens TE, Biederman J, Millstein RB, Wozniak J, Hahesy AL, Spencer TJ. Risk for substance use disorders in youths with child- and adolescent-onset bipolar disorder. *J Am Acad Child Adolesc Psychiatry* 1999;**38**:680–685.

33. Shaffer D, Gould MS, Fisher P, *et al.* Psychiatric diagnosis in child and adolescent suicide. *Arch Gen Psychiatry* 1996;**53**:339–348.

34. Clingempeel WG, Britt SC, Henggeler SW. Beyond treatment effects: Comorbid psychopathologies and long-term outcomes among substance-abusing delinquents. *J Orthopsychiatry* 2008;**78**:29–36.

35. Garrison CZ, Addy CL, McKeown RE, *et al.* Nonsuicidal physically self-damaging acts in adolescents. *J Child Fam Stud* 1993;**2**:339–352.

36. McCarthy DM, Tomlinson, KL, Anderson KG, *et al.* Relapse in alcohol and drug-disordered adolescents with comorbid psychopathology: Changes in psychiatric symptoms. *Psychol Addict Behav* 2005;**19**:28–34.

37. Kaplow JB, Curran PJ, Angold A, Costello EJ. The prospective relation between dimensions of anxiety and the initiation of adolescent alcohol use. *J Clin Child Psychol* 2001;**30**:316–326.

38. Rohde P, Lewinsohn PM, Seeley JR. Psychiatric comorbidity with problematic alcohol use in high school students. *J Am Acad Child Adolesc Psychiatry* 1996;**35**:101–109.

39. Wilens TE, Biederman J, Abrantes AM, Spencer TJ. Clinical characteristics of psychiatrically referred adolescent outpatients with substance use disorder. *J Am Acad Child Adolesc Psychiatry* 1997;**36**:941–947.

40. Goldstein BI, Strober MA, Birmaher B, *et al.* Substance use disorders among adolescents with bipolar spectrum disorders. *Bipolar Disord* 2008;**10**:469–478.

41. Neighbors B, Kempton T, Forehand R. Co-occurrence of substance abuse with conduct, anxiety, and depression disorders in juvenile delinquents. *Addict Behav* 1992;**17**: 379–386.

42. Mason WA, Hawkins JD, Kosterman R, Catalano RF. Alcohol use disorders and depression: Protective factors in the development of unique versus comorbid outcomes. *J Child Adolesc Subst Abuse* 2010;**19**:309–323.

43. Hair EC, Park MJ, Ling TJ, Moore KA. Risky behaviors in late adolescence: co-occurrence, predictors, and consequences. *J Adolesc Health* 2009;**45**:253–261.

44. George SM, Connor JP, Gullo MJ, Young RMcD. A prospective study of personality features predictive of early adolescent alcohol misuse. *Pers Indiv Differ* 2010; **49**:204–209.

45. Colder CR, Chassin L. Affectivity and impulsivity: Temperament risk for adolescent alcohol involvement. *Psychol Addict Behav* 1997;**11**:83–97.

46. Rowney J, Hermida T, Malone D. Anxiety disorders. Cleveland Clinic, Center for Continuing Education, 2010. Available from: http://www.clevelandclinicmeded.com/medicalpubs/diseasemanagement/psychiatry-psychology/anxiety-disorder [accessed 11 March 2011].

47. Ford T, Goodman R, Meltzer H. The British Child and Adolescent Mental Health Survey 1999: the prevalence of DSM-IV disorders. *J Am Acad Child Adolesc Psychiatry* 2003;**42**:1203–1211.

48. Canino G, Shrout PE, Rubio-Stipec M, *et al.* The DSM-IV rates of child and adolescent disorders in Puerto Rico: prevalence, correlates, service use, and the effects of impairment. *Arch Gen Psychiatry* 2004;**61**:85–93.

49. Centers for Disease Control and Prevention. Youth Risk Behavior Surveillance United States 1999. *MMWR Surveillance Summaries* 2000;**49**:1–96.

50. Kilpatrick DG, Ruggiero KJ, Acierno R, Saunders BE, Resnick HS, Best CL. Violence and risk of PTSD, major depression, substance abuse/dependence, and comorbidity: results from the National Survey of Adolescents. *J Consult Clin Psychol* 2003;**71**:692–700.

51. Wagner KD, Brief DJ, Vielhauer MJ, Sussman S, Keane TM, Malow R. The potential for PTSD, substance use, and HIV risk behavior among adolescents exposed to Hurricane Katrina. *Subst Use Misuse* 2009;**44**:1749–1767.

52. Macdonald A, Danielson CK, Resnick HS, Saunders BE, Kilpatrick DG. PTSD and comorbid disorders in a representative sample of adolescents: The risk associated with multiple exposures to potentially traumatic events. *Child Abuse Negl* 2010;**34**:773–783.

53. Rowe CL, La Greca AM, Alexandersson A. Family and individual factors associated with substance involvement and PTS symptoms among adolescents in greater New Orleans after Hurricane Katrina. *J Consult Clin Psychol* 2010;**78**:806–817.

54. Franken IH, Hendriks VM, Haffmans PM, van der Meer CW. Coping style of substance-abuse patients: effects of anxiety and mood disorders on coping change. *J Clin Psychol* 2001;**57**:299–306.

55. Sonntag H, Wittchen HU, Hofler M, Kessler RC, Stein MB. Are social fears and DSM-IV social anxiety disorder associated with smoking and nicotine dependence in adolescents and young adults? *Eur Psychiatry* 2000; **15**:67–74.

56. Blumenthal H, Leen-Feldner EW, Frala JL, Badour CL, Ham LS. Social anxiety and motives for alcohol use among adolescents. Psychology of addictive behaviors. *J Soc Psychol Addict Behav* 2010;**24**:529–534.

57. McFarlane AC, Browne D, Bryant RA, *et al.* A longitudinal analysis of alcohol consumption and the risk of post-traumatic symptoms. *J Affect Disord* 2009;**118**:166–172.

58. Lederman CS, Dakof GA, Larrea MA, Li H. Characteristics of adolescent females in juvenile detention. *Int J Law Psychiatry* 2004;**27**:321–337.

59. Deykin EY, Buka SL. Prevalence and risk factors for posttraumatic stress disorder among chemically dependent adolescents. *Am J Psychiatry* 1997;**154**:752–757.

60. Devlin M, Jahraus J, Dobrow I. Eating disorders. In: Levenson J (ed.), *Textbook of Psychosomatic Medicine*. Washington, DC: American Psychiatric Association, 2005; pp. 311–334.

61. National Eating Disorders Association. Statistics: eating disorders and their precursors. NEDA, 2005. Available from: http://www.nationaleatingdisorders.org.

62. The National Center on Addiction and Substance Abuse (CASA) at Columbia University. *Food for Thought: Substance Abuse and Eating Disorders*. New York: The National Center on Addiction and Substance Abuse (CASA) at Columbia University, 2003.

63. Pisetsky EM, Chao YM, Dierker LC, May AM, Striegel-Moore RH. Disordered eating and substance use in high-school students: results from the Youth Risk Behavior Surveillance System. *Int J Eat Disord* 2008;**41**:464–470.

64. Lewinsohn PM, Seeley JR, Moerk KC, Striegel-Moore RH. Gender differences in eating disorder symptoms in young adults. *Int J Eat Disord* 2002;**32**:426–440.

65. National Eating Disorders Association. Research results on eating disorders in diverse populations. NEDA, 2005. Available from: https://www.nationaleatingdisorders.org.

66. National Eating Disorders Association. Males and eating disorders: research. NEDA, 2005. Available from: https://www.nationaleatingdisorders.org.

67. Root TL, Pisetsky EM, Thornton L, Lichtenstein P, Pedersen NL, Bulik CM. Patterns of co-morbidity of eating disorders and substance use in Swedish females. *Psychol Med* 2010;**40**:105–115.

68. Holderness CC, Brooks-Gunn J, Warren MP. Co-morbidity of eating disorders and substance abuse review of the literature. *Int J Eating Dis* 1994;**16**:1–34.

69. Calero-Elvira A, Krug I, Davis K, Lopez C, Fernandez-Aranda F, Treasure J. Meta-analysis on drugs in people with eating disorders. *Eur Eat Disord Rev* 2009;**17**: 243–259.

70. Conason AH, Sher L. Alcohol use in adolescents with eating disorders. *Int J Adolesc Med Health* 2006;**18**:31–36.
71. Vastag B. What's the connection? No easy answers for people with eating disorders and drug abuse. *JAMA* 2001; **285**:1006–1007.
72. Blinder BJ, Cumella EJ, Sanathara VA. Psychiatric comorbidities of female inpatients with eating disorders. *Psychosom Med* 2006;**68**:454–462.
73. Bulik CM. Eating disorders in adolescents and young adults. *Child Adolesc Psychiatr Clin N Am* 2002;**11**: 201–218.
74. Field AE, Austin SB, Frazier AL, Gillman MW, Camargo CAJr, Colditz GA. Smoking, getting drunk, and engaging in bulimic behaviors: in which order are the behaviors adopted? *J Am Acad Child Adolesc Psychiatry* 2002;**41**: 846–853.
75. Measelle JR, Stice E, Hogansen JM. Developmental trajectories of co-occurring depressive, eating, antisocial, and substance abuse problems in female adolescents. *J Abnorm Psychol* 2006;**115**:524–538.
76. Stock SL, Goldberg E, Corbett S, Katzman DK. Substance use in female adolescents with eating disorders. *J Adolesc Health* 2002;**31**:176–182.
77. Root TL, Pinheiro AP, Thornton L, *et al.* Substance use disorders in women with anorexia nervosa. *Int J Eating Dis* 2010;**43**:14–21.
78. Fischer S, leGrange D. Comorbidity and high-risk behaviors in treatment-seeking adolescents with bulimia nervosa. *Int J Eat Disord* 2007;**40**:751–753.
79. Sysko R, Hildebrandt T. Cognitive-behavioural therapy for individuals with bulimia nervosa and a co-occurring substance use disorder. *Eur Eat Disord Rev* 2009;**17**: 89–100.
80. O'Brien KM, Vincent NK. Psychiatric comorbidity in anorexia and bulimia nervosa: nature, prevalence, and causal relationships. *Clin Psychol Rev* 2003;**23**:57–74.
81. Lock J, Couturier J, Bryson S, Agras S. Predictors of dropout and remission in family therapy for adolescent anorexia nervosa in a randomized clinical trial. *Int J Eating Dis* 2006;**39**:639–647.
82. Krahn DD. The relationship of eating disorders and substance abuse. *J Subst Abuse* 1991;**3**:239–253 [review].
83. Arendt M, Sher L, Fjordback L, Brandholdt J, Munk-Jorgensen P. Parental alcoholism predicts suicidal behavior in adolescents and young adults with cannabis dependence. *Int J Adolesc Med Health* 2007;**19**:67–77.
84. Imran SA, Clark A. Adolescent psychosis: A practical guide to assessment and management. *Psychiatric Times* 2008;**25**:1–7.
85. Reimherr JP, McClellan JM. Diagnostic challenges in children and adolescents with psychotic disorders. *J Clin Psychiatry* 2004;**65** (Suppl. 6):5–11.
86. Roth RM, Brunette MF, Green AI. Treatment of substance use disorders in schizophrenia: a unifying neurobiological mechanism? *Current psychiatry reports.* 2005;**7**:283–291.
87. Cepeda C. *Psychotic Symptoms in Children and Adolescents: Assessment, Differential Diagnosis and Treatment.* New York, NY: Routledge, 2007.
88. Pencer A, Addington J, Addington D. Outcome of a first episode of psychosis in adolescence: a 2-year follow-up. *Psychiatry Res* 2005;**133**:35–43.
89. Large M, Sharma S, Compton MT, *et al.* Cannabis use and earlier onset of psychosis: A systematic meta-analysis. *Arch Gen Psychiatry* 2011;**68**:555–561.
90. Raby WN. Comorbid cannabis misuse in psychotic disorders: Treatment strategies. *Primary Psychiatry* 2009;**16**:29–34.
91. Adalbjarnardottir S, Rafnsson FD. Adolescent antisocial behavior and substance use: longitudinal analyses. *Addict Behav* 2002;**27**:227–240.
92. Semper TF, McClellan JM. The psychotic child. *Child Adolesc Clin N Am* 2003;**12**:679–691.
93. Andreasson S, Allebeck P, Engstrom A, Rydberg U. Cannabis and schizophrenia. A longitudinal study of Swedish conscripts. *Lancet* 1987;**ii**:1483–1486.

17

Risk due to Medical, Neurological, and Neurodevelopmental Conditions

Malena Banks and Matthew Biel

Georgetown University Hospital, Washington DC, USA

INTRODUCTION

Substance use and misuse among young people continues to present a significant health risk. According to the 2009 National Survey on Drug Use and Health, the prevalence of illicit drug use in adolescents was 10%, that of tobacco use was 11.6%, and for alcohol use was 14.6%. An extensive body of research has demonstrated the problematic effects of adolescent substance use upon neurological development, psychological functioning, and academic and vocational achievement. In addition, this exposure may lead to related risky behaviors such as impaired driving, which are explored in more depth in Chapter 12.

However, the prevalence of substance use among youths with chronic medical illness or neurodevelopmental disorders, and any specific effects upon this population, have not been adequately investigated. This lack of empirical research may contribute to false beliefs that chronic medical illness may be a protective factor against substance misuse in youths. In a previous study, Alderman and colleagues [1] found that there were no differences in rates of substance use between healthy adolescents and those with chronic illnesses, and that in fact misuse may be more likely in medically ill youths.

Dramatic advances in recent decades in medical treatments for pediatric disease have improved quality of life and prolonged survival of children and adolescents with chronic and severe illnesses. Among adolescents with chronic and severe illnesses, improved medical outcomes likely have profound effects upon developmental challenges that face these youths as they cope with their illnesses. As they embark upon developmentally crucial tasks, which include moving toward autonomy, separating from parents, and forging individual identities, adolescents with chronic illness are also forced to reckon with the limitations, frustrations, and morbidities associated with their illnesses, and substance use is not infrequently present. Substance experimentation and misuse appears to be a common behavior among adolescents with medical illnesses, with a variety of factors likely contributing to robust prevalence rates. Adolescents may attempt to enhance their self-image and gain peer acceptance to relieve stress and bolster fragile coping skills while engaging in "devil may care" nihilistic behaviors that fly in the face of the constant focus on health that characterizes much of their existence in managing chronic illnesses [2].

Risky behaviors are behaviors that compromise the psychosocial aspects of successful adolescent development [3]. In addition, risky behaviors such as substance use can also potentiate physical morbidity and decrease the efficacy of medical management particularly in those with chronic medical illness. Frequent use of illicit and licit substances can damage current health and present physical and psychosocial issues in adulthood [4]. Another important risky behavior particular to this population is poor adherence to treatment, which can produce a greater negative impact on health status than the illness itself [5].

This chapter reviews existing information about several chronic medical illnesses, namely asthma, sickle-cell disease, cystic fibrosis, cancer, diabetes, fetal alcohol spectrum disorder, and juvenile rheumatoid arthritis. Although the data to review are quite limited, this chapter

Clinical Handbook of Adolescent Addiction, First Edition. Richard Rosner.
© 2013 John Wiley & Sons, Ltd. Published 2013 by John Wiley & Sons, Ltd.

will attempt to take a comprehensive look at the phenomenon of substance use among youths with chronic medical illness. It will examine the prevalence of these comorbidities, some possible reasons behind their substance misuse, and the medical effects of these behaviors.

ASTHMA

According to the Centers for Disease Control and Prevention (CDC) and American Lung Association, asthma is one of the most common chronic diseases among childhood, affecting 7.1 million children under age 18 [6]. Asthma involves chronic inflammation of the respiratory system caused by various types of stimuli, or "triggers," leading to swelling and narrowing of the airways. These processes, if untreated, may cause substantial functional difficulties including difficulty engaging in sports, sleep disturbance, the need to avoid contact with pets and other allergens, and an overall decreased quality of life [7]. Asthma is also one of the leading causes of missed school days and hospitalization, but with advances in asthma management, affected children can live full lives without significant burden.

Observers might imagine that children and adolescents with asthma would attempt to avoid any "triggers" or behaviors that would lead to an exacerbation of their asthma, but some studies have found quite the opposite. For example, cigarette smoke is a powerful initiator of asthma symptoms and respiratory tract inflammation; however, in a study by Zimlichman et al. [8], asthma was not found to be a powerful motivator for smoking prevention in the adolescent population. The prevalence of smoking among asthmatics ranges from 20% to 48% according to the National Longitudinal Study of Adolescent Health [2,9]. Prevalence rates are reported to be as high as 55% in children aged 11 to 15 [10]. These statistics are alarming due to the fact that children and adolescents who smoke are more than four times as likely to experience an asthmatic attack, and are at increased risk of other complications including respiratory failure or arrest. Smoking cigarettes also leads to decreased effectiveness of oral and inhaled steroids used for treatment [8,11]. Alarmingly, children and adolescents who smoke cigarettes can experience a rapid decline in pulmonary function, requiring higher rates of hospitalization and increased rates of intubation [2].

Why would asthmatic youngsters be drawn to cigarette smoking when the evidence is robust for the complications from smoking in asthma? Common psychosocial risk factors may be relevant, including peer pressure, acceptability of smoking among peers, access to cigarettes, depressed mood, stress, and lack of social supports [9]. Having a parent who smokes may be a particularly potent risk factor, increasing rates of smoking among asthmatic youths by 30% [12]. Lack of parental involvement in daily activities may contribute to increased youth autonomy and psychological distress, especially depression, which may subsequently predict smoking initiation in youths [9]. Hublet et al. [7] also found that improved asthma therapeutics may give children a false sense of being "cured," with related thoughts that smoking will not harm them. Some youths may take up smoking in order to demonstrate to others, and to themselves, that they are "normal" despite having asthma. Studies suggest that neglect on the part of physicians may contribute to smoking initiation and lack of smoking cessation: physicians often fail to give adequate guidance about the harmful effects of smoking or about avenues to smoking prevention or cessation [7].

SICKLE-CELL DISEASE

Sickle-cell disease (SCD) and cystic fibrosis (CF) are congenital conditions with onset of symptoms in childhood. They are categorized by some investigators as "invisible" conditions, as the symptoms of both conditions are often not apparent to onlookers. Although affected youths may not have obvious physical abnormalities, they have a shortened lifespan and often experience significant functional impairment as a result of their condition. A psychological burden often accompanies these conditions, and adolescents with SCD and CF may have significant rates of risk-taking behaviors [4].

Sickle-cell disease, or sickle-cell anemia, is named for its sickle-shaped red blood cells; the abnormally shaped cells are prone to destruction within the hematological system, leading to anemia, and also cause impaired blood flow through capillaries, leading to damage to various organ systems. SCD is an autosomal recessive blood disorder caused by a mutation in the hemoglobin gene. In the United States, it mostly affects those of African descent, with a population prevalence of 1 in 5000 individuals; also affected are individuals of Mediterranean, Middle Eastern, and Indian origin. SCD can lead to hematological crises including vaso-occlusive events, hemolytic crisis, aplasia, and splenic sequestration; the condition also predisposes individuals to infections, stroke, kidney and lung damage, and priapism. Cerebrovascular events are of particular neuropsychiatric interest, as cognitive and emotional effects may result [11].

According to one study, adolescents with SCD had significant rates of substance use: the most common drug of use was alcohol (36.9%), followed by cannabis (16.8%) and cigarette smoking (6.5%) [4]. In addition to posing long-term risks of substance abuse and dependence, use of these substances in individuals with SCD may present several specific medical risks: alcohol can lead to dehydration and precipitate a sickle-cell crisis, cigarette smoking can lead to acute chest syndrome and stroke, and excessive use of alcohol and marijuana may lead to episodes of priapism [11,13,14].

CYSTIC FIBROSIS

Cystic fibrosis (CF) is a chronic disease caused by an autosomal recessive genetic mutation; it affects exocrine glands of the respiratory and gastrointestinal systems. The defective gene causes an abnormal secretion of thick mucus that builds in these systems, leading to problems with respiration (including pulmonary infections), chemical breakdown of food, and gastrointestinal absorption of nutrients. CF patients may suffer from impaired oxygenation of tissues, recurrent pneumonia, compromised nutritional status, delayed onset of puberty, impaired growth, and decreased exercise tolerance [11]. CF is typically diagnosed by the age of 2 years, and affects 30 000 persons in the United States, especially Caucasians of northern or central European descent; 1000 new cases are diagnosed in the United States each year.

Britto *et al.* [4] assessed substance use in adolescents with CF and found rates similar to or greater than the age-matched non-CF population. They found alcohol to be the most common reported substance of abuse, with a prevalence of 45.5%, followed by marijuana (9.7%) and cigarette smoking (2.6%) [4]. These authors propose that adolescents affected by "invisible" conditions such as SCD and CF may be at risk for higher rates of substance use and abuse compared with adolescents affected by more physically visible conditions such as cancer [4].

Cigarette and marijuana use is of particular concern in CF patients given the precariousness of the pulmonary system in the disease. In one study, most patients with CF who smoked were aware that smoking would have a negative effect on their health, but initiated or continued smoking despite this knowledge. Of those patients who reported smoking initiation, their major influences were peer groups and "being sociable;" for those who continued to use cigarettes, they reported doing so out of "habit" [15]. Smoking worsens clinical outcomes in CF, with evidence of a dose-dependent relationship between number of cigarettes smoked and disease severity [15]. Smoking decreases the clearance of foreign bodies in respiratory airways, increases cough, decreases exercise tolerance and cardiopulmonary fitness, and increases mucus production, thereby increasing risk of bacterial infections and subsequent hospitalizations. Marijuana may have a brief bronchodilatory effect in some patients, but long-term effects include increased airway obstruction, granuloma formation, and bronchiectasis [15].

CANCER

In the United States, cancer is the second leading cause of death among children and adolescents. The most common types of cancer among children are the leukemias (33%), brain cancer (21%), soft tissue sarcomas (10%), renal cancers (5%), and non-Hodgkin's lymphoma (4%). In the last two decades, huge advances in cancer therapeutics have revolutionized pediatric oncology and led to enormous gains in long-term survival rates: the mean 5-year survival rate among those diagnosed with pediatric cancers between 1999 and 2005 was 81%, compared with a 5-year survival rate of 58% among those diagnosed from 1975 to 1977 [16].

With these major advances in long-term survival, new risks have emerged for cancer survivors, leading to consideration of "late effects" of cancer. Late effects are any side effects that may occur more than 5 years after receiving cancer treatment. These effects may manifest as damage to organs including the liver, heart, and lungs [17,18]. Other late effects include cognitive impairment and psychological symptoms including depression, anxiety, post-traumatic stress disorder, and substance abuse. Substance abuse is a particularly concerning area as cancer survivors may be particularly susceptible to negative medical consequences as a result of these behaviors.

The prevalence of cigarette smoking among 10–19-year-old cancer survivors may range from 5% to15%, and 2% of adolescents may smoke cigarettes during active cancer treatment [11]. Hollen *et al.* [18] reported significant rates of alcohol (49%), tobacco (25%), and marijuana use (16%). Notably, rates of substance use were lower among those who were actively receiving treatment versus healthy controls. This may be explained by under-reporting or hypervigilant parents, or secondary to decreased peer interaction because of intensive and long-term treatment [18,19]. However, some reports describe prevalence rates of alcohol and illicit drug use as high as 84% amongst cancer survivors, which is not significantly different from age-matched controls [20,21].

The most studied substance of abuse in adolescent cancer patients has been tobacco. Cigarette smoking can compromise antineoplastic therapies, especially chemotherapy and radiation, and can lead to more severe respiratory problems, restrictive lung disease, decreased efficacy of the treatment, and greater risk of developing a secondary tumor or disease recurrence [11]. The adolescent cancer patients most at risk of substance use and abuse are those who were older when diagnosed with cancer, had lower household incomes, and were less educated [11]. Higher rates may also be seen in cancer survivors whose treatment was not pulmonary related and who did not receive brain irradiation [11].

Why do youths who are either actively fighting cancer, or who have recently emerged from treatment, engage in substance use at such significant rates? Perhaps as a part of normal maturation and development, these adolescents strive to "fit in" and feel "normal" among their peer groups. They may perceive that the use of illicit drugs is a normative behavior among their age cohort [22]. In turn, they might try to "make up for lost time" as they emerge from the relative quarantine of active cancer treatment. After months or years of missed school and missed social engagements as a result of very intense treatment for cancer, survivors may pursue activities such as substance use that they perceive as normative activities for "normal" teens. Additionally, unrecognized or untreated emotional distress such as depression or PTSD may play a role in increased rates of substance use. Clinicians must pay particular attention to these health behaviors and provide focused anticipatory guidance for cancer patients and survivors around risks related to substance use and abuse in this population.

DIABETES

Diabetes mellitus (DM) is a chronic metabolic disorder, affecting millions of young people per year, characterized by excessively high glucose concentration in the blood. Glucose is needed by the body to provide energy to the brain, muscles, and other tissues. Insulin is a hormone produced by cells in the pancreas that responds to high levels of glucose by facilitating its uptake into cells. In diabetes mellitus, this uptake doesn't occur, leading to various health problems.

Type I diabetes mellitus, formerly known as insulin-dependent or juvenile-onset diabetes mellitus, occurs when the beta cells of the pancreas are destroyed by unknown mechanisms, and the pancreas is unable to produce insulin. Type II diabetes mellitus, formerly known as adult-onset diabetes, occurs as a result of insulin resistance or inadequate use of insulin by the organs. Both forms of DM, when not properly treated, can lead acutely to polyuria, polydipsia, polyphagia, weight loss, fatigue, blurred vision, ketoacidosis or coma; when not managed well, chronic DM leads to an array of pathologics affecting brain, nerves, eyes, heart, and kidneys.

The diagnosis of DM involves the detection of high circulating glucose in the blood. Once detected, DM can be controlled via dietary modifications, exercise, administration of insulin, and other medications. Proper control of both type I and type II diabetes involves modifications in behaviors and life rhythms that can be very challenging for patients to maintain. Adolescents may be particularly at risk for poor management of DM, as various developmental and psychological factors, including struggles for autonomy and rebellion against authority, the quest for identity and assimilation with peers, and feelings of invulnerability, run directly counter to the daily discipline and self-control required to maintain appropriate health behaviors to manage DM [23,24].

Risky behaviors that commonly emerge among adolescents, including misuse of legal and illegal substances, may further contribute to inadequate diabetes management. Several studies suggest that the most common substances of abuse in this population are cannabis, cocaine, stimulants/ecstasy, and nicotine, though reports of prevalence of substance use in this population are rare. One study [11] records prevalence for nicotine abuse to be 8–26% amongst diabetic adolescents. Possible explanations for the frequency of smoking include difficulties adjusting to the emotional strain of having a chronic illness, poor social support, sensation-seeking and rebellion, poor academic performance, low self-esteem, and anxiety [25]. Adolescent smokers with parents who smoke, and those who see smoking as part of their identity (including those smoking in order to become part of an "attractive" group of peers), are at higher risk of developing problematic nicotine abuse [26].

Substance misuse may contribute to poor diabetes control, risk of hyperglycemic crises, increased risk of infection, and compromised liver and kidney function [5]. More specifically, alcohol increases the risk for ketosis and dysregulation of glucose levels via inhibition of glucose formation, stimulation of fat breakdown, and nocturnal hypoglycemia [25]. Smoking increases the risk of cardiovascular and peripheral vascular disease, retinal disease, and kidney dysfunction. Opioids can lead to hyperglycemia, impaired insulin secretion, diabetic ketoacidosis, and death [27]. Diabetic ketoacidosis, in addition to marked hyponatremia and seizures, may be provoked with use of ecstasy and ketamine [28]. Cocaine can lead to dangerous elevations in glucose [28].

Youths with DM have an additional risk of substance misuse: inappropriate use of insulin in order to regulate weight. Adolescent females may be particularly prone to this phenomenon. Optimal care for type I diabetic patients involves a strict dietary regime and daily doses of exogenous insulin [29,30]. Patients may develop insulin resistance from these daily insulin injections, with subsequent weight gain, which then leads to recommendations for more strict insulin regimes to improve glycemic control. To combat weight gain, some teens learn to underuse or even omit use of their insulin, which prompts deterioration in glycemic control and increased risk of complications [31]. Some investigators suggest a strong relationship between type I diabetes and disturbed eating, insulin misuse, and poor glycemic control that may persist beyond adolescence and into young adulthood [30].

JUVENILE RHEUMATOID ARTHRITIS

Juvenile rheumatoid arthritis (JRA) is a chronic inflammatory disorder that affects approximately 50,000 youth ages 6 months to 16 years in the United States each year. The immune system attacks healthy tissues, causing systemic symptoms involving the joints, heart, liver, and spleen.

Substance use has been found in some adolescent patients who are diagnosed with JRA. A study of 52 teens with JRA reported that the most common substance of abuse was alcohol [32]; 19.2% reported experimentation while 11.2% identified themselves as frequent users. Nicotine was found to be the second most commonly used substance, with 11.6% and 3.8% being experimenters and frequent users, respectively. No marijuana use was reported; however, other illicit drugs (barbiturates, psychedelics, inhalants, and amphetamines) were used overall among 1.9% of frequent users.

As with other conditions discussed previously, substance misuse in JRA may specifically worsen medical outcomes. Cardiovascular disease is a common complication of JRA, and alcohol may accelerate cardiac complications. Additionally, when alcohol use occurs in patients taking methotrexate, a commonly prescribed chemotherapy agent in JRA, the risk of hepatotoxicity is increased [33]. Tobacco use has also been associated with cardiovascular risks, vasculitis, vessel wall damage, systemic immune system dysfunction, and increasing circulating autoimmune markers [11].

Many patients with JRA have more frequent contact with rheumatologists than with primary care physicians, and the use of anticipatory guidance around adolescent-onset risk behaviors such as substance abuse may occur less regularly among pediatric specialists. Similarly, specialists may neglect to interview adolescents alone, limiting opportunities to encourage accurate reporting of substance use from teens [32].

FETAL ALCOHOL SPECTRUM DISORDER/ FETAL ALCOHOL SYNDROME

Several developmental disorders are notable for creating risk for substance misuse. Ones that have been well studied are those related to fetal alcohol exposure and the syndrome or spectrum of disorders that follow. Fetal alcohol syndrome (FAS) occurs in approximately

1–3 per 1000 live births generally, and as high as 1 in 100 births in some higher risk populations [34]. Typical signs of fetal alcohol syndrome include low birthweight, growth deficiency with delayed motor development, mental retardation and learning problems, and other less severe fetal alcohol behavioral effects. Fetal alcohol spectrum disorder is a term that reflects acceptance of the variety of signs that may occur rather than the full FAS [34]. Clinical descriptions of patients with FAS found that 35% developed alcohol or drug problems by the time they reached adulthood [35]. Many with FASD may be missed because they do not fit traditional eligibility criteria for mental health and developmental disability services. FASD is not a diagnosable mental illness in the *Diagnostic and Statistical Manual of Mental Disorders, Fourth Edition* (DSM-IV) but individuals with FASD typically experience cognitive impairment that significantly affects social, educational, and vocational functioning.

CONCLUSION

This chapter presents information on the risks of substance use that arise in the context of five different chronic childhood medical conditions; all are examples of dynamic situations that can be compounded by exposure to these toxic substances and by the behaviors inherent in substance use. Medical conditions are not protective factors against substance use, and substance use can have deleterious effects on the underlying condition. As critical improvements in medical care prolong the lives of young people living with chronic medical conditions, particular attention must be paid to psychosocial risk factors that come to affect these youths' lives. Additional research is needed to better characterize the specific substance use behaviors of adolescents with chronic medical conditions, and specific interventions should be developed that prevent onset of substance use disorders and limit the negative effects of these risky behaviors upon the lives of young people already facing significant challenges to leading healthy and full lives.

References

1. Alderman E, Lauby J, Coupey S. Problem behaviors in inner-city adolescents with chronic illness. *Dev Behav Pediatr* 1995;**16**:341–344.
2. Zbikowski SM, Klesges RC, Robinson LA, Alfano CM. Risk factors from smoking among adolescents with asthma. *J Adolesc Health* 2002;**30**:279–287.
3. Jessor R. Risk behavior in adolescence: a psychosocial framework for understanding and action. *J Adolesc Health* 1991;**12**(8):597–605.

4. Britto MT, Garret JM, Duglis MA, *et al.* Risky behavior in teens with cystic fibrosis or sickle cell disease: a multi-center study. *Pediatrics* 1998;**101**:250–256.

5. Frey MA, Guthrie B, Loveland-Cherry C, Soo Park P, Foster C. Risky behavior and risk in adolescents with IDDM. *J Adolesc Health* 1997;**20**:38–45.

6. Bloom B, Cohen RA, Freeman, G. Summary Health Statistics for U.S. Children: National Health Interview Survery, 2010. National Center for Health Statistics. *Vital Health Stat* 2011;**10**:250. http://www.cdc.gov/nchs/data/series/sr_10/sr10_250.pdf

7. Hublet A, De Bacquer D, Boyce W, *et al.* Smoking in young people with asthma. *J Public Health* 2007;**29**:343–49.

8. Zimlichman E, Mandel D, Mimouni F, Schochat T, Grotto I, Kreiss Y. Smoking habits in adolescents with mild to moderate asthma. *Pediatr Pulmonol* 2004;**38**:193–197.

9. Tercyak KP. Psychosocial risk factors for tobacco use among adolescents with asthma. *J Pediatr Psychol* 2003;**28**:495–504.

10. Forero R, Bauman A, Young L, Booth M, Nutbeam D. Asthma, health behaviors, social adjustment and psychosomatic symptoms in adolescence. *J Asthma* 1996;**33**:157–164.

11. Tyc V, Throckmorton-Belzer L. Smoking Rates and the State of Smoking Interventions for Children and Adolescents with Chronic Illness. *Pediatrics* 2006;**118**:e471–e487.

12. Wang MQ, Fitzhugh E, Green B, Turner L, Eddy J, Westerfield R. Prospective social-psychological factors of adolescent smoking progression. *J Adolesc Health* 1999;**24**:2–9.

13. Davies SC, Oni L. Management of patients with sickle cell disease. *BMJ* 1997;**15**(7109):656–60.

14. Rogers ZR. Priapism in sickle cell disease. *Hematol Oncol Clin North Am* 2005;**19**(5):917–28.

15. Verma A, Clough D, McKenna D, Dodd M, Webb AK. Smoking and cystic fibrosis. *J Roy Soc Med* 2001;**94** (Suppl.):29–34.

16. American Cancer Society. *Cancer Facts & Figures 2010.* Atlanta: American Cancer Society; 2010. Available at: http://www.cancer.org/acs/groups/content/@epidemiolo-gysurveilance/documents/document/acspc-026238.pdf

17. Emmons K, Li F, Whitton J, *et al.* Predictors of smoking initiation and cessation among childhood cancer survivors: a report from the Childhood Cancer Survivor Study. *J Clin Oncol* 2002;**20**:1608–1616.

18. Hollen P, Hobbie W, Donnangelo S, Shannon S, Erickon J. Substance use risk behaviors and decision-making skills among cancer-surviving adolescents. *J Pediatr Oncol Nurs* 2007;**24**:264.

19. Tercyak KP, Britto MT, Hanna KM, *et al.*Prevention of tobacco use among medically at-risk children and adolescents: clinical and reasearch opportunities in the interest of public heatlth. *J Pediatr Psychol.* 2008;**33**:119–132.

20. Verrill J, Schafer J, Vannatta K, Noll R. Aggression, antisocial behavior, and substance abuse in survivors of pediatric cancer: possible protective effects of cancer and its treatment. *J Pediatr Psychol* 2000;**25**:493–502.

21. Carpentier M, Mullins L, Elkin T, Wolfe-Christensen. Prevalence of Multiple Health-Related Behaviors in Adolescents with Cancer. *J Pediatr Hematol Oncol* 2008;**30**:902–907.

22. Suris JC, Parera N. Sex, drugs and chronic illness: health behaviours among chronically ill youth. *Eur J Public Health* 2005;**15**:484–488.

23. Ferguson C. Teenagers with diabetes – management challenges. *Aust Fam Physician* 2006;**6**:386–390.

24. Shaw R, DeMasso D. *Clinical Manual of Pediatric Psychosomatic Medicine: Mental Health Consultation with Physically Ill Children and Adolescents.* American Psychiatric Publishing, Inc.2006.

25. Martìnez-Aguayo A, Araneda JC, Fernandez D, Gleisner A, Perez V, Codner E. Tobacco, alcohol and illicit drug use in adolescents with diabetes mellitus. *Pediatr Diabetes* 2007;**8**:265–271.

26. Regber S, Berg Kelly K. Missed opportunities – adolescents with a chronic condition (insulin dependent diabetes mellitus) describe their cigarette-smoking trajectories and consider health risks. *Acta Pediatr* 2007;**96**:1770–1776.

27. Lee P, Greenfield JR, Campbell LV. Managing young people with Type I diabetes in a 'rave' new world: metabolic complications of substance abuse in Type I diabetes. *Diabetic Med* 2009;**26**:328–333.

28. Ng RS, Darko DA, Hillson RM. Street drug use among young patients with Type I diabetes in the UK. *Diabetes Med* 2003;**21**:295–296.

29. Drash AL, Becker DJ. Behavioral issues in patients with diabetes mellitus, with special emphasis on the child and adolescent. In: *Ellenberg and Rifkin's Diabetes Mellitus: Theory and Practice*, 4th Ed. 1990. New York: Elsevier Science, p 922–934.

30. Peveler R, Bryden K, Neil A, *et al.* The relationship of disordered eating habits and attitudes to clinical outcomes in young adult females with Type I diabetes. *Diabetes Care* 2005;**28**:84–88.

31. Bryden K, Neil A, Mayou R, Peveler R, Fairburn C, Dunger D. Eating habits, body weight, and insulin misuse. *Diabetes Care* 1999;**22**:1956–1960.

32. Nash AA, Britto MT, Lovell DJ, Passo MH, Rosenthal SL. Substance use among adolescents with juvenile rheumatoid arthritis. *Arthritis Care Res.* 1998;**2** (8618):1028.

33. Sawyer SA, Drew S, Yeo M, Britto MA. Adolescents with a chronic condition: challenges living, challenges treating. *Lancet* 2007;**369**:1481–1489.

34. Institute of Medicine. *Fetal Alcohol Syndrome: Research Base for Diagnostic Criteria, Epidemiology, Prevention, and Treatment.* Washington, DC: National Academy Press, 1995.

35. Streissguth AP, Bookstein FL, Barr HM, Sampson PD, O'Malley K, Young JK. Risk factors for adverse life outcomes in fetal alcohol syndrome and fetal alcohol effects. *J Dev Behav Pediatr* 2004;**25**:228–238.

Section Four
Clinical Conditions

Edited by Charles Scott

18

Adolescent Alcohol Use

Karen Miotto, Andia Heydari, Molly Tartter, Ellen Chang, Patrick S. Thomas and
Lara A. Ray

Department of Psychiatry and Biobehavioral Sciences, UCLA, Los Angeles, CA, USA

INTRODUCTION AND EPIDEMIOLOGY

Experimentation with substance use is common during the adolescent years, predominantly with substances that are easily accessible. In 2008, the Monitoring the Future Study found that 39% of 8th-graders, 62% of 10th-graders, and 72% of 12th-graders reported having tried alcohol, with 92% of 12th-graders feeling that "it is or would be fairly easy or very easy to get alcohol" [1]. Most young people report that they obtain alcohol from their family or friends. Some parents permit underage drinking, while the majority of parents are an unwitting source of alcohol. For example, data from the National Survey on Drug Use from 2006 to 2009 indicates that 93.4% of adolescents who drank in the past month obtained their alcohol for free, and 44.8% of these adolescents obtained it from family members or from their own homes [2]. For this reason, family involvement is especially important to consider when looking at this prevalent problem. The sources of alcohol and patterns of early use often have prognostic importance: the younger the onset of alcohol use, the greater the risk of developing addiction. Data from a longitudinal study have shown that adolescents with an age of drinking onset (not counting sips or small tastes) of 12 years or younger were found to have a 40% prevalence of lifetime alcohol dependence. Individuals who initiated alcohol use at 18 years of age were found to have a 16.6% prevalence of lifetime alcohol dependence, whereas those who delayed drinking until 21 years of age have a lifetime prevalence of 10.6% [3].

Adolescent binge drinking constitutes a public health concern. Binge drinking is defined as four or more standard drinks for a female and five or more standard drinks for a male within a 1-hour period [4]. The Monitoring the Future Survey found that 10% of 8th-graders, 22% of 10th-graders, 26% of 12th-graders, and 40% of college students reported binge drinking within 2 weeks prior to the date of the questionnaires [1]. Drinking peaks during college years, with more than 30% of college students meeting a *Diagnostic and Statistical Manual of Mental Disorders-IV* (DSM-IV) diagnosis of alcohol abuse or alcohol dependence [5]. It is commonly assumed that young people will outgrow college drinking patterns. However, Jackson *et al.* found that binge-drinking college students had a correlation with heavy drinking at age 29–30 ($r = 0.29$), alcohol consequences ($r = 0.35$), as well as symptoms of alcohol dependence ($r = 0.38$) [6].

Distinguishing between normal and abnormal adolescent alcohol experimentation requires information from a biopsychosocial assessment. In contrast to adults, where a pattern of use such as "needing an eye opener" in the morning is often predictive of alcoholism, information on a confluence of risk factors is necessary in order to assess the level of severity of alcohol use in youth. These risk factors include individual factors (such as depression and anxiety symptoms, poor self-control, and high sensation seeking), family factors (such as family addiction, permissive parents, or disruptive family relationships), school factors (such as lack of academic success), and peer factors. These different types of factors have been shown to increase the likelihood of crossing over from normative adolescent alcohol use to more serious alcohol-related problems. Fortunately, the majority of adolescents who experiment with alcohol do not develop later life addiction. Alcohol experimentation is consistent with other age-appropriate behaviors, including challenging authority, experimenting with adult behaviors, and risk taking. Early motivations for drinking include social facilitation, peer influence, and novelty seeking.

Adolescence is a critical time during which unique cognitive, physical, genetic, social, and academic

Clinical Handbook of Adolescent Addiction, First Edition. Richard Rosner.

influences integrate. Early onset of alcohol use can disrupt this integration and change a person's life trajectory by contributing to a host of problems [7]. A few examples of the perils of alcohol experimentation include personal injury, accidents involving others, unsafe or unwanted sexual activities, legal charges, and incarceration. Adolescents lack the experience and cognitive ability to accurately estimate the probability of harmful alcohol-related consequences, thereby increasing the risk of accidents or even fatality.

INFLUENCES ON ADOLESCENT ALCOHOL USE

Social Determinants

The constant endorsement of alcohol by the media influences young people's beliefs and behaviors regarding drinking. In the United States, alcohol use is promoted through radio, television, billboards, and the internet [8]. A study by Primack *et al.* found that one out of every three of the most popular songs contains either social, sexual, financial, or emotional endorsements for alcohol [9]. Aggressive marketing of flavored beverages that mask the taste of alcohol targets an increasingly younger population. For example, the American Medical Association released a report on the marketing of "alcopops" – fruit-flavored malt beverages. The article cites a rise in adolescent girls' drinking, with the average age on having the first drink now 13 years. Teenage girls report more exposure to advertisements for these drinks than women over 21, and were found to drink alcopops more often than women over 21, despite the alcohol industry's claim that they market only to legal age drinkers [10,11].

The types of drinks geared toward young consumers are predominantly sweet, fizzy, "ready to drink," or premixed alcoholic beverages such as alcopops. Alcopops are a potential risk for the inexperienced drinker because the sweet flavor hides the taste of alcohol, making it easier to become intoxicated. Furthermore, young people have been shown to perceive alcopops as being less harmful than other types of alcohol [12], suggesting that they may be comfortable with drinking more of them, resulting in greater and/or quicker intoxication.

Popular caffeinated alcoholic drinks are also currently being investigated as a source of danger for the young alcohol consumer. The caffeine can counteract the sedating effects, which would normally protect the consumer against overdrinking. Caffeinated drinks are sold as premixed products, or can be made by mixing energy drinks with various forms of alcohol. The Centers for Disease Control and Prevention report that drinkers who mix alcohol and energy drinks are three times more likely to binge drink than those who do not [13]. In addition, those who consume caffeinated alcoholic drinks are three times more likely to leave an event highly intoxicated (breath alcohol level $\geq 0.08\,g/210\,L$) and are four times more likely to intend to drive upon leaving compared to drinkers who did not consume caffeine with their alcoholic drinks [14]. Sweet and caffeinated alcohol drinks in trendy packaging are designed to attract young people; such consumers often lack the knowledge or experience to anticipate the hazards that can occur at various levels of intoxication.

School-Based Substance Abuse Prevention Programs

School-based substance abuse prevention programs provide young people with information that seeks to counter the marketing devices and glamorization of alcohol in the media. Thirty-nine US states require, and all states recommend, that schools provide students with substance use prevention programs [15]. Designing and evaluating programs that prevent substance use is complex and costly; a review of the different school-based programs can be found on the National Institute of Drug Abuse website [16]. Most of the programs advocate that providing information about the more immediate short-term health risks in conjunction with other prevention approaches is more effective than focusing on long-term risk factors. Examples of other prevention approaches include social resistance skills training, normative education about alcohol use, as well as competence enhancement skills training. Social resistance training seeks to increase teens' awareness about the advertising techniques used to sell alcohol and tobacco products and to resist the allure of media pressures in addition to offers of alcohol or drugs from peers. Teens learn how to identify and avoid situations where there is likely to be pressure to drink, and practice realistic and effective ways of communicating refusal to peers. In normative education, adolescents learn about the prevalence of alcohol and drug use. Many adolescents may drink alcohol as a result of the unfounded belief that most of their peers and all those around them are drinking. Normative education is an important technique to correct misperceptions by emphasizing that there are large numbers of young people who drink modestly or do not drink at all. Competence enhancement involves teaching adolescents social skills, such as decision-making and self-control, and enables them to apply these general skills when confronted with an alcohol- or drug-related situation. Teens with poorly developed social and coping skills often turn to drugs or alcohol as a method of facilitating social interaction [17,18]. An active area of research is computer-delivered school-based prevention programs in keeping with the increased utilization of technology. One study found that a series of computer-delivered secondary prevention programs reduced alcohol use for teens transitioning to college [19]. Clinicians will recognize many of these prevention strategies because they are based on common therapeutic interventions used with young people, aimed at helping them develop social-cultural awareness, social skills, and problem-solving capabilities.

Family Influences

Another part of the continuum of factors that contribute to a young person's desire to drink is the influence of their family. Popular federal and state prevention campaigns often read, "Teens that eat dinner with their family are less likely to drink alcohol." Indeed, greater parental involvement in an adolescent's life acts as a form of preventive intervention for substance use. Parental attitudes about substance use have a significant impact when the adolescent endorses family connectedness and high parental supervision. Family connectedness incorporates the extent to which an adolescent feels that their family bonds and communicates with each other [20].

Increased teen drinking is noted at both ends of the family economic spectrum: low income and low parental education are associated with high levels of teen drinking, whereas high parental education and income are both associated with binge drinking in adolescents [21]. Available spending money and low parental monitoring may enable adolescents from these families to purchase alcohol more frequently and experience unsupervised drinking opportunities. These findings highlight the importance of the public health message to parents, emphasizing parental inquiry about a young person's use of spending money, monitoring alcohol in the household, and keeping track of children's whereabouts, not only by asking the young person, but also by confirming plans and locations with the parents of their child's friends.

Parents can potentially pass on their alcohol use patterns in a number of ways, such as modeling the behavior for their child, or promoting or aggravating behaviors associated with alcohol use, such as conduct problems. Parental modeling has been shown to influence adolescent drinking, with a correlation between increased parental drinking during a child's middle childhood (mean age − 10.4 years) and increased frequency of intoxication during middle adolescence (mean age = 16.5 years) [22]. An adolescent's drinking behavior may be a psychological and environmental response to the alcohol use disorder of the caregiver or parent. Consequently, obtaining a family substance use history is essential when treating an adolescent; however, it may be difficult to obtain accurate information from the parent due to shame, guilt, or lack of appreciation of the problem itself. If the drinking caregiver denies the substance use revealed by the teen, this creates an opportunity for the skilled therapist to try to address the "family secret." The assessment requires the use of non-judgmental questions, such as inquiring about drinking *patterns* as opposed to drinking *problems* in the family. Anchoring questions about substance use to a particular point in time in the family's life such as, "Did you drink when you were in the military or after the divorce?" may also be helpful. Motivating an addicted parent to look at the role that their own substance use plays in their child's problem may prove to be a life-altering intervention for an adolescent who is acting out their distress as exemplified by the following vignette.

> Robin said that the school counselor referred her to a psychiatrist. She told the psychiatrist about the chaos in her family and her father's drinking. Robin said that she was not drinking nearly as much as her friends. The psychiatrist wanted to have a family meeting but her father refused; however, he did go in to see the psychiatrist alone. Robin said that she never saw the psychiatrist again and her schoolwork improved. She wanted to thank the psychiatrist because soon after the meeting, her father went into treatment for his alcoholism and she was finally able to have a relationship with her Dad.

The social and psychological dysfunction that results from growing up in a home with an addict parent may promote substance use. Parental addiction also often leads to decreased monitoring of the child, high levels of family conflict, low bonding, and abuse [23]. According to the Substance Abuse and Mental Health Services Administration (SAMHSA), an estimated 8.3 million children in the United States currently live with a parent who meets criteria for a substance use disorder. A large proportion of children with addicted and alcoholic parents are resilient. These children often obtain positive attention from other people and develop adequate communication skills, caring attitudes, desires to achieve, and beliefs in self-help. A common factor found in resilient youths is intelligence greater than or equal to the average [24].

Children significantly impacted by maternal alcoholism may be suffering from fetal alcohol spectrum disorders. Fetal alcohol exposure is a leading known cause of intellectual disability in the United States and Europe [25,26]. Moderate and heavy alcohol use during pregnancy is associated with a spectrum of disorders that involve physical, mental, behavioral, and learning disabilities. Fetal alcohol syndrome (FAS) is characterized by particular physical and mental/neurological defects, including abnormal facial features, reduced or slowed physical growth, a small head, and slowed intellectual or behavioral development. Approximately 1.9 in every 1000 babies worldwide are born with FAS [25]. The incidence of fetal alcohol spectrum disorders (FASD) – describing individuals who do not have all the characteristics of FAS but have still had prenatal alcohol exposure – is estimated to be at least three times that amount [27]. Children with FASD carry a substantial risk of developing early addiction due to genetic vulnerability, cognitive and behavioral problems, and environmental stresses associated with having a potentially addicted mother. A longitudinal study by Baer *et al.* [28] found an association between *in utero* alcohol exposure and higher levels of alcohol use and problems of the offspring at 14 years of age, even after controlling for family history and environmental factors. A similar study by Alati *et al.* [29] of 4363 adolescents also found a link between maternal alcohol use and increased adolescent drinking. Mothers who drank three or more drinks on each drinking occasion during pregnancy were found to have offspring who were at an increased risk of binge drinking during their adolescent years. A follow-up study assessed this cohort at 21 years of age and found a strong relationship between maternal binge drinking in early pregnancy and offspring alcohol use disorders later in life [29].

Information about resources to screen for FASD are readily available at the Fetal Alcohol Disorders Society website [30]. A positive fetal alcohol exposure screen gives the clinician more information about the adolescent's presentation and consequently allows for more tailored treatment. To obtain information about a mother's drinking history, clinicians should show sensitivity. It is recommended to initially inform the mother that half of all women are unaware that they are pregnant until 3 months into their pregnancy, then proceed to ask if she was drinking during this phase when she was unaware of the pregnancy [31]. More indirect, non-judgmental questions such as these will aid in obtaining an accurate family history, thus potentially revealing more about the unique adolescent's path to substance use.

Genetic Risk Factors

Aside from the psychological and environmental risks for developing alcohol use disorders, genetic factors account for approximately 50–60% of the risk, with recent heritability estimates based on twin and adoption studies [32]. Family, twin, and adoption studies have

highlighted that environmental factors, such as substance availability, are often required before any genetic and biological vulnerability can be phenotypically expressed. Specifically, a large twin study of alcoholism [33] found that the concordance rate for male monozygotic (MZ) twin pairs was 77%, as compared to 54% for male dizygotic (DZ) twins. This study estimated the heritability of early-onset alcoholism (before 20 years of age) in males at $72.5 \pm 17.5\%$, with the remaining variation due to environmental factors. Results of twin studies of alcoholism among females generally provide weaker support for the role of genetic factors underlying the risk for alcoholism in women [32]. In addition, twin studies have shown that a number of alcohol-related traits, or phenotypes, such as alcohol sensitivity [34,35], alcohol metabolism [36], and alcohol use [37] are also heritable. Analysis of these phenotypes indicates that children of alcoholic parents have decreased reactions to the negative effects of alcohol, especially during initial usage, which can increase the risk for developing alcohol use disorders [38].

In addition to twin studies, adoption studies have provided support for the role of genetic factors as determinants of alcoholism risk. Specifically, studies have shown that the rate of alcoholism in adopted (i.e., reared away) male children of alcohol-dependent parents ranged between 18% and 63%, in contrast to generally lower rates for adopted children of non-alcohol-dependent parents, ranging between 5% and 24% [39]. These studies generally concluded that adopted sons of alcohol-dependent parents were 1.7 to 6.5 times more likely to develop alcoholism, as compared to adopted sons of controls. Studies of adopted daughters of alcohol-dependent parents indicated odds ratios with a large range between 0.5 and 8.9 [39]. In summary, twin and adoption studies have indicated that approximately 50% of the variance in risk for developing substance abuse and dependence can be explained by genetic factors [40].

Notably, research has found that the effect of genetic factors on adolescent behavior varies significantly across development. For example, an interesting body of research on Finnish twins found that genetics accounted for only 18% of the variance in drinking initiation at age 14. However, at age 16, genetic factors accounted for one-third of the variability in drinking patterns, and by age 18, genetic factors accounted for half of the variability in drinking behavior [41]. In other words, the genetic risk for alcoholism is expressed more fully as individuals reach adulthood. Delaying early alcohol use has been discussed as an important preventive strategy in this chapter; however, it is imperative not to overlook heavy drinking in the later teenage years as "just part of the college experience," and instead to consider the possibility it may be a manifestation of a lifelong disorder, particularly in genetically susceptible individuals. Such a teen may strongly deny an alcohol problem, but when the teenager is asked "What would it mean to have an alcohol problem?" the clinician might learn any of the following beliefs from the adolescent:

"I cannot have an alcohol problem; I am nothing like my alcoholic father."
"I can control my drinking."
"My friends drink more than I do."

SCREENING

Pediatricians comprise the frontlines of screening for adolescent substance use. The American Academy of Pediatrics advises pediatricians to take an active role in screening for alcohol and drugs during general visits and to ensure that they have the training necessary to identify at-risk adolescents and refer them to qualified healthcare professionals for further assessment and treatment [42]. However, access to this screening treatment needs to be expanded. For instance, a study of rural communities in several different countries found that although 92% of primary care providers felt that screening for adolescent alcohol use should start at age 14, only 32% actually screened all patients [43]. Barriers to this screening included lack of screening tools and adolescents' worry that their physicians would not maintain confidentiality. To overcome these barriers, the National Institute on Drug Abuse (NIDA) has provided interactive electronic training tools and educational resources to foster communication between adolescents and clinicians on its NIDAMED website [44].

Screening instruments are more accurate in identifying adolescents' risk level than a clinician's impression alone, making them an important tool in alcohol use prevention. Because adolescents are unlikely to answer substance use questions truthfully or aloud in the presence of a parent or to an adult, paper or computer screening instruments allow for a greater level of privacy and more accurate answers. In addition, they also open an avenue for increased communication with the healthcare provider. When using a screening instrument, it is important to ask the parents to leave the room and to explain confidentiality policies with the adolescent. An explanation of the confidentiality policy is essential in creating a trusting and productive physician-patient relationship. Adolescents must be assured that their answers will be kept confidential and made aware of the possibilities for breaching that confidentiality, such as information that may be a safety risk for themselves or others. Good clinical judgment must be employed for the safety of the youth. Lack of confidentiality can inhibit minors from disclosing sensitive information and create barriers that prove counteractive to attempts aimed at serving young patients and their parents. Furthermore, it is important to inform the adolescent that if there are concerns, the clinician may utilize other venues of information gathering, such as interviewing a parent or guardian, to gain a greater understanding of their situation.

Screening Tools

Some specific screening tools that have been developed for healthcare providers working with adolescent populations can be reviewed in more detail in Table 18.1 . Initial assessments include written screens, such as the Alcohol Use Disorders Identification Test (AUDIT), as well as oral screens (such as the CRAFFT). The CRAFFT is the most commonly used oral screening tool for substance abuse in adolescents. Prior to administration of the CRAFFT, the following three preliminary questions should be asked with regard to the adolescent's behavior over the past 12 months:

1. Did you drink any alcohol (more than a few sips)?
2. Did you smoke any marijuana or hashish?
3. Did you use anything else to get high? [45]

If the answer to any of these three questions is "yes," the six CRAFFT questions summarized in Table 18.2 should be asked before determining whether further screening is necessary.

Even if the adolescent answered "No" to all three of the preliminary screening questions, the clinician must keep in mind that reinforcement for this positive behavior may be just as important as intervening if an alcohol use problem becomes apparent. Offering praise and encouragement for remaining abstinent will help enforce continuation of the adolescent's positive behavior. This positive reinforcement may prove to be a preventive measure in itself.

Both written and oral assessments have their respective advantages and disadvantages related to time, privacy, etc., and can be used as preliminary screens before more individualized plans for care can be followed. Other screens, such as the Adolescent Drinking Inventory (ADI) and the Rutgers Alcohol Problem Index (RAPI), have shown very high internal consistency (0.93–0.95 and 0.92, respectively), specifically for adolescent alcohol use. For instance, in a 7-year longitudinal study, high RAPI scores in 18-year-old adolescents were found to be highly correlated with alcohol use disorder diagnoses at 25 years of age [46]. Apart from these types of screening tools, a physical

Table 18.1 Screening instruments for adolescent alcohol use.

Screening tool	Target	Length	Administration method	Focus of screening tool	Further information
AUDIT	All age groups	10 items; 5 minutes	Written assessment	Screen for substance abuse, as well as mental health and behavioral disorders	Santis et al. [62]
CRAFFT	Adolescents	6 items; 5 minutes	Interview format	Alcohol and drug use and problem severity for adolescents referred for behavioral or emotional disorders	Knight et al. [63]
Adolescent Drinking Inventory (ADI)	Adolescents	24 items; 5 minutes	Interview format	Investigates adolescent drinking by examining psychological, physical, and social symptoms	Harrell and Wirtz [64]
Rutgers Alcohol Problem Index (RAPI)	Adolescents	23 items; 10 minutes	Interview format	Measures consequences of alcohol use related to social and familial problems, psychological and physical problems, and delinquency	White and Labouvie [65]

exam or laboratory screen administration to check for use of drugs other than alcohol may also prove beneficial, as the results have the potential to drastically change treatment paths. Full details are available in *Treatment Improvement Protocol, Screening and Assessing Adolescents for Substance Use Disorders* [47].

CLINICAL PRESENTATION

In some unfortunate cases (e.g., if an adolescent arrives in an emergency room with alcohol poisoning), preventive screening is not an option. In these cases, ideally the individual is referred for a psychological evaluation after the acute crisis has resolved. Acute intoxication, when moderate, may alter mental status and coordination. However, severe alcohol intoxication may result in

seizure, hypothermia, coma, and death. Adolescents are particularly vulnerable to the effects of severe alcohol intoxication. The blood alcohol content (BAC) of adolescents who succumb to coma tends to be lower than the BAC of adults in coma due to alcohol poisoning. The BAC associated with certain clinical presentations can be found in Table 18.3 .

Adolescents are also more likely to binge drink, which is highly associated with alcohol poisoning. Furthermore, as previously mentioned, adolescents are more likely to drink caffeinated alcoholic beverages, which counteract the sedative effects of alcohol. These caffeinated alcoholic beverages pose a problem for peers and clinicians, since alcohol poisoning, which is normally characterized by vomiting, sedation, and lethargy, is not as readily recognizable because the patient is restless or agitated due to the caffeine.

Table 18.2 CRAFFT screening questions [45].

C Have you ever ridden in a CAR driven by someone (including yourself) who was "high" or had been using alcohol or drugs?

R Do you ever use alcohol or drugs to RELAX, feel better about yourself, or fit in?

A Do you ever use alcohol or drugs while you are by yourself, or ALONE?

F Do you ever FORGET things you did while using alcohol or drugs?

F Do your family or FRIENDS ever tell you that you should cut down on your drinking or drug use?

T Have you ever gotten into TROUBLE while you were using alcohol or drugs?

Because alcohol poisoning is an easily preventable risk for adolescents, parents should be encouraged to speak to their children about the dangers of alcohol poisoning. They should emphasize the importance of contacting the emergency response service or going to an emergency room in cases where their peers are not easily arousable, or may be vomiting profusely. Oftentimes in a social situation, adolescents will choose to call a sibling rather than risk calling a parent in the case of apparent alcohol poisoning. The sibling may have little further insight into the situation, and may not realize that the poisoned individual's BAC may still be rising due to recently ingested alcohol that has not been absorbed. Many adolescents fear the harsh consequences of receiving an underage drinking citation if presenting in an emergency room while intoxicated, but the reality is that hospitals cannot disclose underage drinking to authorities due to privacy laws [48]. Unfortunately, the fear of police citation persists if an ambulance is called, since in some instances the police arrive with an ambulance [49]. For this reason, it is valuable for the caregiver to have an agreement with a young person beforehand to contact a parent, adult, or the emergency response service for assessment of a situation where a peer is vomiting or is difficult to arouse. This message is being increasingly reinforced by prevention programs, mental healthcare providers, and pediatricians.

Table 18.3 Blood Alcohol Content (BAC) chart [66].

BAC level (% by vol.)	Effects of dosage
0.02–0.03	No loss of coordination and slight euphoric effect; depressant effects are perceptible. Reduces nervousness or introversion and increases sociability
0.04–0.06	Lowers inhibitions and produces feelings of well-being; euphoria. Slight memory and reasoning impairment while actions are more exaggerated or intensified
0.07–0.09	Impaired fine muscle coordination, balance, speech, reaction time, attention span, and hearing. Flushed appearance and overall improvement in mood; euphoria
0.10–0.125	Inhibited judgment as well as significant impairment of motor coordination. Speech may be slurred; ataxia
0.13–0.15	Sedative and lethargic effects. Blurred vision and motor coordination condition worsens. Sense of euphoria is decreased, dysphoria begins to appear
0.16–0.19	Dysphoria predominates, impaired memory and comprehension. Possible nauseous effects
0.20–0.24	Profound confusion and disorientation; analgesia. Possible vomiting (emesis) or death due to inhalation of vomit. Blackouts are likely to occur
0.25–0.29	Physical, mental, and sensory functions are severely impaired. Increased risk of asphyxiation from choking on vomit and of serious injuries due to impairment
0.30–0.34	Blackout and passing out; anterograde amnesia. Lapses in and out of consciousness or unconsciousness
0.35–0.39	Possible coma; level of surgical anesthesia. Depressed reflexes, decreased heart rate, urinary incontinence, and vomiting
0.40+	Onset of coma; marked and life-threatening respiratory depression. Level at which most deaths due to alcohol poisoning occur

BRIEF INTERVENTION

The recent federal and healthcare initiative to provide addiction screening and brief intervention by primary care doctors has been adopted by many pediatricians. The brief intervention performed by pediatricians after obtaining a positive screening is aimed at reducing alcohol-related harm through identification of the problem as well as tailored advice and support concerning the risk of hazardous alcohol use. Brief interventions focus on providing feedback and negotiating behavioral change. One such technique that can be employed is to ask the adolescent to promise not to ride with a drunk driver, asking them to "make arrangements ahead of time for safe transportation." The clinician can also involve parents by asking them to promise to provide a safe ride with no questions asked, as adolescents may fear punishment for their whereabouts if they ask for a safe ride from their parents. In addition to the pediatricians' office, screening and brief intervention can be performed when an adolescent presents to the emergency department. A recent randomized controlled study of brief intervention for adolescents with alcohol use problems and aggression delivered in emergency departments found that it reduced aggression and negative alcohol consequences [50]. Meta-analyses have also concluded that brief interventions are superior to no-treatment controls, but should not replace specialist-delivered extended treatment approaches [51].

Adolescents at high risk may be referred by pediatricians to a child psychiatrist or other mental health provider to participate in a targeted intervention, involving several meetings or more intense treatment depending on the severity of substance use. Targeted interventions typically involve individual motivational enhancement or group-oriented motivation with cognitive-behavioral therapy to encourage behavioral change. The mental health provider may choose to repeat the same screening measures administered by the primary care physician and/or adjust the instructions of the measures to address more limited time frames (i.e., rather than assessing alcohol use in the last 12 months, assess use in the past 4 weeks). Repeating these measures on multiple visits can assess changes in substance use. Beyond the initial screening, an evaluation involves a relatively comprehensive assessment of the young person's condition and specific problems or needs, including medical, psychiatric, and psychosocial status as well as collateral information from teachers and caregivers.

DIAGNOSTIC CRITERIA

Beyond screening for problematic alcohol use, the challenge of diagnosing alcohol addiction involves getting the drinker to acknowledge the existence of a problem. It is not uncommon for a young person not to meet diagnostic criteria based on a self-report; however, collateral information obtained from teachers and caregivers can reveal the extent of alcohol use problems. Adolescents lack a mature capacity for judgment, reasoning, and problem-solving. Therefore, adolescents are less likely to recognize the potential hazards and consequences of their actions under the influence of alcohol.

Alcohol abuse and dependence are diagnosed using criteria from the DSM-IV-TR, which were developed based on adult data, and are consistent for all substance use disorders. DSM-IV-TR criteria define alcohol abuse as a maladaptive pattern of substance abuse that can lead to clinical impairment if certain conditions are manifested within a 12-month period. These conditions are: recurrent substance use that results in failure to fulfill major obligations; recurrent substance use in situations that are physically hazardous; encountering recurrent legal problems in regard to the substance; or continued substance use even with the emergence of social or interpersonal problems that develop as a result of substance use. If one of the above conditions is met, the DSM-IV-TR classifies this as substance abuse. DSM-IV-TR criteria further define substance dependence as a maladaptive pattern of substance abuse that can lead to clinical impairment. When any three of seven conditions are satisfied, the substance use would be categorized as substance dependence. The conditions used to define dependence include: tolerance; withdrawal; difficulty in controlling use of the substance; a persistent desire or unsuccessful attempts to control or cut down on substance use; spending a great amount of time and effort to obtain, use, conceal, or plan use of the substance; sacrificing important social, occupational, or recreational activities for use of the substance; and recurrent negative physical or psychological consequences that develop and persist due to use of the substance. Because the distinction between alcohol and other substances has recently been emphasized, the DSM-V, projected to be published in 2012 or 2013, has sought to create criteria that are unique to each substance, and to diagnose disorders based on a range of severity, indicated by the number of symptoms endorsed [52].

Other limitations in applying these criteria to the adolescent population also exist. For example, some of the symptoms, such as withdrawal and alcohol-related medical problems, may only occur after years of heavy alcohol use [53], which adolescents do not have. Hazardous use, such as driving under the influence of alcohol, is only applicable to adolescents who have access to automobiles [54]. Furthermore, alcohol abuse is defined as less severe than alcohol dependence, yet oftentimes in adolescents, dependence criteria, such as tolerance, are met before abuse criteria [55,56].

COMORBID DISORDERS

Adolescent alcohol problems do not typically develop in isolation, as mental health providers tend to see many young people with multiple challenges and psychiatric symptoms. Substance use problems are most often accompanied by other problematic behaviors such as drug use, early sexual activity, academic problems, and antisocial behaviors. These behaviors may cluster because of a genetic and environmental predisposition to deviant behavior, and may be affected by early life experiences such as physical or sexual abuse [57]. Thus, adolescents may begin on a path toward problem use due to individual and environmental factors. This path may then be maintained by continued use of alcohol and further exposure to poor environments with reinforcement of maladaptive personality traits [57].

Depression, anxiety, attention deficit, and conduct disorders are common dual diagnoses observed in adolescents with alcohol use disorders, and affect both the course and treatment of alcohol use disorders. The diagnosis of a comorbid mental illness poses several challenges to treatment. A second diagnosis may be the result of alcohol use, or it may have preceded and increased the risk of alcohol use. Differential diagnosis may affect treatment decisions. The earlier the age of alcohol use onset, the more difficult it is to decipher if alcohol use preceded the psychological symptoms or vice versa. In addition, *prior* diagnosis of a mental illness may speed the transition from alcohol use to an alcohol use disorder. For example, social phobia and externalizing disorders have been associated with an expedited transition to problem drinking, even when controlling for other mental illness [58].

Early substance use among children may be a sign of the development of behaviors associated with conduct disorder [59]. The risk factors for the development of overlapping conduct disorder and addiction include traumatic life experiences, lack of academic success, and genetic vulnerability as well as the teratogenic effects of fetal alcohol exposure. In fact, it has been postulated that conduct disorder represents an early adolescent manifestation of the same genetic loading that influences adult alcohol dependence later in life [60]. This genetic loading may include a spectrum of behaviors such as impulsivity and risk taking [61]. Adolescents with impulsive behaviors are generally those who receive attention from their surrounding adults and are referred to healthcare professionals for assessment. This association emphasizes the importance of helping adolescents when the initial signs of conduct problems are manifest, before their identity becomes entrenched as the "bad kid," where no intervention helps.

SUMMARY

In conclusion, though alcohol experimentation in adolescents is common, it is important to make an effort to prevent and to monitor at-risk drinking behavior. School-based prevention programs should provide education about the glamorization of alcohol by the media and facilitate the development of social-cultural awareness, social skills, and problem-solving capabilities. Although school-based programs are helpful in preventing adolescent alcohol use, there are many influences, including social determinants, family, and individual factors, that contribute to an adolescents' use of substances outside of school. A parent's substance-abusing behavior can also place children at biological, psychological, and environmental risk for alcohol use. To prevent their children from adopting drinking habits, parents must establish their own intervention, which includes monitoring both access to alcohol and unsupervised social gatherings. Parents should also utilize their pediatricians to take active roles in screening for signs and symptoms of problem alcohol use in a fashion tailored to adolescents. These pediatricians should advise parents on how best to communicate with their children about safe drinking behavior. Mental health care providers should also be able to evaluate and treat children with a constellation of social and psychiatric risk factors for alcoholism. The screening tools reviewed in this chapter are useful instruments to assess patterns of use in the context of a relationship where confidentiality is discussed.

References

1. Johnston LD, O'Malley PM, Bachman JG, Schulenberg JE. Monitoring the Future national survey results on drug use, 1975–2009. Volume I: Secondary school students. Bethesda, MD: National Institute on Drug Abuse, 2010.
2. National Survey on Drug Use and Health Data Spotlight. Center for Behavioral Health Statistics and Quality, 2011. Available from: http://oas.samhsa.gov/spotlight/Spotlight 022YouthAlcohol.pdf.
3. Grant BF, Dawson DA. Age at onset of alcohol use and its association with DSM-IV alcohol abuse and dependence: results from the National Longitudinal Alcohol Epidemiologic Survey. *J Subst Abuse* 1997;9:103–110.
4. Wechsler H, Davenport A, Dowdall G, Moeykens B, Castillo S. Health and behavioral consequences of binge drinking in college. A national survey of students at 140 campuses. *JAMA* 1994;**272**:1672–1677.

5. Knight JR, Wechsler H, Kuo M, Seibring M, Weitzman ER, Schuckit MA. Alcohol abuse and dependence among U. S. college students. *J Stud Alcohol* 2002; **63**:263–270.

6. Jackson KM, Colby SM, Sher KJ. Daily patterns of conjoint smoking and drinking in college student smokers. *Psychol Addict Behav* 2010;**24**:424–435.

7. Griffin KW, Botvin GJ. Preventing substance abuse among children and adolescents. In: Ries RK, Fiellin DA, Miller SC, Saitz R (eds), *Principles of Addiction Medicine*, 4th edn. Philadelphia: Lippincott Williams & Wilkins, 2009; pp. 1375–1381.

8. Tye JB, Warner KE, Glantz SA. Tobacco advertising and consumption: evidence of a causal relationship. *J Public Health Policy* 1987;**8**:492–508.

9. Primack BA, Dalton MA, Carroll MV, Agarwal AA, Fine MJ. Content analysis of tobacco, alcohol, and other drugs in popular music. *Arch Pediatr Adolesc Med* 2008;**162**: 169–175.

10. TRU. Survey by Teenage Research Unlimited of teenagers aged 12–18 between October 13–18, 2004. 2004; Available from: http://www.teenresearch.com/.

11. Girlie Drinks . . . Women's Diseases. Interactive H. Survey by Harris Interactive of adults between November 4-8, 2004. Available from: http://www.alcoholpolicymd.com/pdf/girlie_drinks_survey%20.pdf.

12. Hasking P, Shortell C, Machalek M. University students' knowledge of alcoholic drinks and their perception of alcohol-related harm. *J Drug Educ* 2005;**35**:95–109.

13. Centers for Disease Control and Prevention, Division of Adult and Community Health. Fact sheets – caffeinated alcoholic beverages. CDC, 2010. Available from: http://www.cdc.gov/alcohol/fact-sheets/cab.htm.

14. Thombs DL, O'Mara RJ, Tsukamoto M, *et al.* Event-level analyses of energy drink consumption and alcohol intoxication in bar patrons. *Addict Behav* 2010;**35**:325–330.

15. National Association of State Boards of Education. Healthy schools. NASBE, 2010. Available from: http://nasbe.org/healthy_schools/hs/bytopics.php?topicid=1160&catExpand=acdnbtm_catA.

16. Kumpfer KL. Identification of Drug Abuse Prevention Programs. Available from: http://www.drugabuse.gov/sites/default/files/preventingdruguse.pdf.

17. Botvin GJ. Preventing drug abuse in schools: social and competence enhancement approaches targeting individual-level etiologic factors. *Addict Behav* 2000;**25**:887–897.

18. Day NL, Goldschmidt L, Thomas CA. Prenatal marijuana exposure contributes to the prediction of marijuana use at age 14. *Addiction* 2006;**101**:1313–1322.

19. Carey KB, Scott-Sheldon LA, Elliott JC, Bolles JR, Carey MP. Computer-delivered interventions to reduce college student drinking: a meta-analysis. *Addiction* 2009;**104**: 1807–1819.

20. Sale E, Sambrano S, Springer JF, Turner CW. Risk, protection, and substance use in adolescents: a multi-site model. *J Drug Educ* 2003;**33**:91–105.

21. Humensky JL. Are adolescents with high socioeconomic status more likely to engage in alcohol and illicit drug use in early adulthood? *Subst Abuse Treat Prev Policy* 2010; **5**:19.

22. Cranford JA, Zucker RA, Jester JM, Puttler LI, Fitzgerald HE. Parental alcohol involvement and adolescent alcohol expectancies predict alcohol involvement in male adolescents. *Psychol Addict Behav* 2010;**24**:386–396.

23. Mason WA, Hawkins JD. Adolescent risk and protective factors: psychosocial. In: Ries RK, Fiellin DA, Miller SC,

Saitz R (eds), *Principles of Addiction Medicine*, 4th edn. Philadelphia: Lippincott Williams & Wilkins, 2009; pp. 1383–1390.

24. Werner EE. Resilient offspring of alcoholics: a longitudinal study from birth to age 18. *J Stud Alcohol* 1986;**47**: 34–40.

25. Abel EL, Sokol RJ. Incidence of fetal alcohol syndrome and economic impact of FAS-related anomalies. *Drug Alcohol Depend* 1987;**19**:51–70.

26. Abel EL, Sokol RJ. Fetal alcohol syndrome is now leading cause of mental retardation. *Lancet* 1986;**ii**:1222.

27. Sampson PD, Streissguth AP, Bookstein FL, *et al.* Incidence of fetal alcohol syndrome and prevalence of alcohol-related neurodevelopmental disorder. *Teratology* 1997;**56**: 317–326.

28. Baer JS, Barr HM, Bookstein FL, Sampson PD, Streissguth AP. Prenatal alcohol exposure and family history of alcoholism in the etiology of adolescent alcohol problems. *J Stud Alcohol* 1998;**59**:533–543.

29. Alati R, VanDooren K, Najman JM, Williams GM, Clavarino A. Early weaning and alcohol disorders in offspring: biological effect, mediating factors or residual confounding? *Addiction* 2009;**104**:1324–1332.

30. FASlink. Fetal Alcohol Disorders Society home page. Available from: http://www.faslink.org.

31. Floyd RL, Decoufle P, Hungerford DW. Alcohol use prior to pregnancy recognition. *Am J Prev Med* 1999;**17**: 101–107.

32. Heath AC, Bucholz KK, Madden PA, *et al.* Genetic and environmental contributions to alcohol dependence risk in a national twin sample: consistency of findings in women and men. *Psychol Med* 1997;**27**:1381–1396.

33. McGue M, Pickens RW, Svikis DS. Sex and age effects on the inheritance of alcohol problems: a twin study. *J Abnorm Psychol* 1992;**101**:3–17.

34. Heath AC, Martin NG. The inheritance of alcohol sensitivity and of patterns of alcohol use. *Alcohol Alcohol Suppl* 1991;**1**:141–5.

35. Viken RJ, Rose RJ, Morzorati SL, Christian JC, Li TK. Subjective intoxication in response to alcohol challenge: heritability and covariation with personality, breath alcohol level, and drinking history. *Alcohol Clin Exp Res* 2003; **27**:795–803.

36. Martin NG, Perl J, Oakeshott JG, Gibson JB, Starmer GA, Wilks AV. A twin study of ethanol metabolism. *Behav Genet* 1985;**15**:93–109.

37. Koopmans JR, Boomsma DI. Familial resemblances in alcohol use: genetic or cultural transmission? *J Stud Alcohol* 1996;**57**:19–28.

38. Schuckit MA, Smith TL. An 8-year follow-up of 450 sons of alcoholic and control subjects. *Arch Gen Psychiatry* 1996;**53**:202–210.

39. McGue M. Phenotyping alcoholism. *Alcohol Clin Exp Res* 1999;**23**:757–758.

40. Kendler KS, Neale MC, Heath AC, Kessler RC, Eaves LJ. A twin-family study of alcoholism in women. *Am J Psychiatry* 1994;**151**:707–715.

41. Rose RJ, Dick DM, Viken RJ, Kaprio J. Gene–environment interaction in patterns of adolescent drinking: regional residency moderates longitudinal influences on alcohol use. *Alcohol Clin Exp Res* 2001;**25**:637–643.

42. Jacobs EA, Joffe A, Knight JR, Kulig J, Rogers D, Abuse CS. Alcohol use and abuse: A pediatric concern. *Pediatrics* 2001;**108**:185–189.

43. Gordon AJ, Ettaro L, Rodriguez KL, Mocik J, Clark DB. Provider, patient, and family perspectives of adolescent

alcohol use and treatment in rural settings. *J Rural Health* 2011;**27**:81–90.

44. National Institute on Drug Abuse. Resources for medical and health professionals. Available from: http://www.nida.nih.gov/nidamed/.

45. Massachusetts Department of Public Health Bureau of Substance Abuse Services. (2009) Provider Guide: Adolescent Screening, Brief Intervention, and Referral to Treatment Using the CRAFFT Screening Tool. Boston, MA: Massachusetts Department of Public Health, 2009. Available from: http://www.mcpap.com/pdf/CRAFFT%20Screening%20Tool.pdf.

46. Dick DM, Aliev F, Viken R, Kaprio J, Rose RJ. Rutgers Alcohol Problem Index scores at age 18 predict alcohol dependence diagnoses 7years later. *Alcohol Clin Exp Res* 2011;**35**:1011–1014.

47. Winters KC. *Screening and Assessing Adolescents for Substance Use Disorders: A Treatment Improvement Protocol*. Rockville: Center for Substance Abuse Treatment, 1999.

48. Prevention and Wellness Services – Alcohol and Drug Consultation, Assessment and Skills, Program. Alcohol 101: What to do in an Alcohol Emergency. ADCAS, 2006. Available from: http://www.wwu.edu/chw/preventionandwellness/AODWebPDFs/AlcoholEmergencies.pdf.

49. Nusser H. Hospital visit for underage drinking can lead to citation. *BG Views News*, 2010.

50. Walton MA, Chermack ST, Shope JT, *et al*. Effects of a brief intervention for reducing violence and alcohol misuse among adolescents: a randomized controlled trial. *JAMA* 2010;**304**:527–535.

51. Moyer A, Finney JW, Swearingen CE, Vergun P. Brief interventions for alcohol problems: a meta-analytic review of controlled investigations in treatment-seeking and non-treatment-seeking populations. *Addiction* 2002;**97**:279–292.

52. American Psychiatric Association. DSM-5 Development. Available from: http://www.dsm5.org/.

53. Martin CS, Winters KC. Diagnosis and assessment of alcohol use disorders among adolescents. *Alcohol Health Res World* 1998;**22**:95–105.

54. Lagenbucher JW. Alcohol abuse: adding content to category. *Alcohol Clin Exp Res* 1996;**20** (8 Suppl.):270A–5A.

55. Martin CS, Langenbucher JW, Kaczynski NA, Chung T. Staging in the onset of DSM-IV alcohol symptoms in adolescents: survival/hazard analyses. *J Stud Alcohol* 1996;**57**:549–558.

56. Brown SA, D'Amico EJ. Outcomes of alcohol treatment for adolescents. *Recent Dev Alcohol* 2001;**15**:307–327.

57. Brown TG, Dongier M, Ouimet MC, *et al*. Brief motivational interviewing for DWI recidivists who abuse alcohol and are not participating in DWI intervention: a randomized controlled trial. *Alcohol Clin Exp Res* 2010;**34**:292–301.

58. Behrendt S, Beesdo-Baum K, Zimmermann P, *et al*. The role of mental disorders in the risk and speed of transition to alcohol use disorders among community youth. *Psychol Med* 2011;**41**:1073–1085.

59. Glaser B, Shelton KH, van den Bree MB. The moderating role of close friends in the relationship between conduct problems and adolescent substance use. *J Adolesc Health* 2010;**47**:35–42.

60. Dick DM, Bierut L, Hinrichs A, *et al*. The role of GABRA2 in risk for conduct disorder and alcohol and drug dependence across developmental stages. *Behav Genet* 2006;**36**:577–590.

61. deWit H. Impulsivity as a determinant and consequence of drug use: a review of underlying processes. *Addict Biol* 2009;**14**:22–31.

62. Santis R, Garmendia ML, Acuna G, Alvarado ME, Arteaga O. The Alcohol Use Disorders Identification Test (AUDIT) as a screening instrument for adolescents. *Drug Alcohol Depend* 2009;**103**:155–158.

63. Knight JR, Sherritt L, Harris SK, Gates EC, Chang G. Validity of brief alcohol screening tests among adolescents: a comparison of the AUDIT, POSIT, CAGE, and CRAFFT. *Alcohol Clin Exp Res* 2003;**27**:67–73.

64. Harrell A, Wirtz PW. *Adolescent Drinking Index: Professional Manual*. Odessa: Psychological Assessment Resources, 1989.

65. White HR, Labouvie EW. Towards the assessment of adolescent problem drinking. *J Stud Alcohol* 1989;**50**:30–37.

66. . Class IoCoV. (2010) Drunk Driving – Facilitator Guide. In:Corrections SoMDo, editor.: Office of Restorative Justice.

67. American Psychiatric Association. *Diagnostic and Statistical Manual of Mental Disorders, Fourth Edition, Text Revision: DSM-IV-TR*. Arlington, VA: APA, 2000.

19

Stimulants

John W. Tsuang[1] and Kathleen McKenna[2]

[1]Dual Diagnosis Treatment Program; Department of Psychiatry, UCLA; Harbor-UCLA Medical Center, Department of Psychiatry, Torrance, CA, USA
[2]Child and Adolescent Psychiatry Fellowship; UCLA; Harbor-UCLA Medical Center, Department of Psychiatry, Torrance, CA, USA

INTRODUCTION

Adolescence is a period of time for exploration, including experimenting with drugs, and stimulants are among the classes of drugs most commonly used and abused by adolescents [1–4]. Multiple factors are involved with adolescents' stimulant use, and clinical sign and symptoms associated with stimulant misuse can be confusing and difficult to diagnose. The longitudinal course and prognosis of those who misuse these drugs can vary, and in severe cases may lead to catastrophic results with permanent physiological and/or psychological damage or death. In this chapter we present epidemiological data on the prevalence of stimulant abuse by adolescents. The diagnostic criteria for stimulant abuse/dependence, signs and symptoms of stimulant use, and clinical vignettes to demonstrate common presenting problems will be shared. Relevant clinical issues specific to cocaine, amphetamine, and medical stimulants will be reviewed. In addition, we explore the complex issue of youths with attention-deficit/hyperactivity disorder (ADHD) and the potential for stimulant misuse or diversion.

We have included college age students along with adolescents in this chapter for two important reasons. First, brain imaging studies demonstrate that myelin maturation of the brain is not completed until the early to mid-twenties [5,6]. Second, from a psychosocial perspective, college students are in a special stage of adolescence and therefore may be regarded as adolescents both biologically and psychologically [5–7].

EPIDEMIOLOGY

Cocaine

According to the 2006 Substance Abuse and Mental Health Services Administration (SAMHSA) National Survey on Drug Use and Health, 35.3 million Americans older than 12 years have used cocaine at least once in their lifetime, with 8.5 million having used crack cocaine [8]. The survey also reported that in 2006, 2.4 million people over the age of 12 were current cocaine users [8]. In the 2009 SAMHSA survey, 0.3% of youths aged 12–17 years and 1.4% of those aged 18–25 years were current cocaine users, with a total of 1.6 million cocaine users among youths. It is critical to note the declining trend of initial cocaine use among persons aged 12 or older: the 1 million first-time users reported in 2002 had decreased to 617 000 first-time users in 2009 [9]. The 2009 SAMHSA survey also highlights the decline of initial crack cocaine use among youths, with 337 000 first-time users in 2002 as compared to 94 000 first-time users in 2009 [9]. Such data suggest that cocaine and crack cocaine use has recently declined among adolescents.

Cocaine Studies

The initiation of cocaine usually occurs at high-school age or later, which is older than that seen with other illicit drugs [10]. One study showed a later onset of initial use, with first cocaine use at 23 years of age, and 26.3 years as the average age of first regular use [11]. The majority of powder cocaine users are white males, with black males

Clinical Handbook of Adolescent Addiction, First Edition. Richard Rosner.
© 2013 John Wiley & Sons, Ltd. Published 2013 by John Wiley & Sons, Ltd.

representing the majority of crack cocaine users [11]. Major reasons cited for cocaine use include: "to see what it is like, to get high, and to have a good time with friends" [10]. Adolescents perceive cocaine as a drug that is more harmful compared to prescription amphetamine. In addition, its use is also met with less approval among high-school seniors. Adolescents at risk for cocaine use include: those who are single; non-college-bound high-school seniors; those from a higher socioeconomic status; and those living in metropolitan areas [10,12]. They are more likely to be heavy drinkers, consume marijuana, and have prior legal and psychiatric problems [13]. For most people, a higher frequency of marijuana use in adolescence is the crucial risk factor for progression to cocaine use when young adulthood is reached [10,14]. Fortunately, most cocaine users in high school do not develop dependence later in life [10].

Amphetamines/Methamphetamine

According to the 2006 SAMHSA survey, an estimated 1.2 million Americans aged 12 years or older used stimulants in the past month [8]. More specifically, 0.7 million people over the age of 12 used methamphetamine during the past month. The survey also indicated that the rate of lifetime use in 2006 was 5.8% of the population, which was lower than the lifetime use of 6.5% during the 2002 survey [9].

Methamphetamine (MA) use in 2006 by persons aged 12 and older was highest in the western United States (1.6%) and lowest in the northeast (0.3%). In the United States, the overall national prevalence of MA use among high-school seniors was 1.5% in 2001, which had declined to 1.1% in 2006. The Youth Risk Behavior Survey of 9th- to 12th-graders shows lifetime prevalence of MA use declining from 9.8% in 2001 to 4.4% in 2007 [15]. According to the 2009 SAMHSA survey, the number of past-month methamphetamine users aged 12 years or older decreased from 731 000 in 2006 to 502 000 in 2009. The survey results also indicated that initial methamphetamine use among persons aged 12 or older also declined, from 299 000 in 2002 to 154 000 in 2009 [9]. These surveys indicate that overall methamphetamine use among adolescents has decreased over the years.

Methamphetamine Studies

Methamphetamine tends to be a drug used by a younger population, with average age at first use of 19.6 years, and age at first regular use of 21.1 years [11]. In a 2004 survey study, "MA use was highest among young adults aged 18–25 years old" [16]. The data also indicate that in rural areas, MA use is highest among whites, working class and heterosexuals [11,17–20]. In the US West Coast and Pacific Islands, where MA is cheap and use is rampant, rates of MA use are highest for Native Hawaiians, Pacific Islanders, and other minority youths [20]. For adolescent boys, prior histories of antisocial behaviors, risky sexual practices, alcohol and illicit drug use, and history of depression put them at higher risk for MA misuse [21–23]. Compared to other illicit drugs, there is less of a gender difference, with one study showing that 54% of MA users are boys [11]. If girls used MA at a younger age compared to boys, they were more likely to use MA as part of weight loss attempts [21,24–27]. MA use is more common in rural regions compared to cocaine, and its use is prevalent among the homosexual communities in urban areas [17,24,28]. The majority of MA users report that their motivations for use include: "experimentation (34%), peer pressure (25%), and to get high (18%)" [24]. The MA use pattern showed that first-time users are more similar to crack cocaine addicts rather than powder cocaine users in that they tend to escalate their use rather rapidly and become addicted much more quickly [29,30]. MA use can precipitate a psychotic state similar to schizophrenia, which may last for months even when the user remains abstinent [31]. Of particular concern, recent brain imaging studies demonstrate that MA use can also lead to chronic brain damage [32].

Prescribed Stimulants

According to the Centers for Disease Control and Prevention (CDC), as of 2003, 2.5 million children aged 4 to 17 years were being treated with stimulant medications [3]. The 2009 SAMHSA survey showed that 7.0 million people over the age of 12 years had used stimulants for non-medical reasons in the past month. The survey emphasized that the percentage of usage for those aged 12 to 17 years declined from 4.0% in 2002 to 3.1% in 2009. However, for those in age range 18–25 years, the rate of prescribed stimulant use rose from 5.5% in 2002 to 6.3% in 2009 [9]. Studies of the illegal use of stimulant medications on college campuses showed that 4–35% of college students have illicitly used these medications [33]. The prevalence of non-medical amphetamine use has increased among young adults: 6% of non-college students and 7% of college students used amphetamine non-medically in the last year, while 8.3% of undergraduates had misused prescription stimulants in their lifetime [34,35].

ADHD and Substance Use

One topic that is most relevant for clinicians assessing and treating adolescents is the safety profile of psychostimulants and the potential for stimulant abuse and diversion [1,36,37]. There are case reports of adolescents taking stimulants and subsequently suffering adverse consequences, such as myocardial infarction or psychosis [32,38]. A recent poison center study showed that calls related to adolescent abuse of prescription ADHD medication rose by 76% from 1998 to 2005 [39]. This dramatic increase compared to other poison center calls suggests a rising problem with teen and stimulant medication abuse [39–41].

Numerous studies indicate that the risk of a substance use disorder (SUD) among patients with ADHD is high. In addition, ADHD patients who have a comorbid SUD also have a poorer prognosis as compared to those without a SUD [42–46]. The presence of comorbid disorders such as conduct disorder with ADHD may account for this increased prevalence of SUD [46–50]. Some studies suggest that using stimulant medications may increase the risk of substance abuse later on, but this finding is not consistently seen [51–56]. In fact, when ADHD is well treated, other studies demonstrate that the risk of SUD is actually reduced [57,58].

Stimulant Medication Misuse

In general, college students who use illicit prescription medications are more likely to be white males, have a grade point average less than 3.5, belong to social fraternities, and live off campus [59]. They are more likely to attend colleges with more competitive admission standards and are also more likely to use alcohol, cigarettes, marijuana, ecstasy, and cocaine, as well as engage in other risky behaviors [57,60–63]. A study of high-school students showed that stimulant medication misuse tended to be more frequent for those students who have no plans for attending college and for those with higher rates of alcohol and drug abuse [3,64,65]. African-American youths and other minorities are less likely to be prescribed stimulant medications than white youths and also less likely to abuse these medications when they are prescribed [61,66].

Studies support the fact that illicit ADHD medications used in college are more likely to be for academic than recreational reasons [4,33,60]. In one collegiate study, "65.2% of students reported the use of stimulant medication to help them concentrate, 59.8% to help them study, and 47.5% to increase their alertness, while only 31% reported to use stimulants to get high" [4,57]. Studies indicate that high-school students are more likely to use stimulant medications for recreational reasons and weight loss [4,61].

Stimulant medications are more likely to be misused because they are readily available, less stigmatized, and because there is a myth that these drugs are safer than illicit drugs [3,33,67]. The misuse typically begins earlier and usually involves only a single type of medication as compared to MA users, who are more likely to use an additional drug concurrently [68]. Among abusers of stimulant drugs, males are more likely than females to misuse methylphenidate, but are less likely to use other types of amphetamines [23]. Sixty-six percent of middle- and high-school students obtained the drugs from a family member or friends, and more than half of patients on stimulant medications were approached to divert their medicine [59,64,65,69]. Most adolescents appear to misuse stimulant medications episodically rather than daily, and with the easy availability and the misperception regarding their safety, stimulant medication misuse is more common than people realize.

DIAGNOSTIC CRITERIA

Different Types of Stimulants

When assessing a potential diagnosis of a stimulant use disorder, the clinician should be aware of a wide range of substances that qualify as "stimulants." In addition to amphetamine and amphetamine-like substances such as cocaine, there are other substances that are structurally different from the classic amphetamine compound but nevertheless have amphetamine-like action. Such substances include methylphenidate, plant stimulants, and caffeine.

Amphetamines (AMP) are synthetic compounds that are longer acting and cheaper to produce compared to cocaine. It has been known for many years that AMP can have energizing and euphorogenic properties. Initially, AMP were given to military personnel during WWII to increase their energy [30]. The medical uses of AMP later expanded and included the treatment of narcolepsy, Attention Deficit Hyperactivity Disorder (ADHD), depression, and weight loss [3]. More recently, AMP have been diverted to students to improve their academic performances and to truckers to assist them on long hauls.

The different types of AMP are based on their method of manufacture and their strength [30]. Prescription AMP were popular in the 1960–70s until the Controlled Substance Act of 1970, which classified AMP as Schedule II drugs thereby discouraging their use. However, this decline of prescription AMP was unfortunately replaced by an increased recreational popularity of MA during the 1980s. With the recent development of the different types of MA, such as "crank" (methamphetamine sulfate), "crystal" (methamphetamine hydrochloride), and "ice" (smokable form of methamphetamine), there has been a further resurgence in their use [30].

Cocaine is produced from the cocoa bush plant and humanity has known its psychoactive properties for centuries. Cocaine is the only naturally occurring topical anesthetic, with powerful vasoconstrictive effects, and has been used for many different anesthetic purposes. In the United States, cocaine epidemics occur every few generations, with the latest explosion occurring in the 1970s–80s, when smokable cocaine (crack) became available [30]. Crack cocaine is a cheaper version of cocaine. Because crack cocaine is smoked, it is more readily absorbed by fat cells in the brain and therefore produces a more intense and longer-lasting high [30]. Between the late 1980s and early 1990s, crack cocaine use crossed all social and economic barriers and this epidemic became associated with many of the ills of our society, including gang violence, crime, and HIV infections [30]. Thus, cocaine use not only negatively affected users physically and psychologically, but also had devastating economic and social ramifications. Recently, the experimentation and casual use of cocaine have declined but hardcore use of cocaine has remained strong.

Cocaine and AMP have similar physical and mental effects, but their duration of effect, methods of use, and pattern of use are different [70,71]. Cocaine has a short duration of action, with a half-life of about 60–90 minutes, compared with AMP (4–6 hours) and MA (up to 12 hours) [70]. Crack cocaine users and MA addicts are more likely to report binge patterns of use, while AMP users typically use it fewer times per day [71]. The cost of these drugs may differ depending on the quality of the drugs, though cocaine is generally more expensive than AMP [30]. Some people report that cocaine produces a much "higher high" whereas AMP offers a greater amount of energy. Smoking crack cocaine has been shown to be more likely to cause dependence than snorting powder [72]. Table 19.1 summarizes the comparison of cocaine and AMP.

Prescription stimulant medications include methylphenidate (Ritalin/Concerta), dextroamphetamine (Dexedrine), and mixed-salts amphetamine (Adderall) and their derivates [61]. They are considered to be the first-line medications for treatment of ADHD, as well as for narcolepsy. These medications are Schedule II controlled substances, with Adderall and Ritalin commonly abused or diverted [30,39,61,73]. Other concerns regarding prescription stimulant medications include

their potential long-term effects on children and potential interactions with illicit street drugs.

Methods of use for all these drugs are similar. AMPs are mainly snorted or injected while MAs are smoked. The most popular ways of using powder cocaine are snorting or injecting, whereas crack cocaine is smoked. Alternative methods of use include being absorbed through any mucous membranes such as sublingually, rectally, or vaginally [21,28,74]. ADHD medications are mainly orally ingested, but some adolescents crush the tablets to snort or inject them, while others dissolve the tablets in water and inject the mixture [4,75]. The subjective stimulant high precipitated by these drugs is linked to the rate of absorption, with intravenous, intranasal, or inhalational routes of administration being the most rapidly absorbed.

Because most stimulant-like substances have similar psychoactive properties, the DSM-IV-TR (*Diagnostic and Statistical Manual of Mental Disorders, Fourth Edition, Text Revision*) diagnostic criteria for cocaine and amphetamine dependence and abuse are the same. Furthermore, there are no established differences in diagnostic criteria between adults and adolescents for substance abuse or dependence [76]. Some researchers have proposed that adolescents should not be diagnosed as having a substance use disorder using adult criteria, but this approach has not been universally accepted. There are seven DSM-IV-TR dependence criteria, of which three or more must be met within the 12-month period to fulfill the diagnosis of dependence. The seven dependence criteria include tolerance; withdrawal; taking the substance often in large amounts or over a longer period than intended; having a persistent desire or making unsuccessful efforts to cut down or control use; devoting a great deal of time in activities needed to get the substance, use the substance, or recover from its effects; giving up or cutting down on important social, occupational, or recreational activities because of substance use; and continuing to use a substance despite knowing one has persistent or recurrent physical or psychological problems [76].

In order to meet criteria for amphetamine abuse, at least one out of four of the maladaptive behaviors must occur within a 12-month period. Amphetamine abuse

Table 19.1 A comparison of cocaine and amphetamine (AMP).

	Cocaine	AMP
Duration	Shorter duration of action	Longer duration of action
Half-life	60–90 minutes	4–6 hours
Patterns of use	Binge	Few times per day
Cost	Expensive	Cheaper
Effects	Produces "higher high"	Offers greater energy

criteria include: recurrent use of a substance resulting in a failure to fulfill major role obligations at work, school, or home; recurrent use of a substance in situations where it is physically hazardous; recurrent substance-related legal problems; and continuing to use a substance despite having persistent or recurrent social or interpersonal problems caused by its use [76].

Stimulants produce similar symptoms of intoxication and withdrawal. In the DSM-IV-TR, the same diagnostic criteria are used for all AMP-like substances [76]. The criteria for stimulant intoxication comprise:

- Recent use of substance.
- The development, during or shortly after substance use, of clinically significant maladaptive behavioral or psychological changes.
- The development, during or shortly after substance use, of two or more of the following symptoms: tachycardia or bradycardia; pupillary dilation; elevated or lowered blood pressure; perspiration or chills; nausea or vomiting; evidence of weight loss; psychomotor agitation or retardation symptoms; muscular weakness, respiratory depression, chest pain, or cardiac arrhythmias; confusion, seizures, dyskinesias, dystonias, or coma.
- Symptoms are not caused by a general medical condition or another mental disorder.

The criteria for stimulant withdrawal are as follows:

- Cessation of (or reduction in) heavy and prolonged stimulant use.
- The development, within a few hours to several days after use, of dysphoric mood and at least two of the following physiological changes: fatigue; vivid, unpleasant dreams; insomnia or hypersomnia; increased appetite; or psychomotor retardation or agitation.
- Clinically significant distress or impairment in social, occupational, or other important areas of functioning are caused by the above symptoms.
- The symptoms are not caused by a general medical condition or another mental disorder [76].

In 2013 DSM-V will be published, and under the current proposal, substance abuse and dependence criteria will be combined together to form the diagnosis of Substance Use Disorder. Though not fully agreed as yet, newly proposed criteria include the following:

- The "recurrent substance-related legal problems" criterion from DSM-IV-TR abuse section will be eliminated and "Craving or a strong desire or urge to use a specific substance" will be added to make up the new 11 criteria.

- To meet criteria for Substance Use Disorder, one must have two (or more) of the criteria within a 12-month period. Cocaine Use Disorder as well as Amphetamine Use Disorder will follow the above criteria.
- No changes in criteria for acute intoxication or withdrawal for either cocaine or amphetamine have been proposed at this time [77].

CLINICAL PRESENTATION

Patients rarely present to a doctor's office with typical symptoms of stimulant intoxication or withdrawal. Usually individuals using amphetamines or related substances only come to the attention of mental health clinicians because of the accompanying psychiatric symptoms and/or behavioral issues. Nevertheless, one needs to be familiar with symptoms associated with stimulant use. Acute stimulant effects include euphoria and feelings of well-being, increased energy, and increased alertness. Persons using stimulants commonly report having a heightened libido, feelings of invincibility, lowered inhibition, and psychosis [3,21,32,74,75,78].

Chronic stimulant use has been associated with reported mental and physical exhaustion, anxiety, insomnia, irritability, anorexia, and confusion. Feelings of depression, panic, inability to concentrate, anhedonia, and even suicidal thoughts have also been described [29,32,74,78–83]. Drug tolerance, formication (a sensation that bugs are crawling under one's skin), and drug-induced hallucinations and/or psychoses are other associated symptoms that can occur [3,28,30,84].

Stimulant withdrawal is usually characterized by an acute phase that can last up to 2 weeks. Commonly described symptoms of stimulant withdrawal in this initial phase include increased sleeping and decreased appetite, depression, anxiety, and drug craving. Many individuals report a more prolonged chronic stimulant withdrawal where the withdrawal symptoms remain at lower levels for months [85]. Although adolescents may experience amphetamine withdrawal symptoms, there is usually an absence of significant physiological changes [86].

Physical signs and symptoms due to stimulant use are quite common but non-specific. For example, patients may present with hypertension, increased respiration and heart rate, pupil dilation, tremor, diaphoresis, dental erosions, weight loss, and seizures [29]. Chronic use of stimulants has been associated with choreoathetotic movements, rhabdomyolysis, damaged cardiac muscles and coronary arteries, hyperthermia, myocardial infarction, acute coronary syndromes, stroke, cardiac arrhythmia, and even death [3,21,32,74,75,78]. More specifically, the active metabolite of cocaine, cocaethylene, seems more likely than AMP to induce cardiac conduction abnormalities [30].

Clinical Vignettes

The common comorbidities associated with stimulant abuse can be various types of psychiatric symptoms, including psychosis, anxiety, depression, and maladaptive behaviors. We will summarize some potential presentations with the following vignettes followed by key "take home" points.

Psychosis as the Primary Presenting Symptom

Jose, a 17-year-old male, presented to the emergency room with complaints of hearing voices for several weeks. He stated that the voices taunt him with derogatory remarks. He had had difficulty falling asleep because he needed to check the doors and windows to be sure he was safe. His parents reported that he often asks them if they think someone is following him. Upon questioning, Jose admitted that he had used methamphetamine several weeks ago but strenuously denied using drugs since that time. Urine toxicology was negative. Jose's mother was very worried because she has a brother and uncle who have schizophrenia. She was worried that Jose may be developing the same illness.

This vignette illustrates several important points. First, the symptoms of amphetamine psychosis, particularly in an adolescent, can closely mimic an emerging schizophrenic or other primary psychotic illness. Psychotic symptoms such as paranoia and hallucinations are common to both amphetamine-induced psychosis and a primary thought disorder. Second, because amphetamines are rapidly metabolized in the body, a negative urine drug screen does not rule out the possibility that amphetamine use is the primary culprit for the presenting symptom. The evaluator should attempt to determine the type, amount, and route regarding the last use of the stimulant to help evaluate any causal link to the reported symptoms. Particular attention to any physical signs of amphetamine intoxication, such as dilated pupils or a rapid heartbeat, should be noted. Rapid resolution of psychotic symptoms over a period of weeks, particularly in the absence of antipsychotic medication treatment, is more consistent with amphetamine use rather than a primary thought disorder. Third, a family history of schizophrenia may indicate an underlying vulnerability to a psychotic thought process. However, a family history alone does not automatically exclude the strong possibility of amphetamine use, particularly in this age range. Fourth, a significant number of individuals with primary mental disorders (such as schizophrenia and/or

bipolar disorder) have a comorbid substance use disorder. The clinician should evaluate if both diagnoses are present as such comorbidity has important implications for both treatment and long term prognosis.

Behavioral Problems as the Primary Presenting Symptom

18-year-old Marcy was brought to the outpatient psychiatry clinic by her parents. Mother and Father were concerned that she has developed a "bad attitude" toward school and her family. Beginning about two years ago, Marcy had begun associating with a new peer group, one known to skip school and to take drugs. Her mother reported that Marcy's interest in the new group occurred shortly after a friend transferred to a new high school and a boyfriend informed Marcy that he was no longer interested in her. She has been treated twice for chlamydia, has lost 15 pounds, seems irritable and, when her parents don't agree to her demands, she becomes enraged, throwing furniture and pushing them. She has slapped her 8-year-old sister several times. She frequently stays up all night using the computer and then can't get up for school in the morning so her parents let her stay home to get some rest. Although during her intake session she denied using drugs, she later acknowledged on a written survey that she has been smoking crack cocaine and drinking alcohol with her new friends. She thinks she is addicted to the cocaine and wishes she could stop. She has exchanged sex for cocaine and is bothered by what her gynecologist told her about frequent chlamydia infections causing infertility. She would like to stop but has felt quite depressed when she tried.

This vignette focuses on various behavioral problems associated with substance abuse. Most adolescents are concerned about being accepted by a peer group and are often willing to engage in maladaptive behaviors to be considered part of the group. Narcissistic injuries, disappointments, loss of previously meaningful relationships, academic or social problems, and stresses at home can precipitate a change in peer group. Affiliation with a group that uses substances can provide an easy path to acceptance since often the substance abuse is the common denominator in the group. For many teens, it is not long before they begin to feel that the drugs provide relief from their problems. Unfortunately, a myriad of other problems often are precipitated by the drug use. As with Marcy, adolescents who use stimulants often use other drugs. The use of cocaine can lead to aggression and mood problems, family conflicts and rapid dependence on the drug. Particularly in the case of females, cocaine can increase risky sexual behaviors, not only because the drug alters the ability to monitor behavior but also because sexual favors are used to procure the drugs. As in this case, attempts to stop using cocaine can lead to depression. While it is important for the clinician to address the substance abuse in its own right, it is crucial to help the teen improve coping skills to deal with the disappointments of life. Family stresses, both those caused by drug use and those that may have predisposed the adolescent to using drugs, need to be explored and ameliorated. Parents need help in knowing how to deal with the adolescent. In this case, the mother has allowed Marcy to sleep late in the mornings and also did not set limits on her evening use of the computer, thus allowing Marcy to associate with drug-using peers in the evenings. The clinician should address the need for the adolescent to develop social skills, including how to make new friends and seek acceptance by a desired peer group. The illicit use of stimulants is often intertwined with an adolescent's developmental challenges. Treatment should include attention to the behavioral challenges as well as to the substance abuse in order to optimize outcome.

ADHD as the Presenting Symptom

The mother of Maria, age 16, and Luz, age 14, brought both her daughters to the outpatient clinic saying, "We just can't go on like this." Maria has been obsessed with losing weight and her mother wonders if she has anorexia. In particular, Maria's weight has dropped from 135 pounds to 108 pounds. According to her mother, Maria has become "difficult to manage," leaves home without permission, argues constantly with her parents and sister, and stays up at night using her computer. She no longer wants to be with her friends, preferring on-line fantasy games. Luz, who has been diagnosed with ADHD in the past, is not doing well in school. She has been taking prescribed methylphenidate (Ritalin), 10 mg three times a day, but her ADHD now seems to be worsening. Her teachers report that Luz is talking in class, does not hand in her homework, and doesn't seem to be paying attention. Luz acknowledges that she does skip her medication but accuses her mother of not getting it refilled on time. Mother agreed that she often loses track of filling her daughter's prescription since she works and her husband is disabled and needs her help. A psychiatrist evaluated both girls and discovered that Maria has been taking Luz's methylphenidate to lose weight and to help her concentrate. She also gives the pills to some of her friends who use them to be able to party longer on the weekends. She does this in order to enhance her popularity. Luz was switched to a longer-acting formulation that is less likely to be abused. Mother is now keeping track of the medications and supervises Luz taking the medications at home. Since

Luz does not need the medication when she is not in school, the psychiatrist now writes for 20 pills a month instead of 30. Maria is making progress in therapy and sees a dietician regularly.

This vignette emphasizes the relationship between ADHD and stimulant abuse. Stimulants are readily available to adolescents and they are usually obtained from friends or relatives. Females often obtain stimulants for use in weight control. As this case illustrates, patients with ADHD may participate in diversion, whether through inattention, the desire to please someone, or for profit. While some patients with ADHD will ask for specific pills, such as short-acting forms of stimulants that are easier to abuse, others may inadvertently provide an opportunity for drug-seekers by not taking their prescribed dose regularly. Some parents fail to keep track of when their adolescent takes their prescribed medications and when a new refill is due. Other parents deliberately seek to increase their teen's dosage in order to divert some of the pills. Clinicians should keep track of prescriptions and maintain a healthy skepticism should a patient or caregiver report frequent losses of prescriptions or insist on higher quantities of medications, particularly of short-acting stimulants that can be injected, smoked, or snorted. Clinicians need to take a careful history of ADHD symptoms in the family. Some caregivers and siblings take diverted prescribed stimulants to treat undiagnosed ADHD and would be better served by an adequate assessment for ADHD followed by appropriate treatment.

Depression as the Presenting Symptom

Luke, age 15, had been in therapy for a year to deal with his depression. He recently told his therapist that he is gay. When asked if he had acted on his attraction to men, he told her that he had begun a relationship with a man in his twenties. Upon questioning, he revealed that he takes methamphetamine given to him by his new friend. Luke has found that this makes him more at ease having sex and less concerned about feeling "different." He is concerned that his parents will ask him to leave the house if they find out he is gay. He is also worried that he will become HIV positive if he keeps having unprotected sex but doesn't want to displease his friend by insisting on a condom. He used to use meth only when having sex but recently he has used it when he feels down.

This vignette demonstrates that amphetamines are often used in the gay community and are associated with sexual activities at high risk for HIV transmission. In this case, an adolescent's exploration of sexual orientation places him in a situation where drugs are not only available but their use is encouraged. While exploring his sexuality, Luke is at risk not only for addiction but also for sexually transmitted disease. While addressing the drug use, the clinician must also be aware of the need to help the adolescent deal with the risks posed by unsafe sexual practices, which can be significantly increased by the use of amphetamines. The clinician must also be aware that gay, lesbian, bisexual, and transgendered teens have unique stresses as they struggle to take their place in society. They are at high risk for depression and suicide, which can further complicate their assessment and treatment.

Anxiety, Post-Traumatic Stress and Bipolar Symptoms as Presenting Symptoms

Monique, age 13, has been treated for post-traumatic stress disorder (PTSD). When she was 12, she was raped by her uncle and has since had a difficult time, especially when she had to testify against him. Her symptoms have improved but recently she has been angry at home, has stopped associating with her friends, and just goes to her room at home. Her grades have also deteriorated. She has resumed cutting herself, an activity that she had stopped last year. She has had several anxiety attacks and has told her mother repeatedly that she would like to die. Her mother asked the doctor if Monique could have bipolar disorder. Monique can be quite cheerful and full of energy only to become depressed, angry, and self-injurious on the same day. Her therapist asked her if anything could account for her current problems, and Monique replied that a friend told her that her uncle would likely be released in a few years. She denied any drug and alcohol use but her urine test was positive for cocaine. Later Monique revealed that she has been using cocaine, which she bought using money stolen from her father's wallet.

This vignette shows that distinguishing between the effects of substance abuse and clinical conditions such as anxiety, PTSD, and bipolar disorder can be difficult. Symptoms of mood instability, sleep problems, and increased energy can result from drug use or other psychiatric conditions. The clinician needs to pay particular attention to gaining information from the caregiver about accompanying symptoms such as change in pupil size, lack of appetite, problems sleeping, and pressured speech. In this vignette the adolescent is experiencing anxiety attacks and has resumed cutting herself, signaling an increase in stress and dysphoria. Her mother is appropriate to question whether her daughter also has bipolar disorder, given the mood lability she is exhibiting. Most adolescents with bipolar disorder experience more pervasive mood disturbance than Monique's mother describes. While teenagers with a "mixed" picture of bipolar disorder can present with a combination of manic and depressed symptoms such as grandiosity and pressured speech accompanied by

irritability and suicidality, in this case Monique vacillates from euthymic mood to depression and anxiety. She does not demonstrate typical manic, depressed, or mixed symptoms. Rather, her presentation is more likely due to waxing and waning anxiety about the upcoming release of her uncle with exacerbation of PTSD symptoms or she is experiencing the agitation and subsequent mood dysregulation associated with cocaine use. The adolescent is probably the best source of information about thoughts and feelings that immediately precede the fluctuations in behavior as well as the correlation of the symptoms with drug use. The latter is important since amphetamines cause symptoms consistent with psychiatric conditions and the withdrawal from the drug can also mimic psychiatric conditions. A strong alliance with the teen will allow the clinician to gain the information necessary to clarify the etiology of the patient's difficulties. In Monique's case, it is likely that she has only recently started using cocaine. The clinician has an opportunity to intervene early, helping the teen control her symptoms of PTSD, learn healthier ways to deal with anxiety, and stop cocaine use before psychological or physical dependence on the drug is experienced. Early recognition of substance use is crucial for preventing more devastating sequelae of addiction, health problems, overall decline in functioning, and destruction of healthy social relationships.

ASSESSMENT

When assessing adolescents in the medical office, the clinician must strive to develop an alliance with the patient. Often, the adolescent is accompanied by an adult who is either desperate for assistance, unwilling to deal with more consequences of drug use, or ignorant regarding the teen's drug use. Feelings of mistrust and anger between the involved parties are common. The youth is often in denial regarding their drug use and frequently minimizes the impact of their substance use. Therefore, it is important to try to develop the youth's trust while maintaining some healthy skepticism regarding the teenager's self-report during the initial assessment.

For the initial evaluation, the evaluator needs to obtain a good psychiatric and comprehensive substance use history. Significant information regarding any family history of substance use disorders and psychiatric disorders, as well as medical diagnosis, social and education information, and cognition are essential data needed for the assessment. Use of semi-structured interviews or validated rating scales for ADHD and addiction severity may also be helpful [87,88]. Additional information from a resource person such as a family member or friend is essential. Objective

measures like a physical exam, screening blood tests –
including blood urea nitrogen (BUN), creatine (Cr), and
creatine phosphokinase (CPK) – and body fluid toxicology test (either from urine or blood), are vital parts of the
initial assessment. The clinician must be fully aware of
the possibility of receiving an altered specimen. The
consequences, such as being grounded, loss of privileges
and/or allowances, or more drastic measures, of a positive toxicology test must be clear to all parties involved.
For youths who are sexually active, the clinician may
also use this opportunity to discuss with the youth testing
for any potential sexually transmitted disease, to include
specific testing for HIV.

When examining a complex case, a cross-sectional
examination is often insufficient; thus, a longitudinal
history and clinical course are essential to determine
the correct diagnosis. In addition, the clinician will
need to re-evaluate psychiatric symptoms after a
period of abstinence to determine whether they are
substance induced. Overall, the development of trust
during the initial assessment and the procurement of
accurate information is an essential but difficult process for adolescents with suspected stimulant use
problems.

The use of validated screening instruments for substance abuse disorders in adolescents such as CRAFFT
(Car, Relax, Alone, Forget, Friends, Trouble) [89],
Drug Use Screening Inventory-Adolescent Version
[90], and Teen Addiction Severity Index [91] might
be helpful. Other psychological scales might be used to
assist in obtaining a psychiatric diagnosis such as the
Psychotic Symptoms Assessment Scale (PSAS) for
psychosis [92], ADHD Rating Scale-IV and Connors
Ratings Scales-Revised for ADHD [93], Adolescent
Young Mania Rating Scale (YMRS) for bipolar disorder [94], and Kutcher Generalized Social Anxiety
Disorder Scale for Adolescents (K-GSADS-A) for
anxiety disorder [95].

TREATMENT

The treatment of amphetamine use disorders is not the
focus of this chapter; therefore, we will only briefly
review some basic drug treatment strategies among this
population. First, it is always advisable to involve family
whenever possible for support and assistance in monitoring medications and substance use. There are no US
Food and Drug Administration (FDA) approved pharmacological agents for the treatment of stimulant dependence, but behavioral modalities like self-help groups,
relapse prevention, contingency management, cognitive
behavioral therapy, and concurrent urine testing are the
most effective treatments currently. For treatment of
ADHD patients, especially those who may have

potential for addiction, one should consider using newer
formulations of stimulants like transdermal agents
(methylphenidate transdermal system, or MTS) and
prodrug (lisdexamfetamine) or second-line agents
such as atomoxetine, bupropion, or guanfacine [87].
Long-acting and newer medications are less likely to
be associated with diversion than short-acting stimulants
[87]. Clinicians should be suspicious of lost prescriptions or early refill requests, and adequate information
about earlier symptoms and evidence of ADHD is
necessary prior to initial prescribing for this population
[96].

SUMMARY

Stimulant misuse by adolescents is a common problem
with serious emotional and physical consequences. Fortunately, the prevalence of stimulant use by youths has
stabilized in more recent surveys. Although an adolescent may present without any typical signs of stimulant
misuse when being evaluated by a physician, there are
often classic accompanying psychiatric or behavioral
problems. We have given several vignettes highlighting
some common presenting problems with stimulant
dependence. The DSM-IV-TR diagnostic criteria for
stimulant abuse and dependence are precise, but obtaining sufficient data in order to make such diagnosis can
be quite difficult. Information obtained from assorted
sources, including family and friends, urine toxicology
testing, and psychological screening instruments is
essential in making the diagnosis. One must also be
careful regarding the diversion or misuse of stimulant
medications by ADHD patients. Finally, since stimulant
misuse and addiction can cause permanent physical and
psychological damage, prevention and early intervention are extremely important.

Acknowledgement

The authors want to thank Holly M. Yong for her
assistance in writing this chapter.

References

1. Driscoll-Malliarakis K. Teen prescription and over-the-
counter drug abuse. *Medscape Public Health & Prevention*
2009. Available at: http://www.medscape.com/viewar-
ticle/713306.
2. Lessenger JE, Feinberg SD. Abuse of prescription and
over-the-counter medications. *J Am Board Fam Med*
2008;**21**:45–54.
3. Apa-Hall P, Schwartz-Bloom RD, McConnell ES. The
current state of teenage drug abuse: trend toward prescription drugs. *J School Nursing* 2008. Available at: http://

www.nasn.org/Portals/0/resources/pd_toolkit_nurses_
supplement.pdf.

4. Teter CJ, McCabe SE, LaGrange K, Cranford JA, Boyd CJ. Illicit use of specific prescription stimulants among college students: prevalence, motives, and routes of administration. *Pharmacology* 2006;**26**:1501–1510.

5. Keniston K. *The Uncommitted: Alienated Youth in American Society*. New York: Harcourt, Brace & World, Inc., 1965.

6. Bartzokis G. Brain myelination in prevalent neuropsychiatric developmental disorders: primary and comorbid addiction. *Adolesc Psychiatry* 2005;**29**:55–96.

7. Johnson SB, Blum RW, Giedd JN. Adolescent maturity and the brain: the promise and pitfalls of neuroscience research in adolescent health policy. *J Adolesc Health* 2009;**45**:216–221.

8. Substance Abuse and Mental Health Services Administration (SAMHSA). *Results From the 2006 National Survey on Drug Use and Health: National Findings*. Office of Applied Studies, NSDUH Series H-32, DHHS Publication No. SMA 07-4293. Rockville, MD: SAMHSA, 2007.

9. Substance Abuse and Mental Health Services Administration (SAMHSA). *Results From the 2009 National Survey on Drug Use and Health: Volume I. Summary of National Findings*. Office of Applied Studies, NSDUH Series H-38A, HHS Publication No. SMA 10-4586 Findings. Rockville, MD: SAMHSA, 2010.

10. National Institute on Drug Abuse. Cocaine use in America: epidemiologic and clinical perspectives. NIDA Research Monograph 61. NIDA, 1985.

11. Hser YI, Huang D, Brecht ML, Li L, Evans E. Contrasting trajectories of heroin, cocaine, and methamphetamine use. *J Addict Dis* 2008;**27**:13.

12. Bachman JG, Johnston LD, O'Malley PM. Smoking, drinking, and drug use among American high school students: Correlates and trends, 1975–1979. *Am J Public Health* 1981;**71**:59–69.

13. National Institute on Drug Abuse. The epidemiology of cocaine use and abuse. NIDA Research Monograph 110. NIDA, 1991.

14. Kandel DB, Yamaguchi K. Developmental patterns of the use of legal, illegal and medically prescribed psychotropic drugs from adolescence to young adulthood. In: *Etiology of Drug Abuse: Implications for Prevention*. NIDA Research Monograph 56, 1985; pp. 193–235.

15. Embry D, Hankins M, Biglan A, Boles S. Behavioral and social correlates of methamphetamine use in a population-based sample of early and later adolescents. *Addict Behav* 2010;**34**:343–351.

16. Office of Applied Studies. The NSDUH Report: methamphetamine use, abuse, and dependence: 2002, 2003, and 2004. SAMHSA, 2005. Available at: http://oas.samhsa.gov/2k5/meth/meth.cfm.

17. Iritani BJ, Hallfors DD, Bauer DJ. Crystal methamphetamine use among young adults in the USA. *Addiction* 2007;**102**:1102–1113.

18. Wu LT, Schlenger WE, Galvin DM. Concurrent use of methamphetamine, MDMA, LSD, ketamine, GHB, and flunitrazepan among American youths. *Drug Alcohol Depend* 2006;**84**:102–113.

19. Furr CDM, Delva J, Anthony JC. The suspected association between methamphetamine ('ice') smoking and frequent episodes of alcohol intoxication: data from the 1993 National Household Survey on Drug Abuse. *Drug Alcohol Depend* 2000;**59**:89–93.

20. Centers for Disease Control and Prevention. Fact Sheet: Methamphetamine use and risk for HIV/AIDS. CDC, 2007. Available at: http://www.cdc.gov/hiv/resources/factsheets/meth.htm.

21. Embry D, Hankins M, Biglan A, Boles S. Behavioral and social correlates of methamphetamine use in a population-based sample of early and later adolescents. *Addict Behav* 2009;**34**:343–351.

22. Yen CF. Relationship between methamphetamine use and risky sexual behavior in adolescents. *Kaohsiung J Med Sci* 2004;**20**:160–165.

23. Wu LT, Pilowsky DJ, Schlenger WE, Galvin DM. Misuse of methamphetamine and prescription stimulants among youths and young adults in the community. *Drug Alcohol Depend* 2007;**89**:195–205.

24. Shrem MT, Halkitis PN. Methamphetamine abuse in the United States: contextual, psychological and sociological considerations. *J Health Psychol* 2008;**13**:669–679.

25. Dluzen DE, Liu B. Gender differences in methamphetamine use and responses: A review. *Gender Med* 2008;**5**:24–35.

26. Biglan A. Sexual coercion. In: Mattaini MA, Thyer BA (eds), *Finding Solutions to Social Problems: Behavioral Strategies for Change*. Washington, DC: American Psychological Association, 1996; pp. 289–316.

27. Brecht ML, O'Brien A, Mayrhauser CV, Anglin MD. Methamphetamine use behaviors and gender differences. *Addict Behav* 2004;**29**:89–106.

28. Russell K, Dryden DM, Liang Y, *et al.* Risk factors for methamphetamine use in youth: a systemic review. *BMC Pediatr* 2008;**8**:48.

29. Sommers I, Baskin D, Baskin-Sommers A. Methamphetamine use among young adults: health and social consequences. *Addict Behav* 2006;**31**:1469–1476.

30. Inaba DS, Cohen WE. *Uppers, Downers, All Arounders, Physical and Mental Effects of Psychoactive Effects*, 4th edn. Medford, OR: CNS Publications, 2004.

31. Glasner-Edwards S, Mooney LJ, Marinelli-Casey P, Hillhouse M, Ang A, Rawson R, the Methamphetamine Treatment Project Corporate Authors. Clinical course and outcomes of methamphetamine dependent adults with psychosis. *J Subst Abuse Treat* 2008;**35**:445–450.

32. Barr AM, Panenka WJ, MacEwan GW, *et al.* The need for speed: an update on methamphetamine addiction. *J Psychiatry Neurosci* 2006;**31**:301–313.

33. DeSantis AD, Webb EM, Noar SM. Illicit use of prescription ADHD medications on a college campus: a multimethodological approach. *J Am Coll Health* 2008;**57**:315–324.

34. Merkel RL, Kuchibhatla A. Safety of stimulant treatment in attention deficit hyperactivity disorder: Part I. *Expert Opin Drug Saf* 2009;**8**:655–668.

35. Herman-Stahl MA, Krebs CP, Kroutil LA, Heller DC. Risk and protective factors for methamphetamine use and nonmedical use of prescription stimulants among young adults aged 18 to 25. *Addict Behav* 2006;**32**:1003–1015.

36. Greenhill LL, Pliszka S, Dulcan M, *et al.* Practice parameter for the use of stimulant medications in the treatment of children, adolescents, and adults. *J Am Acad Child Adolesc Psychiatry* 2002;**41** (Suppl. 2): 26S–49S.

37. Wilens TE, Gignac M, Swezey A, Monuteaux MC, Biederman J. Characteristics of adolescents and young adults with ADHD who divert or misuse their prescribed medications. *J Am Acad Child Adolesc Psychiatry* 2006;**45**:408–414.

38. Gandhi PJ, Ezeala GU, Luyen TT, Tu TC, Tran MT. Myocardial infarction in an adolescent taking Adderall. *Am J Health Syst Pharm* 2005;**62**:1494–1497.

39. Setlik JG, Bond R, Ho M. Adolescent prescription ADHD medication abuse is rising along with prescriptions for these medications. *Pediatrics* 2009;**124**:875–880.

40. Wilens TE, Adler LA, Adams J, *et al.* Misuse and diversion of stimulants prescribed for ADHD: a systemic review of the literature. *J Am Acad Child Adolesc Psychiatry* 2008;**47**:21–31.

41. Brauser D. Prescription ADHD medication abuse by adolescents on the rise. *Medscape Medical News* 2009. Available at: http://www.medscape.com/viewarticle/708037.

42. Schubiner H, Tzelepis A, Milberger S, *et al.* Prevalence of attention-deficit/hyperactivity disorder and conduct disorder among substance abusers. *J Clin Psychiatry* 2000;**61**:244–251.

43. Wilens TE, Biederman J, Mick E, Faraone SV, Spencer T. Attention deficit hyperactivity disorder (ADHD) is associated with early onset substance use disorders. *J Nerv Ment Dis* 1997;**185**:475–482.

44. Biederman J, Wilens T, Mick E, Milberger S, Spencer TJ, Faraone SV. Psychoactive substance use disorders in adults with attention deficit hyperactivity disorder (ADHD): Effects of ADHD and psychiatric comorbidity. *Am J Psychiatry* 1995;**152**:1652–1658.

45. Flory K, Milich R, Lynam DR, Leukefeld C, Clayton R. Relation between childhood disruptive behavior disorders and substance use and dependence symptoms in young adulthood: Individuals with symptoms of attention-deficit-/hyperactivity disorder and conduct disorder are uniquely at risk. *Psychol Addict Behav* 2003;**17**:151–158.

46. McGough JJ, Smalley SL, McCracken JT, *et al.* Psychiatric comorbidity in adult attention deficit hyperactivity disorder: Findings from multiplex families. *Am J Psychiatry* 2005;**162**:1621–1627.

47. Barkley RA, Fischer M, Edelbrock CS, Smallish L. The adolescent outcome of hyperactive children diagnosed by research criteria: I. An 8-year prospective follow-up study. *J Am Acad Child Adolesc Psychiatry* 1990;**29**:546–557.

48. Biederman J, Wilens T, Mick E, *et al.* Is ADHD a risk factor for psychoactive substance use disorders? Findings from a four-year prospective follow-up study. *J Am Acad Child Adolesc Psychiatry* 1997;**36**:21–29.

49. Katusic SK, Barbaresi WJ, Colligan RC, Weaver AL, Leibson CL, Jacobsen SJ. Psychostimulant treatment and risk for substance abuse among young adults with a history of attention-deficit/hyperactivity disorder: A population based, birth cohort study. *J Child Adolesc Psychopharmacol* 2005;**15**:764–776.

50. Wilens TE, Biederman J, Millstein RB, Wozniak J, Hahesy AL, Spencer TJ. Risk for substance use disorders in youths with child- and adolescent-onset bipolar disorder. *J Am Acad Child Adolesc Psychiatry* 1999;**38**:680–685.

51. Huss M, Lehmkuhl U. Methylphenidate and substance abuse: A review of pharmacology, animal, and clinical studies. *J Attention Dis* 2002;**6** (Suppl. 1): S65–S71.

52. Lambert NM, Hartsough, CS. Prospective study of tobacco smoking and substance dependencies among samples of ADHD and non-ADHD participants. *J Learn Disabil* 1998;**31**:533–544.

53. Biederman J, Wilens T, Mick E, Spencer T, Faraone SV. Pharmacotherapy of attention-deficit/hyperactivity disorder reduces risk for substance use disorder. *Pediatrics* 1999;**104**:e20.

54. Mannuzza S, Klein RG, Moulton JLIII. Does stimulant treatment place children at risk for adult substance abuse? A controlled, prospective follow-up study. *J Child Adolesc Psychopharmacol* 2003;**13**:273–282.

55. Wilens TE, Faraone SV, Biederman J, Gunawardene S. Does stimulant therapy of attention-deficit/hyperactivity disorder beget later substance abuse? A meta-analytic review of the literature. *Pediatrics* 2003;**111**:179–185.

56. Faraone SV, Biederman J, Wilens TE, Adamson J. A naturalistic study of the effects of pharmacotherapy on substance use disorders among ADHD adults. *Psychol Med* 2007;**37**:1–10.

57. Kollins SH. ADHD, substance use disorders, and psychostimulant treatment. *J Attention Dis* 2008;**12**:115–125.

58. Schubiner H. Substance abuse in patients with attention-deficit hyperactivity disorder. *CNS Drugs* 2005;**19**:643–655.

59. Garnier LM, Arria AM, Caldeira KM, Vincent KB, O'Grady KE, Wish ED. Sharing and selling of prescription medications in a college student sample. *J Clin Psychiatry* 2010;**71**:262–269.

60. McCabe SE, Knight JR, Teter CJ, Wechsler, H. Non-medical use of prescription stimulants among US college students: prevalence and correlates from a national survey. *Addiction* 2005;**100**:96–106.

61. McCabe SE, Teter CJ, Boyd CJ. The use, misuse and diversion of prescription stimulants among middle and high school students. *Subst Use Misuse* 2004;**39**:1095–1116.

62. Teter CJ, McCabe SE, Boyd CJ, Guthrie SK. Illicit methylphenidate use in an undergraduate student sample: prevalence and risk factors. *Pharmacotherapy* 2003;**23**:609–617.

63. McCabe SE, Teter CJ, Boyd CJ. Medical use, illicit use and diversion of prescription stimulant medication. *J Psychoactive Drugs* 2006;**38**:43–56.

64. Boyd CJ, McCabe SE, Cranford JA, Young A. Adolescents' motivations to abuse prescription medications. *Pediatrics* 2006;**118**:2472–2480.

65. Friedman RA. The changing face of teenage drug abuse – the trend toward prescription drugs. *N Engl J Med* 2006;**354**:1448–1450.

66. Herman-Stahl MA, Krebs CP, Kroutil LA, Heller DC. Risk and protective factors for methamphetamine use and nonmedical use of prescription stimulants among young adults aged 18 to 25. *Addict Behav* 2007;**32**:1003–1015.

67. Office of National Drug Control Policy, Executive Office of the President. Prescription for danger: a report on the troubling trend of prescription and over-the-counter drug abuse among the nation's teens. 2008. Available at: http://www.theantidrug.com/pdfs/prescription_report.pdf.

68. Wu LT, Blazer DG, Patkar AA, Stitzer ML, Wakim PG, Brooner RK. Heterogeneity of stimulant dependence: a national drug abuse treatment clinical trials network study. *Am J Addict* 2009;**18**:206–218.

69. Goldsworthy RC, Mayhorn CB. Prescription medication sharing among adolescents: prevalence, risks, and outcomes. *J Adolesc Health* 2009;**45**:634–637.

70. Hill KP, Sofuoglu M. Biological treatments for amphetamine dependence: recent progress. *CNS Drugs* 2007;**21**:851–869.

71. Simon SL, Richardson K, Dacey J, *et al.* A comparison of patterns of methamphetamine and cocaine use. *J Addict Dis* 2002;**21**:35–44.

72. Estroff TW. *Manual of Adolescent Substance Abuse Treatment.* Washington, DC; London: American Psychiatric Publishing, Inc., 2001.

73. Heal DJ, Cheetham SC, Smith SL. The neuro-pharmacology of ADHD drugs in vivo: insights on efficacy and safety. *Neuropharmacology* 2009;**57**:608–618.

74. Wells KM. The short- and long-term medical effects of methamphetamine on children and adults. In: Covey HC (ed.), *Methamphetamine Crisis: Strategies to Save Addicts, Families, and Communities*. Westport, CT: Praeger Publishers, 2007; pp. 57–74.

75. National Institute on Drug Abuse. (2008) Stimulant ADHD medications: methylphenidate and amphetamine. Available at: www.education.com/reference/article/ref_stimulant_adhd_medication.

76. American Psychiatric Association. *Diagnostic and Statistical Manual of Mental Disorders, Fourth Edition, Text Revision* (DSM-IV-TR) Washington, DC: APA, 2000.

77. American Psychiatric Association. DSM-5 development [website]. Available at: www.dsm5.org.

78. National Institute on Drug Abuse Research Report Series. Prescription Drugs Abuse and Addiction. Available at: http://www.drugabuse.gov/publications/research-reports/prescription-drugs.

79. Barr AM, Markou A. Psychostimulant withdrawal as an inducing condition in animal models of depression. *Neurosci Biobehav Rev* 2005;**29**:675–706.

80. Barr AM, Markou A, Phillips AG. A crash course on psychostimulant withdrawal as a model of depression. *Trends Pharmacol Sci* 2002;**23**:475–482.

81. Allcott JV, Barnhart RA, Mooney LA. Acute lead poisoning in two users of illicit methamphetamine. *JAMA* 1987;**285**:510–511.

82. Anglin MD, Burke C, Perrochet B, Stamper E, Dawud-Noursi S. History of the methamphetamine problem. *J Psychoactive Drugs* 2000;**32**:137–141.

83. Nordahl TE, Salo R, Leamon M. Neuropsychological effects of chronic methamphetamine use on neurotransmitters and cognition: a review. *J Neuropsychiatry Clin Neurosci* 2003;**15**:317–325.

84. Durell TM, Kroutil LA, Crits-Christoph P, Barchha N, VanBrunt DL. Prevalence of nonmedical methamphetamine use in the United States. *Subst Abuse Treat Prev Policy* 2008;**3**:19.

85. McGregor C, Srisurapanont M, Laobhripatr S, Wongtan T, White JM. The nature, time course and severity of methamphetamine withdrawal. *Addiction* 2005;**100**:1320–1329.

86. Schuckit MA. *Drug and Alcohol Abuse, A Clinical Guide to Diagnosis and Treatment*. New York and London: Plenum Medical Book Co., 1995.

87. Upadhyaya HP. Substance use disorder in children and adolescents with attention-deficit/hyperactivity disorder: implications for treatment and role of the primary care physician. *Prim Care Companion J Clin Psychiatry* 2008;**10**:211–221.

88. Wilens TE. Attention-deficit/hyperactivity disorder and the substance use disorders: the nature of the relationship, subtypes at risk, and treatment issues. *Psychiatr Clin N Am* 2004;**27**:283–301.

89. Center for Adolescent Substance Abuse Research. The CRAFFT Screening Tool. 2009. Available at: http://www.ceasar-boston.org/CRAFFT/index.php.

90. Sweet RI, Saules KK. Validity of the Substance Abuse Subtle Screening Inventory-Adolescent Version (SASSI-A). *J Subst Abuse Treat* 2003;**24**:331–340.

91. Kaminer Y, Bukstein O, Tarter RE. The Teen-Addiction Severity Index: rationale and reliability. *Int J Addict* 1991;**26**:219–226.

92. Mahoney JJrd, Kalechstein AD, De LaGarza R2nd, Newton TF. Presence and persistence of psychotic symptoms in cocaine-versus methamphetamine-dependent participants. *Am J Addict* 2008;**17**:83–98.

93. Murphy KR, Adler LA. Assessing attention-deficit/hyperactivity disorder in adults: focus on rating scales. *J Clin Psychiatry* 2004;**65** (Suppl. 3): 12–17.

94. Sysko R, Walsh BT. A systematic review of placebo response in studies of bipolar mania. *J Clin Psychiatry* 2007;**68**:1213–1217.

95. Brooks SJ, Kutcher S. The Kutcher Generalized Social Anxiety Disorder Scale for adolescents: assessment of its evaluative properties over the course of a 16-week pediatric psychopharmacotherapy trial. *J Child Adolesc Psychopharmacol* 2004;**14**:273–286.

96. Mannuzza S, Klein RG, Truong NL, *et al*. Age of methylphenidate treatment initiation in children with ADHD and later substance abuse: prospective follow-up into adulthood. *Am J Psychiatry* 2008;**165**:604–609.

20

Cannabis Use Disorders

Jan Copeland and John Howard

National Cannabis Prevention and Information Centre, University of New South Wales, Sydney, NSW, Australia

INTRODUCTION

Cannabis is the most common illicit drug of dependence in the Western world [1]. The effects of cannabis dependence on health and psychosocial functioning are often under-recognized, and under-treated, in primary healthcare settings and in specialist drug treatment services. Although the short-term negative consequences of cannabis use are fairly well known, the long-term effects of regular cannabis use are less so. Determining the long-term effects of cannabis has been difficult, due to many factors, including high rates of multiple drug use, a long lead time for long-term effects to become apparent, and a lack of literature examining harmful use, although this is now changing.

This evidence base is emerging at a time when there is increasing debate in many countries regarding the regulation of cannabis. A number of jurisdictions have provided for loosely regulated medicinal use of cannabis, some have increased its level of regulation, and some have decriminalized its recreational use. Adolescents are not unaware of the above, or of high-profile sportspeople, entertainers and even politicians making their views and histories of use known. Another consideration of relevance is the past and present use of cannabis by the parents and older siblings of adolescents, and of those who work with them, including health professionals. Much of this reinforces a view that cannabis is a "soft drug" with minimal negative impact on the physical and mental health of individuals. Such views often ignore significant changes in the patterns of cannabis use over the past 30 to 40 years, which include a declining age of initiation of cannabis use, an increase in potency of cannabis due to seed production designed to increase levels of THC at the expense of CBD (see below), use of indoor growing techniques (frequently known as hydroponic but usually involving soil), sinsemilla (growing without seeds and female only plants) [2], and more frequent and heavier use patterns alone and with peers. It is no wonder, therefore, that adolescents receive confusing messages, yet are expected to make informed choices.

TOXICOLOGY AND PHARMACODYNAMICS

Herbal cannabis (known in the United States as marijuana) contains in excess of 300 compounds including more than 60 cannabinoids. The pharmacology of most of these cannabinoids is largely unknown; however, the most potent psychoactive cannabinoid (Δ^9-tetrahydrocannabinol typically abbreviated to THC) has been isolated, synthesized and much studied [3]. THC and other important cannabinoids such as cannabinol (CBN) and cannabidiol (CBD) can have additive, synergistic, or drug opposite effects to THC; making cannabis an extremely complex drug. Cannabinoids interact with the body's endogenous cannabinoid systems and in turn with other neurotransmitters such as the dopaminergic system. It is their actions on these receptor systems that cause dose-related impairment of psychomotor performance, learning and memory, and psychotic symptoms.

In common with other psychoactive drugs, the effects of cannabis depend on the dose, the ratio of THC:CBD, the individual, and the setting. In general, low doses produce a mixture of stimulatory and depressant effects, and high doses are mainly depressant and may be hallucinogenic. The effects of cannabis include euphoria, relaxation, and a feeling of well-being. In addition, there are perceptual distortions such as apparently sharpened senses and altered time sense. Memory, cognition,

Clinical Handbook of Adolescent Addiction, First Edition. Richard Rosner.
© 2013 John Wiley & Sons, Ltd. Published 2013 by John Wiley & Sons, Ltd.

and skilled task-performance are impaired, although subjects may feel confident and highly creative. Peripheral effects include tachycardia, vasodilatation (especially evident in the conjunctiva), hypotension, and initially bronchodilatation. Cannabis also stimulates the appetite and may be antiemetic.

EPIDEMIOLOGY

Population-based studies have consistently revealed that cannabis is the most widely used illicit substance in communities around the world, particularly among young adults aged 20–29 years [1]. It is also the most common illicit drug of dependence in those communities [4,5]. While use appears to be increasing, particularly in developing countries, some developed countries have reported a stabilization of use at lower rates since 2000 after a peak in use during the 1990s [6]. Two consistent correlates of cannabis use are gender and age, with cannabis users typically being younger males. However, gender differences appear to be diminishing among more recent cohorts of users [7]. Two important age-related trends have also become apparent – a decrease in the age of initiation to cannabis use and an apparent prolongation of risk of initiation to cannabis use beyond adolescence [8]. Indigenous communities in the United States [9] and Australia [10] appear to have markedly higher levels of cannabis use, particularly daily use, than the non-indigenous members of their communities. The epidemiology of cannabis use amongst these groups, however, is at an early stage of development.

Since the 1980s, a number of large-scale epidemiological studies internationally have produced estimates of cannabis use disorders. Data from the National Epidemiologic Survey on Alcohol and Related Conditions (NESARC) study show the prevalence of 12-month and lifetime DSM-IV (*Diagnostic and Statistical Manual of Mental Disorders, Fourth Edition*) cannabis abuse (1.1% and 7.2%) and dependence (0.3% and 1.3%) [11]. Using data from two large representative samples, Compton and colleagues claim that despite the stability in the overall prevalence of use, the prevalence of cannabis use disorder in the United States in 2001–02 was greater than in 1991–92 most notably in young black men and women and young Hispanic men [8]. The most recent Australian study of cannabis use disorder in the community reported the prevalence of lifetime and 12-month cannabis abuse to be 3.8% and 0.5%; and the prevalence of lifetime and 12-month cannabis dependence to be 2.7% and 0.5%. Cannabis dependence was significantly higher in males, younger adults, and those who were never married. Cannabis abuse was more prevalent among men and younger adults [12].

On the basis of such studies it has been estimated that approximately 1 in 10 people who had ever used cannabis will become dependent; risk increases markedly with frequency of use, with 50% of daily users likely to become dependent [13]. Rates of dependence tend to be higher among young people [8,10], who may be significantly more likely than adults to develop cannabis dependence for a given dose; early initiators may be particularly at risk. It has been estimated that among young people who have used cannabis, one in six or seven will become dependent [14].

Relatively little is known about the natural history of cannabis dependence. The onset of dependence most commonly occurs in adolescence or young adulthood, within 10 years of initiation [11,14]. Studies have documented the onset of clinical symptoms, commencing with symptoms of loss of control and continued use despite harm, with withdrawal experienced at a later age by relatively fewer users [15].

POTENTIAL HARMS ASSOCIATED WITH CANNABIS USE

While cannabis has a very low acute toxicity and is only a minor contributor to drug-related mortality, its major public health significance resides in its association with morbidity [16]. While cannabis dependence is the most obvious harm, there is a growing body of evidence of subtle cognitive impairment affecting attention, memory, and the organization and integration of complex information as a result of cannabis use [17]. As cannabis is almost always smoked, there is an obvious risk of adverse respiratory effects, such as chronic bronchitis. Some studies have also identified changes in lung tissue that may be precursors to cancer [18]. In addition, many smokers mix cannabis with tobacco, and are regular tobacco smokers, and there is evidence that some of the negative respiratory effects of cannabis and tobacco may be additive [19]. This coexisting cannabis and tobacco use may complicate the management of smoking cessation, where cannabis use prompts relapse to tobacco use, with the reverse also reported in cannabis treatment populations.

Certain groups and life stages may be at a higher risk of developing the adverse acute and chronic effects of cannabis. These include adolescence, pregnancy, those with respiratory or cardiovascular disease, or those with a comorbid mental health disorder [20]. The issue of the comorbidity with other substance use disorders (e.g. cannabis and alcohol use disorders), or substance use and other mental health disorders (e.g. substance use disorders and anxiety or depression) is a clinical concern and occurs relatively commonly [21,22]. There is increasing agreement that cannabis plays a "component cause" role that is neither sufficient nor necessary in the development and course of schizophrenia and other psychotic disorders [23]. That is, there is not yet compelling evidence that there is a direct causal association between cannabis use and schizophrenia or other psychoses. Recent prospective studies among clinical populations, however, do demonstrate that cannabis use is associated with an adverse course of psychotic symptoms in schizophrenia, and vice versa, even when other clinical, substance use, and demographic characteristics are considered [24].

It is clear, however, that early onset, and frequent and heavy use of cannabis exacerbate underlying mental health conditions, including schizophrenia, manifesting as increased symptom number and severity, non-compliance with treatment, and more frequent hospitalizations. Given the confusing media and lobby group materials concerning the potentially antipsychotic and anxiolytic properties of CBD (which is typically at very low levels in street cannabis [2]) adolescents may be led to attempt to find relief from their symptoms via "natural" means despite also recognizing that this often comes at a significant cost to their mental health and well-being as they increase exposure to THC.

DIAGNOSTIC CRITERIA

Assessing dependence and abuse can be an important clinical tool for communicating with other professionals, communicating the nature of the issue to the client, and assessing outcomes. It can be done using structured clinical interviews and questionnaires.

Acute Cannabis Use

The diagnostic systems each describe cannabis intoxication. According to the *DSM-IV-TR intoxication*, the essential feature of cannabis intoxication is the development of behavioral and psychological disturbances (e.g., impaired motor coordination, euphoria, anxiety, sensation of slowed time, impaired judgment, social withdrawal) during, or shortly after, cannabis use. In addition, there are characteristic signs and symptoms, two (or more) of which develop within 2 hours of cannabis use, including: conjunctival injection; increased appetite; dry mouth, or tachycardia – none of which are due to a medical disorder [25].

The pattern of onset and duration of cannabis intoxication is variable. If cannabis is smoked, intoxication usually occurs within minutes and lasts approximately 3–4 hours. When cannabis is consumed orally, onset may take hours and the effects may be longer lasting. The DSM-IV-TR notes that the magnitude of effects will vary with dose, administration route, and personal

characteristics, such as tolerance of and sensitivity to cannabis.

Importantly, the DSM-IV-TR adds a qualifier, "with perceptual disturbances," to cannabis intoxication in which the individual experiences hallucinations with intact reality testing, or in whom auditory, visual, or tactile illusions occur in the absence of a delirium. In other words, this qualifier is noted only when the user realizes that the perceptual disturbances are induced by cannabis use. This experience is distinguished from substance-induced psychotic disorder [25].

ICD-10 acute intoxication: Acute intoxication is a transient condition that follows the administration of alcohol or other psychoactive substance and results in disturbances in level of consciousness, cognition, perception, affect, behavior, or other psychophysiological functions. The *International Classification of Diseases, 10th Revision* (ICD-10) specifies that this diagnosis should be a main diagnosis only in cases in which intoxication occurs in the absence of more persistent alcohol- or drug-related problems. When such problems exist, precedence should be given to diagnoses of harmful use (f1x.1), dependence syndrome (f1x.2), or psychotic disorder (f1x.5) [26].

The diagnostic criteria for cannabis use disorders are set out in the two major classification systems. These criteria are identical to other psychoactive substance use disorders (except that they relate to the individual's cannabis use) and are discussed in other chapters. It should be noted that the DSM-IV-TR includes a disorder specific to cannabis use, whereas the ICD-10 specifies only a generic diagnosis.

Clinical studies over the last decade have produced evidence for a cannabis withdrawal syndrome. Currently, these symptoms are not documented in the DSM-IV-TR or the ICD-10 although this syndrome is expected to be addressed in the next version of DSM. The proportion of clients reporting cannabis withdrawal in treatment studies has ranged from 50% to 95% [24]. Symptoms typically emerge after 1–3 of days of abstinence, peak between days 2 and 6, and typically last from 4 to 14 days [27], with sleep difficulties often taking some weeks to ameliorate. The most common symptoms include nightmares and strange dreams, difficulty getting to and staying asleep, night sweats, irritability, and diminished appetite. The severity of withdrawal symptoms has been linked with difficulty achieving abstinence [24,28,29]. Discussing withdrawal may therefore be an important aspect of treatment. The use of psychoeducation to identify typical withdrawal symptoms and patterns, so that dealing with withdrawal can be incorporated into a treatment plan, is recommended. The first valid and reliable measure of cannabis withdrawal, the Cannabis Withdrawal Scale[30], has now been developed and is available for clinical and research purposes.

Adolescence and Cannabis Dependence

Longitudinal studies of young cannabis users through adolescence to their early twenties have reported that weekly cannabis use in adolescence marked a threshold for increased risk of daily and dependent use at 20 years [31]. In addition, even occasional use in early adolescence is associated with later drug use and poorer educational outcomes [32].

Among adolescents (aged 13–19 years) presenting to an emergency department for a non-substance-related injury, a US study reported that 7.5% met criteria for cannabis use disorder and a further 7.9% for alcohol and cannabis use disorders. The frequency of cannabis use was the best predictor of meeting criteria for disorder [33].

CLINICAL PRESENTATION AND RELEVANT ASSESSMENT ISSUES

Adolescent cannabis users rarely present for specialist treatment [6]. As they are more likely to be seen in educational, criminal justice, or general healthcare settings, screening for the presence of cannabis-related problems is important for the following reasons:

1. Cannabis users may seek assistance for problems, such as poor sleep, anger, depression, anxiety, relationship issues, or respiratory problems, and not mention that they use cannabis.
2. Early detection of cannabis-related issues is important in preventing escalating problems.
3. Only a small minority of cannabis users actively seek some form of intervention to address their cannabis use. Although many cannabis users have only minor problems with cannabis, a significant proportion do experience significant dependence and related harms that affect them and others.
4. Cannabis use is very common in the community, especially among 15- to 30-year-olds and individuals using other illicit substances, and those with mental health conditions. Patients presenting with new persistent respiratory conditions such as a wheeze or cough should be screened for cannabis use as a contributing factor.

A valid and reliable screening tool specifically designed for the detection of current and 12-month cannabis use-related problems, such as the Cannabis Use Problems Identification Test (CUPIT), is recommended [34]. Additional tools for the management of adolescent cannabis-related problems and monitoring of treatment outcome include the five-item Severity of Dependence Scale (SDS) [35] and the adolescent version of the Cannabis Problems Questionnaire (CPQ-A) [36]. These measures may be downloaded at www.ncpic.org.au.

The assessment of adolescents who use substances has been covered extensively in other chapters. In addition to any standardized assessment protocols and procedures, it is helpful to ensure that the pattern of substance use of the adolescent is considered within a broad understanding of the context within which the adolescent lives their life. Important domains to investigate when evaluating an adolescent's cannabis use include:

- What they get from cannabis use – initially and currently, and the "less good" things they experience from their cannabis use.
- Context of use patterns – percentage of use alone and with others, times of day, locations of use, age mix of those they use with, any coercion, any rituals.
- Risks associated with their cannabis use – location, mix of co-users, means of use – bong, or joint.
- Triggers for use: moods/feeling, people (family, friends, peers, others – conflict); places; odors, for example, room and clothing not cleaned; implements and waste around; visual stimuli such as posters or mixing bowls.
- Any perceived benefits that might come from reduction/cessation of use, perceived barriers/losses in making a change.

Below are two common case presentations from very different perspectives; one in a sexual health clinic setting and the other a specialist residential drug treatment setting. While the micro skills to address the clinical issues raised are discussed elsewhere a brief checklist that outlines key issues in these vignettes is included for consideration.

Clinical Vignette 1

"Melissa" is a 14-year-old female who lives with her parents and an older sister and a younger brother. She decided to see a doctor at a youth health service to obtain contraception. She became sexually active at age 13. She told her doctor that she had been using cannabis and did not see it as problematic. Her doctor did not share this view, but when she began to explore Melissa's cannabis use, Melissa became rather hostile and attempted to close off the issue. Employing a motivational enhancement style of interviewing, the doctor was able to engage with Melissa, who revealed that she liked cannabis, feeling it made her more sociable and relaxed. She was using four or five times a week with other similarly aged young women and a group of boys aged 14 to 19, and said she had about two joints on average each time she used. She often stayed over with friends, with parental approval, where she and her friends had parties, and roamed streets and parks. Her "boyfriend" was a 19-year-old male who appeared to be cannabis dependent and unwilling to use condoms. She believed she had no difficulties with her cannabis use, and that she was still doing well at school, even if her grades were not quite as good as they had been.

Her parents had used cannabis in their youth and regarded themselves as "modern" parents who could relate at the level of their children. They appeared to have a *laissez-faire* view of parental control, limit setting, and behavior. They knew that Melissa had tried cannabis and was sexually active, but not the extent of either activity. They had both been sexually active at her age, and had begun drug experimentation at that time. They believed that cannabis was a "soft drug," but did caution their children not to let drugs dominate their lives.

This case raises a number of issues including:

- Child protection – is there a mandatory reporting issue in your jurisdiction for under-age sexual activity?
- Exploring Melissa's relationship with her "boyfriend," his irresponsibility, and their peer group.
- What approach to use to engage Melissa in a more detailed exploration of her cannabis use and beliefs about cannabis?
- Whether to opt for: work only with Melissa using cognitive-behavioral therapy (CBT); a family intervention alone; both family work in addition to individual work with Melissa; or work at times with the whole family, at others with the parents, and at times with Melissa (e.g., Multi-Dimensional Family Therapy (MDTF) or other multi-system approach).
- Gaining Melissa's agreement to meet with her family, irrespective of any child protection service involvement.
- Exploring and addressing the cannabis use of her parents.

Clinical Vignette 2

"Sam" is a 17-year-old male from an Arabic-speaking background who was referred by a youth drug court. He was assessed as meeting criteria for cannabis dependence (SDS score of 13) and methamphetamine and alcohol use. He had no significant physical health concerns. He lives with his mother, who speaks little English, and older brother, who also uses cannabis; his parents separated when he was 8 years old. His father had a history of substance use, gambling and mental health problems, and made inconsistent contact with his sons. Sam said he loved his mother, but said that she knew little about him or his activities, and that she had minimal control over him. As his behavior led to increasing involvement by police and youth justice officers, Sam's mother appears to have become significantly depressed, with frequent weeping and admonitions for Sam to "be good," but becoming incapable of influencing him away from negative peers, drug use, and crime.

Sam liked school, but began to be regarded as very distractible, with poor concentration and frequent unexplained absences. He was asked to leave his school at age 15, and was in casual employment sporadically. He began using cannabis at age 12 and methamphetamines at 14. At assessment he reported daily use of cannabis – smoking about 70 cones (water pipes) a day. He binged on crystal methamphetamine about once a month, and drank alcohol on average 4 days a week. Sam had a long history of criminal offences including robbery, assault, and drug possession.

During his initial assessment, Sam reported experiencing depression, anxiety, sleep difficulties, and, in the past, some auditory and visual hallucinations. He reported that cannabis helped to calm him. Soon after admission to the residential program, Sam indicated that he was hearing things, reported a significant increase in paranoia, a high level of agitation, and erratic moods. He reported vivid dreams. Auditory and visual hallucinations had returned and increased and were telling him not to talk to counselors. Some of his symptoms were consistent with withdrawal from his heavy cannabis use, but also with a psychotic condition. Sam was provisionally diagnosed with drug-induced psychosis by a psychiatrist, but with the view that paranoid schizophrenia was more likely.

Sam's Care Plan issues include:

- Clarification of mental health diagnosis/diagnoses.
- Need for completion of withdrawal to obtain clarity regarding persisting symptoms.
- What medication(s) might be most appropriate to assist him manage his mental health diagnoses and concerns, including sleep?
- Helping Sam to accept his diagnosis and comply with treatment, including medication.
- How to ensure safety for Sam, staff, and other young people in the residential setting when his symptoms are more acute, and clarifying helpful responses for staff and other residents.
- How to engage the family members, if possible, and address issues of culture, language, mental health, and who should and could provide such an intervention.

TREATMENT

Despite these high levels of problem use, as with other illicit drugs, only a minority seek assistance from a health professional [11]. The demand for treatment for cannabis use disorder, nonetheless, is increasing internationally, particularly among adolescents. Adult cannabis users who seek professional help typically report numerous problems related to their use, some clearly related to core dependence criteria, such as an inability to stop or cut down and withdrawal symptoms, and others such as relationship, family, and financial difficulties, health concerns, and poor life satisfaction [37,38].

While there is an extensive literature on the epidemiology of cannabis use, the evidence base on the management of cannabis use disorder is embryonic compared with that for nicotine, alcohol, and opioids. There have been so few randomized controlled trials (RCTs) that no meta-analyses have been conducted on the question. There are two population groups for which the issue of interventions for cannabis use disorder is especially problematical. Cannabis use is most commonly initiated in adolescence, when heavy, regular use is of concern, and voluntary treatment-seeking is rare. Second, those with psychotic disorders are also particularly vulnerable to the effects of cannabis and are difficult to engage, retain, and successfully treat for cannabis dependence [6].

In recent years increased attention has been given to developing general substance use treatment models that take cognizance of the issues and developmental stage of young people, rather than simply generalizing (potentially age-inappropriate) adult programs to this group [28]. Manualized therapies have become available for dissemination to the field, and evidence is emerging for the efficacy of a number of treatment models including structured, family-based therapies, and motivational enhancement and cognitive-behavioral interventions [38].

The largest randomized trial for adolescent cannabis use, the Cannabis Youth Treatment (CYT) study, was a multi-site intervention study of 600 young cannabis users aged between 12 and 18 years who reported one or more DSM-IV cannabis abuse or dependence criteria [39]. Participants received one of five outpatient interventions of various types, ranging from a relatively brief five sessions of motivational enhancement therapy coupled with cognitive-behavioral therapy (MET/CBT) to up to 22 sessions of Family Support Network therapy that included aspects of CBT, family therapy, and additional case management contact. Overall, the clinical outcomes were similar across conditions. All five CYT interventions showed significant pre-/post-treatment effects; compared with baseline, at 12 months there was an increase in reported abstinence, and decreases in symptoms of cannabis abuse and dependence [40].

Researchers are also investigating the use of Contingency Management(CM) in combination with MET-CBT for adolescents with cannabis-related problems. Preliminary data from an initial RCT suggest that the MET/CBT + CM improved cannabis abstinence rates post-treatment compared with MET/CBT combined with weekly parental psychoeducation [41]. This outcome supports the findings of other studies reporting positive outcomes for CM incorporated in multi-systemic therapy or MET/CBT among juvenile offenders [42–44]. Multidimensional Family Therapy (MDFT) is another approach with an evidence base, much of which comes from trials and RCTs with young offenders, often from minority and disadvantaged groups with multiple and complex needs. MDFT therapists form numerous therapeutic alliances; engage with the adolescent, the parents, the whole family, and even the adolescent and their peer groups. The interventions are intensive and time limited, usually 4–6 months [45].

The studies above relate to adolescents or young adults who present for treatment, albeit most via some coercion from family, schools, juvenile justice systems, police, or courts. This population represents a very small percentage of young people who use substances and may constitute a more troubled population. There is a need for active secondary prevention efforts targeting young people at an early stage of their cannabis-using career in an effort to minimize problematic use, promote problem recognition, and facilitate informed choice regarding cannabis use and its potential consequences.

There have been a number of studies exploring brief, opportunistic, motivational interventions among UK college students. While initially encouraging, these non-cannabis-specific interventions did not maintain an effect over time [46]. In the United States and Australia, studies of brief (2–3 sessions) MET interventions, the Teen Marijuana Check-up [47] and the Adolescent Cannabis Check-up [48,49], have been reported. The school-based Teen Marijuana Check-up [47] was compared with a 3-month assessment-only waitlist control, and showed reductions in cannabis use, but no significant differences between groups. The Adolescent Cannabis Check-up (ACCU) recruited from the general community and was compared with a 3-month waitlist control group. At the 3-month follow-up, there were significant between-group differences in levels of cannabis use and dependence that favored the ACCU group [49]. A limitation of the current brief intervention literature is that follow-up periods have been relatively short and it remains unclear whether multiple iterations of the intervention over a relatively long period would aid to entrench or support the short-term gains observed. While the findings of adolescent interventions are encouraging, as with adults, the rates of continuous abstinence are low. There is much yet to be learned about effective and sustainable interventions for adolescents with cannabis-related problems and dependence.

Primary Healthcare Settings

Young, dependent cannabis users are heavy consumers of healthcare services, with around one-third of the participants in one study having seen a medical practitioner in the preceding 2 weeks, and 19% having been hospitalized in the last year [50]. This presentation pattern shows that nurses and other primary healthcare providers have high rates of contact with people experiencing severe cannabis dependence and are ideally placed for opportunistic assessment and intervention. In most cases, individuals will not present in these settings requesting help for cannabis. This is where screening tools and making enquiries about lifestyle issues (which include drug use) that may contribute to presenting health concerns are important. Whilst some clients may avoid conversations about their drug use, others will be relieved that they did not have to bring it up. In addition, clinicians and general practitioners may need to look out for signs that clients are making subtle inquiries to see whether it is safe to talk about cannabis use. At a minimum, such settings are encouraged to provide pamphlets, and basic screening and detection are strongly encouraged [51]. Examples of psychoeducational materials and related materials can be accessed at the National Cannabis Prevention and Information Centre (www.ncpic.org.au).

Much can be done to begin to engage with an adolescent presenting with cannabis use-related difficulties in primary healthcare, and also in settings, such as youth-serving organizations, by frontline workers. A brief motivational approach can be utilized, which aims at engaging with an adolescent around his or her cannabis use, within a conversational style. If it is within the role of the health or other professional, use of any of the evidence-informed therapeutic approaches briefly outlined above could follow; however, it is likely that such approaches will be more effective if initial attention is paid to engaging with the adolescent.

Rationale for a Motivational Approach

Health professionals may feel ill-prepared to engage in meaningful conversations with adolescents accessing their services with regard to reduction or cessation of cannabis use. A motivational enhancement approach can assist in opportunistic interactions with out-of-home/school young people (ones with multiple and complex needs) aged 14 to 24 who might be considering quitting or reducing their cannabis use.

The Approach

In general conversation, the topic of cannabis use may arise and what is said might indicate some possible difficulties associated with its use. At that stage, a health worker may choose to move to a more "motivational enhancement" approach. This, in the main, involves consideration of five key questions within as normal a conversational flow as possible. These "Five Key Questions" are outlined in Box 20.1.

Box 20.1   Five key questions in motivational interviewing

1. *What do you like/enjoy about your use of cannabis*? [exhaust reasons]

2. *OK, and what do you like less about your use of cannabis*? [attempt to discount some, and give appropriate information as necessary]

3. *You say you like . . . ., but are less happy about* . . . . [summary] . . . .*have you thought about what could be good about making a change in your use of cannabis*?

4. *OK, but what might be some less good things about making a change in your use of cannabis*?

5. If the adolescent is not interested in change at this stage: *So, you don't seem too keen on making a change in your use of cannabis at this stage. Here is some info that you might find interesting or useful. Also I am wondering what might lead you to rethink this decision at some stage*?

Add: Before we finish, I would like to give you some info that you might find helpful and some contacts where you might get some help if you reconsider your decision, and remember I am happy to talk with you again about this if you want.

OR

If young person is interested in change: *So we talked a lot about what you like and don't like so much about your use of cannabis, and what you might gain and lose from changing your use. Before we finish, I would like to give you some info that you might find helpful and some contacts where you might get some help in making the changes you are thinking about.*

If is it part of the health worker's role to provide brief interventions for adolescents wishing to address their cannabis use-related issues, the worker could then continue the conversation as follows:

We did not actually talk about how much cannabis you actually use . . . so, can you tell me how many days a week you use?

Naturally, the actual wording of the questions will be determined by the real world "style" of the health worker and take into account the setting and the situation of the adolescent. However, there should be an attempt to ensure respect and empathy and to indicate that the adolescent's use of cannabis is not mindless and that they recognize the benefits and "less good" aspects of its use. The approach also indicates that the health worker understands that change is difficult, and while possibly bringing benefits (never guaranteed) there are "costs" associated with the change process [52].

Pharmacotherapy for Cannabis Use Disorders

Studies on medications for treating cannabis use disorders are even more sparse than those for behavioral treatments. There are no published RCTs of pharmacological interventions for cannabis use disorders among treatment-seeking cannabis-dependent individuals. As a result there are no US Food and Drug Administration (FDA)-approved medications specifically for the management of cannabis use disorder. A small number of human laboratory studies and a small clinical trial exploring the potential of various medications have been conducted [53]. The focus of these studies has largely been withdrawal management.

To date, the most promising findings have been with an agonist medication, oral THC. Both inpatient and outpatient laboratory studies have shown that oral THC dose-dependently reduces or suppresses cannabis withdrawal symptoms [42,54]. One study with a CB1 selective cannabinoid receptor antagonist, SR141716 (rimonabant), demonstrated that it successfully blocks the acute psychological and physiological effects of smoked cannabis and is well tolerated [55]. This drug is no longer licensed in most jurisdictions. Additional agents that have been tested in lab studies or open-label trials include atomoxetine [56], nefazodone, buspirone,

divalproex [53], lithium carbonate [57], and the combination of oral THC and lofexidine (an orphan drug) [58]. Of these studies, only the findings from the THC and lofexidine combination study show substantial promise.

In addition to these promising medications, future adjunctive pharmacotherapies might focus on the neurophysiology of cannabis withdrawal and craving, and also explore medications that target comorbid disorders such as depression and psychosis. Medications containing THC and CBD (*Sativex*) via buccal spray are also extremely promising and are being currently trialed.

Treatment and Comorbid Mental Health Conditions

One of the most challenging clinical issues is the management of comorbid schizophrenia and cannabis dependence [59]. Moreover, the few studies of interventions among this group have not been specific to adolescents. With little evidence-based pharmacotherapy for comorbid schizophrenia and cannabis dependence, the use of psychological interventions and shared care with mental health and substance use disorder treatment services is central to their optimal management [60].

A study of patients with first episode schizophrenia randomized participants to either a cannabis-focused intervention using a combined cannabis and psychosis therapy (CAP) or a clinical control condition of psychoeducation (PE). There were no significant differences between the CAP and PE groups for cannabis use at end of treatment and 6 months post-intervention. Similarly, there were no significant group differences for psychopathology and functional ratings at follow-up [61].

It appears, therefore, that this is an especially challenging group to engage and retain in treatment, with poorer prognoses should cannabis smoking be maintained [62]. In conclusion, clinical recommendations for the management of substance use in the context of severe and persistent mental illness rest with integrated shared care or dual diagnosis services, in which the critical components are assertive outreach, motivational interventions, skilled counseling, social support interventions, a comprehensive and long-term perspective, and cultural sensitivity and competence.

SUMMARY POINTS

There is a growing demand for the treatment of cannabis use disorders and a paucity of evidence on best practice interventions. The targeted screening of high-risk individuals such as clients of mental health services, patients presenting with respiratory and other smoking-related complaints to general medical practices, juvenile justice populations, and those with other substance use disorders would be useful to identify those with earlier stage cannabis use problems for motivational and brief cognitive-behavioral interventions. Clinicians are sometimes reluctant to intervene with cannabis use disorders. A small study in the United Kingdom [63] designed to stimulate general practitioners' incorporation of cannabis-related clinical enquiry in their practice, found that a brief motivational interview led to more positive attitudes and greater clinical activity up to 3 months later.

For those seeking treatment, relatively brief CBT and CM have strong evidence of success for adolescents, and structured, family-based interventions may increase the potency of these interventions for adolescents. Among those involved in the juvenile justice system and those with severe, persistent mental illness, longer and more intensive therapies provided by interdisciplinary teams may be required.

Acknowledgements

The National Cannabis Prevention and Information Centre, at the University of New South Wales, is funded by the Australian Government. There is no conflict of interest to declare.

References

1. United Nations Office on Drugs and Crime. *2010 World Drug Report*. New York: United Nations, 2010.
2. Potter DJ, Clark P, Brown, MB. Potency of D9-THC and other cannabinoids in cannabis in England in 2005: Implications for psychoactivity and pharmacology. *J Forensic Sci* 2008;**53**:1–5.
3. Ashton CH. Pharmacology and effects of cannabis: a brief review. *Brit J Psychiatry* 2001;**178**:101–106.
4. Anthony J, Warner L, Kessler R. Comparative epidemiology of dependence on tobacco, alcohol, controlled substance and inhalants: basic findings from the National Comorbidity Survey. *Exp Clin Psychopharmacol* 1994;**2**:244–268.
5. Swift W, Hall W, Tesson M. Cannabis use and dependence among Australian adults: results from the National Survey of Mental Health and Wellbeing. *Addiction* 2001;**96**:737–748.
6. Copeland J, Swift W. Cannabis use disorder: epidemiology and management. *Int Rev Psychiatry* 2009;**21**:96–103.
7. Degenhardt L, Chiu W-T, Sampson N, *et al.* Toward a global view of alcohol, tobacco, cannabis, and cocaine use: Findings from the WHO World Mental Health Survey. *PLoS Med* 2008;**5**:12–24.
8. Compton WM. Grant BF, Colliver JD, *et al.* Prevalence of marijuana use disorders in the United States: 1991–1992 and 2001–2002. *JAMA* 2004;**291**:2114–2121.
9. Beauvais F, Jumper-Thurman P, Helm H. Surveillance of drug use among American-Indian adolescents: patterns over 25 years. *J Adolesc Health* 2004;**34**:393–500.
10. Clough AR, Lee KSK, Caurney S, *et al.* Changes in cannabis use and its consequences over 3 years in a remote indigenous population in northern Australia. *Addiction* 2006;**10**:696–705.
11. Stinson FS, Ruan WJ, Pickering R, Grant BF. Cannabis use disorders in the USA: prevalence, correlates and co-morbidity. *Psychol Med* 2006;**3**:1447–1460.
12. Slade T, Johnston A, Teesson M, *et al.The Mental Health of Australians 2 Report on the 2007 National Survey of Mental Health and Wellbeing*. Canberra: Department of Health and Ageing, 2009.
13. Hall W, Pacula RL. *Cannabis Use and Dependence: Public Health and Public Policy*. Cambridge: Cambridge University Press, 2003.
14. Anthony J. The epidemiology of cannabis dependence. In: Roffman RA, Stephens RS (eds), *Cannabis Dependence: Its Nature, Consequences and Treatment*. Cambridge: Cambridge University Press, 2006.
15. Rosenberg MF, Anthony JC. Early clinical manifestations of cannabis dependence in a community sample. *Drug Alcohol Depend* 2001;**6**:123–131.
16. Degenhardt L, Hall WD, Lynskey M, *et al.* Should burden of disease estimates include cannabis use as a risk factor for psychosis? *PLoS Med* 2009;**6**:e10000133.
17. Solowij N. *Cannabis and Cognitive Functioning*. Cambridge: Cambridge University Press, 1998.
18. Tashkin DP. Cannabis effects on the respiratory system. In: Kalant H, Corrigall W, Hall W, Smart R (eds), *The Health Effects of Cannabis*. Toronto: Centre for Addiction and Mental Health, 1999.
19. Taylor D, Fergusson D, Milne B, *et al.* A longitudinal study of the effects of tobacco and cannabis exposure on lung function in young adults. *Addiction* 2002;**97**:1055–1061.
20. Swift W, Copeland J, Lenton S. Cannabis and harm reduction. Harm Reduction Digest. *Drug Alcohol Rev* 2000;**19**:101–112.
21. Andrews G, Hall W, Teeson M, Henderson S. *The Mental Health of Australians National Survey of Mental Health and Well-being Report 2*. Canberra: Mental Health Branch, Commonwealth Department of Health and Aged Care, 1999.
22. Degenhardt L, Hall W, Lynskey M. Testing hypotheses about the relationship between cannabis use and psychosis. *Drug Alcohol Depend* 2003;**71**:37–48.
23. D'Souza D, Sewell RA, Ranganathan M. Cannabis and psychosis/schizophrenia: human studies. *Eur Arch Clin Neurosci* 2009;**259**:413–431.

24. Budney, AJ, Hughes JR., The cannabis withdrawal syndrome. *Curr Opin Psychiatry* 2006;**19**:233–238.

25. American Psychiatric Association. *Diagnostic and Statistical Manual of Mental Disorders, 4th edition, Text Revision*. Washington, DC: APA, 2000.

26. World Health Organization. The ICD-10 classification of mental and behavioral disorders: diagnostic criteria for research. Geneva: WHO, 1993.

27. Budney AJ, Moore B, Vandrey RG, Hughes JR. The time course and significance of cannabis withdrawal. *J Abnorm Psychol* 2003;**112**:393–402.

28. Stephens RS, Roffman RA, Simpson E. Adult cannabis users seeking treatment. *J Consult Clin Psychol* 1993;**61**:1100–1104.

29. Copeland J, Swift W, Roffman R, Stephens R. A randomised controlled trial of brief cognitive-behavioural interventions for cannabis use disorder. *J Subst Abuse Treat* 2001;**21**:55–64.

30. Allsop D, Norberg M, Copeland J, Fu S, Budney AJ. The Cannabis Withdrawal Scale development: patterns and predictors of cannabis withdrawal and distress. *Drug Alcohol Depend* 2011;**119**:123–129.

31. Coffey C, Carlin JB, Lynskey M, *et al*. Adolescent precursors of cannabis dependence: findings from the Victorian Adolescent Health cohort study. *Brit J Psychiatry* 2003;**102**:330–336.

32. Degenhardt L, Coffey C, Carlin CR, *et al*. Outcomes of occasional cannabis use in adolescence: 10 year follow up study in Victoria, Australia. *Brit J Psychiatry* 2010;**196**:290–295.

33. Chung T, Colby SM, O'Leary TA, Barnett NP, Monti PM. Screening for cannabis use disorders in an adolescent emergency department sample. *Drug Alcohol Depend* 2003;**70**:177–186.

34. Bashford J, Flett R, Copeland J. The Cannabis Use Problems Identification Test (CUPIT): development, reliability, concurrent and predictive validity among adolescents and adults. *Addiction* 2010;**105**:615–625.

35. Martin G, Copeland J, Gates P, Gilmour S. The Severity of Dependence Scale (SDS) in an adolescent population of cannabis users: Reliability, validity and diagnostic cut-off. *Drug Alcohol Depend* 2006;**83**:90–93.

36. Martin G, Copeland J, Gilmour S, Swift W. The Adolescent Cannabis Problems Questionnaire: psychometric properties. *Addict Behav* 2006;**31**:2238–2248.

37. Copeland J, Swift W, Rees V. Clinical profile of participants in a brief intervention for cannabis use disorder. *J Subst Abuse Treat* 2001;**20**:45–52.

38. Pumariega AJ, Rodriguez L, Kilgus MD. Substance abuse among adolescents: current perspectives. *Addict Dis Treat* 2004;**3**:145–155.

39. Waldron HB, Turner CW. Evidence-based psychosocial treatments for adolescent substance abuse. *J Clin Child Adolesc Psychol* 2008;**37**:238–261.

40. Dennis M, Godley SH, Diamond G, *et al*. The Cannabis Youth Treatment (CYT) study: main findings from two randomized trials. *J Subst Abuse Treat* 2004;**27**: 197–213.

41. Kamon JL, Budney AJ, Stanger C. A contingency management intervention for adolescent marijuana abuse and conduct problems. *J Am Acad Child Adolesc Psychiatry* 2005;**44**:513–521.

42. Henggeler SW, Halliday-Boykins CA, Cunningham PB, et al. Juvenile drug court: enhancing outcomes by integrating evidence-based treatments. *J Consult Clin Psychol* 2006;**74**:42–54.

43. Carroll KM, Easton CJ, Nich C, *et al.* The use of contingency management and motivational/skills-building therapy to treat young adults with marijuana dependence. *J Consult Clin Psychol* 2006;**74**:955–966.

44. Sinha R, Easton C, Renee-Aubin L, Carroll KM. Engaging young probation-referred marijuana-abusing individuals in treatment: a pilot trial. *Am J Addictions* 2003;**12**:314–323.

45. Liddle H, Dakof G, Turner R, Henderson C, Greenbaum P. Treating adolescent drug abuse: a randomized trial comparing multidimensional family therapy and cognitive behaviour therapy. *Addiction* 2008;**103**:1660–1670.

46. McCambridge J, Slym RL, Strang J. Randomized controlled trial of motivational interviewing compared with drug information and advice for early intervention among young cannabis users. *Addiction* 2008;**103**:1809–1818.

47. Walker DD, Roffman RA, Stephens RS, *et al.* Motivational enhancement therapy for adolescent marijuana users: a preliminary randomized controlled trial. *J Consult Clin Psychol* 2006;**74**:628–632.

48. Martin G, Copeland J, Swift W. The Adolescent Cannabis Check-up: feasibility of a brief intervention for young cannabis users. *J Subst Use Treat* 2005;**29**:207–213.

49. Martin G, Copeland J. The Adolescent Cannabis Check-up: randomised trial of a brief intervention for young cannabis users. *J Subst Use Treat* 2008;**34**:407–414.

50. Copeland J, Rees V, Swift W. Health concerns and help-seeking among a sample entering treatment for cannabis dependence.Correspondence. *Aust Fam Physician* 1999;**28**:540–541.

51. Copeland J, Frewen A, Elkins K. *Management of Cannabis Use Disorder and Related Issues: a Clinician's Guide*. Sydney: National Cannabis Prevention and Information Centre, 2010.

52. National Cannabis Prevention and Information Centre. Young people and cannabis use training package. Available from: http://ncpic.org.au/workforce/alcohol-and-other-drug-workers/young-people-training-package/.

53. Hart C. Increasing treatment options for cannabis dependence: a review of potential pharmacotherapies. *Drug Alcohol Depend* 2005;**80**:147–159.

54. Haney M, Hart C, Vosburg S, *et al.* Marijuana withdrawal in humans: effects of oral THC or divalproex. *Neuropsychopharmacology* 2004;**29**:158–170.

55. Huestis M, Gorelick D, Heishman S, *et al.* Blockade effects of smoked marijuana by the CB1-selective cannabinoid receptor antagonist SR141716. *Arch Gen Psychiatry* 2001;**58**:322–328.

56. Tirado A, Goldman M, Lynch K, Kampman K, O'Brien C. Atomoxetine for treatment of marijuana dependence: a report on the efficacy and high incidence of gastrointestinal adverse events in a pilot study. *Drug Alcohol Depend* 2008;**94**:254–257.

57. Winstick A, Lea T, Copeland J. Lithium carbonate in the management of cannabis withdrawal in humans: an open label trial. *Psychopharmacology* 2009;**23**:84–93.

58. Haney M, Hart C, Vosburg S, Comer SD, Reed SC, Foltin, RW. Effects of THC and lofexidine in a human laboratory model of marijuana withdrawal and relapse. *Psychopharmacology* 2008;**197**:157–168.

59. Drake R, Essock S, Shaner A. Implementing dual diagnosis services for clients with severe mental illness. *Psychiatric Services* 2001;**52**:469–476.

60. Drake R, Muesner K. Managing comorbid schizophrenia and substance abuse. *Curr Psychiatr Rep* 2001;**3**:418–422.

61. Edwards J, Elkins K, Hinton M, *et al.* Randomized controlled trial of a cannabis-focused intervention for young people with first-episode psychosis, *Acta Psychiatrica Scandinavica* 2006;**114**:109–117.

62. Foti D, Kotov R, Guey L, Bromet E. Cannabis use and the course of schizophrenia: 10 year follow-up after first hospitalization. *Am J Psychiatry* 2010;**167**:987–993.

63. McCambridge J, Strang J, Platts S, Witton J. Cannabis use and the GP: brief motivational intervention increases clinical enquiry by GPs in a pilot study. *Brit J Gen Pract* 2003;**53**:637–639.

21

Hallucinogens and Related Compounds

Charles S. Grob[1] and Marlene Dobkin de Rios[2]

[1] Harbor-UCLA Medical Center, Torrance, CA, USA
[2] University of California, Irvine; California State University, Fullerton, CA, USA

INTRODUCTION

Hallucinogens consist of a diverse group of biologically active compounds that are among the oldest class of drugs known to humanity. In plant form, they were utilized by many prehistoric and early civilizations as integral components of their religious, healing, and initiation rituals. More than 100 species of plant hallucinogens have been cataloged, the majority in the Western hemisphere and possessing a history of use within indigenous ceremonial practices [1]. In the modern era, the prototype semi-synthetic hallucinogen has been lysergic acid diethylamide (LSD), an extremely potent alkaloid with psychoactive properties evident at microgram doses. LSD was serendipitously discovered during World War II by Swiss natural products chemist and ergot alkaloid investigator, Albert Hofmann, and it and other hallucinogens were avidly studied by research psychiatrists from the 1950s to early 1970s, initially as tools to explore the subjective range of mental illness (the psychotomimetic model) and later as a catalyst for an entirely new and novel psychotherapeutic treatment (the psycholytic and psychedelic models). By the 1960s, however, vast supplies of LSD were clandestinely circulating through society, where they achieved their greatest popularity among adolescents and young adults.

Given the users' relative lack of knowledge and understanding of the range of effects of these potent compounds, and often disregarding essential safeguards, the use of hallucinogens by young people was capable of causing psychological injury, particularly to those individuals with pre-existing vulnerabilities. Because of perceived risks to public health, as well as the suspected role hallucinogens had played in catalyzing social change and cultural turmoil, by the late 1960s the federal government had enacted legislation placing them in the most restrictive use category, Schedule I. An unfortunate and unintended consequence of scheduling hallucinogens was the several decades-long neglect of promising clinical research leads that had been identified by early investigators, including treatment models for psychiatric conditions that are often minimally responsive to conventional therapies [2,3]. Nevertheless, over the past decade formal efforts to explore the range of effects of hallucinogens in normal volunteer and select patient populations have resumed [4–7].

Because of the important role that plant hallucinogens played in many cultures, they aroused interest among anthropologists, medicinal chemists, health practitioners, and others. In the late nineteenth century, Western science had developed the laboratory technology and intellectual interest to explore the biochemical constituents of plant hallucinogens still used by native peoples in various locations around the world. Notable among this work was Arthur Heffter's discovery of mescaline as the active alkaloid of the peyote cactus, *Lophophora williamsii*, used in religious rituals among the Native Indian tribes of the American Southwest. The renowned toxicologist Louis Lewin later isolated harmine from the *Banisteriopsis caapi* vine, which was used to prepare the legendary ayahuasca brew from the Amazon forest of South America. Many years later, in the 1950s, the existence of an extant hallucinogenic mushroom cult was discovered in the village of Huautla de Jimenez in the hills of Oaxaca, Mexico, by amateur mycologist R. Gordon Wasson. Over time Wasson established a strong connection to a Mazatac shaman, Maria Sabina, who eventually allowed him to participate in (and photograph) an all-night healing ceremony. Wasson later published his account in a widely disseminated *Life* magazine article entitled "The Discovery Of Mushrooms That Cause Strange Visions" [8], catalyzing the

Clinical Handbook of Adolescent Addiction, First Edition. Richard Rosner.
© 2013 John Wiley & Sons, Ltd. Published 2013 by John Wiley & Sons, Ltd.

dawning of public awareness and interest in hallucinogens. Shortly after his return from Mexico, Wasson shipped a specimen of the mushroom *Stropharia cubensis* to Albert Hofmann in Switzerland, who isolated and identified psilocybin as the active alkaloid.

During the turbulent 1960s these potent hallucinogens, both natural and synthetic, were commonly referred to as psychedelics, from the Greek prefix *psyche* and the suffix *dellos*, referring to the process of revealing, revelation, or manifestation [9]. Early investigators noted that the effects of these novel compounds at times shared qualities similar to dreams, spontaneous religious epiphanies, and psychotic states, although usually with preservation of orientation, memory, and ego identity. Terminology has frequently been debated, with an often bewildering alternative nomenclature proposed for hallucinogens over the last 100 years, including although not necessarily limited to, deliriants, delusionegens, eidetics, entheogens, misperceptinogens, mysticomimetics, phanerothymes, phantasticants, psychedelics, psychodysleptics, psychogens, psychointegrators, psychosomimetics, psychotaraxics, psychoticants, psychotogens, psychotomimetics, and schizogens. Nevertheless, the most commonly used term, particularly from a scientific perspective, has been hallucinogen. This name has been challenged because of its obvious association with hallucination, which is defined as a false perception. Nonetheless, the etymological root of the term hallucinogen derives from the Latin *alucinari*, which translates as "mind wandering" or "mind traveling." Although no universal consensus as yet exists for a terminology to communicate the distinctive nature of the range of psychological effects, hallucinogen has nevertheless remained the commonly accepted appellation within the medical context.

The classic hallucinogens produce an altered state of consciousness that is characterized by changes in perception, cognition, and mood in the presence of an otherwise clear sensorium, along with visual illusions and internal visionary experience (though rarely frank hallucinations), states of ecstasy, dissolution of ego boundaries, and the experience of union with others and with the natural world. Most hallucinogens have chemical structures similar to endogenous neurotransmitters such as serotonin and dopamine. Many of the more commonly known hallucinogens, including LSD, psilocybin and DMT (*N,N*-dimethyltryptamine), contain an indole nucleus, as does serotonin, and primarily activate serotonergic neurotransmitter receptors, particularly the 5-HT_{2A}, 5-HT_{2C}, and 5-HT_{1A} receptor systems. Although the phenethylamine hallucinogen mescaline bears some structural resemblance to catecholamines, it nevertheless also exerts its effects through serotonergic systems. Recent behavioral and neuroimaging investigations have demonstrated that hallucinogens modulate neural circuits implicated in mood regulation and appear to effect glutamate neurotransmission as well [10]. With many of the more commonly used classic hallucinogens, including LSD, mescaline, psilocybin, and ayahuasca (consisting of plants containing harmala alkaloids and the potent hallucinogen, DMT), impairment of intellectual functioning and memory are minimal, stupor, narcosis, or excessive stimulation are not generally present, and addictive craving is absent [11]. With most classic hallucinogens, tolerance very quickly develops, such that even with increased doses the drug effect is lost within 4–5 days. Most experienced hallucinogen users, whether from indigenous tribal settings or in modern society, have learned to maintain extensive drug-free periods over time in order periodically to experience an optimal hallucinogen-induced alteration of consciousness.

Over the past few decades new patterns of drug use in contemporary culture have emerged, particularly among young people. One compound that has achieved vast popularity has been MDMA (3,4-methylenedioxymethamphetamine, also called "ecstasy"), which possesses chemical structural similarities to both the hallucinogen mescaline, and to amphetamine. MDMA has been widely used as a so-called "club drug," popular among youths who attend mass gatherings known as "raves," and dance for extended periods of time to rapid-paced (120 beats per minute) "techno" music. Similar to the history of the classic hallucinogens 50 years ago, MDMA was initially utilized to enhance the psychotherapy process. Owing to its strong effects facilitating intrapsychic states of empathy, along with a heightened capacity to articulate feelings, it was thought to be an ideal vehicle for the drug-facilitated psychotherapy model that had previously held such promise and yet had never been sufficiently explored because of the cultural reaction evoked by hallucinogen use among young people years before. Replicating the history of LSD and the 1960s, however, MDMA during the late 1980s and 1990s rapidly achieved notoriety as a new counterculture drug popular among youth, and was quickly given Schedule I status, making it extremely difficult to conduct human research. Recently, however, an approved pilot research study was successfully conducted evaluating a putative MDMA treatment model in patients with chronic, refractory post-traumatic stress disorder [12].

Another "club drug" that has achieved popularity as a drug of abuse among young people, but that has also recently been shown to have a potential clinical treatment application, is the dissociative anesthetic ketamine. Similar in receptor mechanism to the drug phencyclidine (PCP), ketamine blocks the *N*-methyl-D-aspartate (NMDA) type of glutamate receptor. Utilized as a valuable anesthetic because of its minimal respiratory depression effects, in recreational users ketamine is reported to induce a sensation of leaving one's body and encountering other planes of existence. Although some "psychonauts" inject the drug intramuscularly, the preferred mode of administration among young "clubbers" is to nasally insufflate ketamine with the desired goal of inducing an intrapsychic state referred to as the "k-hole." A surprising occurrence within mainstream psychiatric research over the last several years, however, has been the development of a new model using injected ketamine for the rapid treatment of severe, refractory depression [13], suggesting a potential advantage over conventional antidepressant medication, which often takes days to weeks to achieve its therapeutic effect.

Interest in the plant *Salvia divinorum* and its psychoactive compound, salvinorin A, has also recently grown, along with concern over its potential to induce psychological disturbances in young, novice users. Native only to a small mountainous region of Oaxaca, Mexico, it has traditionally been used by the native Mazatac people as part of their healing rituals. It is administered by the native people by placing 15–20 compressed salvia leaves in the back of the mouth and allowing for gradual dissolution and absorption of the active compound through the buccal mucosa. Using this method, it has a gradual onset and a sustained plateau altered state of consciousness, with users fully cognizant of their surroundings with eyes closed, encountering mythic deities of their culture in the service of individual and collective healing. The existence of salvia as part of healing and divination ceremonies by the native Mazatac people remained a secret from modernity, long after their use of psychoactive mushrooms was revealed to Western explorers such as Wasson. Over the past two decades the salvia plant has been finally subjected to rigorous laboratory investigation, and the active di-terpene salvinorin A, a highly selective kappa opioid receptor agonist, was isolated. Among young people, with little patience or inclination to allow for the slow (and distasteful) process of gradual oral absorption, the common new method of self-administration is to smoke the leaves of the plant augmented with minute quantities of the extraordinarily potent salvinorin A. Common responses to this form of rapid drug delivery are often reported as being quite bizarre, including the sense of becoming or merging into objects (e.g., the leg of a chair), encountering a two-dimensional world ("flat land"), loss of the body and/or identity, varying sensations of motion, overlapping realities, and uncontrollable hysterical laughter [14]. It is not considered to be addictive, and indeed many users report they had no interest in using it again after their initial experience, yet short videos of adolescents under the influence of salvia recently have become popular postings on You Tube, and have led to increased over-the-counter sales and consequent use of this as yet unscheduled drug [15]. Because of its effects as an opioid receptor modulator, salvia has also aroused interest among researchers as a potential therapeutic agent for psychiatric disorders (including Alzheimer's disease, mood disorders, and drug addiction) and in the treatment of pain [16].

EPIDEMIOLOGY

Hallucinogen use in modern culture was virtually nonexistent until the 1960s, when it rapidly emerged into mainstream society, achieving particular popularity among adolescents and young adults. Although precise data were not kept during that period of sudden awareness and surging interest, it was widely believed that a sizable proportion of the younger-aged population, especially during the late 1960s and early 1970s, had been exposed to LSD. By the mid-1970s, however, use patterns had noticeably dropped from their peak during the "Psychedelic Sixties." From yearly national surveys that began in 1975 until the mid-1990s, the annual prevalence of LSD use among 12th-graders remained below 10%. Subsequently, while a mild resurgence of use did occur – lifetime use peaking at almost 14% in 1997 with annual use reported to be at 8.8% [17] – there has been a perceptible decline since; the most recent lifetime LSD prevalence data for the same age group in 2010 was measured at 4.0%, with 7.7% reporting the use of other hallucinogens; annual use prevalence was 2.6% and 4.8%, respectively [18]. Examining the US population as a whole, a 2008 nationwide survey conducted by the National Survey on Drug Use and Health (NSDUH) found that 23.5 million US citizens (9.4% of the population aged 12 or older) reported lifetime use of LSD [19].

Since the mid-1990s, public health concerns with ecstasy (MDMA) have led to its inclusion in epidemiological data surveyed by the federal government on adolescent drug use. The National Institute on Drug Abuse *Monitoring the Future* annual estimate has reported that among 12th-grade students, lifetime prevalence of ecstasy use has trended from an initial 6.1% in 1996, to a peak of 11.7% in 2001 and then subsided to 7.3% in 2010, the most recently collected data, with annual prevalence reported at 4.6% in 1996, 9.2% in 2001, and 4.5% in 2010 [18]. Females are significantly more likely than males to be new MDMA users [20]. MDMA users also are at greater risk for using cigarettes, alcohol, and cannabis [21]. Younger hallucinogen and MDMA users also were more likely to engage in polysubstance use [22,23].

Although other hallucinogens have not been as rigorously studied as LSD, periodic national data are available. A 2006 NSDUH survey [20] found that among 12–17-year-olds, past year use of ketamine was 0.1%, and among youths aged 18–25 it was 0.2%. For salvia,

12–17-year-olds had a 0.6% annual prevalence, and among 18–25-year-olds 1.7% reported use in the past year. While there are no available data on more recent patterns of ketamine use, growing public concern and attendant media and internet publicity focused on interest in salvia by young people likely reflects actual increased use of the salvia plant and its active chemical constituent, salvinorin A. Validating that concern, for the first time in 2009 the annual *Monitoring the Future* survey [18] included 12th-grade use data on salvia, with 5.7% of 12th-grade high-school students reporting past year use. The other plant hallucinogens that are believed to be maintaining if not increasing in popularity are psilocybin-containing mushrooms, although confirmatory data are thus far lacking. For all of these drugs, whites comprise the ethnic majority of 12th-grade users.

DIAGNOSTIC CRITERIA

As with other substances, formal diagnostic criteria for abuse of hallucinogens are applied when there is a maladaptive pattern of use that has led to clinically significant levels of impairment and/or distress and that has manifested in recurrent and significant adverse consequences [24]. Drug dependence is characterized as a pattern of neuroadaptation, maladaptive cognitions, and impaired control related to drug use. With classic hallucinogens, physiological withdrawal does not occur; however, tolerance has been observed to develop rapidly to the euphoric and psychedelic effects, although not to autonomic effects, such as pupillary dilation, increased blood pressure, tachycardia, increased body temperature, piloerection, and hyperreflexia. Cross-tolerance does exist between various hallucinogens (e.g., LSD, mescaline, and psilocybin), but does not extend to other drugs, including cannabis and PCP.

Individuals who are acutely intoxicated with a hallucinogen generally experience perceptual changes occurring in the fully alert and awake state, including subjective intensification of perceptions, depersonalization, derealization, illusions, hallucinations, and synethesias (a condition in which one type of sensory stimulation evokes the sensation of another, as when the hearing of a sound produces the visualization of a color). Physiological signs may include the presence of pupillary dilation, tachycardia, sweating, palpitations, blurred vision, tremors and incoordination.

Individuals who present with psychological distress after having taken a hallucinogen, and who are experiencing in the colloquial parlance a "bad trip," often manifest with varying degrees of anxiety, depression, ideas of reference, fear of losing one's mind, paranoid ideation, and impaired judgment.

Table 21.1 MDMA vs. other hallucinogens.

Increased risk of:
- Developing clinical dependence
- Developing physical dependence
- Experiencing drug use-related consequences with law enforcement
- Exhibiting compulsive drug-seeking behaviors

A large national survey of recent-onset hallucinogen use, examining young people aged 12 to 21, found that 2% of recent-onset users met criteria for a hallucinogen dependence syndrome, with another 10% considered at risk or at an early stage of dependence [25]. Of greater concern is an apparent stronger association between MDMA use and excess risk of developing clinical dependence, relative to users of classic hallucinogens. More than one in five MDMA users (23%) met criteria for a hallucinogen abuse disorder, with an additional 16% demonstrating sub-threshold dependence. MDMA users also were three times as likely as users of other hallucinogens to exhibit signs of dependence. Furthermore, MDMA users more often reported drug use-related consequences with law enforcement, physical dependence, and compulsive drug-seeking behaviors [26]. Table 21.1 summarizes the increased risks of MDMA compared with users of other hallucinogens.

CLINICAL VIGNETTES

Four cases of young individuals who encountered varying degrees of difficulty with hallucinogens will be presented, two published reports and two patients who were seen for evaluation by one of the authors (CSG):

Clinical Vignette #1

Paulzen and Grunder [27] have reported on the case of A, an 18-year-old young woman without a history of known major mental illness, who presented with acute onset of agitation, disorganization, and hallucinations, purportedly after smoking cannabis. Subsequently, treatment personnel were informed that the cigarette A had smoked had actually contained leaves of *Salvia divinorum* that had been fortified with potentized salvia extract, although apparently she had been unaware of that at the time. Following hospital admission, A's condition rapidly deteriorated with worsening psychotic symptoms, including disordered thinking, thought blocking, derealization, delusions, and self-mutilating behaviors. Despite standard of care treatment with antipsychotic medications, the patient's status did not improve. Instead, her course continued to deteriorate, and was further marked by stupor and catatonic excitement, neuroleptic-induced elevation of creatinine kinase, and traumatic amputation of a 1 cm × 1 cm part of her tongue occurring while in an acutely agitated state, with subsequent aspiration requiring temporary intubation and ventilation. Further medical complications included hypotension, elevated temperature, peritonitis, and small bowel necrosis requiring surgical resection. While A's near-catastrophic medical course was likely attributable to the medical treatment of her severe psychotic state, the psychosis itself was clearly triggered by the unwitting administration of the potent salvia preparation. Following emergency surgical intervention, A's psychiatric (and medical) status eventually improved, her psychotic symptoms disappeared and she was discharged to the care of her parents.

Clinical Vignette #2

A case published in the lay literature by Reitman and Vasilakis [28] portrays another dimension of the range of risk young people may incur while under the influence of a hallucinogen. In this presentation, B was an 18-year-old male student at an elite urban east coast university who was without a formal psychiatric history other than frequent use of cannabis. On the surface he appeared well adjusted with numerous friends, functioned well academically, and had recently engaged in self-experimentation with hallucinogenic mushrooms. One week after an initial experience, which appeared to have occurred without evident adverse effects, B decided to take an unknown dose of mushrooms. Accompanied by two acquaintances, neither of whom were under the influence, B walked for some time through the streets of the city before entering the large campus library. Once inside the building B expressed a wish to take the elevator to the 10th floor, where a month previously another student (with whom B had no known association) had committed suicide by jumping over a balcony to his death.

After exiting the elevator, B sat on the floor, telling his friends he was "not comfortable" and "frightened." As the other two students turned to take the elevator down to the ground level, B got to his feet, walked to the balcony, put his hands on the railing and vaulted over the side, jumping to his death. Subsequent investigation found no contributory factors to the suicide other than acute intoxication with hallucinogenic mushrooms and cannabis. Given the obvious inability to interview the deceased after the event, it was not possible to establish whether B had harbored and kept secret a deep-seated depression with the suicide occurring as the result of intense demoralization triggered by the mushroom experience or whether he was in the throes of a confusional state precipitated by the intoxication, which may have led to severe disorientation and impaired judgment with fatal consequences. Beyond the unpredictable nature of the hallucinogenic mushroom effect itself, having taken these powerful psychoactive compounds in a setting of sensory overload (city streets and buildings) and without the presence of a trained facilitator who could guide him through the challenging inner terrain of the experience, B's state of vulnerability and consequent risk for adverse outcome were greatly enhanced, leading to the catastrophic outcome described.

Clinical Vignette #3

Two adolescent patients presenting within a week of one another for clinical evaluation exemplify the potential range of experience young people may have with hallucinogens. The first case, C, was a 16-year-old boy who presented with a recent history of arrest and incarceration for antisocial behavior. When asked about his use of substances, C reported that his weekend activities often included getting together with several friends, with whom he would ingest LSD, smoke marijuana, and drink a bottle of whiskey. They would then go for extended automobile drives on the local highways, where "everything would be fine until the double lines on the highway turned into snakes and attacked the windshield." Fortunately, C reported no automobile accidents had occurred during these episodes. Further inquiry elicited that the patient had an extensive psychiatric history, with long-standing attentional problems, mood lability, and temper dysregulation, although he had received only minimal mental health treatment interventions in the past. C presents an example of recreational hallucinogen use by an adolescent in a polysubstance abuse context. Apparently motivated by the goal of achieving states of excessive sensory stimulation, C's use of LSD is obviously one replete with severe potential risk not only for the user but for innocent bystanders as well.

Clinical Vignette #4

D was a 19-year-old young man who presented with his father shortly after the beginning of his second year of college. D had begun his higher education with the intention of majoring in pre-engineering and after graduate school joining his father (an immigrant from southeastern Europe) in the successful family engineering firm. During the summer between his first and second year of college, D and a close friend had had several experiences with hallucinogenic mushrooms. They had prepared for the experiences by reading from the available literature on how to optimize set and setting for a psychedelic experience, which included studying selections from esoteric eastern religion and philosophy tracts. The actual settings for the experiences were in nature and away from the distractions and potential interferences of normative daily life. D also reported that he and his friend alternated roles during each session, with one of them consuming the mushrooms and the other remaining sober, providing security and reassurance as needed. During his experiences under the influence of the mushrooms D reported having what he described were states of profound spiritual transcendence, with heightened awareness and appreciation of the natural world. D denied having any adverse psychological events during or after his experiences.

At the end of the summer, however, D confided to his father what he had done and that he planned to change his academic major from pre-engineering to fine arts. This decision led to a protracted conflict with his father, who had assumed that his son would follow his professional path and become an engineer, hopefully with the family firm. Although D, who apparently had a psychologically healthy background, was able to tolerate the mushroom experiences without difficulty, a severe family conflict did ensue in the wake of his radically altered view of himself and his plans for the future. This case therefore provides an illustrative example of how even apparently optimal hallucinogen outcomes in adolescents may evoke understandable levels of anxiety and consternation in parents who are convinced that their child had incurred injury to themselves by their use of such socially unacceptable substances and paths for self-exploration.

ASSESSMENT AND TREATMENT

Although the use of hallucinogens in the clinical research setting has been determined to have a fairly safe range of action [29,30], it is another matter altogether when these highly potent compounds are utilized outside of an approved and carefully monitored treatment context. Outcomes may be unpredictable and ultimately have more dangerous consequences, particularly when naïve and ill-prepared young people take hallucinogens in poorly controlled recreational settings, often combining them with alcohol and other drugs. Going back to the 1960s, when hallucinogens' popularity among adolescents and youth was at its highest point, transient anxiety states were often observed among novice users. Although the levels of anxiety experienced were often very high, they usually resolved quickly with gentle reassurance and reduction of sensory stimuli. In more challenging clinical situations, however, when a

medication intervention is considered necessary, treatment with a benzodiazepine is recommended (e.g., diazepam 20 mg by mouth), as it facilitates a relatively rapid and salutary effect, with bad trips usually resolving in about 30 minutes [31]. Administration of neuroleptics, however, is often contraindicated as they have been observed to amplify the dysphoric nature of the experience, further compounding the patient's distress and prolonging recovery time [32]. Some users of LSD in particular also have reported particular sensitivity to anxiety episodes and symptoms resembling paranoid psychosis toward the latter part of the 8–12-hour experience. Neuropharmacologist David Nichols (personal communication) has suggested that this phenomenon may be attributable to an active metabolite of LSD that reaches a relevant plasma concentration around 6 hours after ingestion. For individuals who suffer prolonged psychosis after taking a hallucinogen, clinical experience has found most of these patients to have had significant levels of premorbid psychopathology. Some investigators have concluded that in certain vulnerable individuals, particularly those with genetic loading for serious mental illness, hallucinogens may act as psychotogens [33].

During the 1960s concern was raised over the phenomenon of LSD-induced flashbacks [34], which were described as consisting of perceptual distortions, spontaneous imagery, and recurrent unbidden images, often beginning days, weeks, or even months following hallucinogen experience. The use of the term flashback has been supplanted by the diagnostic condition termed hallucinogen persisting perception disorder (HPPD), and is currently utilized by the DSM-IV as the generally accepted clinical term [24]. To meet DSM-IV criteria for HPPD, symptoms must cause clinically significant impairment or distress and must not be explainable by other medical conditions. Symptoms may be intermittent or constant, and have been reported by some patients as occurring almost on a daily basis for years [35]. HPPD is a relatively uncommon condition, identified among 4.2% of hallucinogen users in one recent internet survey [36]. The likelihood of developing HPPD increases, however, with multiple exposures and temporally coincident drugs, particularly hallucinogenic mushrooms, MDMA, and dextromethorphan.

One study of 123 LSD users examined patients presenting with visual disturbances, primarily geometric pseudohallucinations, false fleeting perceptions in the peripheral fields, flashes of color, and positive after-imagery [37,38]. The visual disorder persisted in half of the sample over the 5-year follow-up period, with identified precipitants including stress, fatigue, anxiety, a dark environment, intention, marijuana and neuroleptic use. Depression was often comorbidly present and the condition could be catalyzed by only a single dose of LSD. Clinical recognition of the post-hallucinogen perceptual disorder is often delayed, and effective treatment limited. Benzodiazepines ameliorate but do not eliminate the symptoms. Supportive psychotherapy is frequently indicated, to help demoralized patients accommodate to their chronic visual distractions, and to address the common concern of "brain damage." Additional treatment, often including pharmacotherapy, is generally indicated for comorbid conditions, such as depression, psychosis, and panic disorder [31].

Over the past two decades, greatest public health concern has been over the recreational use of MDMA among young people. Sold as ecstasy, illicit MDMA-containing compounds are often adulterated with other drugs [39], some of which have serious potential medical risks; these include para-methoxyamphetamine (PMA), which has been responsible for some deaths attributed to ecstasy. Although facilitators of MDMA psychotherapy prior to the scheduling of the drug in 1986 reported a fairly safe profile of action when administered to patients in controlled treatment settings, once the drug was introduced to the dance club and rave scene serious potential dangers became apparent. One of the greatest concerns has been the risk of developing malignant hyperthermia, manifested by rapid temperature escalation (up to 105–106 °F, or 40.5–41.0 °C), disseminated intravascular coagulation (DIC), kidney and liver failure, seizures, and death. Virtually all known hyperthermia deaths associated with MDMA have occurred under conditions likely to raise core body temperature, including hot tubs and especially the rave dance setting, where individuals frenetically dance in crowded settings for protracted periods of time, often without breaks and without adequate access to hydration. Other causes of fatalities have included severe hyponatremia and water intoxication in individuals (mostly female) who drink excessive amounts of fluids while not engaging in physical activity, and cardiac arrhythmias in individuals with underlying vulnerability in their cardiac conduction system. Recent research also has demonstrated clear gender differences associated with response to MDMA. Although female users are more sensitive than males to the acute and subacute psychological and physical adverse effects of MDMA, as well as long-term alterations in particular aspects of serotonin neurotransmitter function, males are more sensitive to the acute physiological effects of the drug [40]. An additional concern specific to female MDMA users is the risk of (accidental) gestational exposure in women of childbearing age, which may lead to congenital defects and/or increased risk for abnormal neurodevelopment [41,42]. Table 21.2 summarizes potential adverse effects associated with MDMA use.

Table 21.2 MDMA associated adverse effects.

- Malignant hypothermia
- Severe hyponatremia
- Cardiac arrhythmia
- Congenital defect in exposed fetus

Although the medical dangers of recreational MDMA use among young people are undisputed, controversy persists over whether the drug causes neurotoxicity. Many high-profile studies have had important inherent methodological problems. Questionable interpretations of laboratory and clinical data and even questions about accuracy in reporting have pervaded the MDMA research literature from its outset, thus obfuscating the genuine consequences of MDMA use on central nervous system function [43–45]. Concern is justified, however, over the impact of repeated use of MDMA on cognitive function and mood regulation, particularly when other stimulants, cannabis and alcohol, are also utilized, as is often the case. Given the widespread pattern of polydrug use among young MDMA enthusiasts, significant neuropsychiatric risks are likely to manifest over time, including subtle deficits in episodic memory and learning abilities as well as mood and anxiety dysregulation [46].

Since 1985 the professional and lay literature has been particularly preoccupied with the observed effects of high-dose, repeated MDMA administration in laboratory animals, which causes changes in the serotonergic neurotransmitter system. Animal studies strongly suggest that the formation of free radicals is an important factor and that hyperthermia amplifies both the formation of free radicals and the neurotoxic effects of MDMA. The effects on laboratory and clinical models of MDMA neurotoxicity of other drugs commonly consumed in the rave setting also are being studied. Although amphetamines other than MDMA will predictably exacerbate the neurotoxicity profile, cannabis may actually have an unexpected ameliorative effect. As recent investigators have discovered, at the cellular level cannabinoids have neuroprotective actions, including the apparent capacity to block MDMA-induced neurotoxicity, at least in laboratory animals [47]. Given the vast numbers of young people who have self-experimented over the past two decades, along with the highly publicized concerns over long-term deleterious effects of MDMA, it is likely that this field will continue to receive more investigation, which will hopefully lead to more definitive answers in the future.

Although youthful interests in various psychoactive drugs and affiliations with particular social movements tend to ebb and flow over time, the persistent popularity of MDMA and its identification with the rave scene along with its predominant message of "peace and love" are reminiscent of the countercultural ethos of the late 1960s when LSD assumed the role of collective sacrament [48]. Observing its full expression within the context of festival celebration also allows identification of the post-modern mass dance phenomenon as a variant of more archaic expression linked to music and dance among aboriginal cultures where semi-hypnotic trance states are achieved, often aided by ingesting various intoxicating vapors and plant compounds. The anthropologist Mircea Eliade has explored the association of shamanic trance dances among indigenous tribal people with their primordial rituals and celebrations of spiritual expression, worship, fertility rites, and healing [49]. In many respects raves have become the re-enactment of such primitive gatherings, and have similarly achieved the status of great personal and collective significance within these very distinct cultures, separated from one another by vast distances of time and geography.

Further understanding of the function of adolescent hallucinogen use comes from anthropological data investigating the use of various plant hallucinogens by indigenous cultures [50]. We have previously explored cross-cultural perspectives of modern youth and initiation rituals among several aboriginal tribal groups that use plant hallucinogens as integral components of their pubertal initiation rites [51,52]. The analysis of data collected from observations of plant hallucinogens used in the initiation of aboriginal males from the central Australian desert, Tshogana-Tsonga African females of Mozambique, and Chumash Indian youths of central and southern California allows us to identify clear contrasts with abusive patterns of drug use found among modern adolescents. The key findings from these tribes include the extant process of managed altered states of consciousness where plant hallucinogens are administered by elders to youths as part of an intensive, short-term socialization for religious and pedagogical purposes. The use of hyper-suggestibility as a cultural technique to "normalize" youth in tribal societies under study is contrasted to the pathological patterns of drug ingestion patterns among American adolescents.

In non-Western aboriginal cultures of the world where drug use among adolescents may not be viewed as problematic, it is often incorporated into near-universal transition rituals that mark passage into adulthood. Plant hallucinogens historically have played a major role in the transformation of pubertal boys and girls into fully participating members of adult society. By contrast to that are contemporary patterns of adolescent drug abuse in Euro-American societies where abuse rather than salutary use patterns prevail in the face of dysfunctional family life, widespread dysphoria, and self-medication.

Legal constraints on drug use reflect the values of modern society in contrast with ritualistic use observed in traditional tribal societies around the world. This difference allows us to understand the role of managed altered states of consciousness facilitated by tribal elders for adolescents, both male and female, as a culturally accepted, didactic device to prepare youth for new adult roles. In industrial societies there are no integrative rituals in adolescence to address endemic societal problems of alienation, economic disenfranchisement, social status ambiguity, and lack of meaning.

A psychological characteristic of altered states of consciousness induced by hallucinogens is the phenomenon of suggestibility. Simon [53] has written about the selective advantage of bounded rationality. In Euro-American society, suggestibility is also at work; however, it is not managed by tribal elders but rather is part of the complement of drug-induced suggestibility and rock and rap lyrics by distant god-like figures, rock stars, whose frequent antinomian messages are often received by youth high in drug-suggestible states as they listen to such lyrics through electronic media or personally attend concerts and raves. In Western society, the lack of a salutary role played by elders (parents, etc.) is a critical factor contributing to the undeniably damaging consequences of much contemporary drug use.

Not all contemporary hallucinogen use among young people need be seen in an entirely negative light. In research conducted by the authors in Brazil [54], the effects of the plant hallucinogen decoction, ayahuasca, was studied in adolescent members of a syncretic religion which has had formal sanction from the federal government to consume ayahuasca in ritual ceremony since the mid-1980s. Containing the active alkaloid and classic hallucinogen dimethyltryptamine (DMT) from the *Psychotria viridis* plant along with harmala alkaloids from *Banisteriopsis caapi*, which enables the oral activation of DMT (which is otherwise not active when taken by mouth), ayahuasca exerts a powerful 4-hour visionary experience that was much prized by the native people of the Amazon Basin and later appropriated by modern Brazilian culture for use as a psychoactive sacrament within new religious structures [55]. The range of effects and parameters for safe use in adult adherents of the ayahuasca religion, Uniao do Vegetal (UDV), has previously been studied [56], with the adolescent study subsequently requested by the Brazilian judiciary to determine the range of salutary versus injurious effect caused by ayahuasca. Eighty-four adolescents from UDV churches in three Brazilian cities along with matched non-ayahuasca-using controls were recruited into the study. No significant differences between the two groups were found on neuropsychological testing, whereas on formal psychiatric assessment the UDV ayahuasca-exposed adolescents were found to have considerably less anxiety, healthier body image, fewer attentional problems, and significantly less alcohol use histories than their non-ayahuasca-using matched controls [57–60]. The participation of adolescents and youths in religious ceremonies using ayahuasca as a psychoactive sacrament represents a contemporary model for a phenomenon observed previously among tribal people, that of the elder-facilitated, culturally sanctioned, and collective participation in highly meaningful religious rites of initiation.

SUMMARY POINTS

While hallucinogens have a long history of use among indigenous peoples, their emergence in modern culture in the twentieth century led to serious misuse and abuse by vulnerable youths. Early research with hallucinogens, including promising therapeutic models for difficult-to-treat psychiatric disorders, was prematurely halted because of cultural reactions and concerns over a perceived crisis in public mental health. Over the past 20 years new compounds have emerged within youth culture, including the stimulant-hallucinogen, MDMA (ecstasy), and the dissociative hallucinogens, ketamine and salvia. The most common adverse effect caused by hallucinogens is transient anxiety, which can usually be addressed through reassurance, moving the individual to a quiet environment, and if necessary, the administration of a benzodiazepine. Poor attention to set and setting will increase the likelihood of an adverse outcome.

Long-term adverse psychological effects of hallucinogens usually occur in young individuals with significant premorbid psychopathology and genetic loading for serious mental illness. Frequent use may induce a "hallucinogen persisting perception disorder" (HPPD), which may be chronic, disabling, and difficult to treat. Potentially life-threatening adverse health effects of MDMA (ecstasy) include malignant hyperthermia, water intoxication, and cardiac arrhythmias.

While the long-term impact of MDMA on central nervous system function is still not fully understood, frequent use of MDMA along with other drugs (particularly methamphetamine) will lead to varying degrees of cognitive impairment.

The anthropological perspective allows for examination of aboriginal models of hallucinogen administration as part of culturally sanctioned rites of initiation, which are in clear contrast to modern patterns of misuse and abuse. The study of the plant hallucinogen decoction ayahuasca, taken in sanctioned religious contexts in Brazil, offers the opportunity to learn of the short- and long-term psychophysiological effects of these ancient compounds in modern youth.

References

1. Schultes RE, Hofmann A. *Plants of the Gods: Their Sacred, Healing and Hallucinogenic Powers*. Rochester, VT: Healing Arts Press, 1992.
2. Grinspoon L, Bakalar JB. *Psychedelic Drugs Reconsidered*. New York: Basic Books, 1979.
3. Grob CS. Psychiatric research with hallucinogens: What have we learned? *Heffter Rev Psychedelic Res* 1998;**1**:8–20.
4. Griffiths RR, Richards WA, McCann U, Jesse R. Psilocybin can occasion mystical type experiences having substantial and sustained personal meaning and spiritual significance. *Psychopharmacology* 2006;**187**:268–292.
5. Moreno FA, Wiegand CB, Taitano EK, Delgado PL. Safety, tolerability and efficacy of psilocybin in 9 patients with obsessive-compulsive disorder. *J Clin Psychiatry* 2006;**67**:1735–1740.
6. Grob CS. The use of psilocybin in patients with advanced cancer and existential anxiety. In: Winkelman MJ, Roberts TB (eds), *Psychedelic Medicine: New Evidence for Hallucinogenic Substances as Treatments*. Westport, CT: Praeger, 2007; pp. 205–216.
7. Grob CS, Danforth AL, Chopra GS, *et al.* Pilot study of psilocybin treatment for anxiety in patients with advanced-stage cancer. *Arch Gen Psychiatry* 2011;**68**:71–78.
8. Wasson RG. Seeking the magic mushroom Teonanacatl. *LIFE* 1957;**42**:100–120.
9. Osmond H. A review of the clinical effects of psychotomimetic agents. *Ann N Y Acad Sci* 1957;**66**:418–434.
10. Vollendweider FX, Kometer M. The neurobiology of psychedelic drugs: Implications for the treatment of mood disorders. *Nat Rev Neurosci* 2010;**11**:642–651.
11. Hollister LE. *Chemical Psychoses*. Springfield, IL: Charles C. Thomas, 1968.
12. Mithoefer MC, Wagner MT, Mithoefer AT, *et al.* The safety and efficacy of 3,4-methylenedioxymethamphetamine-assisted psychotherapy in subjects with chronic, treatment-resistant posttraumatic stress disorder: The first randomized, controlled pilot study. *J Psychopharmacol* 2011;**25**:439–452.
13. Zarate CA, Singh JB, Carlson PJ, *et al.* A randomized trial of an N-methyl-D-aspartate antagonist in treatment-resistant major depression. *Arch Gen Psychiatry* 2006;**63**:856–864.
14. Turner DM. *Salvinorin: The Psychedelic Essence of Salvia Divinorin*. San Francisco: Panther Press, 1996.
15. Lange JE, Daniel J, Homer K, *et al.* Salvia divinorin: Effects and use among You Tube users. *Drug Alcohol Depend* 2010;**108**:138–140.
16. Johnson MW, MacLean KA, Reissig CR, Prisinzano TE, Griffiths RR. Human psychopharmacology and dose-effects of salvinorin A, a kappa opioid agonist hallucinogen present in the plant Salvia divinorum. *Drug Alcohol Depend* 2011;**115**:150–155.
17. Johnston LD, O'Malley PM, Bachman JG, Schulenberg JE. *Monitoring the Future National Results on Adolescent Drug Use: Overview of Key Findings, 1998*, Bethesda, MD: National Institute on Drug Abuse, 1999.
18. Johnston LD, O'Malley PM, Bachman JG, Schulenberg JE. *Monitoring the Future National Results on Adolescent Drug Use: Overview of Key Findings, 2009*, Bethesda, MD: National Institute on Drug Abuse, 2010.
19. Substance Abuse and Mental Health Services Administration. *Results from the 2008 National Survey on Drug Use*

and Health: National Findings. Rockville, MD: Office of Applied Studies, Substance Abuse and Mental Health Services, 2009.

20. Substance Abuse and Mental Health Services Administration. *The NSDUH Report: Patterns of Hallucinogen Use and Initiation.* Rockville, MD: Office of Applied Studies, Substance Abuse and Mental Health Services, 2007.

21. Wu LT, Schlenger WE, Glavin DM. Concurrent use of methamphetamine, MDMA, LSD, ketamine, GHB and flunitrazepam among American youth. *Drug Alcohol Depend* 2006;**84**:102–113.

22. Rickert VK, Siqueira LM, Dale T, Wiemann CM. Prevalence and risk factors for LSD use among young women. *J Pediatr Adolesc Gynecol* 2003;**16**:67–75.

23. Yacoubian GS. Correlates of ecstasy use among students surveyed through the 1997 College Alcohol Study. *J Drug Educ* 2003;**33**:61–69.

24. American Psychiatric Association. *Diagnostic and Statistical Manual of Mental Disorders*, 4th edn. Washington, DC: American Psychiatric Association, 2000.

25. Stone AL, Storr CL, Anthony JD. Evidence for a hallucinogen dependence syndrome developing soon after onset of hallucinogen use during adolescence. *Int J Methods Psych Res* 2006;**15**:116–130.

26. Wu LT, Ringwalt CS, Weiss RD, Blazer DG. Hallucinogen-related disorders in a national sample of adolescents: The influence of ecstasy/MDMA use. *Drug Alcohol Depend* 2009;**104**:156–166.

27. Paulzen M, Grunder G. Toxic psychosis after intake of the hallucinogen salvinorin A. *J Clin Psychiatry* 2008;**69**: 1501–1502.

28. Reitman J, Vasilakis J. The lost freshman. *Rolling Stone* 2004;**944**: 3/18.

29. Cohen S. Lysergic acid diethylamide: Side effects and complications. *J Nerv Ment Dis* 1960;**130**:30–40.

30. Strassman RJ. Adverse reactions to psychedelic drugs: A review of the literature. *J Nerv Ment Dis* 1984;**172**: 577–592.

31. Abraham HD, Aldridge AM, Gogia P. The psychopharmacology of hallucinogens. *Neuropsychopharmacology* 1996;**14**:282–298.

32. Schwartz C. Paradoxical responses to chlorpromazine. *Psychosomatics* 1967;**8**:210–211.

33. Bowers M. Acute psychosis induced by psychotomimetic drug abuse. *Arch Gen Psychiatry* 1972;**27**:437–440.

34. Horowitz MJ. Flashbacks: Recurrent intrusive images after the use of LSD. *Am J Psychiatry* 1969;**126**:565–569.

35. Abraham HD, Duffy FH. EEG coherence in post-LSD flashback. *Psychiatry Res* 2001;**107**:151–163.

36. Baggott MJ, Coyle JR, Erowid E, Erowid F. Abnormal visual experiences in individuals with histories of hallucinogen use: A web-based questionnaire. *Drug Alcohol Depend* 2011;**114**:61–67.

37. Abraham HD. Visual phenomenology of the LSD flashback. *Arch Gen Psychiatry* 1983;**40**:884–889.

38. Abraham HD. LSD flashback. *Arch Gen Psychiatry* 1984;**41**:632–633.

39. Cole JC, Bailey M, Sumnall HR, *et al.* The content of ecstasy tablets: Implications for the study of their long-term effects. *Addiction* 2002;**97**:1531–1536.

40. Allott K, Redman J. Are there sex differences associated with the effects of ecstasy/3,4-methylenedioxymethamphetamine (MDMA)? *Neurosci Behav Rev* 2007;**31**: 327–347.

41. McElhatton PR, Bateman DN, Evans C, *et al.* Congenital anomalies after prenatal ecstasy exposure. *Lancet* 1999; **354**:1441–1442.

42. Broening HW, Morford LL, Inman-Woof S, *et al.* 3,4-methylenedioxymethamphetamine (ecstasy)-induced learning and memory impairments depend on the age of exposure during early development. *J Neurosci* 2001;**21**:3228–3235.

43. Grob CS. Deconstructing ecstasy: The politics of MDMA research. *Addiction Res* 2000;**8**:549–588.

44. Grob CS. The enigma of ecstasy: implications for youth and society. *Adolesc Psychiatry* 2005;**29**:97–117.

45. Grob CS, Poland RE. MDMA. In: Lowinson JH, Ruiz P, Millman RB, Langrod JG (eds), *Substance Abuse: A Comprehensive Textbook*, 4th edn. Philadelphia: Williams & Wilkins, 2005; pp. 274–286.

46. Soar K, Turner JD, Parrotte AC. Problematic versus non-problematic ecstasy/MDMA use: The influence of drug usage patterns and pre-existing psychiatric factors. *J Psychopharmacology* 2006;**20**:417–424.

47. Goubzoulis-Mayfrank E, Daumann J. The confounding problem of polydrug use in recreational ecstasy/MDMA users: A brief overview. *J Psychopharmacology* 2006;**20**: 188–193.

48. MacDonald S, Newrith C, Blyth F, Winship G. Adolescent transition and the use of hallucinogens: A subcultural analysis. *Brit J Psychother* 1998;**15**:240–248.

49. Eliade M. *Shamanism: Archaic Techniques of Ecstasy.* Princeton, NJ: Princeton University Press, 1964.

50. Dobkin de Rios M. *Hallucinogens: Cross-Cultural Perspectives.* Albuerquerque, NM: University of New Mexico Press, 1984.

51. Grob CS, Dobkin de Rios M. Adolescent drug use in cross-cultural perspective. *J Drug Issues* 1992;**22**:121–138.

52. Dobkin de Rios M, Grob CS. Hallucinogens, suggestibility and adolescence in cross-cultural perspective. *Yearbook of Ethnomedicine* 1994;**3**:113–132.

53. Simon HA. A mechanism for social selection and successful altruism. *Science* 1990;**250**:1665–1668.

54. Dobkin de Rios M, Grob CS. Ayahuasca use in cross-cultural perspective. *J Psychoactive Drugs* 2005;**37**:119–121.

55. Grob CS. The psychology of ayahuasca. In: Metzner R (ed.), *Ayahuasca: Human Consciousness and the Spirits of Nature.* New York: Thunder's Mouth Press, 1999.

56. Grob CS, McKenna DJ, Callaway JC, *et al.* Human psychopharmacology of hoasca, a plant hallucinogen used in ritual context in Brazil. *J Nerv Ment Dis* 1996;**184**:86–94.

57. Doering-Silveira E, Lopez E, Grob CS, *et al.* Ayahuasca in adolescence: A neuropsychological assessment. *J Psychoactive Drugs* 2005;**37**:123–128.

58. Silveira DX, Grob CS, Dobkin de Rios M, *et al.* Ayahuasca in adolescence: A preliminary psychiatric assessment. *Journal of Psychoactive Drugs* 2005;**37**:129–133.

59. Dobkin de Rios M, Grob CS, Lopez E, *et al.* Ayahuasca in adolescence: qualitative results. *J Psychoactive Drugs* 2005;**37**:135–139.

60. Doering-Silveira E, Grob CS, Dobkin de Rios M, *et al.* Report on psychoactive drugs use among adolescents using ayahuasca within a religious context. *J Psychoactive Drugs* 2005;**37**:141–144.

61. American Psychiatric Association. *Diagnostic and Statistical Manual of Mental Disorders*, 4th edn, Text Revision. Washington, DC: American Psychiatric Association, 2000.

22

Opioids and Sedative-Hypnotics

Ann Bruner,[1] Asad Bokhari,[2] and Marc Fishman[3]

[1]Johns Hopkins University Student Health and Wellness Center; Mountain Manor
Treatment Center, Baltimore, MD, USA
[2]Chesapeake Treatment Centers; Mountain Manor Treatment Center, Baltimore, MD, USA
[3]Department of Psychiatry and Behavioral Sciences, Johns Hopkins University School of Medicine;
Mountain Manor Treatment Center, Baltimore, MD, USA

OVERVIEW

These two classes of drugs, opioids and sedative-hypnotics, have important similarities: they are central nervous system (CNS) depressants, they have additive CNS effects with other sedative drugs, tolerance is common, and their withdrawal syndromes are clinically significant with substantial morbidity. Importantly, drugs in both classes are often not illicit in their origins even when they are taken illicitly; they are prescribed medications, readily available, frequently inexpensive, and commonly used. Clinical indications include pain, anxiety, insomnia, and seizures. Federal law regulates their manufacture, importation, possession, use, and distribution. However, individuals can also obtain these drugs ("pharming") online without prescriptions, obtain multiple prescriptions from different providers, steal drugs that were prescribed for someone else, or buy them on the street. The non-medical use of prescription medications has increased 162% in the past decade [1], and an estimated 20% of Americans have misused prescription medicines in their lifetime [2]. Table 22.1 summarizes trends in the lifetime prevalence of misuse of prescription drugs among 12th-graders.

In 2010, one in four teens reported that they knew a peer who abuses prescription drugs, a 19% increase since 2007 [3]. Data from the 2009 National Survey on Drug Use and Health (NSDUH) indicate that 3.1% of youths aged 12 to 17 years reported non-medical use of prescription medications in the past month. Figure 22.1 summarizes the past-month use of selected illicit drugs for youths aged 12 to 17 between 2002 and 2009.

Rates of abuse were highest among the 18–25 age group (6.3%). The 2009 Youth Risk Behavior Surveillance survey found that 20% of high-school students have abused a prescription medication (lifetime prevalence) [4]. Prescription drug abuse is related to other use of illicit drugs: 63% of youths who had used prescription drugs non-medically in the past year had also used marijuana in the past year, compared with 17% of youths who had not used prescription drugs non-medically in the past year [2]. Among the youngest group surveyed, aged 12–13, a higher percentage reported using psychotherapeutics (1.8%) than marijuana (1.0%) [2]. In fact, adolescents and young adults have the fastest growing rates of abuse of prescription drugs – one-third of all new abusers of prescription drugs in 2005 were 12–17-year-olds [5]. There was a four-fold increase in patients entering treatment who reported prescription opiate abuse between 1998 and 2008 [6]. Adolescents seem to believe that because these are prescription medications, they are "safer" than illicit drugs, and the perceived harmfulness of prescription medications has substantially decreased over time [7].

OPIOIDS

Introduction

Natural opiates, derived from alkaloids in the resin of the opium poppy (*Papaver somniferum*), include morphine, codeine, and thebaine. Table 22.2 notes the brand and street names of commonly abused medications.

Semi-synthetic opioids, produced from natural opiates, include hydromorphone, hydrocodone, oxycodone,

Clinical Handbook of Adolescent Addiction, First Edition. Richard Rosner.
© 2013 John Wiley & Sons, Ltd. Published 2013 by John Wiley & Sons, Ltd.

Table 22.1 Trends in lifetime prevalence of misuse of prescription drugs among 12th-graders [11].

	1991	2000	2009
Narcotics other than heroin	6.6%	9.9%	13.2%
Tranquilizers/benzodiazepines	7.2%	8.9%	9.3%
Sedatives/barbiturates	6.2%	9.2%	9.3%

Reproduced with permission from Johnston LD, O'Malley PM., Bachman JG, Schulenberg JE. *Monitoring the Future national survey results on drug use, 1975-2009. Volume I: Secondary school students* (NIH Publication No. 10-7584). Bethesda, MD: National Institute on Drug Abuse, 2010; 734 pp.

diacetylmorphine (heroin), and buprenorphine. Opioids such as fentanyl, methadone, and tramadol are fully synthetic. There are three primary classes of opioid receptors (mu, kappa, and delta) located mainly in the CNS but also in the gastrointestinal system. Activation of these receptors results in analgesia, sedation, euphoria, dependence, and respiratory depression (mu); cough suppression, dysphoria, dissociation, and psychosis (kappa), and analgesia (delta) [8]. Different opioids have various levels of receptor activity; for example, buprenorphine is a high-affinity partial mu agonist and a kappa antagonist. Heroin is a Schedule I drug, the most potent prescription opiates are classified as Schedule II, and buprenorphine and other lower potency opioid analgesics are Schedule III.

Epidemiology

While the misuse of prescription medicines has always been a problem, the abuse of prescribed narcotics exploded with the introduction of a long-acting form of oxycodone (OxyContin) in 1996. The long-acting formulation delivers a consistent dose and eliminates the need

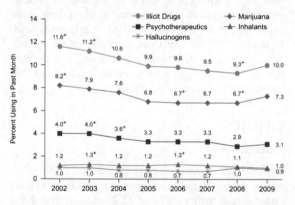

Figure 22.1 Past month use of selected illicit drugs: youths ages 12–17, 2002–2009. Reproduced with permission from Substance Abuse and Mental Health Services Administration. *2009 National Survey on Drug Use and Health: Volume I. Summary of National Findings.* Office of Applied Studies, NSDUH Series H-38A, HHS Publication No. SMA 10-4856 Findings. Rockville, MD: SAMHSA, 2010.

for repetitive dosing for high-potency analgesia – but because of the very high doses they are very desirable for misuse as well. Abusers quickly discovered that simply crushing or chewing the pills deactivates the time-release formulation and affords immediate availability of the full potency. OxyContin is one of the most widely abused prescription drugs of all time, and sales increased six-fold between 1997 and 2005. Initially use was particularly high in rural areas where it was known as "hillbilly heroin." In 2007 some executives of the manufacturer of OxyContin, Purdue Pharma, pleaded guilty to felony charges of misbranding; the company paid almost US$20 million in fines for aggressive marketing and misbranding.

Another factor that may have contributed to the rise in prescription opiate availability (and resultant misuse/abuse) has its roots in a laudable goal: increased emphasis on analgesia as a paramount clinical goal, including the 1992 release of a clinical guideline for pain management by the Agency for Health Care Policy and Research of the US Department of Health and Human Services, followed by the 2001 establishment of Joint Commission on Accreditation of Healthcare Organizations standards for pain assessment and management. But these imperatives have not yet been balanced by the appropriate cautions against the limitations of the effectiveness of opioids for chronic pain, the risks of polypharmacy, or the encouragement of adequate skills for the management of aberrant drug-taking behavior (overuse and/or misuse). There are pending proposed state and federal initiatives aimed at improved, perhaps mandatory, training for responsible opioid prescribing [9].

There has been an increase in prescribing patterns – a controlled medication was prescribed at 6.4% of adolescent visits in 1997 compared with 11.2% of visits in 2007, and in 8.3% of young adult visits in 1997 compared with 16.1% in 2007 [10]. If adolescents can't obtain a prescribed opiate, they have easy access to these drugs since most households contain at least one individual who was once prescribed pain medication (dental procedure, injury, postoperatively) but didn't take all the medicine and didn't destroy the remainder. The source of prescription drugs among those 12th-graders who used in the last year (from 2002 to 2009) is outlined in Table 22.3.

Table 22.2 Commonly abused medications: brand and street names.

Medication	Brand names	Street names
Opioids		
Codeine	Fioricet, Tylenol #1-4, Soma	T-threes, schoolboy, cody
Morphine	MS Contin	M, morph, Miss Emma
Hydromorphone	Dilaudid	Dillies, juice
Meperidine	Demerol	Demmies
Fentanyl	Actiq, Duragesic, Sublimaze	China white, drop dead, TNT
Oxycodone	Percodan, Percocet, Tylox	Percs
	Roxicodone, Roxicet, Endocet	Roxys
	Oxycontin	Oxys, hillbilly heroin, OC
Hydrocodone	Vicodin, Lortab	Vikes
Propoxyphene	Darvon	Pinks
Pentazocine	Talwin	Footballs
Other analgesics		
Tramadol	Ultram, Ultracet	Ultras
Sedative-Hypnotics		
Benzodiazepines	Valium, Xanax, Halcion,	Xanies, Footballs, xany bars, bars,
	Librium, Ativan, Klonopin	candy, downers, benzos,
		tranks, nerve pills
Barbiturates	Phenobarbital, Nembutal, Mebaral	Barbs, yellow jackets
Non-benzodiazepines	Ambien, Sonata, Lunesta	A-, zombie pills, TicTacs
	Rohypnol	Roofies

Table 22.3 Source of prescription drugs[a] among those who used in last year, grade 12, 2007–2009 (entries are percentages).

Where did you get the (insert drug name here) you used without a doctor's orders during the past year? (Mark all that apply.)	Amphetamines		Tranquizers		Narcotics other than heroin	
	2007–2008	2009	2007–2008	2009	2007–2008	2009
Bought on Internet	4.6	3.4	2.4	3.0	2.3	0.0
Took from friend/relative without asking	19.6	10.2	21.1	13.1	24.2	18.6
Took from friend	–	3.9	–	5.7	–	3.6
Took from a relative	–	7.6	–	8.8	–	17.9
Given for free by friend or relative	58.2	55.1	59.8	64.3	50.5	51.5
Given for free by a friend	–	54.5	–	61.7	–	46.1
Given for free by a relative	–	2.9	–	8.8	–	10.1
Bought from friend or relative	45.0	48.8	44.1	39.3	37.1	33.6
Bought from a friend	–	48.8	–	39.3	–	33.6
Bought from a relative	–	1.8	–	0.6	–	2.9
From a prescription I had	15.1	22.9	18.8	15.3	40.2	30.3
Bought from drug dealer/stranger	26.7	21.8	24.2	18.9	18.6	13.0
Other method	18.8	15.1	7.5	12.3	8.5	10.5
Weighted N	201	115	220	94	351	153

[a]In 2009, the response categories were expanded to differentiatie between friends and relatives.

Reproduced from Johnston LD, O'Malley PM., Bachman JG, Schulenberg JE. *Monitoring the Future national survey results on drug use, 1975–2009. Volume I: Secondary school students* (NIH Publication No. 10-7584). Bethesda, MD: National Institute on Drug Abuse, 2010; 734 pp, with permission.

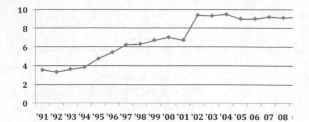

Figure 22.2 Non-medical prescription opioid use: percentage of 12th-graders who used in past 12 months. Beginning in 2002, a revised set of questions on other narcotics use was introduced in which Talwin, laudanum, and paregoric were replaced with Vicodin, OxyContin, and Percocet. Reproduced with permission from Johnston LD, O'Malley PM, Bachman JG, Schulenberg JE. *Monitoring the Future national survey results on drug use, 1975–2009. Volume I: Secondary school students* (NIH Publication No. 10-7584). Bethesda, MD: National Institute on Drug Abuse, 2010, 734 pp.

The 2009 Monitoring the Future (MTF) survey showed that 12th-graders' use of non-heroin opiates increased steeply from an annual prevalence of 3.3% in 1992 to 9.5% in 2004, with rates holding steady around 10% for the past 5 years – total prevalence in all adolescents (MTF only surveys adolescents in school) is presumed to be higher [11]. Figure 22.2 tracks trends in the non-medical prescription opioid use of 12th-graders in the last month, and Figure 22.3 highlights past-month non-medical use of prescription opioids according to age.

There is also illegal, unregulated production of these drugs and diversion making them readily available "on

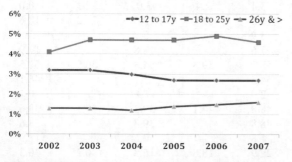

Figure 22.3 Prescription opioids: past-month non-medical users by age: 2002–2007. Reproduced with permission from Substance Abuse and Mental Health Services Administration, Office of Applied Studies. *The NSDUH Report: Trends in Nonmedical Use of Prescription Pain Relievers: 2002 to 2007*. Rockville, MD: SAMHSA, 2009.

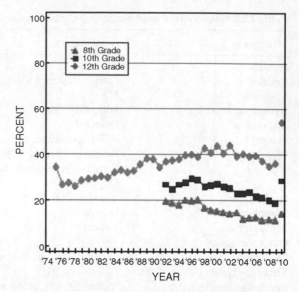

Figure 22.4 Narcotics other than heroin: trends in vailability: percentage saying "fairly easy" or "very easy" to get. Beginning in 2010, a revised set of questions on availability of other narcotics was introduced in which methadone and opium were replaced with Vicodin, OxyContin, and Percocet. Reproduced with permission from Johnston LD, O'Malley PM, Bachman JG, Schulenberg JE. Monitoring the Future national survey results on drug use, 1975–2009. Volume I: Secondary school students (NIH Publication No. 10-7584). Bethesda, MD: National Institute on Drug Abuse, 2010, 734 pp.

the street." Trends in narcotic availability (other than heroin) are presented in Figure 22.4.

In 2009, over one-half of high-school seniors who abused prescription narcotics were given the drugs or bought them from a friend or relative, and an additional 30% reported receiving a prescription for such drugs [12] (see Table 22.3). Vicodin and OxyContin are among the most commonly abused prescription medications; 9.3% of 12th-graders reported using Vicodin without a prescription in the past year, and 5.0% reported using OxyContin [11]. Overall, adolescents and young adults have the highest rates of use of prescription opiates, and these rates are increasing faster than in any other age group [12].

Along with prescription opioids, there has been a rise in heroin use, as indicated in Figure 22.5. The heroin available on the streets today is significantly more potent (50–80% purity today vs. 5% purity decades ago) [13]. Increased potency means that less efficient delivery methods (nasal) can lead to almost the same level of intoxication as intravenous use. While the need for

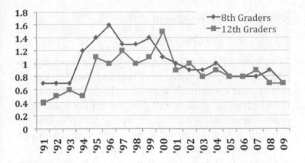

Figure 22.5 Heroin: trends in annual use: percentage who used in past 12 months. Reproduced with permission from Johnston LD, O'Malley PM, Bachman JG, Schulenberg JE. *Monitoring the Future national survey results on drug use, 1975–2009. Volume 1: Secondary school students* (NIH Publication No. 10-7584). Bethesda, MD: National Institute on Drug Abuse, 2010, 734 pp.

injection may have once provided a barrier for initiation, the ease of nasal use has made heroin more acceptable. Rates of heroin use among adolescents have increased according to MTF data [11]. Unlike the adult pattern, with concentration in the inner city, heroin use in youths has primarily been a phenomenon of suburban and rural areas.

While treatment resources remain limited, for adolescents who get to treatment there has been an increase in reported use of opiates. Between 1998 and 2008, there was roughly a 900% increase in the proportion of adolescents and young adults admitted for substance abuse treatment who reported abuse of prescription pain medications: from 0.6 to 5.2% (ages 12–17 years), and 1.5 to 13.7% (ages 18–24 years) [6]. These rates do not reflect patients admitted to medical and psychiatric units for detoxification and then discharged into outpatient treatment programs. Along with increasing rates of dependence there have been increases in overdoses, emergency room visits, and deaths related to prescription opioid abuse.

Diagnostic Criteria

Opiate abuse and dependence are diagnosed using the same criteria as abuse and dependence syndromes with other substances. But the prominence of physiological dependence and withdrawal when use is interrupted is very salient clinically. In addition to the positive reinforcement that comes from the subjective pleasure associated with use, withdrawal produces a potent negative reinforcement of continued use to avoid with-

drawal or alleviate it with a resultant subjective sense of relief. Many patients will describe that such relief cravings are actually more powerful than reward cravings, and they may attribute their use to "getting well more than getting high." Physiological dependence can develop within 4–6 weeks even in patients who appropriately take prescribed opiates over a prolonged period, a pattern seen most commonly in adult pain patients. This rapid development of physiological dependence with withdrawal ("catching a habit"), which worsens over time, typically accelerates the progression of severity, with daily use and overwhelming preoccupation with supply. In this way adolescent opioid use disorders often tend to look more like full addiction (and more like adult pattern addiction) than other non-opioid adolescent substance use disorders. Additionally, because they are sick without opioids, adolescents are often more subjectively aware of their preoccupation and other aspects of the addiction syndrome compared to adolescents with other non-opioid adolescent substance use disorders. In general, opioid dependence denotes an overall higher level of severity in adolescents with substance use disorders. In particular, adolescents with heroin use have higher severity at presentation, poorer response to treatment, and higher rates of relapse than their counterparts who use other substances [14]. Although with opioid dependence adolescents may narrow their repertoire and focus more on opioids, polysubstance abuse is still the rule and continued use of other drugs is associated with poorer outcome and opioid relapse [15].

Clinical Presentation

Vignette

Joan is a 14-year-old girl who is brought to her family physician because her parents are concerned that she is "frequently sick" and often "has the flu." Joan's mother reports that her daughter has requested medications to help with her "sick stomach" and on numerous occasions she has heard her vomiting in the bathroom at home. Joan's father notes that his daughter's academic grades are declining. He adds that she has stayed out past curfew on numerous occasions and has been suspended twice from school in the last 6 months for leaving the school campus. Both parents feel their daughter is depressed and describe her as more isolated and withdrawn with periods of sleeping "like a log" and other times where she is irritable and restless and complains of not being able to sleep.

Adolescents presenting for treatment for opioid dependence often exemplify the typical pattern of an adolescent drug abuser (maladaptive pattern of use with worsening negative consequences including school failure, truancy, opposition, defiance, lying, stealing, breaking curfew, running away, high-risk sexual behaviors, aggression, and/or trouble with the law). But at other times the pattern is different, with the treatment-precipitating crisis less about external consequences and more about withdrawal after loss of access to opioids, or about medical case-identification after overdose. Sometimes the family has been completely unaware of the drug abuse until such withdrawal or overdose. With the latter group, helping the patient and family understand the implications of full physiological dependence, and the difference between "experimentation" and addiction, is difficult but necessary before the patient/family will accept the diagnosis and engage in addiction treatment. Therefore, along with asking the adolescent about drugs used, quantities taken, length of use, patterns of use, maladaptive behaviors, and consequences of use, for opioids in particular it is extremely important to determine if the patient has experienced withdrawal when they didn't/couldn't use. Adolescents may try to attribute opiate withdrawal symptoms to a viral illness, food poisoning, stress, fatigue, or depression as a way of minimizing the severity of opioid dependence.

Many adolescents falsely believe that opiates used nasally or taken by mouth are safe and only intravenous use is dangerous. Some possible signs of abuse/dependence include worsening school/job performance, cessation of previous prosocial activities (i.e., quitting sports teams), decreased involvement in family activities, change in peer group, increasing isolation and withdrawal, mood changes (increased lability, irritability, anger, depression), recurrent/frequent "flu" or other illness (actually related to opiate withdrawal), truancy, curfew violations, and new or increased legal involvement. Abuse can be discovered when families recognize medications have disappeared, or when adolescents are caught buying drugs or engaging in criminal behaviors to get money for drugs. As the adolescent develops tolerance, increasing doses are needed for the youth to experience the desired euphoria/high, which increases the risk of overdose/death because there is less tolerance to respiratory depression. Unusual injuries are suspicious for drug use as a significant proportion of adolescent ER/trauma visits are drug related. Injection site erythema or ecchymoses ("track marks") may bring attention to injection use, as may attempts to hide them by wearing covering clothing such as long sleeves out of season. Occasionally adolescents who abuse opiates may have first clinical presentation with overdose (even fatal overdose) since opiates are potent respiratory depressants that are often combined with alcohol and other sedatives, which potentiate their CNS depressant effects.

Assessment and Treatment

Intoxication and Overdose

Symptoms of opiate intoxication include myosis (pinpoint pupils), drowsiness ("nodding out"), slurred speech, and cognitive impairment. In mild to moderate intoxication, the patient will describe euphoria and often appear sedated. With higher doses patients develop worsening levels of sedation, increasing confusion and cognitive impairment, and ultimately hypotension and respiratory depression that can progress to respiratory arrest. Coma, pinpoint pupils, and respiratory depressions are the classic triad for opiate overdose. If opiate intoxication/overdose is suspected, first-line treatment is intramuscular, intravenous, subcutaneous, or endotracheal administration of the opiate antagonist naloxone. Naloxone displaces already bound opiates from the receptors, reversing the effects of overdose and possibly potentiating withdrawal symptoms. The dose of naloxone may need to be increased for more potent opioids, or repeated/given over a longer time period for opioids with a longer half-life. Because of the high prevalence of opioid use in youths, naloxone should be first-line treatment in any case of unexplained stupor or respiratory depression. In cases of suspected opioid overdose, lack of response should not be seen as evidence that opioids are not involved until multiple doses have been given. When buprenorphine is involved, especially high doses of naloxone are needed because of buprenorphine's high affinity for the opiate receptor. Blood or urine toxicology screens and a blood alcohol concentration should always be obtained when the adolescent is intoxicated to look for other substances of abuse. Patients also may require intravenous hydration and, if withdrawal occurs, additional supportive care measures. Emergency medical treatment for overdose (or other medical sequelae of use) is of course necessary, but never sufficient; initiation of comprehensive treatment for addiction is critical.

Withdrawal/Detoxification

Many adolescents who think they are just "recreational users" realize they are opioid dependent when they first experience withdrawal symptoms when they stop using. Opiate withdrawal has two components: the initial acute phase with marked somatic symptoms, followed by a period of protracted abstinence with persistent but less severe symptoms and prominent cravings.

Acute withdrawal is not life-threatening (in the absence of other severe medical morbidity that might make a hyperdynamic state dangerous), but quitting "cold turkey" is extremely uncomfortable without appropriate pharmacological treatment. As a result, many adolescents resume use because they cannot tolerate withdrawal. The symptoms of opiate withdrawal are the result of lack of activation of the opioid receptor, resulting in a rebound increase in CNS activity previously suppressed by opioids. Onset of symptoms is related to the half-life of the drug used (i.e., 4–6 hours after last heroin use or 1–2 days after last methadone use). Standardized withdrawal assessment protocols are useful tools to assess and monitor withdrawal. Hallmarks of opiate withdrawal include tachycardia, hypertension, mild fever, rhinorrhea, sneezing, pupillary dilation, piloerection, restlessness, irritability, yawning, insomnia, anorexia, nausea, vomiting, and diarrhea. Patients also experience subjective cravings, and the combination of these intense cravings and severe withdrawal symptoms often results in resumption of use. The Clinical Opioid Withdrawal Scale (COWS) is a simple, standardized tool for quantifying and tracking withdrawal severity; it is reproduced in Appendix 22.1 at the end of this chapter [16].

The acute manifestations of opiate withdrawal should be pharmacologically managed. Gradually tapering doses of an opioid agonist is the most effective and physiologically direct method of treatment, and any opioid agonist can be used. Buprenorphine, a high-affinity partial mu agonist, has increasingly become the standard of care for opioid detoxification because of its pharmacological properties, including safety and side effect profile, and ease of transition to maintenance if desired. For detoxification, buprenorphine can be used alone (Subutex) or in the combination product with naloxone (Suboxone), while for maintenance (except in pregnancy) the combination product is preferable to help prevent diversion for injection use. Methadone is sometimes used in adults because of its low cost, but it has the disadvantage of being available only in specialty centers licensed for its use, and it entails some difficulty in transitioning to buprenorphine for maintenance if desired. Clonidine, the sympatholytic alpha-2 agonist, had previously been the mainstay of care prior to the widespread use of buprenorphine, and is still used, though dosing is frequently limited by orthostasis, and it is less effective at reducing symptoms than buprenorphine. In addition, specific symptoms can be targeted: non-steroidal anti-inflammatories like ibuprofen or naproxen for myalgia; dicyclomine (or dicycloverine; Bentyl – an anticholinergic) or bismuth salicylate for cramping and diarrhea; antacids for nausea; diphenhydramine, trazodone, or hydroxyzine for insomnia; and clonidine or diazepam for agitation/irritability and general hyperdynamic state. Care should be taken to delay first administration of buprenorphine for detoxification until moderate withdrawal symptoms have emerged (COWS score >10), in order to avoid the possibility of precipitated withdrawal.

The American Society of Addiction Medicine Patient Placement Criteria (ASAM PPC2-R) recommend that adolescents receive residential care during opiate detoxification that is severe enough to require pharmacological management [17]. Detoxification is an essential first step for treatment, but detoxification alone is never sufficient. Linkage to comprehensive addiction treatment and continuing care is critical to avoid the revolving door of repeated crisis-oriented episodes of detoxifications that punctuate a worsening course.

Medication-Assisted Treatment (MAT)/Medication-Assisted Recovery (MAR)

The second component of withdrawal, after resolution of acute somatic symptoms, is the initial period of abstinence during which time patients report persistent and often severe cravings. Patients are at a very high risk of relapse during this phase, and continued use of relapse prevention medications could diminish cravings and help prevent relapse. The use of medication-assisted treatment (MAT)/medication-assisted recovery (MAR) for opiate addiction is now considered the standard of care for opiate addiction in adults, and has been shown to be effective in adolescent patients. MAR/MAT includes agonists (methadone or buprenorphine) and opioid receptor antagonists (naltrexone). The use of buprenorphine, usually prescribed in the combination product with naloxone to deter diversion (Suboxone), is increasing. Unlike methadone maintenance, which is only available in specially licensed methadone programs, which generally do not have developmentally appropriate treatment components, buprenorphine can be prescribed by any physician certified through easily available training, and is easily linked to adolescent-specific treatment programs. In a multi-site randomized controlled trial, extended treatment with buprenorphine plus counseling has been shown to be more effective in adolescents than detoxification alone plus counseling [18,19]. Opiate antagonist therapy is another pharmacological option. Although poor compliance limits the effectiveness of daily oral naltrexone, in October 2010 the US Food and Drug Administration (FDA) approved a once-a-month extended-release injectable formulation of naltrexone (Vivitrol) for relapse prevention in opioid dependence. Extended-release naltrexone has been shown to be effective in adults, and there is preliminary suggestion of its suitability for adolescents [20]. This long-acting formulation may be particularly appropriate for patients who have had trouble with treatment adherence, or for whom there might be a preference to avoid an agonist. Any maintenance medication should be prescribed as part of a comprehensive recovery treatment plan, which should include group and/or individual and/or family counseling, assessment, and treatment of co-occurring disorders, and appropriate life-skills, educational, or vocational services.

Additional Assessment Issues

When opiate abuse/dependence is suspected or confirmed, the initial step is a thorough assessment, including a medical evaluation/history, with particular attention to educational/vocational issues, family history, psychiatric history, drug history, and social history (peers, romantic/sexual relationships, living arrangements, and agency involvement such as social or juvenile services). Understanding the adolescent's access to opiates is important, in that family and friends need to safely dispose of or secure any prescription narcotics in the home. This can become challenging when a parent/guardian is taking prescribed opiates for chronic pain, or when family or friends are also abusing opiates. Urine toxicology screening is an important tool in a variety of settings, but particularly in acute intoxication or overdose and during treatment/recovery to monitor for relapse. It is important to remember that standard opioid immunoassay screening tests do not typically detect buprenorphine, methadone, or oxycodone. Additionally, naloxone (as contained in Suboxone) and naltrexone (as contained in Vivitrol) can produce false-positive results on the standard qualitative opioid immunoassay screening tests, distinguished by low concentrations on quantitative assays [21].

Patients with substance use disorders tend to engage in other high-risk behaviors resulting in medical complications including sexually transmitted infections (STIs), pregnancy, trauma, and malnutrition. There are numerous associated medical conditions related to opiate use, which must be considered in both acute and chronic use. Complications of injection use include hepatitis (particularly hepatitis C virus, or HCV), HIV, cellulitis, abscesses, and endocarditis. Heroin nephropathy, more common in chronic adult users, is an important cause of end-stage renal disease; whether the nephropathy is secondary specifically to heroin, all opiates, adulterants, or related diseases (hepatitis/HIV) is not clearly understood. Amenorrhea is a common endocrine complication related to the dopaminergic effects of opiates. All patients being evaluated for opioid abuse/dependence should be screened for STIs, offered family planning services, including pregnancy testing, and screened for hepatitis and HIV. Psychiatric assessment is important given the high rates of co-occurring mental health disorders in adolescents with substance use disorders. In one study, 78% of opiate-dependent youths admitted to a SUD treatment program had a clinically significant psychiatric disorder, including

40% with depression [22,23]. Mood disorders and attention-deficit/hyperactivity disorder (ADHD) are two commonly associated mental health disorders both of which can be treated with medications; other associated mental health disorders include conduct disorder and oppositional defiant disorder, which are addressed with behavioral treatments. Concurrent diagnosis and treatment of the addiction and the coexisting psychiatric disorder is more effective than trying to serially manage the disorders.

Summary Points

Prescription opioids are relatively accessible to adolescents, who often consider prescription medications "safer" than illicit drugs. National surveys of drug use demonstrate that prescription opioids are now very common drugs of choice for adolescents, second only to marijuana. Nearly 1 in 10 high-school seniors has abused a prescription opiate, and the morbidity and mortality of opiate abuse is rising. Heroin use is also epidemic with higher purity of street supplies allowing initiation through nasal use. Progression to injection heroin use is an advanced stage of illness, associated with very high severity and morbidity. Withdrawal is a prominent feature of opioid dependence, and detoxification often is a required component of treatment. Residential substance abuse treatment is the standard of care for adolescent opiate detoxification, and a buprenorphine detoxification taper is often utilized. Associated morbidities include HCV, HIV, overdose, and trauma in the context of intoxication. Many adolescents with opiate addiction also have comorbid psychiatric illness such as mood disorders, and they have often engaged in other high-risk behaviors. Assessment should include mental health and STI screening. Relapse prevention pharmacotherapy (medication-assisted recovery) is recommended for opiate-dependent patients as part of a comprehensive treatment plan.

SEDATIVE-HYPNOTICS

Introduction

Sedative-hypnotic is a general term used to describe a wide range of CNS depressants including benzodiazepines, barbiturates, and non-benzodiazepine agents (zolpidem, baclofen, meprobamate, etc.) used to treat anxiety and insomnia or as muscle relaxants (see Table 22.2). Barbiturates and benzodiazepines are gamma-aminobutyric acid (GABA) agonists, and the sedative-hypnotics as a class act on the GABA system, though not exclusively. GABA is an inhibitory neurotransmitter, and sedative-hypnotics potentiate GABA effects. Barbiturates were developed in the early 1900s, and their use decreased with the introduction of benzodiazepines in the 1960s. Benzodiazepines were believed at that time to be safer and less addictive than barbiturates. But while benzodiazepines do have some pharmacological advantages over barbiturates – somewhat less sedating, more effective as anxiolytics, less induction of hepatic metabolism, fewer drug-drug interactions, less dangerous respiratory depression and hypotension in overdose – they have severe side-effect profiles of their own, and certainly substantial addiction risk. Withdrawal from both benzodiazepines and barbiturates can involve life-threatening seizures and delirium.

Diazepam, introduced into the market in 1963 as Valium, was the most prescribed drug in the United States from 1969 until 1982. It was nicknamed "Executive Excedrin" and immortalized in song ("Mother's Little Helper") by the Rolling Stones. Initially benzodiazepines were falsely promoted as nonaddictive and free of side effects, but their addiction risk has since been well established. In the 1980s a large class action lawsuit was filed in Great Britain against the manufacturers alleging prior knowledge of the risk of benzodiazepine dependence. Sedative-hypnotics are prescribed for a variety of conditions including insomnia, anxiety, seizure disorder, skeletal muscle pain and spasm, and alcohol withdrawal. They can be given rectally, orally, or by intravenous or intramuscular injection. Clinically benzodiazepines are extremely effective short-term agents for status epilepticus, acute anxiety, and alcohol detoxification. They have minimal risk of respiratory depression when used orally and alone, but this is increased with parenteral use, and there is considerable risk of deadly potentiation of respiratory depression when combined with alcohol or opioids. In addition to dependence, other side effects include cognitive and psychomotor impairment, and induction or exacerbation of psychiatric conditions, particularly mood disorders [24]. Benzodiazepines are classified as Schedule IV drugs. The debate over the risks versus benefits of benzodiazepine use continues: while some patients tolerate and responsibly manage low doses without dose escalation over time, many others have cumulative side effects and/or aberrant drug-taking behaviors. Any benefits of short-term use are potentially complicated by high rates of dose escalation and side effects, as well as the risks of misuse and all too easy transition to long-term use. Especially high-risk populations include adolescents, patients with history or risk of addiction, and patients with psychiatric disorders. Flunitrazepam (Rohypnol) is a benzodiazepine that is illegal in the United States; also known as the "date rape" drug, "roofies" have rapid onset and strong amnestic properties; assailants may surreptitiously add flunitrazepam to a victim's drink to sedate them, and victims may have no memory of what happened to them. Alprazolam (Xanax), lorazepam (Ativan), clonazepam (Klonopin), and diazepam (Valium) are among the best known and most popular benzodiazepines.

Other related agents used as anxiolytics and/or muscle relaxants are included in the broad class of sedative-hypnotics. These include baclofen, carisoprodol, meprobamate, cyclobenzaprine, and others. Additionally, a newer class of non-benzodiazepine hypnotics was introduced in the 1990s as treatment for insomnia and is marketed as being safer and less addictive then benzodiazepines. Although they are not chemically benzodiazepines, they share the GABA mechanism of benzodiazepines. The "Z-drugs" (zolpidem, zaleplon, zolpiclone, and eszopiclone) are widely prescribed; taken alone they are generally safe but they are unsafe when combined with other CNS depressants. As with benzodiazepines, long-term use is not recommended. They have the typical sedative-hypnotic side-effect profile (cognitive impairment, affective instability, disinhibition), and tolerance, dependence, and withdrawal do occur, although perhaps to a lesser degree than with benzodiazepines. Patients with a history of addiction should not be prescribed these agents given the risk of dependence.

Barbiturates, like benzodiazepines, are classified according to their half-life. Phenobarbital, which has a long half-life, is prescribed for seizures and has been used in alcohol detoxification protocols for the prevention and treatment of delirium tremens. Thiopental is a short-acting barbiturate that can cause disinhibition and was sometimes called "truth serum." Benzodiazepines have replaced most medical uses of barbiturates. When taken alone a barbiturate overdose can be more dangerous than a benzodiazepine overdose; however, when combined with other CNS depressants both can be fatal.

Epidemiology

In 2000, more Americans (over 10%) used benzodiazepines than any other drug class [25]. While in recent years the rise in rates of prescription opiate abuse has garnered lots of media attention, rates of benzodiazepine abuse have also increased. Annual prevalence rates among 12th-graders more than doubled between 1990 and 2002, and since then have remained constant at about 6% [7]. Figure 22.6 highlights trends in benzodiazepine use among young people.

Alprazolam (Xanax) is the most popular and widely abused of the sedative-hypnotics. Benzodiazepines are Schedule IV drugs, a classification that implies that they have less potential for abuse than Schedules I to III substances, but this can be misleading. Barbiturate abuse has remained steady as noted in Figure 22.7.

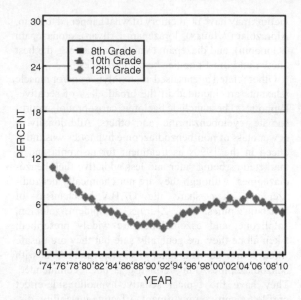

Figure 22.6 Sedatives (benzodiazepines): trends in annual use: percentage who used in past 12 months. Reproduced with permission from Johnston LD, O'Malley PM, Bachman JG, Schulenberg JE. *Monitoring the Future national survey results on drug use, 1975–2009. Volume I: Secondary school students* (NIH Publication No. 10-7584). Bethesda, MD: National Institute on Drug Abuse, 2010, 734 pp.

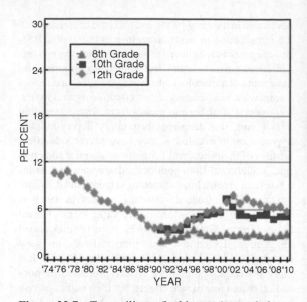

Figure 22.7 Tranquilizers (barbiturates): trends in annual use: percentage who used in past 12 months. Reproduced with permission from Johnston LD, O'Malley PM, Bachman JG, Schulenberg JE. *Monitoring the Future national survey results on drug use, 1975–2009. Volume I: Secondary school students* (NIH Publication No. 10-7584). Bethesda, MD: National Institute on Drug Abuse, 2010, 734 pp.

Diagnostic Criteria

Sedative-hypnotic abuse and dependence are diagnosed using the same criteria as those for abuse and dependence syndromes with other substances, with the core feature represented by the maladaptive pattern of use and worsening negative consequences of use. Most sedative-hypnotic use by adolescents is sporadic, accompanying the abuse of other primary substances of choice. Sometimes they have access to sedative-hypnotics because they live with an individual (parent/guardian) who has been prescribed a benzodiazepine for anxiety/panic attacks. Benzodiazepine use seems to be more common among youths with opioid dependence. Furthermore, some adolescents use sedative-hypnotics to help themselves "come down" or balance the agitating effects of cocaine or methamphetamine. On the other hand, a subgroup of youths develop full physiological dependence on sedative-hypnotics; in these cases the presence of tolerance and withdrawal is clinically significant.

Physiological dependence can develop even in patients who take non-escalating doses of prescribed benzodiazepines over a prolonged period, although this is seen less often in adolescents since they are less likely to be prescribed benzodiazepines. It is much more difficult to assess for abuse/dependence in patients taking benzodiazepines for anxiety/mood disorders or insomnia. While these patients may accept the diagnosis of dependence/addiction for other drugs, they may be less accepting of evidence of impairment associated with benzodiazepines because they have experienced partial relief from their anxiety/panic with benzodiazepines and do not want them discontinued. While they may exhibit signs of withdrawal, the patient may minimize these, convinced that their symptoms are not withdrawal but a re-emergence of their underlying anxiety/mood disorder. The *Diagnostic and Statistical Manual of Mental Disorders, Fourth Edition* (DSM-IV) classification includes Sedative, Hypnotic, or Anxiolytic abuse, dependence, intoxication, or withdrawal, with a variety of subclassifications for psychosis, delirium, hallucinations, dementia, etc. Barbiturate abuse is less common than benzodiazepine and opioid abuse, most likely because barbiturates became less commonly prescribed with the advent of benzodiazepines.

Clinical Presentation

Clinical Vignette

Joe is a 15-year-old boy brought to the emergency room via ambulance after his friends called 911. They noted that he was "way too zombied out" after he had been drinking with them following a high-school football game. His peers report that Joe only drank "three beers" and he started acting increasingly confused and "didn't make sense." On arrival, the paramedics noted that Joe appeared confused and had trouble identifying the date, where he was, and recalling the names of his friends. His speech was grossly slurred and he was ataxic. A search of his backpack revealed an empty prescription bottle of diazepam that had been prescribed for his mother.

Benzodiazepines are highly lipophilic with rapid dissemination into the CNS. Adolescents who abuse sedative-hypnotics may initially exhibit minimal signs of use or they may overdose since they are often combined with alcohol and other sedatives that potentiate their CNS depressant effects. Sedation is also a common presenting symptom of barbiturate use. In general, benzodiazepines and barbiturates are taken along with other licit and illicit drugs, and the clinical presentation is a mixed picture of disinhibition, sedation, cognitive impairment (ranging from mild slowing to confusion or delirium), and physiological changes reflecting multiple substances. Extensive urine and blood toxicology screening is mandatory, and standard management of ABCs (airway, breathing, circulation) is recommended. There are minorities of adolescents who exclusively abuse benzodiazepines, but, unlike adults, adolescents tend to continue to use a wider range of drugs.

Assessment and Treatment

Intoxication/Overdose

Symptoms of sedative-hypnotic intoxication include sedation, ataxia, slurred speech, and cognitive impairment. With higher doses patients can develop stupor or coma, and barbiturate overdose can lead to hypotension, cardiovascular collapse, and respiratory arrest. Death from benzodiazepine overdose alone is uncommon, but many adolescents will have ingested a variety of intoxicants. Alcohol or opioids (including buprenorphine) taken together with benzodiazepines can lead to respiratory depression or arrest. Some patients have a paradoxical reaction to benzodiazepines, exhibiting increased irritability, impulsivity, aggressiveness, and lowering of the seizure threshold. If benzodiazepine intoxication/overdose is suspected, flumazenil should be administered parenterally as a competitive antagonist that can reverse the sedative effects of benzodiazepines. Airway management is integral in any sedative-hypnotic overdose, and gastric lavage and activated charcoal are sometimes used for ingestions. To look for other substances of abuse, blood or urine toxicology screens and a blood alcohol concentration should always be obtained when the adolescent is intoxicated.

Withdrawal/Detoxification

Benzodiazepine withdrawal symptoms include tachycardia, fever, hypertension, anxiety, agitation, delirium, hallucinosis, seizures, insomnia, fatigue, irritability, sensory disturbances, headache, tremor/muscle fasciculations, sweating, dizziness, and inattention. For patients taking benzodiazepines for anxiety, it can be difficult to assess whether some of these symptoms are related to benzodiazepine withdrawal or exacerbation of the anxiety disorder. Benzodiazepines can be grouped into three categories: short-, medium-, and long-acting, depending on their half-life. Determining which category of benzodiazepine the patient has taken is crucial to the successful management of patients presenting with benzodiazepine intoxication or withdrawal. The drug taken, its half-life, dose, and the duration of use/abuse influence the severity and course of withdrawal. Psychiatric comorbidity tends to exacerbate withdrawal symptoms. Pharmacological management is based on substituting a long-acting benzodiazepine, which is then tapered and discontinued. Clonazepam has often been used as a tapering agent for detoxification, with broad cross-reactivity to all benzodiazepines and most other sedative-hypnotics. Although rare now among adolescents, when barbiturate detoxification is needed, generally the most practical agent to use is phenobarbital. Depending on the prior duration of benzodiazepine use, the taper may need to occur over days to weeks. Other useful agents include carbamazepine or gabapentin to mitigate the risk of seizures and possibly allow lower doses of substitute benzodiazepines, antacids for nausea, diphenhydramine or hydroxyzine for agitation/irritability/insomnia, antipsychotics for hallucinations/sensory disturbances, and dicyclomine (an anticholinergic) for diarrhea. Finally, patients with a comorbid mood disorder should be started on an alternative therapy for their anxiety such as a selective serotonin reuptake inhibitor (SSRI).

Additional Assessment Issues

Although sedative-hypnotics are certainly available on the street from anonymous traffickers, like prescription opioids they are most often obtained from a relative or friend; the family medicine cabinet is the most common dealer. Assessment should include investigation of sources, and education about securing enduring supplies in the home. Sometimes modeling of aberrant drug-taking behavior comes from parents who take prescribed sedative-hypnotics, especially on a p.r.n. ("as required") basis. Sedative-hypnotic problems can be iatrogenic. Some adolescents presenting with polysubstance abuse may have had current or past treatment with benzodiazepines for anxiety or panic or other mood disorders. In their attempts to manage difficult comorbidities it is easy for practitioners to get "over their heads" with escalating doses and/or polypharmacy. A typical example might be benzodiazepines added to an expanding regimen in an attempt to offset side effects of stimulant-induced irritability/anxiety/insomnia. Adolescents may also seek treatment for anxiety while not reporting surreptitious street drug use, sometimes even with the complicity of their families. Even if the adolescent has never been prescribed benzodiazepines, the evaluator should determine if there is a component of comorbid anxiety/depression that may sustain their use as a partial "self-medication." The same principle is true of other sedative-hypnotics in relation to their prescription as muscle relaxants for pain.

When abuse with a sedative-hypnotic is suspected, a thorough history is taken, with particular attention to psychiatric history, family history, recent stressors or life changes, educational/vocational issues, drug history, and social history (peers, romantic/sexual relationships, living arrangements, and agency involvement). As with opiates, understanding the adolescent's access to sedative-hypnotics is important; adolescents often take or are offered medications of other people when they have anxiety. Outside prescribing physicians should be involved and an alternative treatment plan for the adolescent's anxiety developed and implemented. Urine toxicology screening is an important tool in a variety of settings, but particularly in acute intoxication or overdose and during treatment/recovery to monitor for relapse. The NIDA-5 panel tests for five common drugs of abuse (cannabinoids, cocaine, phencyclidine, opiates, and amphetamines) but not for benzodiazepines or barbiturates. Again, as in the case of adolescent opiate abuse, patients with substance use disorders tend to engage in other high-risk behaviors resulting in medical complications including sexually transmitted infections (STIs), pregnancy, trauma, and malnutrition. Psychiatric assessment is important given the high rates of co-occurring mental health disorders in adolescents with substance use disorders; in particular, adolescents with a history of benzodiazepine abuse often have persistent or new-onset anxiety and irritability once the drug is discontinued. If benzodiazepine detoxification is needed, residential treatment for substance abuse is the most appropriate setting, where the adolescent can be supported and provided with pharmacological treatment as needed. In addition, adolescents with underlying anxiety/panic disorders can be more smoothly transitioned to an alternative psychopharmacological agent.

Summary Points

Rates of prescription drug abuse have been increasing, particularly among adolescents and young adults. Sedative-hypnotics, and particularly benzodiazepines, are commonly prescribed for anxiety, panic attacks, and insomnia and are readily available in many homes. Many adolescents use sedative-hypnotics sporadically, mixed with a variety of other substances of abuse. These drugs are potent CNS depressants and, while not usually fatal when taken alone, can be lethal when combined with other drugs, especially alcohol or opioids. Adolescents who are using or have been prescribed these agents for management of anxiety or panic can develop benzodiazepine tolerance and dependence. These patients have a difficult time agreeing to stop using the drugs because they are so potently reinforcing. Patients are often adamant that benzodiazepines are the "only" medicine that has ever helped them. SSRIs are a commonly used alternative for the treatment of anxiety, and residential treatment may be necessary to taper and discontinue the benzodiazepine while initiating alternative treatments. Similar to adolescent opioid users, adolescents with sedative-hypnotic abuse often have comorbid psychiatric illness and are engaged in other high-risk behaviors; assessment should include mental health and STI screening. A comprehensive recovery treatment plan should include group or individual substance abuse counseling, individual and/or family therapy, and appropriate life-skills, educational, or vocational services.

APPENDIX 22.1: CLINICAL OPIATE WITHDRAWAL SCALE

For each item, circle the number that best describes the patient's signs or symptom. Rate on just the apparent relationship to opiate withdrawal. For example, if heart rate is increased because the patient was jogging just prior to assessment, the increased pulse rate would not add to the score.

Patient's Name:_____ Date and Time _____/_____/_____ : _____

Reason for this assessment: _____

Resting Pulse Rate:_____beats/minute
Measured after patient is sitting or lying for one minute
0 pulse rate 80 or below
1 pulse rate 81-100
2 pulse rate 101-120
4 pulse rate greater than 120

GI Upset: *over last $^1/_2$ hour*
0 no GI symptoms
1 stomach cramps
2 nausea or loose stool
3 vomiting or diarrhea
5 Multiple episodes of diarrhea or vomiting

Sweating: *Over past $^1/_2$ hour not accounted for by room temperature or patient activity*
0 no report of chills or flushing
1 subjective report of chills or flushing
2 flushed or observable moistness on face
3 beads of sweat on brow or face
4 sweat streaming off face

Tremor *Observation of outstretched hands*
0 no tremor
1 tremor can be felt, but not observed
2 slight tremor observable
4 gross tremor or muscle twitching

Restlessness *Observation during assessment*
0 able to sit still
1 reports difficulty sitting still, but is able to do so
3 frequent shifting or extraneous movements of legs/arms
5 unable to sit still for more than a few seconds

Yawning *Observation during assessment*
0 no yawning
1 yawning once or twice during assessment
2 yawning three or more times during assessment
4 yawning several times/minute

Pupil size
0 pupils pinned or normal size for room light
1 pupils possibly larger than normal for room light
2 pupils moderately dilated
5 pupils so dilated that only the rim of the iris is visible

Anxiety or irritability
0 none
1 patient reports increasing irritability or anxiousness
2 patient obviously irritable or anxious
4 patient so irritable or anxious that participation in the assessment is difficult

---

Bone or joint aches *If patient was having pain previously, only the additional component attributed to opiates withdrawal is scored*
0 not present
1 mild diffuse discomfort
2 patient reports severe diffuse aching of joints/muscles
4 patient is rubbing joints or muscles and is unable to sit still because of discomfort

Gooseflesh skin
0 skin is smooth
3 piloerection of skin can be felt or hairs standing up on arms
5 prominent piloerection

Runny nose or tearing *Not accounted for by cold symptoms or allergies*
0 not present
1 nasal stuffiness or unusually moist eyes
2 nose running or tearing
4 nose constantly running or tears streaming down cheeks

Total Score _____

The total score is the sum of all 11 items
Initials of person
completing Assessment:_____

Score: 5–12 = mild; 13–24 = moderate; 25–36 = moderately severe; more than 36 = severe withdrawal

References

1. Manchikanti L, Singh A. Therapeutic opioids: a ten-year perspective on the complexities and complications of the escalating use, abuse, and nonmedical use of opioids. *Pain Physician* 2008;**11**:S63–S88.

2. National Institute on Drug Abuse. *NIDA Research Report: Prescription Drug Abuse and Addiction.* NIH Publication Number 05-4881 [revised 2005].

3. The National Center on Addiction and Substance Abuse at Columbia University. *National Survey of American Attitudes on Substance Abuse XV: Teens and Parents.* New York:National Center on Addiction and Substance Abuse at Columbia University, 2010.

4. Centers for Disease Control. Youth Risk Behavior Surveillance – United States, 2009. *MMWR: Morbidity and Mortality Weekly Report* 2010;**59** (SS-5):1–142.

5. Substance Abuse and Mental Health Services Administration, Office of Applied Studies. *The TEDS Report: Substance Abuse Treatment Admissions Involving Abuse of Pain Relievers: 1998 and 2008.* Rockville, MD:Substance Abuse and Mental Health Services Administration, Office of Applied Studies, 2010.

6. Office of National Drug Control Policy, Executive Office of the President. *Teens and Prescription Drugs: An Analysis of Recent Trends on the Emerging Drug.* Washington DC:Office of National Drug Control Policy, 2007.

7. Johnston LD, O'Malley PM, Bachman JG, Schulenberg JE. *Monitoring the Future: National Results on Adolescent Drug Use: Overview of Key Findings, 2010.* Ann Arbor: Institute for Social Research, The University of Michigan, 2011.

8. Cox BM, Borsodi A, Caló G, *et al.* Opioid receptors. Introduction. IUPHAR database (IUPHAR-DB). Available at: http:// www.iuphar-db.org/ DATABASE/ FamilyIntroductionForward?familyId=50.

9. Okie S. A flood of opioids, a rising tide of deaths. *N Engl J Med* 2010;**363**:1981–1985.

10. Fortuna RJ, Robbins BW, Caiola E, Joynt M, Halterman JS. Prescribing of controlled medications to adolescents and young adults in the United States. *Pediatrics* 2010;**126**:1108–1116.

11. Johnston LD, O'Malley PM, Bachman JG, *et al.* *Monitoring the Future: National Results on Adolescent Drug Use: Overview of Key Findings, 2009.* Ann Arbor, MI: Institute for Social Research, The University of Michigan, 2010.

12. Substance Abuse and Mental Health Services Administration. *Results from the 2009 National Survey on Drug Use and Health: Volume I. Summary of National Findings.* Rockville, MD:Substance Abuse and Mental Health Services Administration, Office of Applied Studies, 2010.

13. Salter J, Caldwell AA. Cheap, ultra-potent heroin is causing rise in deaths. Salon, 24 May 2010. Available from: http://www.salon.com/news/feature/2010/05/24/us_drug_war_mexican_heroin.

14. Clemmey P, Payne L, Fishman M. Clinical characteristics and treatment outcomes of adolescent heroin users. *J Psychoactive Drugs* 2004;**36**:85–94.

15. Branson C, Clemmey P, Harrell P, Subramaniam G, Fishman M. Polysubstance use and heroin relapse among adolescents following residential treatment. *J Child Adolesc Subst Abuse* 2012;**21**:3.

16. Wesson DR, Ling W. The Clinical Opiate Withdrawal Scale (COWS). *J Psychoactive Drugs* 2003;**35**:253–259.

17. Mee-Lee D, Shulman GD, Fishman M, Gastfriend D (eds). *ASAM Patient Placement Criteria for the Treatment of Substance-Related Disorders, Second Edition–Revised* (ASAM PPC-2R). Chevy Chase, MD: American Society of Addiction Medicine, Inc., 2001.

18. Woody GE, Poole SA, Subramaniam G, *et al.* Extended vs short-term buprenorphine-naloxone for treatment of opioid-addicted youth: a randomized trial. *JAMA* 2008;**300**:2003–2011.

19. Subramaniam G, Fishman M, Woody G. Treatment of opioid-dependent adolescents and young adults with buprenorphine. *Curr Psych Rep* 2009;**11**:360–363.

20. Fishman M, Winstanley E, Curran E, Garrett S, Subramaniam G. Treatment of opioid dependence in adolescents and young adults with extended release naltrexone: preliminary case series and feasibility. *Addiction* 2010;**105**:1669–1676.

21. Jenkins AJ, Poirier JG, Juhascik MP. Cross-reactivity of naloxone with oxycodone immunoassays: implications for individuals taking Suboxone®. *Clin Chem* 2009;**55**:1434–1436. Available at:http://www.clinchem.org/cgi/reprint/55/7/1434.

22. Subramaniam G, Stitzer M, Woody G, Fishman M, Kolodner K. Clinical characteristics of treatment seeking adolescents with opioid versus cannabis/alcohol use disorders. *Drug Alcohol Depend* 2009;**99**:141–149.

23. Subramaniam G, Stitzer M. Clinical characteristics of treatment-seeking prescription opioid vs. heroin-using adolescents with opioid use disorder. *Drug Alcohol Depend* 2009;**101**:13–19.

24. Robinson DS. Benzodiazepines: clinical use and abuse. Primary Psychiatry. Available at:http://www.primarypsychiatry.com/aspx/article_pf.aspx?articleid=666.

25. Bellenir K. *Drug Abuse Sourcebook.* Detroit:Omnigraphics, 2000, p. 133.

26. Substance Abuse and Mental Health Services Administration, Office of Applied Studies. *The NSDUH Report: Trends in Nonmedical Use of Prescription Pain Relievers: 2002 to 2007.* Rockville, MD:SAMHSA, 2009.

23

Nicotine Use Disorders

Kevin M. Gray,[1] Matthew J. Carpenter,[1] and Himanshu P. Upadhyaya[2]

[1]*Department of Psychiatry and Behavioral Sciences; Hollings Cancer Center, Medical University of South Carolina, Charleston, SC, USA*
[2]*Department of Psychiatry and Behavioral Sciences; Eli Lilly and Company, Indianapolis, IN, USA*

INTRODUCTION

Despite tremendous education and prevention efforts, tobacco smoking continues to be common in adolescents. As the leading cause of preventable death both in the United States and throughout the world, tobacco smoking is among the most important topics for prevention, screening, diagnosis, and treatment in all age groups [1]. Adolescents are of particular concern for several reasons. First, adolescence is a developmental stage characterized by elevated risk-taking, including experimentation with substances including tobacco. Second, emerging evidence suggests that adolescents may be particularly prone to progression from smoking initiation to dependence [2,3]. Third, almost all adult smokers (90%) began smoking by age 18, indicating the potential longstanding nature of adolescent-initiated smoking behavior [4].

Adolescent smoking is rarely a main focus of clinical encounters. Clinicians may be (i) unaware of the high prevalence of smoking within this age group, (ii) unfamiliar with evidence-based methods for screening and assessment, and (iii) under the assumption that adolescent smokers are not interested in quitting and not amenable to smoking cessation interventions. Compounding these issues, adolescent smokers may (i) underreport or fail to report smoking during clinical encounters, (ii) underestimate the potential for personal long-term health consequences of smoking, and (iii) choose to "go it alone" (rather than seeking help) even when motivated to quit smoking, a strategy that is rarely effective [5–7].

Addressing these challenges is daunting, but is critical given the tremendous potential long-term health impact of identifying and assisting adolescent smokers. One-fifth of deaths in the United States result from smoking, a toll greater than those of alcohol, illegal drugs, homicide, suicide, car accidents, and AIDS combined [8]. One might reason that this mortality rate will likely decline in light of improved knowledge among young people about smoking's dangers. However, given that young adults currently smoke at a greater rate than all older age groups, it is likely that without significant advances or changes the devastating burden of tobacco-related illness will remain [9].

Within this chapter, the background on adolescent smoking is provided in the form of an epidemiological overview, detailing tobacco use prevalence by severity/frequency, age, grade level, race/ethnicity, method of administration, and comorbidity. Adolescent attitudes about tobacco use are also explored. Diagnostic criteria for nicotine use disorders are then provided, with review of relevant rating scales and measures validated among adolescent smokers. Next, guidance is provided regarding typical presentations of adolescent tobacco use in clinical practice. Assessment issues are addressed in detail, with a practical guide for clinicians to efficiently and effectively screen, assess, diagnose, and assist adolescent smokers. Specific methods for treatment are detailed in the "Treatment" section of this text.

EPIDEMIOLOGY

While most adult smokers are generally assumed to be habitual daily smokers ("pack a day," etc.), a wide range of smoking rate and frequency is seen in adolescence. This initial lack of any one pattern reflects, in part, the early stages of smoking, with transition from isolated experimentation to occasional and more frequent use. There are, however, some potentially distinct and sustained smoking patterns common in this age group (e.g., "chippers" or "chunk smokers") [10]. "Chippers" are defined as very light smokers who regularly use tobacco without developing dependence, and "chunk smokers" are characterized by smoking only in specific circumstances or settings [11]. For example, while occasional smokers represent 25% of the adult smoking population they comprise 65% of young adult tobacco users [12,13].

The National Survey on Drug Use and Health (NSDUH) provides an overview of tobacco use in adolescence and other age groups [9]. Among individuals 12 to 17 years old, 11.6% use any tobacco products (generally defined as any use in the past 30 days), 8.9% smoke cigarettes, and 2.3% use smokeless tobacco (some of whom are dual users of cigarettes). Of cigarette smokers within this age group, 2.1% smoke daily and 98% do not; only 0.4% smoke one or more packs daily). Cigarette use (again, any use in past month) increases steadily during adolescence, with 1.4% of 12–13-year-olds, 7.5% of 14–15-year-olds, 16.9% of 16–17-year-olds, and 33.1% of 18–20-year-olds currently smoking. Smoking prevalence is now highest in young adults, compared with all other age groups. Gender differences in adolescent (ages 12–17) cigarette smoking are small and not statistically significant, with 9.2% of males and 8.6% of females smoking. Table 23.1 summarizes the smoking prevalence among various racial/ethnic groups.

The Monitoring the Future (MTF) survey provides a similar overview of smoking prevalence rates, though it surveys by grade level (rather than age), includes additional details, and explores attitudes toward smoking [14]. In concordance with NSDUH, MTF reveals an increase in smoking rates from 8th to 10th to 12th grade. Among 8th-graders, 20.1% have ever smoked, 6.5% have smoked in the last month, 2.7% smoke daily, and 1.0% smoke at least half a pack (10 cigarettes) daily. Among 10th-graders, 32.7% have ever smoked, 13.1% have smoked in the last month, 6.3% smoke daily, and 2.4% smoke at least half a pack daily. Among 12th-graders, respective estimates are 43.6%, 20%, 11.2%, and 5%. Differences in smoking rates by

Table 23.1 Smoking prevalence among racial/ethnic groups (ages 12–17) [9].

Racial/ethnic group	Smoking prevalence
American Indians/ Alaskan Natives	11.6%
White	10.6%
Hispanics	7.5%
Blacks	5.1%
Asians	2.5%

educational aspirations exist; of students aspiring to less than four years of college the current rate of smoking is 19.5%, compared with only 5.3% for those aspiring to at least four years of college. Perceived risk of smoking gradually rises with grade level, with 59.1% of 8th-graders, 67.3% of 10th-graders, and 74.9% of 12th-graders believing that smoking at least a pack daily involves "great" risk. Between 82% and 87% of students disapprove of smoking, 75% to 81% prefer to date a nonsmoker, 73% describe smoking as a dirty habit, and 49% to 56% dislike being near a smoker.

Smokeless tobacco includes dip, chew, and snuff. While this form of tobacco is not smoked/inhaled, it still conveys significant health risk, including the risk of oral and throat cancer. MTF data reveal that, among 8th-graders, 9.6% have ever used smokeless tobacco, 3.7% have used it in the last month, and 0.8% use it daily. Among 10th-graders, parallel estimates are 15.2%, 6.5%, and 1.9%, and among 12th-graders, 16.3%, 8.4%, and 2.9%. Between 40% and 45% of students perceive health risks incurred by regular use of smokeless tobacco, and 80% disapprove of using it. A hookah (water pipe) is a single or multi-stemmed instrument for smoking in which the smoke is cooled and passed through water. This tobacco ingestion method is gaining popularity among young people. One recent study estimated ever-usage and past-month usage among middle-school students to be 2% and 1%, and among high-school students to be 10% and 5% [15]. Water pipe use is even more prevalent in young adult (college) populations: 15–48% of college freshman have ever used, and 10–20% report usage in the past month [16–18].

Psychosocial and socioeconomic stress as well as parental and peer smoking are associated with increased risk of adolescent smoking [19]. Psychiatric disorders, including attention-deficit/hyperactivity disorder (ADHD), oppositional defiant disorder, conduct disorder, major depressive disorder, anxiety disorders, and other substance use disorders are all associated with higher rates of tobacco use in adolescents [20,21]. Anxiety disorders, particularly panic disorder, predict development of nicotine dependence, while mood disorders and nicotine dependence appear to share common underlying factors. Disruptive behavior disorders and nicotine dependence possess a bidirectional association (each predicts the other). Other substance use (particularly abuse or dependence) is among the strongest predictors of nicotine dependence in adolescence [20]. This relationship appears to be bidirectional, and debate continues on whether it may be explained as a "gateway effect" or a result of shared vulnerabilities [22,23]. In light of the strong association of psychiatric and substance use disorders with smoking, clinicians should be particularly vigilant about assessing smoking among adolescents presenting with these disorders.

DIAGNOSTIC CRITERIA

The *Diagnostic and Statistical Manual of Mental Disorders, Fourth Edition, Text Revision* (DSM-IV-TR) contains the formal diagnostic criteria for Nicotine Use Disorders, including Nicotine Dependence (305.1), Nicotine Withdrawal (292.0), and Nicotine Use Disorder Not Otherwise Specified (292.9) [24]. Diagnostic criteria for dependence are the same as for other substances (i.e., general substance dependence criteria). Differences in diagnostic assessment of nicotine vs. other substances of abuse, and the implications of these differences for treatment, have been discussed elsewhere [25] and are not within the scope of this chapter. Of note, however, nicotine, unlike other substances, does not have an associated "abuse" diagnosis. As such, individuals presenting with clinically significant symptoms that do not meet criteria for Nicotine Dependence and/or Nicotine Withdrawal may only be diagnosed with Nicotine Use Disorder NOS.

The limits of DSM-IV-TR present a diagnostic conundrum for the clinician evaluating adolescent smokers. To meet nicotine dependence criteria, adolescents must exhibit clinically significant nicotine-related impairment or distress, meeting at least three of seven criteria, such as tolerance, withdrawal, difficulty cutting down or quitting, and continued use despite negative impacts on time, activities, and psychological and physical health.

While some adolescent smokers do meet sufficient criteria for this diagnosis, many (particularly those early in the course of smoking) do not [26]. Given that most adolescent smokers do not smoke daily, it stands to reason that withdrawal (and to some extent tolerance) may not be clinically apparent. Escalating use beyond intended parameters may be restricted by external factors (e.g., limited availability of cigarettes, smoking restrictions in school and other settings). A desire to cut down or cease use may not be present early in the course of smoking. Time engaged in nicotine-related activities may not be perceived as excessive, as nicotine use is not generally associated with acute impairments in sensorium. Important social, occupational, and recreational activities may therefore often continue unabated, even in light of frequent nicotine use. Adolescents may additionally not perceive physical or psychological harm associated with nicotine, as this often requires cumulative exposure over several years of nicotine use. It is important to note that adolescents early in the course of smoking (>100 cigarettes smoked) who meet some nicotine dependence criteria (but not sufficient for formal diagnosis) are more likely to continue smoking than those not meeting any dependence criteria [27]. As such, the threshold for clinical attention to adolescent smoking should be set below the standard of dependence diagnosis. Non-dependent adolescent smokers meeting only one or two dependence criteria may be among the highest-yield targets for early intervention, given their (i) propensity for progression to long-term smoking, and (ii) potential early-stage smoking behavior malleability.

While the Nicotine Use Disorder Not Otherwise Specified (NOS) diagnosis may be employed for adolescent smokers not meeting dependence criteria, the NOS diagnosis is non-specific and lacks descriptive quality that sufficiently reflects a particular adolescent's nicotine-related impairment. To address these limitations, alternative/complementary nicotine-related assessment measures have been developed and validated among adolescent smokers. Of particular value with these measures is the ability to utilize a continuous score, rather than a categorical "yes" versus "no," in evaluating presence and severity of nicotine-related symptoms [28]. Three of these measures are discussed under "Relevant Assessment Issues" below.

A DSM-IV-TR diagnosis of nicotine withdrawal is characterized by at least four of eight signs, such as depressed mood, insomnia, irritability, anxiety, difficulty concentrating, restlessness, decreased heart rate, and increased appetite, causing clinically significant distress or impairment within 24 hours of abrupt cessation or reduction in nicotine use after several weeks of daily nicotine use. Despite the diagnostic requirement for several weeks of daily smoking, clinically significant withdrawal symptoms in non-daily adolescent smokers have been reported [29]. The most commonly used assessment instrument for nicotine withdrawal in adolescent research is the Minnesota Nicotine Withdrawal Scale [30]. This instrument notably adds an item reflecting urge or craving to smoke, a core element of withdrawal omitted from the DSM-IV-TR criteria. Though some adolescent smokers claim withdrawal during abstinence, the vast majority of youth smokers, by nature of their irregular smoking behavior, do not exhibit objective indices of withdrawal, but do report significant craving [31,32]. Finally, clinicians assessing adolescents with psychiatric comorbidity should be aware of potential overlaps between symptoms of withdrawal and those of common psychiatric conditions [33]. For example, depressed mood, insomnia, restlessness, and difficulty concentrating each overlap significantly with other DSM-IV-TR diagnostic categories (depression, ADHD, etc.), and clinicians should be careful not to confuse one with the other.

CLINICAL PRESENTATION

Clinical Vignette

During screening for depression as part of a routine office visit, "Martin" (a 15-year-old patient), reveals symptoms of irritability, particularly during school hours. He mentions in passing that smoking a cigarette on the way home quickly relieves his irritability. Further questioning reveals that Martin typically smokes two to three cigarettes in the afternoon/evening, and one cigarette in the morning on the way to school. On the weekends, especially when socializing with friends, Martin smokes more frequently. However, Martin insists that he is not a "smoker," emphasizing that he is "not hooked," and only smokes to relieve stress and to facilitate social interactions. He acknowledges the associated health risks, but emphasizes that he does not plan to continue smoking long-term.

Because many young smokers do not even identify themselves as smokers [10], identifying them is the first hurdle clinicians may encounter. Many adolescents will downplay their smoking behavior, often minimizing risk. Teens, like adults, may overestimate the general risks of smoking but underestimate the personal risks [34,35]. Examples of self-exempting beliefs of risk include "I don't smoke that much" or "I'll quit before I graduate college or get married" or "I have family members who smoked for years and never had a problem." Though adolescents who smoke may not present clinically with smoking-related physical complaints, several studies have shown that smoking even at low levels can lead to health problems [36–38]. Nonetheless, the principal risk for smoking at this vulnerable stage of adolescence is the progression toward chronic nicotine dependence that will make future quitting even more difficult. Thus, adolescent smokers need to be educated about the nature of dependence and its implications for quitting.

Given their propensity for underestimation of personal risks from smoking, many adolescents may be unmotivated to quit. Some, particularly those who do not smoke daily and/or only smoke in certain contexts, might not even identify themselves as smokers. In this situation, the concept of quitting may appear foreign to an adolescent who considers his/her smoking to be non-habitual. A critical component of assessment is open-ended questioning about ANY (even once) experiences with nicotine use, rather than asking whether or not the adolescent is a smoker. A non-judgmental, open-ended approach is most likely to yield information. Adolescents may additionally be more receptive to screening without a parent/guardian in the room, as parents/guardians may not be aware of any smoking.

However, not all adolescents should be discounted in their desire to quit. One recent review (over 50 studies included) examined the prevalence, frequency, and duration of quit attempts among teen smokers [39]. Among these, estimates of past 6-month, past year,

and ever quit attempts were 58%, 68%, and 74%, respectively. Quit attempts were not restricted to daily smokers, but were common among low-rate smokers as well, a finding that has been replicated elsewhere [40]. The majority of adolescents who do attempt to quit will try again, but the median prevalence of relapse at 1 week, 1 month, 6 months, and 1 year is 34%, 56%, 89%, and 92% [39]. Other studies have shown that variables associated with quit interest vary among regular vs. intermittent smokers [41]. For example, among established smokers, the quantity of cigarettes smoked and time to first cigarette are both inversely associated with making a quit attempt (i.e., more established/early morning smokers are less likely to try to quit). In contrast, among occasional smokers, these traditional markers of dependence were unrelated to making a quit attempt.

RELEVANT ASSESSMENT ISSUES

Most adolescent smokers do not seek out treatment information, and rarely is tobacco use a presenting problem within clinical settings. It is therefore critically important that all clinicians effectively screen for tobacco use. The US Public Health Service guidelines for smoking cessation advise the 5A approach, in which clinicians first Ask about smoking status for all patients [42]. A systematic approach is best, in which embedded chart reminders or electronic red flags prompt comprehensive screening, thus treating tobacco use as a vital sign [43]. Clinicians should then Advise all smokers to quit, and all ex-smokers to remain quit. This message should be clear and unequivocal. It is then incumbent upon clinicians to Assess motivation. There are a number of formal and informal methods to assess motivation to quit (see below), and it is not uncommon for adolescents to be ambivalent about or uninterested in quitting. For those who are ready to quit, the next step in the screening model requires clinicians to Assist. Finally, screening of tobacco use is not a one-time discussion, but should be done repeatedly, and clinicians should remember to Arrange for follow-up, inquiring about status and progress at future visits. Table 23.2 summarizes the 5A approach guidelines for smoking cessation.

Table 23.2 "5A" approach to smoking cessation [41].

1.	Ask about smoking
2.	Advise smokers to quit
3.	Assess motivation
4.	Assist in quitting
5.	Arrange for follow-up

Beyond simple screening and advice to quit, a more formal assessment of smoking behavior will allow clinicians to more effectively identify and treat smoking behavior within adolescents. The first step in this process is to gather a complete history of smoking. At minimum, this will include age of first use, age of first regular use, and frequency and quantity of smoking. It is important to remember that both frequency and quantity are particularly variable in this population. Non-daily and situation-specific smoking are common [10], and many adolescents will go days without smoking, or exhibit "chunk" smoking on certain days of the week (weekends), times of day (before, after school) or specific situations (parties, social events). Thus, simply asking number of days smoked in past week or number of cigarettes smoked per day will likely mask many of the subtleties in smoking behavior. As part of the smoking history, clinicians should also query about prior quit attempts. This too can be challenging, since a period of non-smoking (which is common) should not be confused with a quit attempt (which is less common). The latter is typically defined as an attempt to "stop smoking for one day or longer because you were trying to quit smoking." Adolescents who have tried to quit should be asked further details of each attempt, including when it took place, its duration, and strategies used (behavioral, pharmacological, etc.).

A number of studies question the validity of self-reported cigarette use among adolescents, in part because they engage in inconsistent patterns of smoking that often result in unreliable self-reports [44,45]. For example, two recent studies [46,47] found poor sensitivity and poor-to-moderate specificity of self-reported smoking behavior when compared to urine or saliva cotinine (a metabolite of nicotine). Nonetheless, for clinicians who are interested in more objective measures of smoking behavior, a number of testable biomarkers exist. The easiest to collect is expired carbon monoxide (CO), collected through a breathalyzer and measured in parts per million (ppm). CO is sensitive to recent smoking, and is highly related to smoking topography [48]. Cotinine has a longer half-life (approximately 16 hours) than nicotine (2 hours), and thus lends itself to detection of smoking over a longer period. Cotinine can be detected through urine, serum, saliva, and even hair samples. Other biomarkers exist – e.g., thiocyanate (SCN), anabasine, anatabine [49] – but their utility within adolescent populations is unclear.

Assessment of nicotine dependence among adolescent smokers has received considerable research attention in recent years, particularly in light of some evidence that suggests a steep onset of dependence within this age group [29,50–52]. The two most commonly used adolescent-specific measures of nicotine

dependence are (i) the modified Fagerström Tolerance Questionnaire (mFTQ) [50,53,54] (Table 23.3), which derives largely from the adult literature on assessment of dependence [55], and (ii) the Hooked on Nicotine

Table 23.3 The modified Fagerström Tolerance Questionnaire (mFTQ) [52].

Mftq

1. On the days that you smoke, how many cigarettes do you smoke per day?
   - *Less than a whole cigarette per day* (0)
   - *1 whole cigarette per day* (0)
   - *2–5 cigarettes per day* (0)
   - *6–15 cigarettes per day (about half a pack)* (0)
   - *16–25 cigarettes per day (about 1 pack)* (0)
   - *26–35 cigarettes per day (about $1^1/_2$ packs)* (1)
   - *More than 35 cigarettes per day* (1)
2. How often do you take in smoke or inhale when you smoke?
   - *Always* (2)
   - *Quite often* (1)
   - *Seldom* (1)
   - *Never* (0)
3. How soon after waking up in the morning do you smoke your first cigarette?
   - *Within the first 5 minutes* (1)
   - *Between 6 and 30 minutes* (1)
   - *Between 31 and 60 minutes* (0)
   - *Between 1 and 2 hours* (0)
   - *More than 2 hours* (0)
4. Which cigarette is hardest to give up?
   - *First cigarette in the morning* (1)
   - *Any other cigarette before noon* (0)
   - *Any other cigarette in the afternoon* (0)
   - *Any other cigarette in the evening* (0)
5. Do you find it difficult not to smoke inside places where it is forbidden (for example, inside a school, church, library, movies, etc.)?
   - *Yes, very difficult* (1)
   - *Yes, somewhat difficult* (1)
   - *No, not usually difficult* (0)
   - *No, not at all difficult* (0)
6. Do you smoke even if you are so ill that you are in bed most of the day?
   - *Yes, always* (1)
   - *Yes, quite often* (1)
   - *No, not usually* (0)
   - *No, never* (0)
7. Do you smoke more during the first 2 hours of the day or more during the rest of the day?
   - *More during the first 2 hours of the day* (1)
   - *More during the rest of the day* (0)

Table 23.4 The Hooked on Nicotine Checklist (HONC) [55].

HONC
1. Have you ever tried to quit, but couldn't?
2. Do you smoke <u>now</u> because it is really hard to quit?
3. Have you ever felt like you were addicted to tobacco?
4. Do you ever have strong cravings to smoke?
5. Have you ever felt like you really needed a cigarette?
6. Is it hard to keep from smoking in places where you are not supposed to, like school?

When you tried to stop smoking (or when you haven't used tobacco in a while) . . . .

7. Did you find it hard to concentrate because you couldn't smoke?
8. Did you feel more irritable because you couldn't smoke?
9. Did you feel a strong need or urge to smoke?
10. Did you feel nervous, restless, or anxious because you couldn't smoke?

All items are scored as follows:
- *Yes* (0)
- *No* (1)

Table 23.5 The Autonomy Over Smoking Scale (AUTOS) [58].

AUTOS
1. When I go too long without a cigarette I get impatient
2. When I go too long without a cigarette I get strong urges that are hard to get rid of
3. When I go too long without a cigarette I lose my temper more easily
4. When I go too long without a cigarette I get nervous or anxious
5. I rely on smoking to focus my attention
6. I rely on smoking to take my mind off being bored
7. I rely on smoking to deal with stress
8. I would go crazy if I couldn't smoke
9. When I feel stressed I want a cigarette
10. When I see other people smoking I want a cigarette
11. When I smell cigarette smoke I want a cigarette
12. After eating I want a cigarette

All items are scored as follows:
- *Not at all* (0)
- *A little* (1)
- *Pretty well* (2)
- *Very well* (3)

Checklist (HONC) [56–58] (Table 23.4). The developers of HONC have also recently developed and validated the Autonomy over Smoking Scale (AUTOS) [59] (Table 23.5). The mFTQ is heavily weighted on consumption as a marker of dependence, while HONC and AUTOS are heavily weighted on loss of autonomy, and may be more sensitive to onset of dependence among low-rate smokers [60]. Each measure has its advantages and drawbacks [61,62], which may reflect a larger debate as to whether frequency and/or quantity of smoking are either necessary or sufficient indicators of nicotine dependence. It is perhaps safest to note that no gold standard for the assessment of dependence exists [28].

Another important target of assessment is motivation or readiness to quit. The most ubiquitous assessment tool for motivation is the stages of change algorithm [63–65], though this has received mixed support [66–68]. Based on the transtheoretical model, the stages of change model posits that smokers (including adolescent smokers) progress through a sequence of stages, from precontemplation (not wanting to quit in next 6 months, or not at all), contemplation (wanting to quit in next 6 months but not next 30 days), preparation (wanting to quit in next 30 days), action (active attempts to change smoking behavior), and maintenance (relapse

prevention following successful cessation). Another, similar approach uses a visual analog scale, or ladder, in which smokers can express their motivation to quit on a continuous scale. Such "contemplation ladders" are empirically supported as being predictive of future quitting [69,70].

Clinicians should be mindful to assess other relevant clinical data that have significant bearing on smoking behavior, and adolescents' ability to quit. A number of studies have shown a link between adolescent smoking and depression [71,72], ADHD [73], parental smoking [74], and peer smoking [75], to name a few. Psychosocial influences on adolescent smoking behavior have a sizable research base, and a full discussion is outside the scope of this chapter. The crucial point is that adolescents, like adults, are subject to a wide range of influences on smoking, many of which act as moderators of quitting success, and none of which should be ignored.

Finally, clinicians should be mindful that noncigarette tobacco use is common among adolescents (see above), and assessment of dual use can be challenging. As regards assessment strategies, much of the above still applies, though two exceptions are worth noting. The first relates to measures of dependence. The two aforementioned adolescent nicotine dependence scales (mFTQ and HONC) do not lend themselves to non-cigarette tobacco use. The mFTQ has been adapted for users of smokeless tobacco [76,77], but it is unclear if or how this might apply to adolescents. The second issue relates to testable biomarkers. Only CO and thiocyanate can distinguish between smoked vs. smokeless tobacco (cotinine and nicotine cannot, nor can anabasine and anatabine). SCN is known to be influenced by diet [78], which may leave CO as the only viable option.

An overview of education, screening, evaluation, and assistance within clinical practice is provided in Figure 23.1.

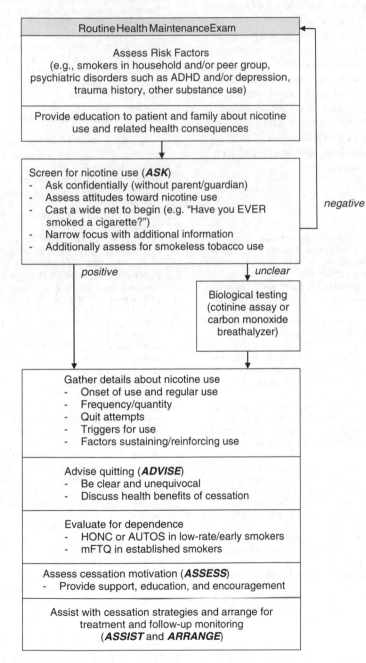

Figure 23.1 Flowchart for assessing adolescent nicotine use in clinical practice.

SUMMARY POINTS

Adolescent smoking is a topic of considerable public health importance. Smoking almost always begins in adolescence, with prevalence rates steadily increasing to about one-third of 18-year-olds. Clinicians must be able to effectively screen for and assess smoking behaviors among their adolescent patients. Since adolescents rarely actively seek information on nicotine or seek help with cessation, clinicians must take the initiative in this process. In the midst of busy day-to-day practice, though, clinicians may focus only on acute presenting concerns and dismiss nicotine use as a "background" issue to be dealt with later. Given the enormous morbidity and mortality associated with nicotine use, and the potentially rapid progression from adolescent smoking initiation to nicotine dependence, screening must be considered a "vital sign" to be performed during all clinical encounters with adolescents. A stepwise approach to education, screening, assessment, and management is feasible and essential.

References

1. Centers for Disease Control and Prevention. *Targeting Tobacco Use: The Nation's Leading Cause of Preventable Death*. CDC, 2007. Available at http://www.cdc.gov/nccdphp/publications/aag/pdf/osh.pdf.
2. Doubeni CA, Reed G, DiFranza JR. Early course nicotine dependence in adolescent smokers. *Pediatrics* 2010;**125**:1127–1133.
3. Kandel DB, Chen K. Extent of smoking and nicotine dependence in the United States: 1991–1993. *Nicotine Tob Res* 2000;**2**:263–274.
4. Backinger CL, Fagan P, Matthews E, Grana R. Adolescent and young adult tobacco prevention and cessation: current status and future directions. *Tobacco Control* 2003;**12**:iv46–iv53.
5. Chassin L, Presson CC, Pitts SC, Sherman SJ. The natural history of cigarette smoking from adolescence to adulthood in a midwestern community sample: Multiple trajectories and their psychosocial correlates. *Health Psychol* 2000;**19**:223–231.
6. Stanton WR, McClelland M, Elwood C, Ferry D, Silva PA. Prevalence, reliability and bias of adolescents' reports of smoking and quitting. *Addiction* 1996;**91**:1705–1714.
7. Zhu SH, Sun J, Billings SC, Choi WS, Malarcher A. Predictors of smoking cessation in U.S. adolescents. *Am J Prev Med* 1999;**16**:202–207.
8. United States Department of Health and Human Services. *NIDA Research Report: Tobacco Addiction*. NIH Publication Number 09-4342. US DHHS, 2009.
9. Substance Abuse and Mental Health Services Administration. *Results from the 2009 National Survey on Drug Use and Health: Volume I. Summary of National Findings*. Office of Applied Studies, NSDUH Series H-38A, HHS Publication No. SMA 10-4586 Findings. Rockville, MD: SAMHSA, 2010.
10. Berg CJ, Parelkar PP, Lessard L, *et al*. Defining "smoker": College student attitudes and related smoking characteristics. *Nicotine Tob Res* 2010;**12**:963–969.
11. Shiffman S. Tobacco "chippers" – individual differences in tobacco dependence. *Psychopharmacology* 1989;**97**:539–547.
12. Centers for Disease Control and Prevention. *Behavioral Risk Factor Surveillance System Survey Data*. Atlanta, GA:Department of Health and Human Services, Centers for Disease Control and Prevention, 2009.
13. Moran S, Wechsler H, Rigotti NA. Social smoking among US college students. *Pediatrics* 2004;**114**:1028–1034.
14. Johnston LD, O'Malley PM, Bachman JG, Schulenberg JE. Smoking continues gradual decline among U.S. teens, smokeless tobacco threatens a comeback. Ann Arbor, MI:University of Michigan News Service, 2009. Available online at:http://www.monitoringthefuture.org.
15. Primack BA, Walsh M, Bryce C, Eissenberg T. Water-pipe tobacco smoking among middle and high school students in Arizona. *Pediatrics* 2009;**123**:e282–288.
16. Eissenberg T, Ward KD, Smith-Simone S, Maziak W. Waterpipe tobacco smoking on a U.S. college campus: prevalence and correlates. *J Adolesc Health* 2008;**42**:526–529.
17. Grekin ER, Ayna D. Argileh use among college students in the United States: An emerging trend. *J Stud Alcohol Drugs* 2008;**69**:472–475.
18. Smith SY, Curbow B, Stillman FA. Harm perception of nicotine products in college freshmen. *Nicotine Tob Res* 2007;**9**:977–982.
19. Schepis TS, Rau U. Epidemiology and etiology of adolescent smoking. *Curr Opin Pediatr* 2005;**17**:607–612.
20. Griesler PC, Hu MC, Schaffran C, Kandel DB. Comorbid psychiatric disorders and nicotine dependence in adolescence. *Addiction* 2011;**106**:1010–1020.
21. Upadhyaya HP, Deas D, Brady KT, Kruesi M. Cigarette smoking and psychiatric comorbidity in children and adolescents. *J Am Acad Child Adolesc Psychiatry* 2002;**41**:1294–1305.
22. Biederman J, Monuteaux MC, Mick E, *et al*. Is cigarette smoking a gateway to alcohol and illicit drug use disorders? *Biol Psychiatry* 2006;**59**:258–264.
23. Vaughn M, Wallace J, Perron B, Copeland V, Howard M. Does marijuana use serve as a gateway to cigarette use for high-risk African-American youth? *Am J Drug Alcohol Abuse* 2008;**34**:782–791.
24. American Psychiatric, Association., *Diagnostic and Statistical Manual of Mental Disorders*, 4th edn, Text Revision. Washington, DC:American Psychiatric Association, 2000.
25. Hughes JR, Weiss RD. Are differences in guidelines for the treatment of nicotine dependence and non-nicotine dependence justified? *Addiction* 2009;**104**:1951–1957.
26. Rose JS, Dierker LC. An item response theory analysis of nicotine dependence symptoms in recent onset adolescent smokers. *Drug Alcohol Depend* 2010;**110**:70–79.
27. Dierker L, Mermelstein R. Early emerging nicotine-dependence symptoms: a signal of propensity for chronic smoking behavior in adolescents. *J Pediatrics* 2010;**156**:818–822.
28. Colby SM, Tiffany S, Shiffman S, Niaura RS. Measuring nicotine dependence among youth: A review of available approaches and instruments. *Drug Alcohol Depend* 2000;**59** (Suppl. 1):S23–S39.
29. Doubeni CA, Reed G, DiFranza JR. Early course of nicotine dependence in adolescent smokers. *Pediatrics* 2010;**125**:1127–1133.
30. Hughes J, Hatsukami D. Minnesota Nicotine Withdrawal Scale. 2003. Available from http://www.uvm.edu/~hbpl.

31. Prokhorov AV, Hudmon KS, Cinciripini PM, Marani S. "Withdrawal symptoms" in adolescents: A comparison of former smokers and never-smokers. *Nicotine Tob Res* 2005;**7**:909–913.

32. Rubinstein ML, Benowitz NL, Auerback GM, Moscicki AB. Withdrawal in adolescent light smokers following 24-hour abstinence. *Nicotine Tob Res* 2009;**11**:185–189.

33. Gray KM, Baker NL, Carpenter MJ, Lewis AL, Upadhyaya HP. Attention-deficit/hyperactivity disorder confounds nicotine withdrawal self-report in adolescent smokers. *Am J Addictions* 2010;**19**:325–331.

34. Al-Delaimy WK, White MM, Pierce JP. Adolescents' perceptions about quitting and nicotine replacement therapy: Findings from the California Tobacco Survey. *J Adolesc Health* 2006;**38**:465–468.

35. Weinstein ND, Marcus SE, Moser RP. Smokers' unrealistic optimism about their risk. *Tobacco Control* 2005;**14**:55–59.

36. Bjartveit K, Tverdal A. Health consequences of smoking 1–4 cigarettes per day. *Tobacco Control* 2005;**14**:315–320.

37. Korhonen T, Broms U, Levälahti E, Koskenvuo M, Kaprio J. Characteristics and health consequences of intermittent smoking: Long-term follow-up among Finnish adult twins. *Nicotine Tob Res* 2009;**11**:148–155.

38. Luoto R, Uutela A, Puska P. Occasional smoking increases total and cardiovascular mortality in men. *Nicotine Tob Res* 2000;**2**:133–139.

39. Bancej C, O'Loughlin J, Platt RW, Paradis G, Gervais A. Smoking cessation attempts among adolescent smokers: A systematic review of prevalence studies. *Tobacco Control* 2007;**16**:e8.

40. Carpenter MJ, Garrett-Mayer E, Vitoc C, Cartmell K, Biggers S, Alberg AJ. Adolescent non-daily smokers: Favorable views of tobacco yet receptive to cessation. *Nicotine Tob Res* 2009;**11**:348–355.

41. Fagan P, Augustson E, Backinger CL, *et al.* Quit attempts and intention to quit cigarette smoking among young adults in the United States. *Am J Public Health* 2007;**97**:1412–1420.

42. Fiore MC, Jaen CR, Baker TB, *et al. Treating Tobacco Use and Dependence: 2008 Update. Clinical Practice Guidelines.* Rockville, MD:United States Public Health Service, 2008.

43. Ahluwalia JS, Gibson CA, Kenney RE, Wallace DD, Resnicow K. Smoking status as a vital sign. *J Gen Intern Med* 1999;**14**:402–408.

44. Dolcini MM, Adler NE, Lee P, Bauman KE. An assessment of the validity of adolescent self-reported smoking using three biological indicators. *Nicotine Tob Res* 2003;**5**:473–483.

45. Rubinstein ML. Who's smoking? Cotinine versus self-report in adolescent populations. *J Adolesc Health* 2008;**43**:205–206.

46. Kandel DB, Schaffran C, Griesler PC, Hu M-C, Davies M, Benowitz N. Salivary cotinine concentration versus self-reported cigarette smoking: Three patterns of inconsistency in adolescence. *Nicotine Tob Res* 2006;**8**:525–537.

47. Malcon MC, Menezes AMB, Assunção MCF, Neutzling MB, Hallal PC. Agreement between self-reported smoking and cotinine concentration in adolescents: A validation study in Brazil. *J Adolesc Health* 2008;**43**:226–230.

48. Moolchan ET, Parzynski CS, Jaszyna-Gasior M, Collins CC, Leff MK, Zimmerman DL. A link between adolescent nicotine metabolism and smoking topography. *Cancer Epidem Biomar* 2009;**18**:1578–1583.

49. Hatsukami DK, Hecht SS, Hennrikus DJ, Joseph AM, Pentel PR. Biomarkers of tobacco exposure or harm: Application to clinical and epidemiological studies. *Nicotine Tob Res* 2003;**5**:384–396.

50. Kandel DB, Hu M-C, Griesler PC, Schaffran C. On the development of nicotine dependence in adolescence. *Drug Alcohol Depend* 2007;**91**:26–39.

51. Rose JS, Dierker LC, Donny E. Nicotine dependence symptoms among recent onset adolescent smokers. *Drug Alcohol Depend* 2010;**106**:126–132.

52. DiFranza JR, Savageau JA, Fletcher K, *et al.* Symptoms of tobacco dependence after brief intermittent use: The Development and Assessment of Nicotine Dependence in Youth-2 study. *Arch Pediatr Adolesc Med* 2007;**161**:704–710.

53. Prokhorov AV, Pallonen UE, Fava JL, Ding L, Niaura R. Measuring nicotine dependence among high-risk adolescent smokers. *Addict Behav* 1996;**21**:117–127.

54. Nonnemaker JM, Mowery PD, Hersey JC, *et al.* Measurement properties of a nicotine dependence scale for adolescents. *Nicotine Tob Res* 2004;**6**:295–301.

55. Heatherton TF, Kozlowski LT, Frecker RC, Fagerström KO. The Fagerström Test for Nicotine Dependence: A revision of the Fagerström Tolerance Questionnaire. *Brit J Addiction* 1991;**86**:1119–1127.

56. DiFranza JR, Savageau JA, Fletcher K, *et al.* Measuring the loss of autonomy over nicotine use in adolescents: The DANDY (Development and Assessment of Nicotine Dependence in Youths) study. *Arch Pediatr Adolesc Med* 2002;**156**:397–403.

57. DiFranza JR, Savageau JA, Fletcher K, *et al.* Susceptibility to nicotine dependence: The Development and Assessment of Nicotine Dependence in Youth 2 study. *Pediatrics* 2007;**120**:e974–e983.

58. Wheeler KC, Fletcher KE, Wellman RJ, DiFranza JR. Screening adolescents for nicotine dependence: The Hooked on Nicotine Checklist. *J Adolesc Health* 2004;**35**:225–230.

59. DiFranza JR, Wellman RJ, Ursprung WW, Sabiston C. The Autonomy Over Smoking Scale. *Psychol Addict Behav* 2009;**23**:656–665.

60. MacPherson L, Strong DR, Myers MG. Using an item response model to examine the nicotine dependence construct as characterized by the HONC and the mFTQ among adolescent smokers. *Addict Behav* 2008;**33**:880–894.

61. Carpenter MJ, Baker NL, Gray KM, Upadhyaya HP. Assessment of nicotine dependence among adolescent and young adult smokers: A comparison of measures. *Addict Behav* 2010;**35**:977–982.

62. Wellman RJ, DiFranza JR, Pbert L, *et al.* A comparison of the psychometric properties of the Hooked on Nicotine Checklist and the modified Fagerström Tolerance Questionnaire. *Addict Behav* 2006;**31**:486–495.

63. DiClemente CC, Prochaska JO, Fairhurst SK, Velicer WF, Velasquez MM, Rossi JS. The processes of smoking cessation: An analysis of precontemplation, contemplation, and preparation stages of change. *J Consult Clin Psychol* 1991;**59**:285–304.

64. Prochaska JO, Redding CA, Evers KE. The transtheoretical model and stages of change. In:Glanz K, Rimer B, Lewis F (eds), *Health Behavior and Health Education: Theory, Research, and Practice.* San Francisco, CA:Jossey-Bass, 2002; pp. 97–122.

65. Norman GJ, Velicer WF, Fava JL, Prochaska JO. Cluster subtypes within stage of change in a representative sample of smokers. *Addict Behav* 2000;**25**:183–204.

66. Bondy SJ, Victor JC, O'Connor S, McDonald PW, Diemert LM, Cohen JE. Predictive validity and measurement issues in documenting quit intentions in population surveillance studies. *Nicotine Tob Res* 2010;**12**:43–52.

67. Riemsma RP, Pattenden J, Bridle C, *et al.* Systematic review of the effectiveness of stage based interventions to promote smoking cessation. *Brit Med J* 2003;**326**:1175–1181.

68. West R. Time for a change: Putting the Transtheoretical (Stages of Change) Model to rest. *Addiction* 2005; **100**:1036–1039.

69. Biener L, Abrams DB. The contemplation ladder: Validation of a measure of readiness to consider smoking cessation. *Health Psychol* 1991;**10**:360–365.

70. Herzog TA, Abrams D, Emmons KM, Linnan L. Predicting increases in readiness to quit smoking: A prospective analysis using the contemplation ladder. *Psychol Health* 2000;**15**:369–381.

71. Audrain-McGovern J, Rodriguez D, Kassel JD. Adolescent smoking and depression: Evidence for self-medication and peer smoking mediation. *Addiction* 2009;**104**:1743–1756.

72. Munafò MR, Hitsman B, Rende R, Metcalfe C, Niaura R. Effects of progression to cigarette smoking on depressed mood in adolescents: Evidence from the National Longitudinal Study of Adolescent Health. *Addiction* 2008;**103**:162–171.

73. Upadhyaya HP, Carpenter MJ. Is attention deficit hyperactivity disorder (ADHD) severity associated with tobacco, alcohol and other drug use among college students? *Am J Addictions* 2008;**17**:195–198.

74. Gilman SE, Rende R, Boergers J, *et al.* Parental smoking and adolescent smoking initiation: An intergenerational perspective on tobacco control. *Pediatrics* 2009;**123**:e274–e281.

75. Go MH, Green HD, Kennedy DP, Pollard M, Tucker JS. Peer influence and selection effects on adolescent smoking. *Drug Alcohol Depend* 2010;**109**:239–242.

76. Ebbert JO, Patten CA, Schroeder DR. The Fagerström Test for Nicotine Dependence-Smokeless Tobacco (FTND-T). *Addict Behav* 2006;**31**:1716–1721.

77. Ferketich AK, Wee AG, Shultz J, Wewers ME. A measure of nicotine dependence for smokeless tobacco users. *Addict Behav* 2007;**32**:1970–1975.

78. Sherer G. Carboxyhemoglobin and thiocyanate as biomarkers of exposure to carbon monoxide and hydrogen cyanide in tobacco smoke. *Health Psychol* 2006;**3**:563–581.

24

Emerging Clinical Conditions

Christopher R. Thompson[1] and Lauren Reba-Harrelson[2]

[1] UCLA Department of Psychiatry, Child and Adolescent Division, Los Angeles, CA, USA
[2] University of Southern California, Institute of Psychiatry, Law, and Behavioral Science;
Keck School of Medicine, Los Angeles, CA, USA

Child and adolescent psychiatry is not a static field. As our knowledge base expands, clinical conditions emerge and gain acceptance or are reconceptualized and disappear (e.g., homosexuality) with regularity. Some of these "emerging clinical conditions" are discussed here. Based on their length of existence, research base, and a variety of other factors, the disorders listed below have achieved varying degrees of acceptance by the psychiatric community. All, however, have two common features. First, they can be loosely construed as impulse control disorders. Second, little scientific evidence is available about almost all facets of these disorders as they relate to children and adolescents.

PATHOLOGICAL GAMBLING

Vignette: Gambling

Robert is a 16-year-old boy who, like many teenagers, spends ample time on the internet. After coming home from his after-school job at a local fast food restaurant, he often logs onto various social networking sites to keep up with friends and school gossip. However, over the past few months, his time spent on the internet has shifted from chatting with friends to playing online poker. After finding out about a poker site from another boy at school, who heard about it from a television commercial, Robert thought he'd try his luck. He had played poker occasionally on the weekend with a group of guys from his school for dollars and he often won 15 to 20 dollars. The guys would meet in his friend's basement and they started drinking a beer or two during the game; it helped that his friend's parents didn't monitor the boys much. However, unlike the weekend "live game," online poker offered Robert the excitement of possibly making thousands of dollars per month,

according to one of Robert's friends. Beside, gambling didn't seem so different than other online games he played in the past, except that he used real money. He justified his behavior by telling himself that he could use the money he made at his job to gamble and that he surely would win additional money.

After he came home from school the next day, Robert created an account on the website he had been frequenting and deposited the 300 dollars he had saved over the summer. He decided that he would start at "low stakes" games so he could practice playing poker without losing too much money. He began to play and was soon "hooked." However, the card game went more quickly than expected, and after 3 hours of play, he had already lost 75 dollars. Around 1 : 00 a.m., he decided that he would quit and resume playing the next day.

Although he was fatigued during school the following morning, Robert could not stop thinking about his new "hobby." He was upset that he had lost money and was determined to win it back. He had trouble concentrating in school because he had slept for only 5 hours and was distracted because he was thinking about various strategies he could use to win at poker. Over the ensuing 3 months, Robert's playing escalated significantly. His 3 hours per night had turned into over 10 hours per day. His playing began to interfere with his schoolwork. His parents started to ask why he wanted to have dinner in his room, seemed increasingly irritable, and didn't seem to hang out as much with his friends on weekends. Although he consistently had been a B- and C-level student in the past, Robert began to receive mostly Cs and Ds in his classes; this was especially troublesome to his family because of his upcoming college applications. Robert didn't seem to care about his parents' concerns and became increasingly focused on how he could get more money to continue playing. His after-school job earnings were no longer enough to finance his habit and he began stealing money from his mother's purse. Although he knew this was wrong, he found this a better option than quitting gaming, which had become his sole source of excitement, enjoyment, and relief from school boredom and the stress of the pending college application process.

Introduction

Legalized and quasi-legalized forms of gambling have increased dramatically over the past 25 years, both in the United States and worldwide. This proliferation has included casinos, state lotteries, and, more recently, internet gambling, with its wide variety of gaming options (sports betting, table games, slot machines, etc.) and questionable efforts to prohibit minors' participation in them. As a result, adolescents have had increased access to numerous forms of gaming.

While both the number and accessibility of gambling options for adolescents has increased exponentially, particularly via the internet, parental disapproval of gambling has diminished markedly. Today, gambling is frequently seen as a rite of passage and is well accepted in Great Britain, the United States, and Canada. It is difficult to extrapolate how other cultures view youth gambling as most research on adolescent gambling has been conducted in these Western countries, in racially homogeneous samples. In fact, in the United States, 75% of children have gambled in their own home [1] and 85% of parents do not object to gambling [2]. Both media and advertisers have attempted to capitalize on this shift in the public's attitude toward gambling (e.g., televising numerous poker tournaments on cable TV, marketing Las Vegas as "a family entertainment spot"), further destigmatizing gambling in our collective cultural mindset.

This confluence of factors has led to gambling's becoming the most prevalent adolescent risk-taking behavior, far outdistancing cigarette, alcohol, and illicit drug use, and even sex. Although most adolescents will gamble sporadically and "responsibly" (if not legally) and will not develop significant psychopathology, a substantial minority will escalate their gambling behaviors and eventually meet formal criteria for pathological gambling (PG). However, in light of this trend, a recent review of research of PG suggests that the extant literature on adolescent gambling remains sparse and has many limitations.

Epidemiology

In the past, perhaps because of most societies' age restrictions on most forms of gaming, PG has generally been thought of as an exclusively adult disorder. However, in reality, this disorder is two to four times more prevalent in adolescent than in adult populations (4–8% vs. 1–3%) [3–5] and tends to have its onset in early to middle adolescence. This statistic is not surprising given adolescents' general impulsivity and decreased ability to engage in socially responsible decision-making [6].

Individuals who develop PG as adolescents differ from individuals who develop PG as adults in several key ways: age of onset of potentially problematic gambling behaviors (10 years of age [2] vs. late adolescence/early adulthood); rapidity of progression from initiation of gambling to pathological gambling (12–24 months vs. 10–20 years) [7,8]; level of impairment (more vs. less) [8]; and refractoriness to treatment (more vs. less) [8].

Research on the natural course of adolescent PG is limited, but should improve as longitudinal data are collected and analyzed. Some researchers believe that the disorder is phasic and that the vast majority of adolescents who develop PG will "grow out of it" as their central nervous systems mature and they gain new responsibilities (e.g., marriage, children). Others propose that the development of PG as an adolescent is an ominous sign that predicts a high likelihood of continued problem-gambling behavior as an adult. Current research focuses, in part, on identifying the traits of individuals at high risk for persistent PG [9].

Diagnostic Criteria

Social Gambling

Individuals involved in "social gambling" appear to enjoy the social aspects of gaming, gamble only for a limited amount of time, have predetermined and acceptable losses (i.e., reasonable for their financial situation), and don't encounter lasting problems because of their gambling. Most (80–85%) adolescents who gamble on a regular basis can be grouped in this category [10]. As of 2000, in the United States and Canada, it has been estimated that more than 15 million adolescents (ages 12–17 years) have gambled [11].

Problem Gambling

Approximately 10% of adolescents are problem gamblers [11] and continue to gamble despite minor problems in their lives. These youths may gamble frequently, lose more money than intended, or give up important activities (e.g., in an adolescent's case, dating, socializing, or sports). Because gambling is starting to affect their quality of life and, potentially, psychosocial development, these adolescents are "at risk" for developing PG. At-risk individuals typically will meet several, but not the required five, *Diagnostic and Statistical Manual of Mental Disorders, Fourth Edition, Text Revision* (DSM-IV-TR) criteria for pathological gambling.

Pathological Gambling

The individuals at the most extreme end of the "gambling spectrum" fall into the category of pathological gambling (4–8% of adolescents) [4,12]. The DSM-IV-TR criteria for PG requires persistent and recurrent maladaptive gambling behavior including five or more of the following characteristics: (1) a preoccupation with gambling; (2) a need to gamble with increasing amounts of money in order to achieve the same level of excitement (similar to tolerance); (3) repeated unsuccessful efforts to control, cut back, or stop gambling; (4) restlessness or irritability when attempting to cut down or stop gambling (similar to withdrawal); (5) gambling to escape problems or relieve dysphoria; (6) continued gambling, even after losing money; (7) lying to family, a therapist, or others to conceal the extent of involvement with gambling; (8) performing illegal acts such as forgery, fraud, theft, or embezzlement) to finance gambling; (9) jeopardizing relationships, job, or education or career opportunities secondary to gambling; or (10) reliance upon others to relieve a desperate financial situation due to gambling [13]. Further, the gambling behavior cannot be better accounted for by a Manic Episode [13].

DSM-IV-TR criteria for PG are loosely modeled on those for substance dependence.

Modeling the criteria for PG on those for substance dependence is obviously not a coincidence. Pathological gamblers share many personality traits with those who abuse substances (e.g., impulsive, easily bored) [14], and the treatment paradigms that have been developed for PG closely resemble those developed for substance dependence (e.g., cognitive-behavioral therapy, motivational enhancement therapy).

Clinical Presentation

Risk-taking is a hallmark of adolescence. Substance use, reckless driving, and unprotected sex are fairly common behaviors for the average teenager. A low to moderate degree of risk-taking can help foster personal growth, differentiation, and development. Indeed, complete abstinence from risk-taking behaviors during adolescence is atypical. Therefore, some degree of recreational gambling may be considered normal.

Adolescent pathological gamblers, on the other hand, tend to be motivated by reasons other than typical adolescent risk-taking. Evans proposed that the theoretical conceptualization common to both adolescent substance abuse and gambling behavior includes social inoculation, reasoned action, planned behavior, and problem behavior theory [7]. Gupta and Derevensky identified four other major reasons why adolescents gamble; some are specific to pathological gamblers, others apply to both recreational and pathological gamblers [15]. These explanations for adolescent gambling include the following:

1. *To "stay in the action."* In contrast to their recreational gambler peers, most adolescent pathological gamblers report that they do not gamble primarily to win money to spend on material items. Rather, their winning is merely a means to continue playing. Ultimately, their desire is to achieve a singular, unmatched gambling success, which will prove their worth to others.
2. *To escape life stresses and control helplessness.* Through the possibility of substantial wins, gambling can provide adolescents an escape from daily stresses and resultant negative emotions. Some pathological gamblers, presumably to avoid these negative emotions, gamble for days on end without rest and experience an almost dissociative state [16].
3. *For excitement or to relieve boredom.* By engaging in a typically adult activity, adolescents can demonstrate that they are willing to take risks and accept challenges.
4. *Social acceptance/competition.* In order to be accepted by peers, adolescents may start gambling. Peer pressure can have a dramatic effect on rates of gambling. In addition, being part of a social group that gambles provides a sense of community and shared experience. Finally, gambling, by its very nature (i.e., there is a winner and a loser), provides competitive youths with a means to prove themselves successful within a specific peer group.

Risk Factors

Numerous potential risk factors have been identified that may increase an adolescent's chance of developing PG. These include the following [8,17]:

1. *Demographic factors.* Adolescents who engage in PG are more likely to be male than female [18]. They are also more likely than non-PG peers to begin gambling at a younger age, to be involved in delinquent or criminal behaviors, to have poor academic records, and to have parents or friends who also engage in problem gambling [18].
2. *Genetic contributions.* These have not been well defined, but a family history of gambling problems, particularly in families with several generations of pathological gamblers, is a strong predictor of development of adolescent PG [11]. Aberrant expression of genes is believed to lead to distorted

perceptions of risk, a heightened response to reward (e.g., winning a bet), and a relative insensitivity to punishment (e.g., losing a bet). These responses are probably mediated through dopaminergic pathways.

3. *Neurodevelopmental considerations.* During adolescence, the frontal lobes are continuing to develop and myelinate. These areas are responsible for planning, response inhibition, abstract thinking, and, to some extent, the ability to maturely evaluate the consequences of one's actions [19]. This neurodevelopmental immaturity leaves adolescents susceptible to engaging in high-risk behaviors, such as gambling.

4. *Psychiatric comorbidity (presumably) preceding pathological gambling.* Individuals with substance use disorders and ADHD are at particular risk for developing PG.

5. *Personality factors.* Adolescents who are extroverted, competitive, rejection sensitive, risk-taking, have low self-esteem, or have difficulty with self-discipline or coping with stressful situations are more likely than their peers to develop PG. Additionally, adolescents with PG manifest numerous cognitive distortions and symptoms of dissociation, though the origin of these is unclear.

6. *Access.* Increased opportunities for gambling lead to gambling-related problems [20]. The combination of internet gambling and the advent of personal digital assistants (PDAs – with continuous online access) has made the opportunities for gambling practically limitless.

7. *Exposure.* Adolescents who are exposed to gambling at an early age are more likely than non-exposed peers to develop pathological gambling behaviors [1]. Similarly, having friends who gamble regularly increases an individual's risk for developing gambling problems [11].

8. *Gambling "versatility."* The more different types of gaming in which an adolescent engages (e.g., sports betting, table games, horse racing), the greater the risk for developing problem gambling.

9. *Cultural issues.* If a youth's culture views gambling positively or optimistically (e.g., some Asian cultures), he or she is more likely to participate in gambling on a regular basis than a peer from a cultural background that disapproves of gambling [21]. Of the few studies that have reported the racial/ethnic compositions of their samples, one reported that 10–12-year-old Caucasians were more likely to gamble than youths of other ethnicities [22]. Another study found no significant differences in gambling behaviors between Native American and non-Native American adolescents [23]. However, when taking high-risk behaviors and self-esteem into consideration, Native American participants were more frequent gamblers, but not more at risk for PG than Caucasian participants. Of note, higher rates of alcohol and marijuana use, as well as parental gambling, predicted that Native Americans would gamble more frequently [23].

Typically, adolescent pathological gamblers are less likely than their adult counterparts to build up substantial gambling debts. This is because most adolescents do not support themselves financially and do not have access to large amounts of money (e.g., checking accounts, lines of credit, credit cards). Most of the money lost tends to be their families' money and was acquired through the adolescents' borrowing, deception, or outright theft.

However, adolescent pathological gamblers experience a host of other problems. They generally have marked disruption in their family relationships, mainly because of their repeated deception with regard to their gambling and their shirking of family duties because of time spent gambling. Their school performance typically deteriorates and they experience delays in achieving developmental milestones because of the time they spend gambling or thinking about gambling (average around 8 hours a week) [24,25].

In addition, adolescent pathological gamblers experience a variety of social difficulties. Not surprisingly, they tend to have few friends, and the friends they do have generally are heavily involved in gambling. They give up extracurricular activities. They also have higher rates of engaging in high-risk behaviors (e.g., drug use, carrying weapons, unprotected sex) than their non-gambling peers. Overall, adolescents who engage in PG have greater difficulty coping with life stressors than those who do not gamble [26]. Perhaps most concerning, they have higher rates of delinquency, aggressive crimes, and other antisocial behavior [10] than their non-PG peers.

Psychiatric Comorbidities

In most cases, adolescent pathological gamblers suffer from comorbid psychiatric disorders. Whether these disorders were caused by the PG, or rather caused or contributed to the development of PG, is unclear. Psychiatric disorders frequently encountered in this population include: substance abuse/dependence, major depressive disorder, attention- deficit/hyperactivity disorder, and personality disorders [27,28]. One recent longitudinal study found that the presence of depressive symptoms increased the odds of future problem gambling four-fold [29]. Adolescents with PG also have higher rates of suicidal ideation and suicide attempts than their age-matched peers [3].

Adolescents with PG also frequently develop problems with a different impulse control disorder (e.g., kleptomania, compulsive shopping), either concomitantly or serially (i.e., after treatment for pathological gambling) [3,30,31]. These findings lend credence to the notion that these different behaviors/diagnoses may be manifestations of the same primary psychopathology.

Relevant Assessment Issues

Adolescents frequently lack insight into their gambling problems. They often underestimate the severity and minimize the consequences of their gambling and tend to view themselves as invincible. For this reason, adolescents will rarely seek treatment for PG until their families insist upon it. Frequently, adolescents are brought in for evaluation for a comorbid psychiatric disorder, and an astute clinician only identifies PG serendipitously. Therefore, screening for PG in both adolescents and collateral contacts in a variety of non-psychiatric settings (e.g., schools, primary care settings) is an extremely important step in identifying problem gambling behaviors at an early stage.

In addition to the clinical interview, there are a variety of screening instruments available to identify potentially problematic gambling behaviors. Most of these were designed for adults, but are presumed to be valid for adolescents. These range from simple screening tools (e.g., the Lie/Bet Questionnaire) to more comprehensive, semi-structured interviews (DSM-IV-J). Some of these are described below:

1. *Lie/Bet Questionnaire* [32]. This screening tool asks two questions: "Have you ever lied to anyone important about how often you gamble?" and "Have you ever had to increase your bet to get the same excitement from gambling?" A positive response to either indicates the need for further exploration of gambling behaviors. This screening instrument appears to be valid in differentiating problem from non-problem gambling in adolescents [32], and may be particularly useful in a time-limited setting.
2. *DSM-IV-J.* This 12-item, semi-structured interview is modeled on DSM-IV-TR criteria for PG. This instrument tends to be less sensitive but more specific than other gambling screens. The DSM-IV-J was later revised to include some multiple response categories (rather than the dichotomous options in the original version), creating the DSM-IV-MR-J [33]. This instrument has been found to discriminate well between problem and non-problem adolescent gamblers.
3. *South Oaks Gambling Screen-Revised for Adolescents (SOGS-RA)* [34]. This screening tool uses self-report data on gambling activities and consequences of gambling to assess severity of gambling behavior over the past 12 months. The items on this screen are based and validated on DSM-III criteria for PG and have dichotomous response options. One study of 13 000 middle- and high-school students in Canada found that this measure had adequate stability and internal consistency reliability [18].
4. *Gamblers Anonymous questionnaire (GA 20)* [35]. This 20-item, "yes/no" screening tool was initially developed by the Gamblers Anonymous organization and focuses on the consequences of gambling activities (social, physical, emotional) rather than actual gambling behaviors in order to determine gambling severity and the need for further treatment. More than seven positive responses indicate likely "compulsive gambling." It has been demonstrated reliable with and has good convergent validity with the SOGS in adolescents [35].
5. *Canadian Adolescent Gambling Inventory (CAGI)* [36]. The Canadian Centre on Substance Abuse (CCSA) and an associated consortium developed this instrument to assess gambling risk and problem gambling in adolescents. Three phases of research of this instrument suggest the CAGI possesses initial estimates of reliability, validity, and classification accuracy [36].

Treatment

Psychotherapy

Unfortunately, there is a dearth of data on treatment of PG in adolescents. Most current treatment modalities are based on anecdotal reports, clinical experience, and extrapolation of treatment principles for adult PG. Perhaps because of this lack of empirically based treatments for adolescent PG, there are few gambling programs designed specifically for adolescents. This is unfortunate because gambling treatment programs targeted at adults generally do not adequately address problems specific to adolescents (e.g., peer pressure, school difficulties, parental conflict). Moreover, a 2010 review of extant treatment studies on adolescent PG found that there is evidence that adolescent problem gamblers often fail to be referred to or seek treatment [17].

Individual Therapy Cognitive-behavioral therapy (CBT) is the most well established and empirically validated form of therapy for adults with PG [24]. Some empirical and case studies suggest that CBT is a valid approach for decreasing gambling frequency in adults [37]. This form of therapy focuses on identifying and correcting cognitive distortions in problem gamblers (e.g., "I'm due to win after all those losses"). It also targets problematic behavioral components of gambling (e.g., teaches money management, stresses developing alternative forms of entertainment) and focuses on relapse prevention (e.g., dealing with triggers, voluntarily excluding oneself from casinos).

Unfortunately, there are few studies examining CBT's effectiveness in adolescents [17]. Applied to PG in adolescents, CBT would focus on identifying gambling-associated cognitive distortions and related emotions that increase one's vulnerability to PG. Further research is needed to address these factors, as well as to teach relapse prevention, assertiveness and gambling refusal, problem-solving, and reinforcement of gambling-inconsistent activities and interests. Psychodynamic psychotherapy, motivational enhancement therapy (MET)/motivational interviewing, and couples therapy have also been used in the treatment of PG, but there are much fewer data to support their use, particularly in adolescents [37,38].

Group Therapy One form of group treatment is Gamblers Anonymous (GA), which operates on principles similar to Alcoholics Anonymous or Narcotics Anonymous and attempts to address problem gambling behaviors through fellowship and support [39]. Members typically must acknowledge the illness (i.e., PG) and attempt to reverse the damage caused by their gambling. At present, there are few GA meetings geared toward adolescents. This is unfortunate because adolescents with PG are subsequently forced to negotiate an adult-oriented setting, despite the fact that they typically lack good social and coping skills.

Although GA is widely accepted as an effective treatment for PG, there is little empirical evidence to support this notion in adolescents. On the contrary, one adult study showed a one-year abstinence rate of only 8% [39]. However, GA is generally accessible, free, and many teens find the support networks they develop invaluable (e.g., sponsors).

Coman and Burrows [40] hypothesized that group treatment may be a superior method to individual treatment for addressing PG because of its provision of extra support, encouragement, and motivation for change. This hypothesis is supported by a study investigating the 12-step versus a group CBT approach, which found a significant improvement in self-efficacy and reduction in gambling episodes that lasted over a 6-month period [37].

Family Therapy As with most psychiatric diagnoses in adolescents, family involvement is crucial to successful treatment. Like group therapy, there are few, if any, empirical data demonstrating the effectiveness of family therapy in treating PG. Family therapy focuses primarily

on reducing the tension between family members and facilitating the adolescent's recovery. This is accomplished in a variety of ways, which include: dealing with the patient's and family's guilt/shame; addressing (often) parents' denial; providing tools for the family to work toward financial recovery; and eliminating enabling behaviors in family members.

Additionally, although not "family therapy" *per se*, collateral information from parents, both at initial assessment and throughout treatment, is critical, particularly because there are no laboratory tests for or physical stigmata of PG. Savvy parents can monitor credit card or bank statements for clues as to whether gambling behaviors persist.

Pharmacotherapy

Currently, there are no FDA-approved medications for the treatment of PG. Although there is a modest literature base on the pharmacological treatment of adult PG, there are virtually no data available regarding pharmacological treatment of PG in adolescents. For this reason, pharmacological treatment approaches have been based on those employed for adult PG or other addictive or impulse-control disorders (e.g., substance abuse).

Because of the questionable efficacy of medications in treating adolescent PG and the lack of data regarding the long-term effects of psychotropics on development and cognition in children and adolescents, pharmacotherapy is reserved for the most severely affected patients, those with significant psychiatric comorbidities, or those who have already failed psychotherapeutic and psychosocial interventions.

Before starting a medication for PG, clinicians should be very clear about the expected effects of the medication, the time course for those effects to be realized, and the medication's limitations. This is extremely important because adolescents with PG tend to be quite impulsive and expect immediate results from any prescribed medication. Perhaps as a result of this, they have a higher rate of discontinuing psychiatric treatment than those with other psychiatric diagnoses [41].

Some of these classes of medications are discussed below, with their order of appearance in the text denoting a general treatment algorithm:

Selective Serotonin Reuptake Inhibitors (SSRIs) Individuals with PG are postulated to be likely to respond to SSRIs because they have psychiatric symptoms similar to individuals with anxiety disorders (e.g., obsessions, anxiety) and these disorders have been treated effectively with SSRIs (e.g., obsessive-compulsive disorder, OCD). The literature is equivocal on the effectiveness of SSRIs in the treatment of PG. In one randomized controlled trial (RCT), Hollander *et al.* demonstrated significant reductions in scores on the Yale–Brown Obsessive-Compulsive Scale modified for Pathological Gambling (Y–BOCS-PG) with fluvoxamine treatment [42]. However, in another RCT, Grant *et al.* did not note any significant difference between paroxetine and placebo in reducing gambling behaviors [43]. If SSRIs are started, dosing strategies are similar to those used in adolescents with depressive or anxiety disorders.

Opiate Antagonists This class of medications has been used in the treatment of adult PG for both theoretical and practical reasons. Theoretically, the opiate system is believed to play an important role in reward and reinforcement. Practically, these agents have demonstrated effectiveness in treating other addictive disorders, such as alcohol dependence. Opiate antagonists should block both the euphoria and craving associated with gambling. However, only one double-blind RCT of naltrexone has been completed [44], though the results were positive (i.e., those subjects taking naltrexone showed a significant improvement on three gambling outcome scales when compared with controls).

Dosing strategies for adolescents with PG are similar to those for adolescents and adults with alcohol dependence. Treatment with naltrexone is generally initiated at 25 mg/day and the dose is increased by 25 mg/week to a target dose of 50–200 mg/day. Liver function tests (LFTs) should be monitored periodically. Medication effects are generally noted approximately 2 weeks after beginning treatment, much like SSRIs.

Mood Stabilizers Medications such as valproic acid, lithium, and carbamazepine have been used to treat PG because some clinicians and researchers feel that the impulsivity typical of pathological gamblers is very similar to the impulsivity seen in individuals with bipolar disorder. Although there are limited data regarding the effectiveness of this class of medications in treating PG, in a single-blind RCT, Pallanti *et al.* did note that individuals treated with lithium or valproate showed a significant decrease in their scores on the Y–BOCS-PG when compared with controls [45]. Topiramate, which has shown effectiveness in treating both binge eating disorder and alcohol dependence, is currently being investigated as a treatment for PG. Dosing strategies for mood stabilizers are similar to those used in the maintenance phase of bipolar disorder.

Prevention Strategies

Although promising treatment options for adolescent PG are on the horizon, prevention remains the best option in reducing the morbidity from PG. Prevention strategies should focus on limiting adolescents' access to gaming, raising public awareness about the negative consequences of PG, educating parents about the dangers of PG, and working to change our culture's perception that gambling is glamorous and completely innocuous.

Summary Points

Adolescent PG is an under-recognized, but potentially devastating psychiatric disorder. Screening by healthcare providers and other adults is critically important in identifying PG early and limiting its morbidity. Currently, there is little empirical evidence on the etiology, phenomenology, and treatment of adolescent PG. Although CBT and certain classes of medications show great promise, prevention remains vital, though this may be difficult in our current cultural milieu. It is also important to consider that most research on adolescent gambling has been conducted in Western cultures with racially homogeneous samples, is primarily prevalence focused, is most often published in one journal (e. g., *Journal of Gambling Studies*), and generally lacks valid and reliable assessment instruments [17]. Future research should address these limitations and help inform identification of adolescents at high risk for developing PG as well as treatment decisions.

BINGE EATING DISORDER

Introduction

Unlike pathological gambling, binge eating disorder (BED) is not a recognized DSM-IV-TR disorder. Rather, it is a clinical entity included in Appendix B of the DSM-IV-TR [13] under the heading "Criteria Set and Axes Provided for Further Study" (i.e., research criteria set). Like many psychiatric disorders in the DSM-IV-TR, the criteria for BED have generally been formulated on adults rather than children and adolescents.

The DSM-IV-TR criteria for BED requires recurrent episodes of binge eating, characterized by both: eating within a two hour period an amount of food larger than most people would eating in such a time period under similar circumstances and a feeling of not being able to control eating during the episode [13]. Further, the episode requires three or more of the following characteristics: (1) eating more rapidly than normal; (2) eating until feeling uncomfortably full; (3) eating large amounts of food when not feeling physically hungry; (4) eating along because of being embarrassed by how much one is eating; (5) feeling disgusted with oneself, depressed, or very guilty after overeating [13]. The individual must also feel significant distress during the episode, which must occur at the frequency of at least 2 days a week for 6 months [13]. Finally, binge eating can neither occur exclusively during the course of anorexia nervosa or bulimia nervosa, nor be associated with regular, inappropriate use of compensatory behaviors, such as purging or fasting [13]. Of note, the method of determining frequency differs from that used for bulimia nervosa. Future research should address whether the preferred method of setting a frequency threshold is counting the number of days on which binges occur or counting the number of episodes of binge eating. Binge eating behavior is not necessarily driven by hunger or metabolic need and individuals with this disorder often eat until they feel uncomfortably full [46,47]. Moreover, they may eat alone because they feel embarrassed about how much they are eating, feel ashamed or disgusted by their behavior during binges, and feel markedly depressed after binges.

Epidemiology

In community samples, binge eating is present in around 5% of U.S. adults at some time in their lives [49,50]. Individuals with BED tend to be overweight or obese, as evidenced by findings from numerous settings (e.g., clinics, community, population-based studies). The rate of BED among overweight individuals is almost double that of the overall population (2.9% vs. 1.5%) [51]. Unlike other eating disorders, BED affects women only slightly more than men (60% vs. 40%) [51].

Typically, BED begins in late adolescence or early adulthood. Somewhat less frequently, it may begin in childhood or early adolescence, particularly in overweight or obese children. Decaluwe and Braet found that 1% of children and adolescents (aged 10–16 years) seeking weight-loss treatment met criteria for BED, according to the eating disorder examination (EDE) [52]. An additional 9% were found to have objective bulimic episodes (OBEs) in which they overate with loss of control. Some data also suggest that individuals who report binge eating before dieting also report that their first episode of binge eating started between ages 11 to 13 [53,54]. Earlier onset of BED may also connote a worse prognosis. In obese women with eating disorders, one retrospective study found that onset of binge eating before age 18 was associated with earlier onset of obesity, eating disorder symptoms, and mood disorders [55].

Data are mixed about the natural course of BED. Fairburn et al. found that BED tended to remit spontaneously over a 5-year span, with only 18% of individuals having any form of eating disorder at the end of this period [56]. In contrast, data from the McKnight longitudinal study showed that without treatment, eating disorder pathology (including BED) persisted over time [57,58]. Examination of wait-list, control-period data has generally been consistent with the McKnight data and suggests that BED is stable and persistent, at least over a 2–6-month period [57].

Biology

Recently, biological evidence has been proposed to better classify binge eating (and other eating disorders). Foulds et al. argue that understanding the biological foundations for binge eating through investigation of existing data about analogous animal behaviors may help clarify the binge eating phenotype in humans [59]. In a 2009 review of the biology of binge eating, the authors note that the precursors to the development of binge eating are similar in animals and humans, and include a history of caloric restriction, stress, food availability, and conditioning to environmental and sensory stimuli. Similar to substance abuse, these findings also suggest that binge eating may result from natural reward system anomalies.

Diagnostic Criteria

Controversy currently exists as to whether BED is a syndrome of clinical significance separate from other eating disorders. Binge eating was first identified by Stunkard in 1959, though BED has not yet gained full diagnostic status in DSM-IV-TR [13]. Current criteria remain controversial in part due to difficulty in defining a binge episode, particularly distinguishing simple overeating from the more pathological diagnostic criterion of "an amount of food that is definitely larger than most people would eat" [60]. This distinction, as well as the "loss of control" criterion, has proved difficult to measure [60].

Wilfley et al., among others, have presented evidence to support BED as a disorder with distinct phenotypic characteristics [61]. Compared to age-matched controls, individuals with BED are more likely to consume more calories at binge meals and non-binge meals [62], display more chaotic and disinhibited eating, demonstrate higher levels of eating psychopathology [63], and have higher rates of psychiatric comorbidity [54]. Distinct comorbid core psychopathology, psychiatric disorders, and physical sequelae associated with BED may also support this contention [58]. Further, notable distinctions exist between BED and bulimia nervosa, including general psychopathology and eating behaviors.

Latner and Clyne reviewed research in order to support or refute current diagnostic criteria for BED [48]. Research findings are varied regarding the appropriateness of the DSM-IV-TR's 2-day-per-week criterion for binge frequency. However, several studies suggest that loss of control is a core feature of binge eating, regardless of the amount of food consumed [48,64]. In turn, the authors suggest that future definitions of BED should include episodes that involve a loss of control over eating even if only consuming a small or moderate amount of food. The study concludes that few studies support additional DSM-IV-TR criteria for BED. This review also notes that regardless of whether an individual meets full BED criteria, sub-threshold binge eating problems may also cause intense distress and impairment. This finding suggests a need also to develop treatments for individuals who demonstrate some symptoms of BED.

Clinical Presentation

Risk Factors

A variety of risk factors for developing BED have been identified. These are presumed to be similar for childhood-, adolescent-, and adult-onset BED, though those for adult-onset BED have been more extensively studied. Striegel-Moore *et al.* found that Caucasian women with BED were more likely to have been sexually or physically abused as children, bullied by peers, or discriminated against because of their race than healthy comparison women [65]. African-American women with BED were more likely to have been sexually or physically abused as children or bullied by peers (but not racially discriminated against) than healthy comparison women [65].

Fairburn *et al.* found that women with BED were more likely to have been subjected to parental depression, vulnerability to obesity, and repeated negative comments about body shape, weight, and eating [66]. However, neither of these studies included males with BED. The presence of overweight or obesity, particularly when co-occurring with psychiatric disorders or low self-esteem, raises concern about the potential presence of BED.

The ways that mothers with eating disorders feed their children may also have an impact on the development of BED or other eating disorders in these children. Fear of binge eating in the mother, which extends to her child, may impact maternal feeding behaviors of mothers with eating disorders (EDs) [67–69], causing these mothers to keep smaller amounts of food in the house than mothers without EDs [69,70]. Large prospective studies of mothers and 36-month-old children have found that mothers who engaged in binge eating were more likely to report restrictive feeding styles and eating problems in their children than mothers without eating disorders [71].

Peer influence may also be associated with binge eating behavior. In a 5-year prospective study of 2516 adolescents, females with friends who dieted at baseline were more likely to engage in binge eating 5 years later [72].

Psychiatric Comorbidities

Because research on BED in children and adolescents is in its early stages, issues of causation are problematic. For example, difficulty arises when trying to distinguish whether psychiatric symptoms or disorders are risk factors for developing BED, are caused by BED, or are comorbid with and independent of BED.

Notwithstanding this concern, the child, adolescent, and adult BED scientific literature has identified several personality traits that are fairly consistent across individuals with BED. Generally, adults with BED show low self-esteem and poor social adjustment [58]. Similarly, children and adolescents with BED show low levels of self-esteem and low levels of body esteem [73,74]. In one study of 1739 females aged 12 to 18, binge eating was associated with loss of overall control in 15% of participants [75]. It was also associated with an increased likelihood of engaging in disordered eating, including self-induced vomiting in 8.2% of participants, diet pills in 2.4%, laxative misuse in 1.1%, and diuretics in 0.6%. Another study, in a sample of 170 adolescent BED patients, found that self-criticism mediated the correlation between a history of emotional abuse and both depressive symptoms and body dissatisfaction [76].

With regard to more "official" psychiatric diagnoses, both community and treatment-seeking samples of adult individuals with BED have consistently demonstrated substantially higher rates of various psychiatric disorders than their weight-matched controls [77]. For example, individuals with BED are three times more likely to suffer from current major depressive disorder than a weight-matched, non-eating-disordered sample [78]. In children, the literature base is more limited and, perhaps not surprisingly, the data more equivocal. One study found that adolescent girls with subclinical binge eating disorder had a higher prevalence of mood disorders (major depression and dysthymia) and anxiety symptoms compared with girls reporting no eating disorders [79]. In another study, Isnard *et al.* found that obese children who demonstrated binge eating symptoms (but did not necessarily meet formal research criteria for BED) also showed significantly higher levels of anxiety and depression than their non-bingeing counterparts [73]. However, Decaluwe *et al.* found that obese binge eaters did not differ from obese non-binge eaters in their degree of depression [74]. In a recent longitudinal study of children with a mean age of 10.4 years, data suggested that, when compared to children with healthy eating behavior, children who displayed symptoms of a loss of control in their eating style were more likely to display these eating patterns into adolescence as well as to have worsening emotional distress over time [80].

Relevant Assessment Issues

Like many psychiatric disorders, BED is most often diagnosed by clinical interview. The initial interview can be supplemented with more structured diagnostic interviews such as the Eating Disorders Examination-Questionnaire (EDE-Q) [81] or the Questionnaire of Eating and Weight Patterns [82]. Over the past decade, multiple self-report assessments have also been developed to assess eating disorders, including the Binge Eating Scale [83], the Three Factor Eating Questionnaire [84], and the Body Shape Questionnaire [85]. However, these measures have been developed and validated in adult populations, and further research is needed to develop reliable assessments that reflect more refined definitions of BED [59]. At present, valid and reliable assessment instruments that diagnose binge eating or BED in children are few. Some studies have used instruments such as the Kids' Eating Disorders Survey [86] and the Eating Symptoms Inventory [87], neither of which assesses loss of control. More recently, the Children's Binge Eating Disorder Scale was developed to measure BED in children using DSM-IV-TR provisional criteria via a brief interview [88]. It has been suggested that this scale may be a useful tool in identifying early-onset BED, including adult obesity and associated symptoms [89]. However, further research in child and adolescent populations remains paramount to develop valid and reliable assessment tools.

Treatment

Psychotherapy

Effective treatment of children and adolescents with binge eating disorder remains elusive. In a 2006 comprehensive review of all treatment studies conducted for BED [90], the authors found that no studies enrolled patients younger than 18 years of age.

In adults, CBT, both individual and group, is the most well-established psychotherapeutic treatment for BED and has consistently proved superior to control groups (e.g., wait-list) and, more recently, fluoxetine in the treatment of this disorder [91–94]. By reducing cognitive distortions related to eating, body shape, and weight, CBT has been found to reduce binge frequency, hunger, and disinhibition in adults [94,95]. However, current data suggest that CBT does not impact changes in body weight seen in BED [89].

Other studies have explored the effect of interpersonal psychotherapy (IPT) and dialectical-behavioral therapy (DBT) for the treatment of BED. IPT aims to improve interpersonal functioning, mood, and self-esteem, deficits of which are hallmarks of BED. DBT focuses on skill development in the areas of mindfulness, emotion regulation, interpersonal effectiveness, and distress tolerance. Wilfley *et al.* showed that binge-eating recovery rates were equivalent for group CBT and group IPT, both immediately post-treatment and at 1-year follow-up [94]. DBT has also been found to be an effective modality to decrease binge eating [96]. In fact, 89% of individuals in the DBT group had stopped binge eating at the end of treatment and 56% of individuals were still not bingeing at 6-month follow-up [96]. However, similar to CBT, neither DBT nor IPT appear to impact weight gain.

Pharmacotherapy

To date, the scientific literature regarding pharmacological treatments for BED (mainly SSRIs) is somewhat equivocal. Of note, this research almost exclusively has been conducted in adult samples. Most commonly, RCTs have focused on second-generation antidepressants (specifically fluoxetine and fluvoxamine), tricyclic antidepressants, anticonvulsants, and sibutramine [46,89,90,97].

Several RCTs have found SSRIs superior to placebo in reducing binge eating [98–101]. However, other studies have called into question the efficacy of SSRIs in treating BED. Grilo *et al.* found that fluoxetine was not significantly superior to placebo in treating the behavioral and psychological features of BED [91]. Similarly, Ricca *et al.* found that the addition of fluoxetine to cognitive-behavioral therapy (CBT) did not provide any clear advantage over CBT alone [92].

Other psychopharmacological options are currently being explored, and some (e.g., topiramate) show promise in the treatment of BED [102]. One study found that topiramate was associated with reduction in binge episodes and in Yale–Brown Obsessive Compulsive Scale for Binge Eating (Y–BOCS-BE) scores [103]. However, topiramate did not differ from placebo with regard to residual severity of BED symptoms or weight gain [103].

In a 2008 review, Reas and Grilo contended that while the evidence base for pharmacotherapy for BED is growing, it continues to be limited to studies lacking follow-up data on both maintenance and "durability of effect" [97]. The authors suggest that antiobesity (sibutramine) and antiepileptic (topiramate) medications may have greater utility than SSRIs in reducing binge eating and impacting weight loss. Further, CBT is recommended over self-help approaches alone, though self-help CBT may provide a useful first step for individuals with BED. Moreover, while binge-eating reduction may not be impacted strongly by the combination of psycho-pharmacological and psychotherapeutic treatment modalities, the combination of specific medications, such as orlistat and topiramate, with CBT may moderately enhance weight loss [91,104]. Finally, the treatment of BED should focus not only on core eating disorder psychopathology, but also on any comorbid psychiatric disorders. Additionally, any medical problems that have resulted from BED (e.g., obesity, diabetes, hypertension) should be addressed while psychiatric treatment is ongoing.

Summary Points

At present, virtually no medication or behavioral intervention trials exist for adolescents with BED. In a 2006 comprehensive review of all treatment studies conducted for BED [90], it was found that no study enrolled patients younger than 18 years old. Future BED research must acquire epidemiological data to determine the extent to which this disorder is a problem for adolescents as well as to explore differential outcomes by age.

Unfortunately, most of the scientific literature on the pathogenesis, phenomenology, and treatment of BED is based on adult studies, much as it is in pathological gambling. The ability to generalize these findings to the assessment and treatment of children and adolescents with BED is unknown. In adult, child, and adolescent populations, further research addressing how best to target both binge eating and weight loss goals, optimal duration of interventions, and prevention of relapse is needed in order to refine and improve treatment options.

OTHER EMERGING CLINICAL CONDITIONS

As our society advances and new technologies are developed, invariably some individuals use them in a maladaptive fashion, negatively impacting their functioning or causing themselves clinical distress. Such is the case with both of the entities discussed below. Neither is a recognized DSM-IV-TR diagnosis or even a "Criteria Set Provided for Further Study," and much controversy exists as to whether either is a true psychiatric disorder. However, for convenience's sake, both are referred to as "disorders" in the text. In the interest of time and space, these disorders are discussed only briefly here.

Internet Addiction Disorder

Clinical Vignette: Internet Addiction

Steven is a 13-year-old boy who has never had many friends at school. Somewhat awkward socially, he is less interested in dating than his older brother was at his age, and he doesn't have much interest in socializing with other kids or participating in after-school activities. Until 5th grade, he was a voracious reader and particularly enjoyed fantasy and science fiction series. However, after his parents got him his first computer at age 11, he became increasingly interested in visiting virtual reality sites. After spending a substantial amount of time surfing the web, he found one site that was of particular interest to him. This site was free to join and allowed him to navigate a complex, imaginary virtual world (which was similar to the worlds in his fantasy books). Although he was required to be 18-years old to join, he easily created a fake log-in and instantly had the opportunity to create his own 3-D avatar and new persona – a 19-year-old man with an athletic physique and ample confidence. This new virtual world was inhabited by millions of other members, with whom he began to socialize, both through texting and speaking. For Steven, this imaginary world was an exciting place in which to exist, and he began spending several hours a day after school on the site. He told his parents that he was involved in a chat-room for teens who enjoyed science fiction. In reality, this world was inhabited by adults and had no restrictions for younger users.

Steven began to make friends on the site with other adult avatars, visited virtual areas with mature themes, and began to spend his allowance purchasing the site's currency, which allowed him to buy virtual gifts for his new online friends. Noticing the amount of time he was spending online, his parents began to encourage him to go outside after school to meet some of the neighborhood boys who often played an inclusive, pick-up basketball game. However, in order to stay online as much as possible, he made the excuses that he had "too much homework" or was chatting with school friends. Although he felt guilty lying to his parents, he was "hooked" on this virtual world in which he could be whoever he wanted, had self-esteem, and would not be mocked by his peers.

Introduction

Since the 1990s, internet addiction has been recognized as a mental health problem with symptoms akin to other established addictions. Internet addiction disorder (IAD) has been defined as an "uncontrollable and damaging use of the Internet and is recognized as a compulsive-impulsive Internet usage disorder" [105–107].

Epidemiology

Given the emerging nature of this disorder, there is also no clear agreement about the prevalence, severity, or natural course of IAD. Research on the epidemiology of IAD suggests that prevalence estimates vary widely, likely an artifact of the lack of a consensus definition of this disorder or associated assessment methodology.

One large-scale telephone survey of over 2500 adults in the United States found that 4–14% of the survey respondents showed evidence of some aspects of problematic internet use [108]. Problematic use included characteristics such as being preoccupied with the internet while offline, being secretive about internet use, and suffering relationship problems as a result of excessive use. Shaw and Black reported that the incidence of IAD was greater in countries with a higher prevalence of internet use, was higher among males, and that its etiology was unknown [109]. Studies in Taiwanese and Chinese college-age populations have found incidence rates of 5.9% and 10.6%, respectively [110,111]. In South Korea, internet addiction is considered one of the country's most serious public health issues [112]. Recently, the South Korean government established various programs designed to treat internet addiction in adolescents, including the popular Jump Up Internet Rescue School, a camp intended to cure children who are considered internet-addicted or online game-addicted [113].

Diagnostic Criteria

At present, there is no accepted set of criteria for IAD listed in the DSM-IV-TR. The criteria researchers have used to diagnose IAD are very similar to the criteria used to diagnose either pathological gambling or substance dependence [114,115], which are also on the impulse control disorder spectrum. Such characteristics may include preoccupation, tolerance, loss of control, withdrawal, escape, dishonesty, crime, and social, academic, or professional harm, each associated with pathological internet usage. Proponents of this diagnosis (i.e., those who believe that it is a bona fide disorder) correctly note that there is a subset of individuals whose internet use is problematic and, to some extent, uncontrollable. Subtypes of pathological internet use have been defined as excessive gaming, sexual preoccupations, and e-mail/text messaging [112,116]. Common features of these proposed subtypes include the following:

- excessive use, often manifested in a loss of sense of time or a neglect of basic drives;
- withdrawal, with feelings of anger, tension, and/or depression when the computer is inaccessible;
- impaired tolerance, including the need for better computer equipment, more software, or more hours of use; and
- negative repercussions, (e.g., arguments, lying, poor achievement, social isolation, and fatigue) [117].

Clinical Presentation

Researchers have attempted to ascertain psychological, social, and behavioral features of those who have been diagnosed as "internet addicts" on different instruments. The results have been fairly consistent, though researchers have noted that there are not yet any clearly defined or well-established symptom clusters that characterize gaming "addiction" [118]. Despite these studies, issues of causality remain problematic [119]. Factors associated with IAD are highlighted in Table 24.1.

Relevant Assessment Issues

Although there are several instruments designed to assess excessive internet use (e.g., Young's Internet Addiction test, Internet Addiction Scale (IAS)), the psychometric soundness of these has been questioned. Across studies, there is little consensus about the definition of "internet addiction" and how much time spent online is problematic.

Treatment

At present there are no evidence-based treatment methods for IAD. Based on the impulse-control deficit characteristics of the disorder, CBT might be a helpful approach. However, empirical support for psychotherapy or pharmacotherapy interventions is currently lacking.

Summary Points

Critics of IAD's designation as a true mental disorder point to numerous shortcomings in both its database and conceptual framework [120]. First, they note that IAD started from an atheoretical framework, is based mainly on exploratory surveys with a fairly homogeneous population set (White or Asian males), and has not addressed issues of causality. They also observe that there is little agreement on the definition of this disorder. Second, they comment that although some individuals certainly spend too much time online, many individuals also spend too much time performing a variety of other activities (e.g., watching television, reading) with a resultant negative impact on their functioning. Yet these activities do not qualify as addictive disorders. Third, they postulate that individuals who have been diagnosed with IAD are driven not by a compulsive need to use the internet, but rather the desire to avoid other problematic or difficult areas of their lives. They also argue that their excessive use of the internet may be phasic (i.e., their internet use is greatest when they are first introduced to the medium and tapers with time). Fourth, they argue that the criteria used to diagnose IAD (i.e., pathological

Table 24.1 Factors associated with internet addiction in adolescents.

Category	Symptoms/factors	References
Male gender		106,109,125
Psychological symptoms	Depression	106,115,123,134–137
	Anxiety	
	ADHD	
	Suicidal ideation	
	Alcohol use	
	Self-injurious behavior	
	Boredom	
	Risk-taking behavior	
Familial and social factors	Family dissatisfaction	106,114,134,138
	Social and familial loneliness	
	Social phobia	
	Recent stressful event	
	Academic difficulties	
	Interpersonal sensitivity	
Patterns of internet use	Internet use between more than 2 hours/day and 55 hours/week	106,123,139,140
	Daily internet use	

gambling criteria) are inappropriate because these behaviors are quite different. Pathological gambling is a single type of antisocial act; internet use is quite varied, generally prosocial, and interactive. Fifth, they point out that most internet use among individuals diagnosed with IAD is designed to correspond with other individuals and that this behavior is not pathological just because the communication occurs online as opposed to over the phone.

Video Game Addiction

Introduction

Video games inarguably are becoming one of the dominant forms of electronic entertainment for both adults and children around the world. In 2007 in the United States, approximately $18.8 billion dollars were spent on video games, and these estimates are rising quickly [121]. Not surprisingly, this phenomenon has led to concerns that video games may lead to both addictive tendencies and sedentary lifestyle in children.

Epidemiology

Similar to IAD, little scientific data exist regarding the incidence, prevalence, distribution/demographics, and natural course of video game addiction (VGA). One recent study found that in a sample of over 1100 U.S. youths aged 8 to 18 years, around 8% of video-game

players exhibited pathological behaviors [122]. Further, the study found that compared to non-VGA youths, VGA youths received poorer grades in school, had attention problems, and played video games around twice as much [122]. One large, longitudinal study of online gamers in the Netherlands found that 1.5% (2008) or 1.6% (2009) of Dutch adolescents aged 13–16 years were "addicted," heavy online gamers [123].

Diagnostic Criteria

As a diagnostic entity, VGA is very similar to IAD. Both are controversial disorders of relatively recent vintage, limited research database, and questionable validity. Additional similar features of VGA to IAD include: seeking to explain certain individuals' problematic behaviors through discovery (or creation) of a psychiatric disorder; lack of consensus regarding the definition of VGA or diagnostic criteria to be used to identify VGA; use of proxy criteria to define the disorder (e.g., substance dependence and pathological gambling criteria); serious questions regarding causality; and scant scientific evidence about the incidence, prevalence, distribution/demographics, and natural course of the disorder.

Clinical Presentation

Proponents of VGA as a diagnostic entity have noted high rates of (up to 20% of children [124]) and numerous negative characteristics associated with excessive video game use in children and adolescents. Chiu et al. reported higher rates of hostility, decreased social skills, and decreased academic achievement in Taiwanese children and adolescents with VGA when compared with the general population [125]. Lo et al. noted that the quality of interpersonal relationships decreased and levels of social anxiety increased with increasing online video game use in college-age individuals [126]. Grusser et al. found that children participating in excessive video game use were less likely to be able to concentrate in class than their peers who did not use video games excessively [127]. A correlation has also been found between a decline in academic performance and video game addiction severity [128]. But, none of the studies directly addressed issues of causality. However, Grusser et al. noted that their data suggested that these individuals used video games as a "coping strategy" for stress and other negative emotions, indicating that excessive video game use was merely an outlet for individuals with pre-existing psychiatric disorders or maladaptive coping styles (e.g., social anxiety disorder, avoidant personality disorder) rather than an independent disorder or cause of psychiatric comorbidity [127].

Relevant Assessment Issues

Well-validated, widely used instruments to assess problem video game playing are lacking. Fisher developed a scale to identify video arcade game addiction in adolescents [129]. Tejeiro Salguero and Moran devised a short scale, the Problem Video Game Playing scale (PVP) [130]. Neither has been used widely or validated in other studies. Of note, a recent bibliometric review of research on video game (and internet) addiction noted that while the number of publications in this area is growing, conducting precise searches of the literature is difficult because of the absence of consistent and clear terminology describing VGA [131].

Treatment

The treatment of VGA in adolescents has not been well studied. In the popular media, China has been identified as the country at the forefront of addressing the treatment of VGA, but little empirical evidence supports the efficacy of their efforts. Of note, the Chinese government operates several clinics to treat those addicted to online games, chatting, and web surfing, many of whom are forced to attend either by parents or the government [132]. Another initiative by the Chinese government has attempted to limit the amount of time adolescents spend playing video games online [133].

Summary Points

Those skeptical of VGA's validity as a diagnostic entity observe that the scientific database for VGA is even more sparse than that for IAD and note other limitations similar to those for IAD. One difference between the two involves the appropriateness of the criteria used to diagnose VGA. Arguably, VGA can be conceptualized as more comparable to pathological gambling than IAD because of the levels of socialization involved in the media (i.e., VGA and pathological gambling have long been regarded as solitary pursuits, as opposed to IAD, which is inherently prosocial, if dysfunctional). This lends credence to the notion of using pathological gambling criteria to diagnose VGA (as opposed to IAD). However, this view may change with the proliferation of online video games, which usually require some form of interaction with other individuals.

SUMMARY

Clearly, research into all of the disorders discussed in this chapter is in its early stages as it relates to children and adolescents. For some of these disorders (e.g., IAD, VGA), more data are needed to determine if they are valid diagnoses. Even those disorders that are recognized DSM-IV-TR diagnoses (e.g., pathological gambling) or are included in the DSM-IV-TR as research criteria sets (e.g., binge eating disorder) lack data regarding their respective etiologies and phenomenologies. Hopefully, future research can help improve our knowledge base in all of these domains and help inform the development of effective treatment paradigms for these potentially devastating disorders.

References

1. Gupta R, Derevensky J. Familial and social influences on juvenile gambling behavior. *J Gambl Stud* 1997;**13**:179–192.
2. Derevensky JL, Gupta R, Winters K. Prevalence rates of youth gambling problems: are the current rates inflated? *J Gambl Stud* 2003;**19**:405–425.
3. Gupta R, Derevensky JL. Adolescent gambling behavior: a prevalence study and examination of the correlates associated with problem gambling. *J Gambl Stud* 1998;**14**:319–345.
4. Derevensky JL, Gupta R. Prevalence estimates of adolescent gambling: a comparison of the SOGS-RA, DSM-IV-J, and the GA 20 questions. *J Gambl Stud* 2000;**16**:227–251.
5. Schofield G, Mummery K, Wang W, Dickson G. Epidemiological study of gambling in the non-metropolitan region of central Queensland. *Aust J Rural Health* 2004;**12**:6–10.
6. Cauffman E, Steinberg L. (Im)maturity of judgment in adolescence: why adolescents may be less culpable than adults. *Behav Sci Law* 2000;**18**:741–760.

7. Evans RI. Some theoretical models and constructs generic to substance abuse prevention programs for adolescents: possible relevance and limitations for problem gambling. *J Gambl Stud* 2003;**19**:287–302.

8. Fong TW. Pathological gambling in adolescents: no longer child's play. Paper presented at Gamblers Anonymous. The Recovery Program. UCLA NPI Grand Rounds; 5 September 2010, Los Angeles, California.

9. Wanner B, Vitaro F, Ladouceur R, Brendgen M, Tremblay RE. Joint trajectories of gambling, alcohol and marijuana use during adolescence: a person- and variable-centered developmental approach. *Addict Behav* 2006;**31**:566–580.

10. Shaffer HJ, Korn DA. Gambling and related mental disorders: a public health analysis. *Annu Rev Public Health* 2002;**23**:171–212.

11. Jacobs DF. Juvenile gambling in North America: an analysis of long term trends and future prospects. *J Gambl Stud* 2000;**16**:119–152.

12. Shaffer HJ, Hall MN. Estimating prevalence of adolescent gambling disorders: a quantitative synthesis and guide toward standard gambling nomenclature. *J Gambl Stud* 1996;**12**:193–214.

13. American Psychiatric, Association. *Diagnostic and Statistical Manual of Mental Disorders*, 4th edn, Text Revision. Washington, DC: APA, 2000.

14. Slutske WS, Caspi A, Moffitt TE, Poulton R. Personality and problem gambling: a prospective study of a birth cohort of young adults. *Arch Gen Psychiatry* 2005;**62**:769–775.

15. Gupta R, Derevensky JL. An Empirical examination of Jacobs' general theory of addictions: do adolescent gamblers fit the theory? *J Gambl Stud* 1998;**14**:17–49.

16. Kofoed L, Morgan TJ, Buchkoski J, Carr R. Dissociative experiences scale and MMPI-2 scores in video poker gamblers, other gamblers, and alcoholic controls. *J Nerv Ment Dis* 1997;**185**:58–60.

17. Blinn-Pike L, Worthy SL, Jonkman JN. Adolescent gambling: a review of an emerging field of research. *J Adolesc Health* 2010;**47**:223–236.

18. Poulin C. An assessment of the validity and reliability of the SOGS-RA. *J Gambl Stud* 2002;**18**:67–93.

19. Chambers RA, Taylor JR, Potenza MN. Developmental neurocircuitry of motivation in adolescence: a critical period of addiction vulnerability. *Am J Psychiatry* 2003;**160**:1041–1052.

20. Toneatto T, Ferguson D, Brennan J. Effect of a new casino on problem gambling in treatment-seeking substance abusers. *Can J Psychiatry* 2003;**48**:40–44.

21. Delfabbro P, Thrupp L. The social determinants of youth gambling in South Australian adolescents. *J Adolesc* 2003;**26**:313–330.

22. Hurt H, Giannetta JM, Brodsky NL, Shera D, Romer D. Gambling initiation in preadolescents. *J Adolesc Health* 2008;**43**:91–93.

23. Peacock RB, Day PA, Peacock TD. Adolescent gambling on a Great Lakes Indian reservation. *J Hum Behav* 1999;**2**:5–17.

24. Ladouceur R, Boisvert JM, Dumont J. Cognitive-behavioral treatment for adolescent pathological gamblers. *Behav Modif* 1994;**18**:230–242.

25. Ladouceur R, Sylvain C, Sevigny S, *et al.* Pathological gamblers: inpatients' versus outpatients' characteristics. *J Gambl Stud* 2006;**22**:443–450.

26. Bergevin T, Gupta R, Derevensky J, Kaufman F. Adolescent gambling: understanding the role of stress and coping. *J Gambl Stud* 2006;**22**:195–208.

27. Carlton PL, Manowitz P, McBride H, Nora R, Swartzburg M, Goldstein L. Attention deficit disorder and pathological gambling. *J Clin Psychiatry* 1987;**48**:487–488.

28. Kaminer Y, Burleson JA, Jadamec A. Gambling behavior in adolescent substance abuse. *Subst Abuse* 2002;**23**:191–198.

29. Lee GP, Storr CL, Ialongo NS, Martins SS. Compounded effect of early adolescence depressive symptoms and impulsivity on late adolescence gambling: a longitudinal study. *J Adolesc Health* 2011;**48**:164–169.

30. Hollander E, Wong CM. Body dysmorphic disorder, pathological gambling, and sexual compulsions. *J Clin Psychiatry* 1995;**56** (Suppl. 4): 7–12; discussion 3.

31. Welte J, Barnes G, Wieczorek W, Tidwell MC, Parker J. Alcohol and gambling pathology among U.S. adults: prevalence, demographic patterns and comorbidity. *J Stud Alcohol* 2001;**62**:706–712.

32. Johnson EE, Hamer RM, Nora RM. The Lie/Bet Questionnaire for screening pathological gamblers: a follow-up study. *Psychol Rep* 1998;**83**:1219–1224.

33. Fisher S. Developing the DSM-IV criteria to identify adolescent problem gambling in non-clinical populations. *J Gambl Stud* 2000;**16**:253–273.

34. Winters KC, Stinchfield RD, Fulkerson J. Toward the development of an adolescent gambling problem severity scale. *J Gambl Stud* 1993;**9**:371–386.

35. Ursua MP, Uribelarrea LL. 20 Questions of Gamblers Anonymous: A psychometric study with population of Spain. *J Gambl Stud* 1998;**14**:3–15.

36. Tremblay J, Wiebe J, Stinchfield R, Wynne H. Canadian Adolescent Gambling Inventory (CAGI). Canadian Centre on Substance Abuse and the Interprovincial Consortium on Gambling Research, 2010. Available from: http://www.ccsa.ca/Eng/Priorities/Gambling/CAGI/Pages/default.aspx.

37. Marceaux J, Melville C. Twelve-step facilitated versus mapping-enhanced cognitive-behavioral therapy for pathological gambling: a controlled study. *J Gambl Stud* 2011;**27**:171–190.

38. Bertrand K, Dufour M, Wright J, Lasnier B. Adapted Couple Therapy (ACT) for pathological gamblers: a promising avenue. *J Gambl Stud* 2008;**24**:393–409.

39. Stewart RM, Brown RI. An outcome study of Gamblers Anonymous. *Br J Psychiatry* 1988;**152**:284–288.

40. Coman GJ, Evans BJ, Burrows GD. Group counseling for problem gambling. *Brit J Guid Couns* 2002;**30**:145–158.

41. Grant JE, Kim SW, Kuskowski M. Retrospective review of treatment retention in pathological gambling. *Compr Psychiatry* 2004;**45**:83–87.

42. Hollander E, DeCaria CM, Finkell JN, Begaz T, Wong CM, Cartwright C. A randomized double-blind fluvoxamine/placebo crossover trial in pathologic gambling. *Biol Psychiatry* 2000;**47**:813–817.

43. Grant JE, Kim SW, Potenza MN, *et al.* Paroxetine treatment of pathological gambling: a multi-centre randomized controlled trial. *Int Clin Psychopharmacol* 2003;**18**:243–249.

44. Kim SW, Grant JE, Adson DE, Shin YC. Double-blind naltrexone and placebo comparison study in the treatment of pathological gambling. *Biol Psychiatry* 2001;**49**:914–921.

45. Pallanti S, Quercioli L, Sood E, Hollander E. Lithium and valproate treatment of pathological gambling: a randomized single-blind study. *J Clin Psychiatry* 2002;**63**:559–564.

46. Brownley KA, Berkman ND, Sedway JA, Lohr KN, Bulik CM. Binge eating disorder treatment: a systematic review

of randomized controlled trials. *Int J Eat Disord* 2007;**40**:337–348.

47. Davis JF, Melhorn SJ, Shurdak JD, *et al.* Comparison of hydrogenated vegetable shortening and nutritionally complete high-fat diet on limited access-binge behavior in rats. *Physiol Behav* 2007;**92**:924–930.

48. Latner JD, Clyne C. The diagnostic validity of the criteria for binge eating disorder. *Int J Eat Disord* 2008;**41**:1–14.

49. Hudson JI, Hiripi E, Pope HGJr, Kessler RC. The prevalence and correlates of eating disorders in the National Comorbidity Survey Replication. *Biol Psychiatry* 2007;**61**:348–358.

50. Grucza RA, Przybeck TR, Cloninger CR. Prevalence and correlates of binge eating disorder in a community sample. *Compr Psychiatry* 2007;**48**:124–131.

51. Smith DE, Marcus MD, Lewis CE, Fitzgibbon M, Schreiner P. Prevalence of binge eating disorder, obesity, and depression in a biracial cohort of young adults. *Ann Behav Me*. 1998;**20**:227–232.

52. Decaluwe V, Braet C. Prevalence of binge-eating disorder in obese children and adolescents seeking weight-loss treatment. *Int J Obes Relat Metab Disord* 2003;**27**:404–409.

53. Spurrell EB, Wilfley DE, Tanofsky MB, Brownell KD. Age of onset for binge eating: are there different pathways to binge eating? *Int J Eat Disord* 1997;**21**:55–65.

54. Grilo CM, Masheb RM. Onset of dieting vs binge eating in outpatients with binge eating disorder. *Int J Obes Relat Metab Disord* 2000;**24**:404–409.

55. Marcus MD, Moulton MM, Greeno CG. Binge eating onset in obese patients with binge eating disorder. *Addict Behav* 1995;**20**:747–755.

56. Fairburn CG, Cooper Z, Doll HA, Norman P, O'Connor M. The natural course of bulimia nervosa and binge eating disorder in young women. *Arch Gen Psychiatry* 2000;**57**:659–665.

57. Agras WS, Telch CF, Arnow B, *et al.* Does interpersonal therapy help patients with binge eating disorder who fail to respond to cognitive-behavioral therapy? *J Consult Clin Psychol* 1995;**63**:356–360.

58. Crow SJ, Stewart Agras W, Halmi K, Mitchell JE, Kraemer HC. Full syndromal versus subthreshold anorexia nervosa, bulimia nervosa, and binge eating disorder: a multicenter study. *Int J Eat Disord* 2002;**32**:309–318.

59. Mathes WF, Brownley KA, Mo X, Bulik CM. The biology of binge eating. *Appetite* 2009;**52**:545–553.

60. Cooper Z, Fairburn CG. Refining the definition of binge eating disorder and nonpurging bulimia nervosa. *Int J Eat Disord* 2003;**34** (Suppl.): S89–95.

61. Wilfley DE, Wilson GT, Agras WS. The clinical significance of binge eating disorder. *Int J Eat Disord* 2003;**34** (Suppl.): S96–106.

62. Guss JL, Kissileff HR, Devlin MJ, Zimmerli E, Walsh BT. Binge size increases with body mass index in women with binge-eating disorder. *Obes Res* 2002;**10**:1021–1029.

63. Brody ML, Walsh BT, Devlin MJ. Binge eating disorder: reliability and validity of a new diagnostic category. *J Consult Clin Psychol* 1994;**62**:381–386.

64. Niego SH, Pratt EM, Agras WS. Subjective or objective binge: is the distinction valid? *Int J Eat Disord* 1997;**22**:291–298.

65. Striegel-Moore RH, Dohm FA, Pike KM, Wilfley DE, Fairburn CG. Abuse, bullying, and discrimination as risk factors for binge eating disorder. *Am J Psychiatry* 2002;**159**:1902–1907.

66. Fairburn CG, Doll HA, Welch SL, Hay PJ, Davies BA, O'Connor ME. Risk factors for binge eating disorder: a community-based, case-control study. *Arch Gen Psychiatry* 1998;**55**:425–432.

67. Fahy T, Treasure J. Children of mothers with bulimia nervosa. *Brit Med J* 1989;**299**:1031.

68. Patel P, Wheatcroft R, Park RJ, Stein A. The children of mothers with eating disorders. *Clin Child Fam Psychol Rev* 2002;**5**:1–19.

69. Russell GF, Treasure J, Eisler I. Mothers with anorexia nervosa who underfeed their children: their recognition and management. *Psychol Med* 1998;**28**:93–108.

70. Stein A, Woolley H, Cooper SD, Fairburn CG. An observational study of mothers with eating disorders and their infants. *J Child Psychol Psychiatry* 1994;**35**:733–748.

71. Reba-Harrelson L, VonHolle A, Hamer RM, Torgersen L, Reichborn-Kjennerud T, Bulik CM. Patterns of maternal feeding and child eating associated with eating disorders in the Norwegian Mother and Child Cohort Study (MoBa). *Eat Behav* 2010;**11**:54–61.

72. Eisenberg ME, Neumark-Sztainer D. Friends' dieting and disordered eating behaviors among adolescents five years later: findings from Project EAT. *J Adolesc Health* 2010;**47**:67–73.

73. Isnard P, Michel G, Frelut ML, *et al.* Binge eating and psychopathology in severely obese adolescents. *Int J Eat Disord* 2003;**34**:235–243.

74. Decaluwe V, Braet C, Fairburn CG. Binge eating in obese children and adolescents. *Int J Eat Disord* 2003;**33**:78–84.

75. Jones JM, Bennett S, Olmsted MP, Lawson ML, Rodin G. Disordered eating attitudes and behaviours in teenaged girls: a school-based study. *Can Med Assoc J* 2001;**165**:547–552.

76. Dunkley DM, Masheb RM, Grilo CM. Childhood maltreatment, depressive symptoms, and body dissatisfaction in patients with binge eating disorder: the mediating role of self-criticism. *Int J Eat Disord* 2010;**43**:274–281.

77. Grilo CM. Recent research of relationships among eating disorders and personality disorders. *Curr Psychiatry Rep* 2002;**4**:18–24.

78. Telch CF, Stice E. Psychiatric comorbidity in women with binge eating disorder: prevalence rates from a non-treatment-seeking sample. *J Consult Clin Psychol* 1998;**66**:768–776.

79. Touchette E, Henegar A, Godart NT, *et al.* Subclinical eating disorders and their comorbidity with mood and anxiety disorders in adolescent girls. *Psychiatry Res* 2011;**185**:185–192.

80. Tanofsky-Kraff M, Shomaker LB, Olsen C, *et al.* A prospective study of pediatric loss of control eating and psychological outcomes. *J Abnorm Psychol* 2011;**120**:108–118.

81. Fairburn CG, Cooper MJ. *The Eating Disorder Examination*, 12th edn. New York: Guilford Press, 1993.

82. Nangle DW, Johnson WG, Carr-Nangle RE, Engler LB. Binge eating disorder and the proposed DSM-IV criteria: psychometric analysis of the Questionnaire of Eating and Weight Patterns. *Int J Eat Disord* 1994;**16**:147–157.

83. Hawkins RC 2nd, Clement PF. Development and construct validation of a self-report measure of binge eating tendencies. *Addict Behav* 1980;**5**:219–226.

84. Stunkard AJ, Messick S. The three-factor eating questionnaire to measure dietary restraint, disinhibition and hunger. *J Psychosom Res* 1985;**29**:71–83.

85. Cooper PJ, Taylor MJ, Cooper Z, Fairburn CG. The development and validation of the Body Shape Questionnaire. *Int J Eat Disorder* 1986;**6**:485–494.

86. Childress AC, Brewerton TD, Hodges EL, Jarrell MP. The Kids' Eating Disorders Survey (KEDS): a study of middle school students. *J Am Acad Child Adolesc Psychiatry* 1993;**32**:843–850.

87. Whitaker A, Davies M, Shaffer D, *et al.* The struggle to be thin: a survey of anorexic and bulimic symptoms in a nonreferred adolescent population. *Psychol Med* 1989;**19**:143–163.

88. Shapiro JR, Woolson SL, Hamer RM, Kalarchian MA, Marcus MD, Bulik CM. Evaluating binge eating disorder in children: development of the children's binge eating disorder scale (C-BEDS). *Int J Eat Disorder* 2007;**40**:82–89.

89. Bulik CM, Brownley KA, ShapiroJr., Diagnosis and management of binge eating disorder. *World Psychiatry* 2007;**6**:142–148.

90. Berkman ND, Bulik CM, Brownley KA, *et al.* Management of eating disorders. *Evid Rep Technol Assess (Full Rep)* 2006 Apr (135): 1–166.

91. Grilo C, Masheb, RM, Wilson, GT. Efficacy of cognitive behavioral therapy and fluoxetine for the treatment of binge eating disorder: a randomized double-blind placebo-controlled comparison. *Biol Psychiatry* 2005;**57**:301–309.

92. Ricca V, Mannucci E, Mezzani B, *et al.* Fluoxetine and fluvoxamine combined with individual cognitive-behaviour therapy in binge eating disorder: a one-year follow-up study. *Psychother Psychosom* 2001;**70**:298–306.

93. Wilfley DE, Agras WS, Telch CF, *et al.* Group cognitive-behavioral therapy and group interpersonal psychotherapy for the nonpurging bulimic individual: a controlled comparison. *J Consult Clin Psychol* 1993;**61**:296–305.

94. Wilfley DE, Welch RR, Stein RI, *et al.* A randomized comparison of group cognitive-behavioral therapy and group interpersonal psychotherapy for the treatment of overweight individuals with binge-eating disorder. *Arch Gen Psychiatry* 2002;**59**:713–721.

95. Hilbert A, Tuschen-Caffier B. Body image interventions in cognitive-behavioural therapy of binge-eating disorder: a component analysis. *Behav Res Ther* 2004;**42**:1325–1339.

96. Telch CF, Agras WS, Linehan MM. Dialectical behavior therapy for binge eating disorder. *J Consult Clin Psychol* 2001;**69**:1061–1065.

97. Reas DL, Grilo CM. Review and meta-analysis of pharmacotherapy for binge-eating disorder. *Obesity (Silver Spring)* 2008;**16**:2024–2038.

98. Arnold LM, McElroy SL, Hudson JI, Welge JA, Bennett AJ, Keck PE. A placebo-controlled, randomized trial of fluoxetine in the treatment of binge-eating disorder. *J Clin Psychiatry* 2002;**63**:1028–1033.

99. Hudson JI, McElroy SL, Raymond NC, *et al.* Fluvoxamine in the treatment of binge-eating disorder: a multicenter placebo-controlled, double-blind trial. *Am J Psychiatry* 1998;**155**:1756–1762.

100. McElroy SL, Casuto LS, Nelson EB, *et al.* Placebo-controlled trial of sertraline in the treatment of binge eating disorder. *Am J Psychiatry* 2000;**157**:1004–1006.

101. McElroy SL, Hudson JI, Malhotra S, Welge JA, Nelson EB, Keck PEJr., Citalopram in the treatment of binge-eating disorder: a placebo-controlled trial. *J Clin Psychiatry* 2003;**64**:807–813.

102. McElroy SL, Guerdjikova AI, Martens B, Keck PE Jr, Pope HG, Hudson JI. Role of antiepileptic drugs in the management of eating disorders. *CNS Drugs* 2009;**23**:139–156.

103. McElroy SL, Arnold LM, Shapira NA, *et al.* Topiramate in the treatment of binge eating disorder associated with obesity: a randomized, placebo-controlled trial. *Am J Psychiatry* 2003;**160**:255–261.

104. Claudino AM, deOliveira IR, Appolinario JC, *et al.* Double-blind, randomized, placebo-controlled trial of topiramate plus cognitive-behavior therapy in binge-eating disorder. *J Clin Psychiatry* 2007;**68**:1324–1332.

105. Shapira NA, Goldsmith TD, Keck PEJr, Khosla UM, McElroy SL. Psychiatric features of individuals with problematic internet use. *J Affect Disord* 2000;**57**:267–272.

106. Lam LT, Peng ZW, Mai JC, Jing J. Factors associated with Internet addiction among adolescents. *Cyberpsychol Behav* 2009;**12**:551–555.

107. Dell'Osso B, Altamura AC, Allen A, Marazziti D, Hollander E. Epidemiologic and clinical updates on impulse control disorders: a critical review. *Eur Arch Psychiatry Clin Neurosci* 2006;**256**:464–475.

108. Aboujaoude E, Koran LM, Gamel N, Large MD, Serpe RT. Potential markers for problematic internet use: a telephone survey of 2,513 adults. *CNS Spectr* 2006;**11**:750–755.

109. Shaw M, Black DW. Internet addiction: definition, assessment, epidemiology and clinical management. *CNS Drugs* 2008;**22**:353–365.

110. Chou C HM. Internet addiction, usage, gratification, and pleasure experience: the Taiwan college students' case. *Comput Educ* 2000;**35**:65–80.

111. Wu H ZK. Path analysis on related factors causing internet addiction disorder in college students. *Chin J Public Health* 2004;**20**:1363–1366.

112. Block JJ. Issues for DSM-V: internet addiction. *Am J Psychiatry* 2008;**165**:306–307.

113. Koo C, Wati Y, Lee CC, Oh HY. Internet-addicted kids and South Korean government efforts: boot-camp case. *Cyberpsychol Behav Soc Netw* 2011;**14**:391–394.

114. Nichols LA, Nicki R. Development of a psychometrically sound internet addiction scale: a preliminary step. *Psychol Addict Behav* 2004;**18**:381–384.

115. Yoo HJ, Cho SC, Ha J, *et al.* Attention deficit hyperactivity symptoms and internet addiction. *Psychiatry Clin Neurosci* 2004;**58**:487–494.

116. Block J (ed.). Pathological computer use in the USA. In: 2007 International Symposium on the Counseling and Treatment of Youth Internet Addiction. Seoul, Korea: National Youth Commission, 2007; p. 443.

117. Beard KW, Wolf EM. Modification in the proposed diagnostic criteria for Internet addiction. *Cyberpsychol Behav* 2001;**4**:377–383.

118. Petry N. Commentary on Van Rooij *et al.* (2011): 'Gaming addiction' – a psychiatric disorder or not? *Addiction* 2011;**106**:213–214.

119. Dong G LQ, Zhou H, Zhao X. Precursor or sequela: pathological disorders in people with internet addiction disorder. *PLoS ONE* 2011;**6**:e14703.

120. Grohol J. Internet Addiction Guide. 2005. Available from: http://psychcentral.com/netaddiction.

121. Riley DM. US video game and PC sales exceed $18.8 billion marking third consecutive year of record-breaking sales [cited 5 September 2010]. Available from: www.npd.com/press/releases/press/080131b.html.

122. Gentile D. Pathological video-game use among youth ages 8 to 18: a national study. *Psychol Sci* 2009;**20**:594–602.
123. Van Rooij AJST, Vermulst AA, Van Den Eijnden RJJM, Van DeMheen, D. Online video game addiction: identification of addicted adolescent gamers. *Addiction* 2011;**106**:205–212.
124. Griffiths MD, Hunt N. Dependence on computer games by adolescents. *Psychol Rep* 1998;**82**:475–480.
125. Chiu SI, Lee JZ, Huang DH. Video game addiction in children and teenagers in Taiwan. *Cyberpsychol Behav* 2004;**7**:571–581.
126. Lo SK, Wang CC, Fang W. Physical interpersonal relationships and social anxiety among online game players. *Cyberpsychol Behav* 2005;**8**:15–20.
127. Grusser SM, Thalemann R, Albrecht U, Thalemann CN. [Excessive computer usage in adolescents – results of a psychometric evaluation]. *Wien Klin Wochenschr* 2005;**117**:188–195.
128. Gentile DA, Lynch PJ, Linder JR, Walsh DA. The effects of violent video game habits on adolescent hostility, aggressive behaviors, and school performance. *J Adolesc* 2004;**27**:5–22.
129. Fisher S. Identifying video game addiction in children and adolescents. *Addict Behav* 1994;**19**:545–553.
130. Tejeiro Salguero RA, Moran RM. Measuring problem video game playing in adolescents. *Addiction* 2002;**97**:1601–1606.
131. Carbonell X, Guardiola E, Beranuy M, Belles A. A bibliometric analysis of the scientific literature on Internet, video games, and cell phone addiction. *J Med Libr Assoc* 2009;**97**:102–107.
132. Sebag-Montefiore P. China's young escape into the web. *Observer* 20 November 2005. Available from: http://www.guardian.co.uk/technology/2005/nov/20/news.china.
133. Lee A. China limits teenage internet gaming. Health Encyclopedia, 2007 [cited 5 September 2010]. Available from: http://www.3-rx.com/ab/more/china-limits-teenage-internet-gaming/.
134. Whang LS, Lee S, Chang G. Internet over-users' psychological profiles: a behavior sampling analysis on internet addiction. *Cyberpsychol Behav* 2003;**6**:143–150.
135. van Hamel A, Derevensky J, Takane Y, Dickson L, Gupta R. Adolescent gambling and coping within a generalized high-risk behavior framework. *J Gambl Stud* 2007;**23**:377–393.
136. Lam LT, Peng Z, Mai J, Jing J. The association between internet addiction and self-injurious behaviour among adolescents. *Inj Prev* 2009;**15**:403–408.
137. Ryu EJ, Choi KS, Seo JS, Nam BW. [The relationships of Internet addiction, depression, and suicidal ideation in adolescents.] *Taehan Kanho Hakhoe Chi* 2004;**34**:102–110.
138. Yoo HJ, Kim M, Ha JH, *et al.* Biogenetic temperament and character and attention deficit hyperactivity disorder in Korean children. *Psychopathology* 2006;**39**:25–31.
139. Ko CH, Yen JY, Chen CS, Yeh YC, Yen CF. Predictive values of psychiatric symptoms for internet addiction in adolescents: a 2-year prospective study. *Arch Pediatr Adolesc Med* 2009;**163**:937–943.
140. Khan M. Emotional and behavioral effects, including addictive potential, of video games. Report of the Council on Science and Public Health, 2007. CSAPH Report 12-A-07. Available at: http://psychcentral.com/blog/images/csaph12a07.pdf.

Section Five

Treatment

Edited by Timothy W. Fong

2 5

Adolescent Substance Abuse Treatment Outcomes

Rachel Gonzales, Mary Lynn Brecht and Richard A. Rawson

Integrated Substance Abuse Programs, University of California Los Angeles, Los Angeles, CA, USA

INTRODUCTION

The problems associated with adolescent substance use abuse and dependence[1] in the United States have been a long-standing public health issue, greatly impacting healthcare, educational, and legal systems. This chapter provides an overview of this problem within substance abuse treatment programs, using the Californian publicly funded system for illustrative purposes. The primary objective of this chapter is to help clinicians develop a better understanding of the treatment challenges associated with substance use disorders among adolescents as well as treatment response to such clinical issues by examining treatment outcome data.

National household survey data approximate that 8% (1.9 million) of adolescents meet criteria for abuse/dependence of illicit drugs [1]. At the treatment front, statistics collected from the national data set of publicly funded substance abuse treatment programs estimate that about 8.5% of admissions were adolescents under 18 years old. Adolescents in substance abuse treatment represent a segment of the population that has received much attention given the risks posed by their substance abuse/dependence. Specifically, 70% of all adolescent mortality (ages 15–24) has been attributed to unintended injuries, homicide, and suicide [2], all of which are mainly associated with substance abuse behaviors [3]. Moreover, substance abuse/dependence among adolescents is related to

high-risk sexual behavior, resulting in major public health issues including unwanted pregnancies, HIV, and other sexually transmitted infections [4].

Given that most adolescent treatment for substance abuse/dependence is provided through public funding, there is considerable interest in ensuring that such programs are using public dollars responsibly and producing effective outcomes. Although research on the effectiveness of adolescent substance abuse treatment is still growing, treatment outcome studies with adolescent populations demonstrate that treatment, in general, produces measurable and desirable changes in substance use and other social behaviors [5,6], as the benefits of treatment continue to be seen in follow-up studies as measured by reductions in substance use and illegal-/criminal behaviors by 40–60% [7,8]. The landscape of adolescent substance abuse problems is a major challenge to treatment programs. Beyond mainstay substances of abuse among adolescent culture, like tobacco, alcohol, and marijuana [9], every generation looks for new ways to get high. The emergence of problematic substance abuse trends in MDMA (methylene dioxymethamphetamine, or ecstasy), inhalants, GHB (gamma-hydroxybutyrate), and other club drugs, as well as prescription and over-the-counter medicines that has occurred over recent years impacts not only the way clinical services are delivered, but also how outcomes are evaluated.

ADOLESCENT TREATMENT SYSTEM IN CALIFORNIA

As part of a State evaluation effort, the Integrated Substance Abuse Programs (ISAP) from the University

---

[1] The term "substance abuse/dependence" will be used interchangeably with "substance use disorders" as these terms are represented by the *Diagnostic and Statistical Manual of Mental Disorders, Fourth Edition, DSM-IV* (American Psychiatric Association, 1994).

Clinical Handbook of Adolescent Addiction, First Edition. Richard Rosner.
© 2013 John Wiley & Sons, Ltd. Published 2013 by John Wiley & Sons, Ltd.

of California Los Angeles (UCLA) analyzed data collected from the California Outcomes Measurement System (CalOMS) during the fiscal year 2006–07 [10]. Examining the public treatment system landscape in California, about 10% of all admissions ($n = 216\ 781$) were for adolescents between the ages of 12 and 17. The average age of adolescent admissions was 16 years. About 35% of adolescent admissions were female and 56% were Latino (with remaining admissions being mainly White and African American, 22% and 14%, respectively, and fewer Asian/Pacific Islander (2.7%) or American Indian/Alaska Native (1%). In terms of educational status, 9th grade was the average grade completed among adolescent admissions. Many of the adolescent admissions had past criminal justice involvement (48%), with 44.4% currently on probation.

Among the adolescent admissions, marijuana was the dominant primary substance reported (63%), followed by alcohol (23%). Nearly 10% of adolescent admissions were for primary methamphetamine abuse. Prescription and over-the-counter drugs were reported as primary drugs of abuse for about 1.5% of total admissions [11,12]. The prescription drugs most commonly abused by adolescents included stimulants (e.g., Adderall, Concerta, Ritalin). Fewer admissions were for cocaine/crack (1.4%) and heroin (less than 1%). The majority of adolescent admissions were from outpatient treatment programs (94%), with only 5% from residential treatment settings (31 days or more). The primary source of referral to treatment for adolescent admissions was "other," which could include healthcare professional, school, or family-/friends (47%), and the criminal justice system (30%), with self-referral accounting for 19%. Roughly 8% of adolescent admissions reported a lifetime history of mental illness. Rates of sexually transmitted infections were minimal among adolescent admissions (<1%).

ADOLESCENT TREATMENT OUTCOMES IN CALIFORNIA

According to the treatment effectiveness literature, outcomes are defined as critical areas of life functioning measured at the client level that are expected to be positively influenced by treatment [13]. At the very core, outcome measurement allows for the evaluation of substance abuse treatment and ability to hold the system accountable for producing "client success" across the following areas deemed important by the federal government: alcohol/drug use, employment/education, criminal involvement, housing, and social connectedness [14]. As such, the CalOMS database is specifically designed to monitor such core outcomes (substance use, criminal/illegal activity, health functioning, employment/education, housing stability, and social support)

as a means to measure and understand treatment effectiveness of public programs in California.

Examining data collected from CalOMS, we present a detailed description of treatment outcomes among adolescents who entered the California publicly funded treatment system during the July 2006 to June 2007 fiscal year. Outcome analyses are based on "treatment episodes," which take the first admission and last discharge record in a treatment episode to allow for adequate assessment of "change" in client functioning. Using episode treatment data, adolescents had significant reductions in any use of their primary substance (in past 30 days) from 60% at admission to 27% at discharge. Also, significant decreases were found in the average number of days of primary substance use (reported in past 30 days) at discharge (33.3%) compared to admission (63.3%). Adolescents also showed significant decreases in the percentage with criminal justice involvement from admission (9.1%) to discharge (3.9%), a drop of 5.2%, and a 3% increase in employment from 6.5% at admission to 9.5% at discharge.

DISCUSSION

In efforts to better understand youth substance use and how to develop effective intervention models, etiological factors of risk and protective factors must be considered. As confirmed by substance use etiological research, youth substance use is influenced by a complex array of cognitive, attitudinal, social, personality, pharmacological, and developmental risk factors.

Psychosocial factors related to substance use behaviors have included: sociodemographic variables, educational achievement, inadequate family bonding and attachment, parental drug use, peer influence, poor school performance, exposure to positive substance use in media and advertising, and personal/personality factors such as perceived competency, self-efficacy, risk-taking, and aggressive behaviors.

The role of the family, the school, and peer clusters have all been extensively examined and supported through research in relation to the etiology of drug use and deviance among adolescent populations. Many studies in the literature consistently show that the *family* is a major force in predicting the initiation, maintenance, and exacerbation of drug use in youths. There have also been a number of studies that have judged *school* factors as having major roles in the initiation of drug use and deviance among youths; for example, students who experienced alienation, lack of success within the school framework, perceptions of racism from teachers, and other problems with deriving rewards from school have a greater tendency toward drug use and deviance. *Peer associations* have also been consistently supported by research over the past five decades, showing that weak bonds with parents and school, are overpowered by the strong ties with peers groups, which can have a major influence on drug use.

Adolescents entering the treatment system in California have a varied set of substance abuse problems, with diverse sociodemographic traits that must be considered when examining treatment outcomes. As the data in our study indicate, racial/ethnic differences exist among youths in California with respect to substance use. Overall, we see this in national data: past 30-day prevalence rates of illicit drug use are more than twice as high among Latinos compared with Asians, with rates for Blacks and Whites fairly comparable.

It is important to consider that such higher rates of alcohol and drug use among Latinos are compounded by environmental factors, including lower socio-economic status, feelings of hopelessness, and lower self-image [15–17]. Although a gap exists in the literature with regards to cultural differences of social norms about substance use among ethnically diverse adolescents, research indicates that different ethnic groups, particularly immigrant populations, bring with them a vital history and a set of cultural norms that may differ in important ways from current US society, which may serve as protective factors to substance use. It appears that ethnic minorities from varying cultures may have buffers that contribute to lower rates of substance abuse. However, significant differences exist between the foreign-born and native populations (e.g., age structure of the populations) and intergenerational conflict affects all ethnic groups. Often young people and their parents do not view the same values and norms of life in the same manner. The literature suggests, for instance, that acculturation stress and intergenerational conflicts can enhance deviant behavior including substance abuse [18]. Hence, it is crucial for substance abuse providers to understand these conflicting issues around social norms to accurately depict ethnic group perceptions, and in turn inform practice.

CONCLUSION

As shown in this chapter, information collected from treatment outcome data can be useful to clinicians to determine treatment priorities and make changes for improved treatment. From a clinical perspective, there are some factors worth considering when examining treatment outcomes among adolescent populations, such as sexual orientation, housing status (i.e., youth runaways), and history with and/or incidence of trauma or abuse. The addition of this type of information is useful to guide the identification of adolescent-specific treatment needs, gaps in service delivery, and what, if any, changes should be made to service delivery to improve treatment.

References

1. SAMHSA. *National Survey on Drug Use and Health: National Findings*. Report No. NSDUH Series H-32, DHHS Publication No. SMA 07-4293. Rockville, MD: Substance Abuse and Mental Health Services Administration (SAMHSA) Office of Applied Studies (OAS), 2006.
2. CDC. *Youth Risk Behavior Survey*. Atlanta, GA:Centers for Disease Control and Prevention, 2009.
3. Solovitch S. Reclaiming futures. In:Isaacs SL, Colby DC (eds), *To Improve Health and Health Care*, vol. XIII. Robert Wood Johnson Foundation, 2009. Available from:http://rwjf.org/files/research/4232.pdf.
4. Centers for Disease Control and Prevention. Youth risk behavior surveillance – United States. Surveillance summaries, 2009. *MMWR* 2010;**59**(SS-5).
5. Grella CE, Hser YI. Drug Abuse Treatment Outcome Studies for Adolescents (DATOS-A) [special issue]. *J Adolesc Res* 2001;**16**(6).
6. Dennis ML, Dawud-Noursi S, Muck R, McDermeit M. The need for developing and evaluating adolescent treatment models. In:Stevens SJ, Morral AR (eds), *Adolescent Substance Abuse Treatment in the United States – Exemplary Models from a National Evaluation Study*. Binghampton, NY:Haworth Press, 2002; pp. 3–56.
7. Dennis ML, Godley SH, Diamond G, *et al.* The Cannabis Youth Treatment (CYT) study: Main findings from two randomized trials. *J Subst Abuse Treat* 2004;**27**(3):197–213.
8. Kaminer Y, Burleson JA, Burke RH. Efficacy of outpatient aftercare for adolescents with alcohol use disorders: A randomized controlled study. *J Am Acad Child Adolesc Psychiatry* 2008;**47**:12.
9. SAMHSA. Treatment Episode Data Set (TEDS). Rockville, MD: US Department of Health and Human Services Substance Abuse and Mental Health Services Administration Office of Applied Studies, 2008.
10. Rawson RA, Gonzales R. Evaluation of the substance abuse treatment system. Los Angeles, CA: CalOMS, UCLA Integrated Substance Abuse Program, 2009.
11. Gonzales R, Anglin DA, Beattie R, Ong CA, Glik DC. Perceptions of chronicity and recovery among youth in treatment for substance use problems. *J Adolesc Health* (in press).
12. Gonzales R, Anglin DA, Beattie R, Ong CA, Glik DC. Understanding recovery barriers: youth perspectives about relapse. *J Health Behav* (in press).
13. McLellan AT, Chalk M, Bartlett J. Outcomes, performance, and quality – what's the difference? *J Subst Abuse Treat* 2007;**32**(4):331–340.
14. SAMHSA. Treatment Episode Data Set (TEDS) Report –Predictors of substance abuse treatment completion and transfer to further treatment, by service type. Rockville, MD:U.S. Department of Health and Human Services Substance Abuse and Mental Health Services Administration Office of Applied Studies, 2009.

15. Botvin GJ, Dusenbury L, Baker E, James-Ortiz S, Kerner J. A skills training approach to smoking prevention among Hispanic youth. *J Behav Med* 1989;**12**:279–296.

16. Lawrence GE, Greta BL. Some determinants of attitudes toward substance use in an urban ethnic community. *Psychol Rep* 1984;**54**:539–545.

17. Penn NE, Kar SB, Kramer J, Skinner J, Zambrana R. Ethnic minorities, health care systems, and behavior. *Health Psychol* 1995;**14**:641–646.

18. De LaRosa M. Acculturation and Latino adolescents' substance use: A research agenda for the future. *Subst Use Misuse* 2002;**37**:429–456.

Translating Evidence-Based Therapies into Outpatient Practice

Ara Anspikian

Semel Institute for Neuroscience and Human Behavior at UCLA, Los Angeles, CA, USA

INTRODUCTION

There are numerous critical junctions in the process of substance abuse treatment, which can significantly alter both its course and prognosis. One can argue that every step from referral, to treatment, to follow-up, and everything in between can be viewed as essential components of determining outcome. Ultimately, there are multiple elements to consider when addressing how to keep adolescent patients engaged in treatment and how to improve outcomes. The following will be discussed in this chapter: family involvement/therapy, timely/appropriate referrals, treatment of comorbidities, appropriateness of the treatment setting, qualities of the clinician, interviewing/assessment techniques, and office-based policies/procedures. The chapter does not intend to review all the evidence-based practices but rather it attempts to bring to light the different issues to consider with regard to engaging and maintaining adolescents in treatment and improving outcomes.

The main intent of substance abuse treatment, or any kind of treatment for that matter, is usually to achieve positive outcomes. Staying in substance abuse treatment is linked to better long-term outcomes and leaving treatment early is linked to increased relapse rates [1,2]. There are also many other significant financial and clinical reasons for providers and programs to monitor how effective they are at engaging and maintaining patients in treatment. Although research demonstrates a relationship between treatment completion and positive outcomes there remain a large number of patients who do not finish their course of outpatient treatment [1]. Information from the Treatment Episode Data Set (TEDS) noted that in 2007, of the nearly 730 000 outpatient discharges for patients aged 12 years

and older, approximately 14% of them discontinued treatment prior to 30 days [1]. Furthermore, 44.5% continued in treatment for at least 90 days, leaving close to 400 000 who did not make the 90-day cut-off for a variety of reasons [1]. Exploring the reasons for why patients do not make it past the initial appointment, or to the third or fourth session, or to 30, 60, and 90 days of treatment is critical to making positive treatment/system changes. Some non-modifiable variables will remain but studying the modifiable factors will help individual clinicians, programs, and systems of care in better understanding the nature of substance abuse and the key elements of treatment that work.

There has traditionally been a dearth of information regarding evidence-based treatments for adolescent substance abuse. Although much has been learned over the last decade and a strong push has been made to rely on science and well-designed studies with well-delineated outcome measures, there continues to be an underwhelming amount of adolescent-specific evidence-based information and treatment. A slightly tangential point is that the term "evidence-based practice" is used loosely in many settings. There is also some debate among professionals about the definition but in general they can be referred to as "programs or practices that are proven to be successful through empirical research study and result in consistently positive results" [3].

The NIATx[1] organization has a very helpful list of "Promising Practices," which are geared toward improving a variety of outcomes. The promising practices that

---

[1] NIATx was formerly the acronym for the Network for the Improvement of Addiction Treatment. NIATx is now part of the University of Wisconsin-Madison's Center for Health Enhancement Systems Studies (CHESS).

are included in this chapter have been summarized under the appropriate sections. Please refer to the NIATx website for further details. Many of the promising practices have multiple examples and easily accessible handouts, checklists, and outlines of how other institutions have implemented these changes into their curriculums. NIATx provides useful tools, research, promising practices, and process improvement models. Their tools can be used to help make healthcare delivery more efficient and cost-effective, and improve retention/access to care [4]. The NIATx model consists of their Aims, Principles, Promising Practices, and Collaborative Model (it can be accessed on their website: www.niatx.net). It is also important to note that the examples cited in this chapter do not necessarily present information specifically for adolescents, as many of the examples are for adults; rather the examples are intended to illustrate the elements that were targeted for change/improvement.

OUTCOMES

Defining outcomes can be a daunting task in itself. For simplicity and so as not to lose track of the big picture, the main outcomes of concern in this text will be retention in treatment and reduction/elimination of substance use. Other notable outcomes to consider include decreased legal consequences, and improved social, occupational, educational, spiritual, and familial domains.

Retention in substance treatment has been notoriously low. It has been reported that approximately 50% of patients in outpatient treatment drop out within the first 4 weeks of treatment [2]. It is further complicated in adolescents because a greater percentage of them tend to be in treatment due to outside influences such as family and the legal system, and hence there is less personal investment in attaining and maintaining sobriety. Conversely, these data can be regarded as encouraging, when considering the ample room for quality improvement. The outpatient setting is an ideal environment in which to enact change and it can greatly benefit from flexibility in regard to quality improvement measures to improve outcomes.

WORKING WITH ADOLESCENTS

Working with an adolescent, whether for substance abuse problems or any other mental health issues, has its own unique set of pitfalls and benefits. By being developmentally aware and incorporating age-appropriate interview techniques, the clinician can considerably improve retention and active participation by the adolescent in his/her care. There are also qualities pertaining to the clinician that can facilitate or hinder this process. Some are inherent to an individual but most can and should be identified and worked on.

Development

Developmental factors are concurrently affected by substance use and influence treatment. Many of the expected developmental tasks of an adolescent, such as dating, marrying, establishing a career, independence, identity, and intimacy can be derailed by substance use [5]. Substance use can alter many aspects of one's interactions and the way one approaches life's challenges; it can therefore distort many aspects of psychological and social development [5]. Emotional and intellectual growth, rewarding personal relationships, and a sense of empowerment are also noted in the literature to be affected by substance use [5].

Substance abuse treatment needs to have firm limits and boundaries. However, giving patients, especially adolescents, some domains of autonomy and choice can go a long way to conveying care, respect, and understanding. Adolescents in particular have to put up with lower social status and social stigma, and are subject to their parents' decisions, conclusions, and expectations. Frequently they do not have the luxury of experiencing the autonomy they are striving to achieve, which is developmentally appropriate for them to seek. Respecting an adolescent's wishes for such things as scheduling appointments, and striving to give them a choice within the constructs of appropriate treatment, can keep an adolescent coming back for more sessions despite many reasons not to. Frequently, in substance abuse treatment, the adolescents have been either explicitly or implicitly "pushed" into treatment [5]. Allowing adolescents an increased and flexible level of choice and autonomy can convert a reluctant patient, waiting for any excuse to discontinue treatment, into the greatest advocate for continued treatment.

During adolescence, it is normal for teens to work toward separating from their parents during the process of developing their own identities. A notable struggle can ensue when parents try to keep too much control and/or when the teen attempts to develop his or her identity too quickly and/or in an extreme fashion. Similarly with substance abuse treatment the teen's feeling of being "controlled" tends to increase. More conflict during this time and increased control by the patient's parents, whether real or perceived, can increase the risk for continued use and discontinuation of treatment. Extra care must be taken to help facilitate and encourage the development of the teen's identity within the controlled environment of substance abuse treatment. It is equally important to educate the parent or guardian about these developmental factors to maximize treatment outcomes and optimize buy-in from the patient.

Adolescents also have a sense of "invincibility" and a notion of "it won't happen to me." These developmentally expected beliefs can not only increase risk-taking behavior, but also lead to the minimization of the potential consequences of risk-taking behavior. Substance use falls under the umbrella of risky behavior, a constellation of decisions/activities that can include sexual risk-taking, along with other types of physical and behavioral risk-taking [5]. It should be noted that some risky activities during adolescence are normal; therefore care should be taken not to label adolescents prematurely with substance abuse/dependence or other diagnostic labels [5]. Labeling the teenager and convincing them that they have a disease that needs treatment can have its own set of deleterious developmental consequences [5].

Peer groups during adolescence are paramount to the types of activities, interests, and behaviors teens participate in. Initially, during early teenage years, the group is mostly of the same sex, whereas toward older adolescence mixed sex groups and relationships begin to become more common and influential. Peer groups are only one target of attachment for the maturing adolescent [5]. They also begin identifying with many other elements such as sports, hobbies, political views, science, and religion. A balance is achieved for each child between their family's values and their own developing set of values/beliefs. Treatment providers should be aware of this phenomenon and also attempt to use it to the benefit of substance abuse treatment (i.e., finding prosocial, healthy groups for the teenager to be involved with).

Practical Development-Based Treatments

How does one practically take these aspects of development into consideration and incorporate them into treatment in the outpatient setting? The following are some simple examples of being developmentally aware in the treatment of adolescents with substance use disorders:

1. Flexibility in scheduling appointments (give them choice).
2. Encourage and expect participation by the young client in their own treatment plan.
3. Spend time asking the adolescent about his or her interests and strengths.
4. Encourage participation in non-drug-related activities of interest and inquire with parents regarding follow-through.

5. Facilitate conversations with the parents in the office, being mindful of developmental issues.
6. Help to facilitate connections with positive peer groups in the community (substance use groups, sports, clubs, volunteer organizations, etc.).

NIATx Promising Practices

Promising Practice: "Ask Clients to Participate in Treatment Planning" [4] According to the NIATx Promising Practice, patients without a personal investment in their own treatment are less likely to stay in treatment. For this reason, asking patients to participate in their own treatment plans, helping to tailor them to their individual needs, should improve engagement. The following is an example by NIATx where this philosophy has demonstrated to be effective. "Mid-Columbia Center in Dalles, Oregon, increased continuation rates from 59 percent to 84.5 percent by having all their clients attend a pre-treatment group after assessment to teach them the rules and expectations of the group and the stages of change. The clients discussed their motivations for being in treatment and created their treatment plans" [4]. Information gathered early in the assessment process can be used for the foundation of the patients' individual treatment plans. Additionally, should disruptive behaviors occur from patients, they could be used as learning opportunities. A relapse is sometimes a basis for early termination in some clinics or programs, but it can instead be treated as a personalized growth opportunity for the patient to practice getting back on track and for constructing a unique treatment plan.

Promising Practice: "Adjust Staff Schedules to Meet Client Demand" [4] Daytime appointments or appointments at certain times of the day may cause difficulty in attendance for some patients, such as students or working adolescents. The treatment provider should consider adjusting the clinic schedule to meet patient demands with the goal of maintaining treatment. A NIATx example included the following: "Bridge House in New Orleans, Louisiana, increased continuation by changing their staff hours from 12–8 p.m. to 2–10 p.m. so that residential patients who worked during the day could meet with their counselors during the evening. Their continuation rate increased from 59.5 percent to 68.2 percent in the first month and continued to increase in subsequent months" [4]. Adding appropriate time slots for appointments when client demand is at its greatest is vital when attempting to increase patient continuation rates.

Promising Practice: "Assign Peer Buddies" [4] A possible problem can ensue when clients start treatment without being connected to other people in the treatment community. The Promising Practice's solution is to assign peer buddies or mentors to help new clients connect with someone who knows what they're going through, and to help orient them to the agency as well as introduce them to others. An example where this has been implemented and found to be effective was at the Women's Recovery Association in Burlingame, California, where they "increased intensive outpatient continuation from 33 percent to 80 percent over the course of a year. They developed an orientation program for new patients, which included a handout written by an individual who had been through the program. New patients also were connected with a peer mentor who oriented them to the program" [4]. Assigning a peer buddy or mentor can also have positive effects for the mentor and help reduce workload for treatment providers by having the mentors explain rules and advise patients from their own experience. Peer buddies are a valuable asset when dealing with clients at risk for leaving treatment.

Interview

Many basic interviewing texts will emphasize rapport building as a key element of a successful assessment and as part of continued treatment. With adolescents in general and especially for those in substance abuse treatment, this aspect of the interview is even more valuable. Adolescents are typically not the ones initiating mental health/substance abuse treatment but rather are usually referred by multiple sources including school, family, pediatric physicians, etc. For addiction treatment, the majority of the referred cases are from the criminal justice system, along with a smaller but significant percentage from families and schools [6]. Adolescents may feel coerced into treatment not just by the law but also by their parents. This coincides with a time in their life where they are trying to challenge authority and develop independence as noted above. The added time spent in rapport building initially, in lieu of extensive data gathering, can help lay a solid foundation for trust, and continued treatment.

An initial interview with an adolescent can be a difficult time to develop rapport. It is important for the patient to feel that the clinician is somewhat of an advocate for them and not an agent of their parent(s) [7]. An adolescent can have reservations about opening up about their personal lives in part because they fear it could be communicated back to the parents; therefore it is a good idea to discuss confidentiality. Laws can vary from state to state regarding limits to confidentiality, and clinicians should be educated on the matter, and also inform parents and the adolescent about what they can expect when it comes to confidentiality [7].

After confidentiality has been discussed the primary focus of the interview should be on the patient's strengths and interests. Generally, an adolescent can convey what interests they have and feel comfortable talking about their strengths, thus "breaking the ice" [7]. By asking open-ended questions, the therapist gives the adolescent a chance to express him or herself, which can help the therapist gain better insight into the adolescent's views. Follow-up questions can be more specific and focused. It is important that the interview feels more like a conversation than an interrogation [7]. If the adolescent is resistant, and answering questions with "I don't know" it is often a sign that he or she is not yet engaged and the therapist may have to spend more time trying various techniques in order to move forward [7]. Dulcan [7] describes the interview as a cycle, consisting of the following: "1) Clinician engages the adolescent and seeks to understand his or her concerns, fears, and hopes. 2) Clinician conveys this understanding to the adolescent. 3) Adolescent begins to feel understood and to see clinician as an ally, leading to clinician's improved ability to collect accurate data. 4) Clinician uses data collection to increase understanding of patient's problems. 5) Clinician conveys this increased understanding to improve engagement with the adolescent."

Another delicate balancing act occurs between coming across as authoritative versus authoritarian. Drawing from the extensive parenting literature, an authoritative parenting style is characterized as high in support and behavioral regulation and an authoritarian style as high in behavioral regulation and low in support [8]. Support is defined as the "empathetic and responsive recognition of the child's perspective," and regulation as including both "supervising and monitoring children's behavior within reasonably set boundaries" and "creating an organized and predictable environment for children by being consistent in disciplining and communicating expectations" [8]. Since children of authoritative parents demonstrate less externalizing and internalizing disorders [8], it is important to model this style to the parents. From experience, parents of substance-abusing teens tend to be low in regulation, or low in support, or low in both. It is especially important for treatment not to come across as excessively high in regulation without taking an equally strong supportive stance.

The effort put into communicating one's expertise about substance abuse and treatment planning can easily cross over to become excessively directive and fit into the same mold as the adolescent's parents' reaction or an authoritarian style. However, being cognizant about appropriate boundaries is also important, so as not to risk coming across more as a friend than a treatment provider in an attempt to be supportive.

Incorporating techniques from Motivational interviewing (MI) can be very useful when working with adolescents, and not only help treatment outcomes but also improve engagement in treatment as some of its core concepts align developmentally with adolescents. Motivational interviewing was first described by Rollnick and Miller and has been developing a strong evidence base in the adult literature [9]. The limited adolescent literature has also been showing some promising results in regard to substance use and behavior change. A recent meta-analysis specifically reviewing motivational interviewing for adolescents with substance use demonstrated a small but significant effect size for motivational interviewing interventions, also suggesting that they may retain their effect over time [10]. The interventions reviewed appeared to be effective across many settings, for a variety of substance use behaviors, for sessions of different lengths, and by providers with different levels of training [10]. Motivational interviewing techniques tend to emphasize a collaborative process, a client-centered approach, and aim to increase motivation to change and resolve the ambivalence [10].

NIATx Promising Practices

Promising Practice: "Use the Spirit of Motivational Interviewing during the First Contact" [4] The promising practice talks about how patients are caught somewhere between not wanting to change and wanting to change, and if engagement does not happen with the therapist, the patient will start to miss appointments. As a solution to this problem, NIATx suggests using motivational interviewing during the first contact as a way to reduce ensuing no-show rates. Open-ended questions and empathetic conversations can help to engage patients in continued care. According to NIATx, clinics in Ohio, California, and Massachusetts incorporated motivational interviewing techniques into their intake process and reduced no-show rates from 58 percent to 14 percent, 36 percent to 10 percent, and an overall reduction of 41 percent respectively.

Promising Practice: "Use Motivational Interviewing During Treatment" [4] The promising practice explains that because patients are stuck between wanting to change and not wanting to change, they need help focusing on their intent to change and maintaining their desire for continued treatment. In addition to using open-ended questions and empathy, it is also important to expect and respect the patient's resistance. Creating discrepancy can help illustrate the dichotomy of the patient's concurrent wanting and not wanting to change. Finally, concluding the session by summarizing the patient's expressed needs and concerns will communicate that the patient has been heard. The promising practice notes the following examples:

1. The Center for Drug Free Living in Orlando, Florida, increased continuation rates to the fourth session of treatment by 27%.
2. The Addiction Research and Treatment Services in Denver, Colorado, increased continuation rates through the first 30 days of treatment for their outpatient opioid maintenance patients by almost 10%.

The treatment provider may want to practice one or two new motivational interviewing techniques on a regular basis to help to seamlessly incorporate these recommendations into day-to-day practice.

Qualities of the Clinician

Adolescents have an uncanny skill at "seeing right through" someone. Therefore, one of the qualities a clinician should practice is "being real," although this is easier said than done and vague as a concept. It takes a certain level of comfort with yourself plus a degree of interpersonal relatedness to be able to convey this sense to the adolescent. It is important to maintain professional boundaries and concurrently be able to treat the patient with empathy and sincerity. Medical terminology is a great conduit for communicating to other professionals and at times an opening for psychoeducation about something the adolescent is going through. Many of the general guidelines and rules about conducting therapy or an interview are also great foundations to build on as a clinician. Unfortunately, a novice provider may fall into the trap of coming across as "fake" by overusing medical jargon and adhering strictly to textbook rules about therapy or interviewing. The other extreme where providers are found crossing boundaries and eroding the therapeutic relationship between patient and clinician is even more perilous. A point of emphasis is that ethical rules and professional boundaries in no way preclude the level of authenticity that a clinician should provide in a therapeutic setting with an adolescent. But these rules and boundaries should never be sacrificed in striving to be "more real." An alternate point is that experienced providers do not escape the risk of being "fake" just because of their experience. It may, in some cases, hinder the true expression of authenticity. The way to conceptualize this point is to firmly remind yourself that the basic tenet of being authentic in your communication is even more paramount with an adolescent because more times than not they are expecting you not to be.

Honesty is another key concept. Being truthful and not sugar coating things can be helpful in engaging and maintaining adolescents in treatment. At times families will pressure clinicians into keeping certain pieces of information from adolescents. Although reticence is sometimes necessary, in general it is good practice to maintain open lines of communication between all involved parties.

Consistency is something that is included as a central concept in many parenting programs. It is no different in a treatment provider-patient relationship. Consistency can apply to a variety of situations including: appointments, phone calls, standards, expectations, etc.

It is important to be aware of one's tone of voice and body language, making sure one does not come across as if talking down to the adolescent. Work on respecting the adolescent's viewpoints without necessarily agreeing with them, and maintain unconditional positive regard for the patient. Refrain from communicating judgment in all forms of communication and being. It is paramount to conduct critical self-appraisal of one's own prejudices and biases and work on displaying acceptance and respect toward the patient.

WORKING WITH FAMILIES

Family-based interventions, including family-involved therapy, family therapy, and family psychoeducation, are gaining a stronger evidence base for many disorders [7,11–13]. Specifically, results have been encouraging for adolescents with substance abuse and conduct disorder [7,12]. Family therapy techniques for adolescents with substance abuse have been outlined in multisystemic therapy (MST) and multidimensional family therapy [12]. It is outside the scope of this chapter to review these and some of the other family-based approaches in detail, but we will touch on some elements and review the related NIATx promising practices. It may not be feasible for the individual provider reading this chapter to conduct family therapy, especially without appropriate training and resources. However, it can be very important to be informed about family therapy and to make use of family therapy-based techniques and knowledge when treating adolescents with substance use disorders [11].

Family therapy can be defined as "a collection of therapeutic approaches that share a belief in family-level assessment and intervention," where the term family is defined as "a system" [11]. Since all parts within a system are usually interrelated, "a change in any part of the system will bring about changes in all other parts" [11]. Family therapy addresses disturbances within the general confines of a family or any interpersonal system. Whereas family therapy targets the family as the therapeutic focus and attempts to make interventions within this system, family-involved therapy generally relies on interventions that aim to educate families about substance abuse, and about the relationship patterns that can contribute (initiation and continuation) to substance abuse. Family psychoeducation (FPE), when described as a formalized process, labels "the illness" as the primary target of the treatment instead of the family [13]. The evidence-based practice KIT (Knowledge Informing Transformation) by SAMSHA (Substance Abuse and Mental Health Services Administration) about family psychoeducation further emphasizes the collaborative nature between treatment providers, families, and patients, with the overarching goal of supporting recovery and providing honest and practical information about the illness in question [13]. Despite many differing formats of education delivery the key elements of the intervention are noted as: education about the illness, providing information resources, skills training, ongoing advice about managing the illness, support (emotion/social), and problem-solving [13].

Family interventions for adolescent substance abuse aim to:

1. provide psychoeducation;
2. assist parents to initiate and sustain their efforts at getting their child into appropriate treatment;
3. assist parents in limit setting, developing structure within the home, and appropriate monitoring of behavior;
4. improving communication;
5. referring family members to treatment; and
6. referring family members to support organizations [7].

Family therapy for substance abuse aims to maximize the family's strengths and utilizes them to find ways to reduce and eliminate substance abuse in the adolescent and in his/her family [11]. It also strives to minimize the impact of the adolescent's substance abuse on the patient and on his or her family [11]. As positive change and improved communication take place within the family system it can not only help to reduce substance abuse in the adolescent in question but also help to prevent future substance-related use and offenses in siblings [11].

Family therapy has the potential to improve engagement and retention in treatment and reduce the adolescent's substance use [11]. The family-based thera-pies that have some positive evidence are multi-dimensional family therapy, multisystemic family therapy, and brief strategic family therapy [12]. Brief strategic family therapy is based on principles that the family is an interdependent system, that patterns of interaction of the family members affect the behavior of the other members, and that interventions need to specifically target these patterns of behavior with prac-tical ways of changing these interactions [14]. Multi-systemic therapy (MST) views substance abuse within the broader context of the social system/outside world and considers it to be multidetermined and multi-variable. Its goals are to empower parents with skills and resources, engage family members, empower teens to cope with family/peer/neighborhood problems, address risk and protective factors, and examine the strengths and needs of the involved systems as they pertain to the problem at hand [11,12]. Some of the interventions include support and skill building, and are intended to encourage responsible actions; they are present-focused, action-oriented, and require consistent effort by the family and responsibility of the therapist to assist in overcoming barriers [11,12]. Multidimensional family therapy (MDFT) views adolescent substance abuse as multidimensional and multidetermined [11]. It is also regarded as a complex problem, which requires addressing multiple personal, familial, interpersonal, and social factors to enact lasting change [15]. It seeks to increase or restore adaptive, developmentally appro-priate functioning, and improve the functioning of the teen and parent in multiple domains [11]. The overall treatment is referred to as being "flexible," with indi-vidual sessions involving the adolescent, the family, and/or the family as a whole [15].

There are manuals and training courses for many of the different forms of family therapy/interventions. What is most important to take away from this section is that substance abuse in the adolescent is a family disease, such that it is both a disease that affects every-one in the family, and the initiation and maintenance of use is a by-product, to some degree, of the maladaptive functioning of the family system. It is imperative to involve the adolescent's family in all treatment modal-ities including education about the disease, methods to improve communication, and encouraging active par-ticipation in family therapy. Without the aforemen-tioned, treatment outcomes and engagement may be limited.

NIATx Promising Practices

Promising Practice: "Include Family and Friends" **[4]** This promising practice suggests including family and friends in the treatment process from the beginning to help strengthen the patient's commitment to treatment and the family's understanding and involvement in the patient's recovery. Inclusion into treatment can start from admission and continue through discharge. NIATx notes that the STEPS program at the Liberty Center in Wooster, Ohio, found higher completion rates of 77.3% at six sessions for patients with family involvement and support. Conversely, patients without family support had a completion rate of 45.5%. Generally, families usually want to help but don't know what to do. Treat-ment providers should make an effort to educate families about what to expect and about what they can do to support recovery. Simple interventions to suggest when working with families also include offering support groups for family members and friends, keeping them informed about the client's progress, offering a direct line for family members to call, and offering family visitation times. Treatment providers may also consider providing families with a factsheet about the treatment process and facts about addiction, or a curriculum for families to be involved in while the patient is in treat-ment. Additional information on how to engage the family can be found in Gosnold's "Becoming Family Informed, Family Involved" (http://www.niatx.net/ toolkits/provider/GosnoldFamilyInformedEngagement .pdf).

RESOURCES AND REFERRALS

A well-developed network of referral sources (both to and from) and resources for your practice and for your patients is invaluable. Such a network can not only make life easier for you but can become one of the critical elements that elevate the standard of care for your patients and improve their engagement in treatment. If regular contact is kept with these sources they can be educated about the scope of the services you provide and will in time make referrals more suited to your skills. Staying in touch with sources that referred patients to you can assist in keeping patients in continued care by facilitating the exertion of the referrer's influence on the patient. In today's age of increasing medical knowledge and specialization of treatment, it is not fair to assume that one person or one setting can necessarily provide the best care for a patient. Having ready access to referral options, which complement the services you provide, can improve care for the patient and their family. Finally, educational resource material can supplement the care provided in the outpatient setting, and organi-zational resources can get families and patients into contact with outside sources that can provide for addi-tional support and services.

The following are just a few of the many available organizations, which have a wealth of information, educational materials, and programs (use discretion to determine the appropriateness of the resources found below):

- Addiction Technology Transfer Centers (ATTC)
- Al-Anon and Alateen
- American Academy of Addiction Psychiatry (AAAP)
- American Society of Addiction Medicine (ASAM)
- National Center for Substance Abuse and Child Welfare (NCSACW)
- National Institute on Alcohol Abuse and Alcoholism (NIAAA)
- National Institute on Drug Abuse (NIDA)
- Substance Abuse and Mental Health Services Administration (SAMHSA)

NIATx Promising Practices

Promising Practice: "Collaborate with Referrers to Motivate Clients" [4] This promising practice attempts to demonstrate the importance of collaborative relationships. Collaborating with referrers who can follow up with patients who miss their appointments can assist the treatment provider's efforts. Sometimes due to a referrer's influence or with the implementation of natural consequences, the referrer encourages patients to attend appointments. According to NIATx, a counseling center in Delaware sent letters to the patient's family service workers and probation officers asking for their collaboration (without penalizing the patients) in re-engaging the patients in treatment. Overall, re-engagement rates went from 45% to 89% over a 3-month period. This example shows that it may prove to be useful to set the standard of acknowledging referrals, notifying referrers when appointments are missed, and keeping referrers in the loop regarding a patient's treatment progress. Patients may be more motivated for treatment with just the knowledge that feedback will be given to the referral source. Two-way communication with referrers can also engage referrers with assisting in problem-solving the barriers to treatment.

KNOWING WHEN TO CHANGE TREATMENT SETTINGS

Treatment engagement and maintenance can sometimes suffer because the patient is not in the appropriate level of care for his or her situation. Knowing when and how to recommend changing the setting of care and developing ways to assess if your particular care setting is the right setting for the patient can be key elements to

improving outcomes. The Center for Substance Abuse Treatment, Treatment Improvement Protocol (TIP) Series 32 [5] provides a very good description of the different levels of care and simple characteristics about the type of patient who is appropriate for each level of care.

NIATx Promising Practices

Promising Practice: "Transition Clients to the Next Level of Care as Soon as they are Ready" [4] NIATx proposes another problem that may interfere with continuing care; too many clients are not moving to the next level of treatment when they are ready, occupying slots that could be used by others. Furthermore, clients may be in an inappropriate level of care thus resulting in their dropping out of treatment altogether. When appropriate, clients should be moved to the next level of care as soon as they are ready. Examples provided by NIATx demonstrate this necessity:

1. "STEP 2 in Reno, Nevada, reduced the waiting time for treatment from 15 days to 10 days by reviewing treatment plans to ensure that clients were at the appropriate level of care. Eligible clients were then transitioned to the next level of care to increase the number of openings for new clients" [4].
2. "The Patrician Movement in San Antonio, Texas, instituted a more aggressive case management system to better track scheduled and completed discharges to ensure that clients remained in treatment the appropriate length of time and that clients ready for discharge were discharged on a timely basis. This change made it possible for clients on the waiting list to access treatment more quickly" [4].

With regard to these examples, it may be appropriate to offer brief treatment with specific endpoints instead of an open-ended course. Finally, going back to the role of coordinating efforts with the referrer, it would be beneficial to include them during client transitions from one level of care to the next.

TREATING AND SCREENING FOR COMORBID CONDITIONS

It is outside the scope of this chapter to review all the methods for screening and treating comorbid psychiatric conditions. It is, however, important to note that dual diagnosis tends to be the rule rather than the exception. Studies demonstrate high, although variable, comorbidity rates, with some reports noting a greater than 50% prevalence of mostly mood, conduct/oppositional, and attention-deficit/hyperactivity disorders [5]. At minimum it would be beneficial to incorporate screening rating scales, targeted diagnostic interviews, and appropriate referrals.

PROCEDURAL AND POLICY-BASED OFFICE INTERVENTIONS

Patients' experience of the "treatment" they are receiving is partly determined by their interaction with the treatment provider, but many providers mistakenly assign a greater value to this aspect and neglect the rest of the patient experience. It is important to note that every element of the process of care is part of the treatment received. The initial phone call, the office and treatment setting, friendliness of front-desk or ancillary staff, cleanliness, follow-up/missed appointments procedures, scheduling of appointments, wait times for intakes or follow-up appointments, and punctuality are just some of these aspects. Although much effort is put into our interviewing and assessment skills, treatment planning, and education, an equal amount needs to be devoted to these procedural and policy practices, which are so often overlooked.

NIATx Promising Practices

Promising Practice: "Use Motivational Incentives" [4]   This particular promising practice suggests using motivational incentives to improve attendance at assessment, intake, and treatment sessions. In order to increase motivation and encourage patients to stick with treatment long enough to achieve and maintain sobriety, one can make use of positive reinforcement and rewards that reinforce the desired positive behavior by the patient. Incentives can be used during treatment and transitions from one level of treatment to another. For example, in the Mid-Columbia Center for Living, Oregon, 10-dollar gift certificates were used after every fourth session of treatment, and group pizza parties after four consecutive 100% attended groups. Concurrently, continuation in treatment increased from 46 % to 73%. Motivational incentives can include individualized incentives that are related to the desired behavior needing reinforcement. The incentives can logically be connected to the desired behavior at stake. For example, the treatment provider may consider a point system, to raise money toward a watch for someone needing to be on time for appointments, or low-cost incentives like certificates for certain accomplishments (e.g., time in treatment, courage, etc.).

Promising Practice: "Remind Clients about Appointments" [4]   Patients may miss appointments solely because they forgot about the session. The promising practice suggests that it would be beneficial to remind patients about upcoming appointments 1–2 days prior to their appointment to help reduce no-shows. In Massachusetts, night staff made phone calls to remind patients about their appointments. This intervention helped reduced no-show rates in intakes by 27% and improved continuation from intake to first appointment by 23%. A simple solution such as reminder calls to patients could greatly increase treatment continuation. The treatment provider may also want to consider if the patient would like to receive a text message in lieu of a reminder call, especially for adolescents.

Promising Practice: "Orient Clients" [4]   Another promising practice advises to orient patients about what is expected from them and of the treatment facility regarding the initial assessment and treatment phases. Orienting patients will assist in alleviating their anxiety and uncertainty about transitioning to another level of care or facility. NIATx reports that in Oregon continuation rates increased from 59% to 84.5% when patients attended a pre-treatment group to teach them the rules and expectations of the group and about the stages of change. Suggested tips regarding orientation include creating a standardized script for staff to use when orienting patients, using videos, providing handouts/-checklists for patients to refer to, developing relationships with providers for the next level of care, and consider having them meet patients to orient them prior to transition.

Promising Practice: "Help Eliminate Barriers to Treatment" [4]   Motivational interviewing concepts can help eliminate barriers to treatment that frequently lead to patients dropping out of treatment despite a desire to continue. The goal is to help patients identify and solve logistical problems (i.e., transportation limitations, childcare, financial limitations, occupational issues, etc.). The Sinissippi Centers in Dixon, Illinois, used a motivational interviewing-inspired conversational approach to reduce no-show rates for the patient's first appointment from 58% to 14%. They found that simply bringing up the topic of barriers to treatment and facilitating the patients' thinking through the logistics helped reduce no-show rates. One of the questions they asked the patient was: "Do you see anything that may prevent you from making your appointment?" They followed the question with reflective listening skills and assisted in problem-solving. The treatment provider should plan to have conversations with patients about potential barriers to treatment on a regular basis and may want to consider providing financial assistance for travel issues (cab voucher, bus pass/tickets, etc.).

Promising Practice: "Follow-up with No-shows" [4]
Another policy-based promising practice suggests follow-up with no-shows to inquire about why they missed the appointment and reschedule the appointment to help reduce overall no-show rates. A program in South Carolina used a staff member with a "good telephone voice" to call patients who did not show up to their appointments. She would ask if anything was "wrong" for them to miss their appointment, if the program could "help," and identified herself as a contact person for future questions/problems. They found that their no-show rates decreased from more than 60% to approximately 40%. Combining phone calls with motivational interviewing skills to engage patients can decrease overall no-show rates.

Promising Practice: "Establish Attendance Policy" [4] Treatment providers should not assume that something as simple as expecting regular attendance is a given. Patients should be given clear communication about the attendance policy and what is expected of them. The promising practice example shows that "Connections Counseling in Madison, Wisconsin, increased attendance in its evening opioid treatment group sessions from 62% to 81% by establishing a clear attendance policy . . . If they had 2 unexcused absences in a row, they had to fill out a Group Absentee Form and were required to meet with their counselor to problem solve about attendance barriers such as transportation and childcare" [4]. Patients will benefit from clear expectations, structure, and consistency.

Promising Practice: "Identify Clients at Risk for Leaving and Intervene" [4] Patients will frequently give signs and make statements that indicate that they are leaning toward quitting treatment. Providers typically do not have policies and procedures to respond to this risk of discontinuation. Providers should practice receiving regular feedback from patients to identify those at risk for discontinuation, find out the problem, and provide appropriate and quick interventions. The following NIATx example illustrates how this promising practice has shown itself to be beneficial: "Bridge House in New Orleans, Louisiana, increased continuation rates from 48 percent to 63 percent by implementing weekly check-ins, asking clients to rate on a scale of 1–10: How willing are you to continue treatment here? How important is it for you to stay in treatment? How motivated are you to stay? How strong has your urge to use been this past week? A high rating on 'How strong has your urge to use been this past week?' was the best predictor that a client would quit treatment" [4]. They intervened by using motivational interviewing

techniques. Treatment providers should expect that their patients will think about quitting treatment and therefore should look for ways to intervene. Take time to analyze your data to determine why patients are leaving treatment and make appropriate changes.

Promising Practice: "Get Client to Commit to Attend the First Four Treatment Sessions" [4] The final promising practice included for procedural and policy-based interventions is to have a commitment from clients to attend the first four sessions and instill that this is expected from them. Two examples illustrated by NIATx follow:

1. "The Jackie Nitschke Center in Green Bay, Wisconsin, increased attendance in their Aftercare program over the first five sessions from 38 percent to 83 percent by creating a policy that requires clients to attend the first five treatment sessions without any absences" [4]. Their own data demonstrated that their clients who attended the first five sessions were more likely to complete the full treatment.
2. "Community Concepts in South Paris, Maine, developed a script recommending that clients try attending four sessions before deciding whether to stay" [4]. During the wrap-up period of the session the treatment provider reminded the client about the provider's request for the client to attend three or four sessions before making his/her decision about continuing or discontinuing treatment. Providers should be confident in expressing their expectations of the patient to commit to the first four sessions of treatment and ask them to reconfirm to come back at the end of each session.

CONCLUSION

The office-based clinician has an enormous task in engaging and maintaining adolescents in substance abuse treatment. Working with adolescents in such a way as to maximize outcomes, demands a thorough understanding of developmental concepts, interviewing skills, and certain qualities of the clinician. Working with families is just as important as the individual work being done with the adolescent when considering the system-based nature of substance abuse and the intricacies of its relationship with the family. Thorough and effective management of the adolescent includes being ready to assess and treat comorbidities, making accurate assessments of the appropriate treatment setting, and having a well-developed and interactive web of referral sources. It is also imperative to critically evaluate and improve office-based procedures and policies with the intent to maximize treatment outcomes. An overall spirit of dedication to quality improvement and seeking evidence-based practices will keep the office-based provider at the forefront of substance abuse treatment for the adolescent.

References

1. Substance Abuse and Mental Health Services Administration (SAMHSA), Center for Behavioral Health Statistics and Quality. *The TEDS Report: Characteristics of Clients Who Left Outpatient Treatment During the First 30 Days*. Rockville, MD: SAMHSA, 2011.

2. Center for Substance Abuse Treatment. *Substance Abuse: Administrative Issues in Outpatient Treatment*. Treatment Improvement Protocol (TIP) Series 46. DHHS Publication No. (SMA) 06-4151. Rockville, MD: Substance Abuse and Mental Health Services Administration, 2006.

3. Gonzalez R. Adolescent Substance Abuse. PowerPoint presentation. UCLA Integrated Substance Abuse Programs, 2009. Available from: NIDA; Institute of Medicine.

4. NIATx website (http://www.niatx.net/promisingpractices/).

5. Center for Substance Abuse Treatment. *Treatment with Substance Use Disorders*. Treatment Improvement Protocol (TIP) Series 32. DHHS Publication No. (SMA) 99-3283. Rockville, MD: Substance Abuse and Mental Health Services Administration, 1999.

6. Dennis ML, Dawud-Noursi S, Muck RD, *et al.* The need for developing and evaluating adolescent treatment models. In: Stevens SJ, Morral AR (eds), *Adolescent Substance Abuse Treatment in the United States: Exemplary Models From a National Evaluation Study*. Binghampton, NY: Haworth Press, 2003; pp. 3–34.

7. Dulcan MK. *Dulcan's Textbook of Child and Adolescent Psychiatry*. Arlington, VA: American Psychiatric Publishing, Inc., 2010.

8. Koen Luyckx EA, Soenens B, Andrews JA, *et al.* Parenting and trajectories of children's maladaptive behaviors: a 12-year prospective community study. *J Clin Child Adolesc Psychol* 2011;**40**:468–478.

9. Miller S, Rollnick S. *Motivational Interviewing: Preparing People For Change*, 2nd edn. Guilford Press, 2002.

10. Jensen CD, Cushing CC, Aylward BS, *et al.* Effectiveness of motivational interviewing interventions for adolescent substance use behavior change: a meta-analytic review. *J Consult Clin Psychol* 2011;**79**:433–440.

11. Center for Substance Abuse Treatment. *Substance Abuse Treatment and Family Therapy*. Treatment Improvement Protocol (TIP) Series, No. 39. DHHS Publication No. (SMA) 04-3957. Rockville, MD: Substance Abuse and Mental Health Services Administration, 2004.

12. Martin A, Volkmar FR. *Lewis's Child and Adolescent Psychiatry, A Comprehensive Textbook*, 4th edn. Philadelphia, PA: Lippincott Williams & Wilkins, 2007.

13. Substance Abuse and Mental Health Services Administration. *Family Psychoeducation: Building Your Program*. HHS Pub. No. SMA-09-4422. Rockville, MD: Center for Mental Health Services, Substance Abuse and Mental Health Services Administration, U.S. Department of Health and Human Services, 2009.

14. National Institute on Drug Abuse. *Brief Strategic Family Therapy for Adolescent Drug Abuse*. NIH Publication Number 03-4751. National Institute on Drug Abuse, 2003.

15. Sherman C. Multidimensional family therapy for adolescent drug abuse offers broad, lasting benefits. national institute on drug abuse. National Institute on Drug Abuse, 2010. Available from: http://www.nida.nih.gov/NIDA_notes/NNvol23N3/Multidimensional.html.

Albert Ellis' Rational Emotive Behavior Therapy[1]

Richard Rosner

*Forensic Psychiatry Residency Program, New York University School of Medicine;
Forensic Psychiatry Clinic, Bellevue Hospital Center, New York, NY, USA*

If you are distressed by anything external, the pain is not due to the thing itself but to your own estimate of it; and this you have the power to revoke at any moment.

Marcus Aurelius

The essential premise of rational emotive behavior therapy (REBT) is that people cause themselves distress and dysfunction by their habitual irrational beliefs, and that these maladaptive thinking patterns can be changed, with resultant improvement in emotional states and functioning. Therapy involves training patients in rational self-analysis to help them become aware of their thought patterns, followed by teaching them how to see their reactions in more constructive (i.e., rational) terms. They then have daily relearning exercises during which they practice their new thinking patterns – termed rational emotive imagery – several times a day.

ALBERT ELLIS, THE FOUNDER OF REBT

Albert Ellis was born in 1913 and died in 2007. His career was remarkable not only because of his prolific publications and contributions to psychology, but because of his productivity throughout his life – he continued writing and publishing in his nineties. He attended the City College of New York, from which he received a bachelor's degree in 1934. After attempting

careers in business and writing, he decided at age 29 to study psychology. He did his graduate studies at Columbia University, receiving his master's degree in 1943 and his doctoral degree in 1947. He obtained training in psychoanalysis and underwent a personal analysis for three years. Ellis practiced marriage, family, and sex counseling, as well as psychoanalysis and psychoanalytically oriented psychotherapy. He worked as chief psychologist for the New Jersey Department of Institutions and Agencies, and taught as an instructor at Rutgers University and at New York University. His certification in clinical psychology was awarded by the American Board of Examiners in Clinical Psychology. He was Executive Director of the Institute for Rational Living, Inc., and was President Emeritus of the Albert Ellis Institute for Rational Emotive Behavior Therapy in New York City at the time of his death [1].

THE ORIGINS AND CORE CONCEPTS OF RATIONAL EMOTIVE BEHAVIOR THERAPY

Ellis had an early interest in philosophy, beginning in his adolescent years, especially stoic philosophy, and describes what a revelation it was to him to realize that people partly constructed their own feelings of anxiety, depression, and rage [2].

Ellis described his development of REBT as follows:

> I began formulating this pioneering form of therapy and counseling in 1953, when I abandoned my practice and teaching of psychoanalysis because I found it to be seriously misinformed about how and why people disturb themselves and

[1]Rational Emotive Therapy. Previously published as "Albert Ellis' Rational-Emotive Behavior Therapy" in Adolescent Psychiatry, Volume 1, pages 82–87, Bentham, 2011, and reproduced here with their kind permission.

what to do about changing with therapy. I realized, as few therapists did at that time, that people are importantly affected by their early and present environment. They are constructivists who not only *get* emotionally upset by their family members and other significant people but *also* have powerful tendencies, both innate and acquired, to construct the sabotaging of their mental and physical health. Fortunately, however, when people destructively deal with themselves and create neurotic behaviors, they also have the power to reconstruct their lives and to significantly improve. It is nice if they dig up the childhood and adolescent influences of the past, but even without doing so, they have amazing propensities for reconstructing the present and the future – that is, if they acknowledge their own disturbability and work at correcting it.

Ellis, 2004, pp. 9–10 [3]

The theory of REBT is based on the following series of psychological premises ([4], pp. 109–110):

1. Human beings are both rational and irrational. When humans act rationally they are more effective and happier than when they act irrationally.
2. Human psychological/emotional disturbance is due to human irrationality. Thoughts and emotions are inextricably linked; thoughts entail emotions, so that irrational thinking is accompanied by irrational (i.e., maladaptive, inappropriate, unrealistic) emotions.
3. Irrational thinking has its origins in early life, particularly in our early experiences with our parents and with our society's culture.
4. Human thinking is symbolic, usually verbal, in nature. Our thoughts are our self-talk, the things we say to ourselves. Because thinking and emotion are linked, what we tell ourselves in our internal self-talk elicits emotions. When we engage in irrational thinking, what we are telling ourselves will elicit irrational (i.e., maladaptive, inappropriate, unrealistic) emotions. When we engage in rational thinking, our self-talk will elicit rational (i.e., adaptive, appropriate, realistic) emotions. Human psychological/emotional disturbance is the result of human irrational thinking. Persistent psychological/emotional disturbance, i.e., neurosis or other mental disorders, results from persistent irrational thinking. To overcome emotional disorders, it is not enough to understand the origins of our irrational thoughts; the irrational thoughts must be extinguished and replaced by rational thoughts.
5. Human psychological/emotional disturbance is not due to external events and circumstances, it is due to the irrational thinking that accompanies those events and circumstances. Our irrational thinking distorts our perception and interpretation of external events. It is what we tell ourselves about external events (not the events themselves) that causes our psychological/ emotional disturbance. Our irrational thoughts elicit our irrational emotions.
6. We can attack, challenge, and refute our irrational thinking (perceptions and interpretations) of external events. By replacing our irrational thoughts about external events with rational thoughts, we can replace our irrational (i.e., maladaptive, inappropriate, unrealistic) feelings with new rational (i.e., adaptive, appropriate, realistic) feelings. Through REBT, a therapist can teach a client to realize that the client's irrational thinking (perceptions and interpretations) of external events causes the client's psychological/emotional disturbance. Through REBT, a client can learn how to attack, challenge, refute his or her irrational thinking (perceptions and interpretations) of external events and replace it with new rational thinking. Through the ongoing practice and application of REBT, clients can reduce their irrationality and improve their effectiveness and happiness.

THE ABCDE TECHNIQUE OF RATIONAL EMOTIVE BEHAVIOR THERAPY

The actual process of REBT is described as a series of five steps: A, B, C, D, and E. The therapist teaches the client that the cause of the client's emotional/psychological disturbance is not due to external events. Rather, the client is taught that (A) **A**ctual external events automatically/habitually elicit (B) **B**eliefs and irrational thoughts (perceptions and interpretations of the external events) that entail (C) **C**onsequent emotions that may be irrational (maladaptive, inappropriate, unrealistic), and that must be (D) **D**isputed, attacked, challenged so that (E) **E**ffective rational thoughts (perceptions and interpretations of the external events) may take their place.

Applying this ABCDE process to the treatment of substance abusers, F. Michler Bishop, Director of Alcohol and Substance Abuse Services at the Albert Ellis Institute of Rational Emotive Behavior Therapy, suggests a five-step approach to clients ([5], pp. 42–45):

1. Start at C: Ask the client what problem behavior or psychological/emotional upset they want to address in the REBT session.
2. Explore the A: Ask the client what actual event apparently activated the problem behavior or psychological/emotional upset.
3. Uncover the B: Ask the client what they were thinking, what they were telling themself, about the actual event, and identify the irrational elements

in the client's perception and interpretation of the actual external event.

4. Encourage D: Help the client to dispute their irrational thoughts.
5. Assist E: Help the client find more effective, rational thoughts about the actual event, so that the client can diminish their behavioral or emotional problems.

Once the client/patient has been taught the ABCDE theory and technique, the therapist can ask that the client/patient practice the technique between scheduled visits to the therapist; that is, keeping a daily log of instances of emotional upset and applying the ABCDE technique to each instance can be a homework assignment ([6], pp. 404–405). Specifically, the client is directed to:

1. keep a daily log of problematic emotional states;
2. for each occasion of a problematic emotional state, record the apparently activating external event;
3. figure out the irrational beliefs/self-talk/thoughts that constituted the (mis)perception and (mis)interpretation of the actual activating external event;
4. dispute the irrational beliefs/self-talk/thoughts;
5. figure out more effective rational beliefs/self-talk/thoughts to replace the disputed irrational thoughts.

RECOGNIZING IRRATIONALITY

Central to REBT is the recognition of irrational (maladaptive, inappropriate, unrealistic) perceptions and interpretations of external events. Ellis has identified many common examples of irrational thinking: ([4], pp. 110–112):

1. I must be loved and approved of by virtually everyone.
2. I must be totally competent and totally successful.
3. Bad people exist and must be blamed and punished for their wickedness.
4. I must have things the way that I want them to be.
5. Unhappiness is due to external events; I have no control over my unhappiness.
6. I must continually be vigilant to guard against the awful dangers in the world.
7. I must avoid difficulties, rather than face them; I must avoid self-responsibility, rather than accepting self-responsibility.
8. I should be able to depend on someone else; someone else should be responsible for protecting and taking care of me; someone stronger should protect me from life's difficulties.
9. Past experiences and external events are the cause of my present behavior; the influence of the past cannot be overcome.
10. Other people's problems and psychological/emotional disturbances should make me upset.

11. I must find the one perfect answer to every single problem that I encounter; every problem has one perfect answer.

According to Ellis, these examples of irrational thinking are widespread in our society. The principle technique of REBT is to bring instances of these irrational beliefs to the attention of a client, so that they can be recognized, refuted, and replaced by rational beliefs.

Bishop has condensed Ellis' 11 types of common irrational thoughts into four main varieties of irrational thinking ([5], pp. 96–97). These include:

1. "Catastrophizing" and "awfulizing" thinking that evaluates actual external events in an exaggerated and negative way.
2. The reaction to the actual external event includes the thought "I can't stand it."
3. The reaction to the actual external event includes "demandingness," i.e., that the client "should" or "must" other than he or she really is, or that the event "should" or "must" not have happened.
4. "Global self-downing," i.e. the client is totally unaccepting of himself or herself.

DISPUTING IRRATIONALITY

In discussing how to (D) dispute, challenge, and attack "awfulizing" beliefs and "should" beliefs, Howard Young, a counselor at the Albert Ellis Institute for Rational Emotive Behavior Therapy, wrote ([7], pp. 21–22):

If you examine any situation closely, you will discover that *nothing is awful*. You might discover that a particular situation is unfortunate or even highly unpleasant and that there may be some realistic disadvantages involved. But it unlikely that anything is truly terrible or horrible.

You question **shoulds** by asking *why should it be – who said so?* The answer to a **should** is, *It doesn't have to be*. Nothing has to be the way you want, and although it might be better if things were the way you want – that doesn't mean they **must, ought** or **should** be that way. ...It is important to recognize that **reality is reality, not what you want it to be**. You are not owed certain desirable satisfactions (such as love, approval, success or prestige) even if you experienced a deprived childhood, suffered many hardships, or someone is doing better than you. YOU DO NOT RUN THE UNIVERSE. THINGS DO NOT HAVE TO GO YOUR WAY!

In discussing how to (D) dispute "I can't stand it itis" and "self-downing", Ellis wrote ([8], pp. 248–249):

> *I can't stand it itis"* is a false position, because if you really *couldn't stand* something, you would die of its existence, or it would be impossible for you to live and be happy *at all*.
>
> Self-downing, or self-hatred, over and above criticizing some of your characteristics, is perhaps the worst form of emotional disturbance. . . . According to REBT, all self-blaming (instead of merely criticizing some of your behaviors) is incorrect and anxiety-producing, and is to be actively and forcefully disputed. For example: *Disputing:* Where is the proof that I, as a person, am rotten or worthless...when I do anything badly or foolishly? *Rational Answer:* Nowhere! The "proof" of my being rotten or worthless is non-existent. I do many stupid, self-defeating *acts* and, as a fallible human, will always do some more. But I am only a *person who* does these things, never a *bad person!* I can usually change my . . . habits. But if I never do, I can still always accept *myself,* my *personhood,* and I still deserve to make myself as happy as I can.

REBT IN CHILDREN AND ADOLESCENTS

Rational emotive behavior therapy is considered by its proponents to be highly effective for children and adolescents [9,10]. REBT does not require much adaptation to be used with adolescents, once a therapeutic alliance has been formed. Especially with teenagers who have achieved formal operational thinking, the therapist can discuss irrational beliefs in general terms. For more intellectually limited adolescents, as for children, the therapist must tie verbal interventions to very concrete specific situations, using role play at times. Basically, implementing the techniques for children and adolescents involves making the disputations less abstract in accordance with the patient's developmental level. For adolescents who have achieved formal operational thinking, it is appropriate to challenge their irrational beliefs in abstract terms – as in the examples given above. A teenager with good intellectual functioning who is depressed and anxious can be challenged with respect to their belief that "I need people to approve of me," whereas a youngster who is more limited would need to have this discussed in terms of their feeling that they are worthless when people tease him or her. For those whose thinking is more concrete, it is necessary to base the discussion in a specific concrete context. Thus, the abstract belief, "everybody should treat me fairly" would be "my teacher, Mr Smith, should treat me fairly."

Case Example

The patient is an 18-year-old female first-year college student who comes for therapy because of social anxiety.

Therapist (T): OK, what is the problem you would like to work on today?

Patient (P): I have a lot of anxiety and feel really dumb whenever I meet someone who seems to be very intelligent.

T: You remember that it is not what happens in the world around you that makes you anxious. What make you anxious are your thoughts about those events, the things you tell yourself about what happens in the world around you. We have already discussed the four most common kinds of unrealistic thinking, or irrational thoughts as they are called in REBT. Do you remember them?

P: Yes: self-downing, awfulizing, should-ing on myself, I-can't-stand-it-itis.

T: Let's see how they apply to your problem. What is it that you are telling yourself that elicits your anxiety when you meet someone who seems to be very intelligent?

P: That I am stupid.

T: Let's dispute what you have been telling yourself. Is it true that you are stupid? Whenever you tell yourself that you are stupid, you can dispute that idea. For example, a stupid person does stupid things all the time, or almost all the time. In contrast, you get to your appointments on time, you dress appropriately, you participate in our therapeutic work together; in those, and many other ways that you can easily think of, you do not act in the way that a stupid person acts. You may not always know as much as you wish to know, but everyone has areas of relative ignorance. You are not stupid, it is just that you have the usual human admixture of greater and lesser knowledge.

T: And what else are you telling yourself?

P: That it's awful that I am stupid.

T: Even if it were true (and it is not true) that you are stupid, would that really be awful? Awful might be the sun going supernova, or somewhat less awful might be global warming wiping out all human life on earth, or still less awful might be an atomic bomb terrorist attack on the USA. In the context of those truly awful events, even if you were stupid (and you are not stupid), that would be unfortunate, but that would not amount to being awful. You have already dealt with many unfortunate facts in the course of your daily experiences, you know how to cope with unfortunate events.

T: Is there something else that you are telling yourself?

P: That I should not be stupid.

T: What is the evidence that you "should not" be stupid. Is it written in the US Constitution, is it in the Bible, did it appear in the *New York Times*, is it taught in some college science course? There is no evidence that you "should not" be stupid. You do not want to be stupid, but that is not the same thing as there being a logical necessity that you (among all the people alive) uniquely are exempt from being stupid. Just because you wish something does not mean that it must be so. Remember the old adage: "If wishes were horses, beggars would ride."

T: Is there anything else that you haven't mentioned yet?

P: Well, that I can't stand being stupid.

T: Is it true that you can't stand being stupid? The last time that you thought that you were stupid, did you die? Did you have a stroke or a heart attack? If not, then you can stand being stupid, you just do not like it one bit.

You have already coped with many things in life that you do not like one bit, you can cope with this too.

P: I guess that the next time I get anxious and feel dumb, you want me to practice disputing my self-downing thoughts, my awfulizing thoughts, my should-ing on myself, and my I can't-stand-it-it is?

T: That is absolutely correct. Practice disputing your unrealistic thoughts. Practice makes perfect.

DISCUSSION

Positive Aspects of REBT

In clinical practice, there are several advantages to using REBT:

1. It appeals to insurance companies and managed care companies because it promises therapeutic results in less time than some other treatments, e.g. supportive therapy, psychoanalytically oriented therapy.

2. Clients/patients are often more interested in relief from their problems than in understanding the childhood roots of their problems.

3. The ABCDE theory and technique of therapy are relatively easy to explain (e.g., as contrasted to psychoanalytic theory and therapy) to clients/patients.

4. The use of homework assignments permits the client/patient to have an active role in the therapy between scheduled visits to the therapist.

5. There is a wealth of printed material generated by Ellis and his colleagues at the Institute for Rational Emotive Behavior Therapy that can be recommended to clients/patients for their self-study and self-application of REBT methods.

6. There are regularly scheduled lectures, seminars, books, tapes, videotapes, and experiential groups available for counselors/therapists who want to learn REBT, leading to certification as an REBT practitioner by the Albert Ellis Institute of Rational Emotive Behavior Therapy.

7. When working with clients/patients who have substance abuse problems, individual and group psychotherapy with a counselor/therapist can be supplemented with free services from the SMART®-Recovery self-help organization; SMART®-Recovery uses the REBT method at its meetings, rather than the 12-Step model of Alcoholics Anonymous.

8. For clients/patients with substance abuse problems, REBT places the locus of control within the client/patient, rather than insisting that the client/patient admit to "helplessness" and place their hope for help in a "higher power." This approach is particularly valuable with adolescents, who are loath to admit to personal helplessness/inadequacy.

9. REBT does not make the client/patient dependent on the therapist to make ongoing progress. Once the patient has been taught the REBT theory and methods, and has had the counselor/therapist supervise them in the practice/application of REBT to problems of daily living, the goal is for the therapist to be dispensable, for the client/patient to become their own therapist. Once the REBT theory and methods have been learned, the client/patient is free to live a (more) rational life now and in the future.

Negative Aspects of REBT

In clinical practice, there may also be disadvantages associated with REBT:

1. REBT is difficult to integrate into the treatment philosophy of 12-Step programs, like that of Alcoholics Anonymous (AA). While AA sees substance abusers as being helpless without a "higher power," REBT does not accept that such helplessness is true. Rather, REBT holds that substance abusers can be taught to gain control of their problem behaviors, i.e., their dependence/addiction to substances.

2. REBT and SMART-Recovery are so different from, and such challenges to, the treatment philosophy of 12-Step programs, that REBT practitioners may have difficulty in being accepted by other counselors committed to the 12-Step approach, and may have difficulty finding employment in organizations that are committed to the 12-Step approach.

3. Although REBT and SMART-Recovery are nationwide programs, there are fewer SMART-Recovery self-help groups than there are 12-Step self-help groups, and it may be more difficult for clients/patients with substance abuse problems to find such services outside major urban areas.

4. REBT requires an active, assertive counselor/therapist, continually challenging and disputing the irrational beliefs of the client/patient. Not all counselors/therapists are characterologically suited to this role. Not everyone can be an effective REBT therapist.

5. Some clients/patients are so psychologically fragile that they cannot tolerate the active/assertive style of REBT counselors/therapists. Some persons with borderline personality disorder may fall into this category.

6. Some patients may be actively psychotic, actively suicidal, dangerously violent, or suffering from organic brain diseases (e.g., Alzheimer's disease); these conditions may prevent effective concentration, attention, and participation in REBT.

7. The type of improvement that REBT offers may fall short of what many patients want. Reducing the intensity of one's upset is not the same as eliminating one's upset. REBT offers hope for the former, not the latter.

8. There is a discrepancy between what many patients want and what REBT offers. Many patients want to be cured by the counselor/therapist, in the same way as a surgeon cures a patient with an inflamed or infected appendix. REBT requires the active participation of the client/patient; it is hard work.

Overall Evaluation of REBT

REBT has not been extensively evaluated in controlled studies. Nonetheless there is a body of knowledge supporting its efficacy and effectiveness, including cost-effectiveness. Lyons and Woods [11] concluded from their meta-analysis of 70 studies that REBT was an effective form of therapy, although they cautioned that there were methodological flaws in the studies they reviewed, such as lack of follow-up data and information regarding attrition rates. The authors of another meta-analysis concluded that the efficacy of REBT appeared to be comparable with both cognitive-behavior therapy (CBT) and systematic desensitization [12]. They found the standard deviation of results was quite large, suggesting considerable variability among individuals in treatment response, raising an interesting question about what kind of person does best with this kind of treatment.

A meta-analysis of REBT in children and adolescents also showed comparable effectiveness with other forms of psychotherapy, with the best results in conduct disorders [13] – an interesting finding, in that conduct disorders are associated with neuropsychological deficits, particularly with executive functioning [14]. Adelman and colleagues [15], working in a residential substance abuse treatment facility for adolescents, found that clients' ability to manage anger improved after the incorporation of REBT into treatment.

Recently Sava and colleagues in Romania [16] compared cognitive therapy, REBT, and fluoxetine for major depressive disorder in a randomized clinical trial. They found significant improvement and comparable results for all three treatments at 6 months follow-up. They addressed the issue of cost-effectiveness by dividing the total cost by the number of depression-free days and quality-adjusted life years. The two psychotherapies were found to be more cost-effective than pharmacotherapy. A recent pilot study [17] evaluated the results of REBT for anger treatment in a small group of adults with a variety of psychiatric disorders. REBT was not used in isolation, but implemented along with a variety of other interventions involving relapse prevention, problem-solving, assertiveness, relaxation, and other techniques. They found significant improvements in measures of anger and depression.

The approach of REBT differs from other forms of therapy in that its goal is a new philosophical outlook, rather than just a different mode of interpreting life events. The main questions raised have to do with the validity of the assumptions underlying REBT; it is important to keep in mind that not all of these have been tested and validated. There is some evidence that irrational beliefs are related to psychological disturbance and maladaptive behaviors. Chang and Bridewell [18] found a significant association between irrational beliefs and pessimism in college students. Ziegler and Leslie [19] found empirical support for the ABC model underlying REBT by using a questionnaire to study college students. They found correlations between high scores on irrational thinking, awfulizing, and low frustration tolerance and the students' reports of experiencing daily hassles (a marker for stress). But we really do not know that people who have only rational beliefs are more effective and happier than people who have both rational and irrational beliefs. Similarly, it simply is not true that all human emotional/psychological illness is unrelated to actual external events: physically traumatic brain injury, exposure to neurotoxins, metabolic diseases, cerebrovascular accidents, and brain tumors are all actual external events that have severe impact on emotional/psychological functioning. Ellis may have overstated his case.

REBT was one of the earliest forms of cognitive therapy. It is difficult to believe now, when cognitive therapies are so well accepted, that it was initially met with criticism and derision. It led to the development of other treatments – for example, cognitive-behavioral therapy (CBT) uses elements derived from Aaron Beck's cognitive therapy as well as Ellis' cognitive restructuring techniques.

Although not suitable for all clients/patients, REBT may be a useful theory and technique for many. Particularly in this period where a cost-benefit analysis of all modalities of care is routine, the promise that REBT offers relatively rapid improvement of many common emotional/psychological problems (e.g., anxiety,

depression, substance abuse) merits giving it serious consideration either as one treatment of first choice, or as an adjunctive supplement to other treatments.

References

1. Anon. About Albert Ellis. The Albert Ellis Institute. Available from: http://www.rebt.org(public(about-albert-ellis.html.
2. Ellis A. Why I (really) became a therapist. *J Clin Psychol* 2005;**61**:945–948.
3. Ellis A. *The Road to Tolerance: the Philosophy of Rational Emotive Behavior Therapy*. New York: Prometheus Books, 2004.
4. Patterson CH. *Theories of Counseling and Psychotherapy*. New York: Harper & Row, 1966.
5. Bishop FM. Helping clients manage addictions with REBT. *J Rational-Emotive Cogn-Behav Ther* 2006;**18**.
6. Corey G. *Theory and Practice of Group Counseling*, 6th edn. Brooks-Cole, CA: Thomson, 2004.
7. Young HS. *A Rational Counseling Primer*. New York: Institute for Rational-Emotive Therapy, 1974.
8. Ellis A, Abrams M, Dengelegi L. *The Art & Science of Rational Eating*. Fort Lee, NJ: Barricade Books, 1992.
9. Bernard M E. Rational-emotive therapy with children and adolescents: treatment strategies. *School Psychol Rev* 1990;**19**:294–303.
10. Bernard ME, Joyce MR. Rational-emotive therapy with children and adolescents. In: Kratochwill TR, Morris RJ (eds), *Handbook of Psychotherapy with Children and Adolescents*. Needham Heights, MA: Allyn & Bacon, 1993; pp. 221–241.
11. Lyons LC, Woods PJ. The efficacy of rational-emotive therapy: A quantitative review of the outcome research. *Clin Psychol Rev* 1991;**11**:357–369.
12. Engels GI, Garnefski N, Diekstra RF. Efficacy of rational-emotive therapy: a quantitative analysis. *J Consult Clin Psychol* 1993;**61**:1083–1090.
13. Gonzalez JE, Nelson JR, Gutkin TB. Rational emotive therapy. *J Emot Behav Disord* 2004;**12**:222–235.
14. Närhi V, Lehto-Salo P, Ahonen T, Marttunen M. Neuropsychological subgroups of adolescents with conduct disorder. *Scand J Psychol* 2010;**51**:278–284.
15. Adelman R, McGee P, Power R, Hanson C. Reducing adolescent clients' anger in a residential substance abuse treatment facility. *Joint Comm J Qual Patient Safety* 2005;**31**:325–327.
16. Sava FA, Yates BT, Lupu V, Szentagotai A, David D. Cost-effectiveness and cost-utility of cognitive therapy, rational emotive behavioral therapy, and fluoxetine (Prozac) in treating depression: a randomized clinical trial. *J Clin Psychol* 2009;**65**:36–52.
17. Fuller JR, Digiuseppe R, O'Leary S, Fountain T, Lang C. An open trial of a comprehensive anger treatment program on an outpatient sample. *Behav Cogn Psychother* 2010;**38**:485–490.
18. Chang EC, Bridewell WB. Irrational beliefs, optimism, pessimism, and psychological distress: a preliminary examination of differential effects in a college population. *J Clin Psychol* 1998;**54**:137–142.
19. Ziegler DJ, Leslie YM. A test of the ABC model underlying rational emotive behavior therapy. *Psychol Rep* 2003;**92**:235–240.

28

Relapse Prevention[1]

Richard Rosner

Forensic Psychiatry Residency Program, New York University School of Medicine;
Forensic Psychiatry Clinic, Bellevue Hospital Center, New York, NY, USA

To say adolescent addiction psychiatry and adolescent addiction medicine is an underserved area is an understatement. It is a difficult area that is avoided by many psychiatrists, even those who treat adolescents. But adolescents with addictive disorders can be treated. As my colleague Dr Robert Weinstock, Clinical Professor of Psychiatry at the University of California at Los Angeles, taught me, "Never confuse the truly impossible with the merely horrendously difficult."

MARLATT AND GORDON'S CONCEPTS

This chapter will provide an introduction to the work of G. Allan Marlatt and Ruth Gordon, whose model of relapse and intervention strategies has been very influential. Their main publication in this field is *Relapse Prevention, Maintenance Strategies in the Treatment of Addictive Behaviors*, published in 1985 [1]. Although a revised edition was published in 2005 [2], the original edition is a classic in the field.

What is relapse prevention all about? Relapse prevention (RP) is a generic term that refers to a wide range of strategies designed to prevent relapse in the area of addictive behavior change. The primary focus of relapse prevention is on the crucial issue of maintenance in the habit change process. The purpose is two-fold: to prevent the occurrence of initial lapses after one has embarked on a program of habit change and/or to prevent any lapse from escalating into a total relapse.

The main emphasis of relapse prevention is on addictive behaviors, which include problem drinking, smoking, substance abuse, eating disorders, and compulsive gambling. The theoretical orientation is that addictive behaviors are best conceptualized as over-learned habit patterns rather than as diseases. A key assumption is that addictive habit patterns can be changed through the application of self-management or self-control procedures. The task of the therapist is to teach every client to be responsible for his or her own maintenance in the habit change process.

Applications of Relapse Prevention

Relapse prevention procedures can be provided as a specific maintenance program to prevent relapse or as a more global program of lifestyle change. In the former case, the goals of the program are to anticipate and to prevent the occurrence of a relapse after the initiation of habit change and to prevent a slip from becoming a full-blown collapse or relapse. These procedures can be used regardless of the theoretical orientation of the practitioner.

The second more general application of the relapse prevention model is to facilitate global changes in personal habits and daily lifestyles so as to reduce the risk of physical disease and psychological stress, to teach the individual to achieve a balanced lifestyle, and to prevent the development of unhealthful habit patterns. At this point it sounds extraordinarily like the goal in dialectical behavior therapy (DBT) – to teach the borderline person to have a life worth living – the goal of relapse prevention is to teach the addict how to have a life worth living again.

[1]Relapse Prevention. Previously published in Adolescent Psychiatry, Volume 2, Bentham, 2011, and reprinted here with their kind permission.

SELF-CONTROL VERSUS DISEASE MODELS

There is controversy in the field of addiction medicine and addiction psychiatry between those who are committed to a disease model for understanding addictions and those who are committed to a self-control model. The disease model has substantial support among organized medicine, in part because calling addiction a disease makes it possible to obtain insurance reimbursement. However, just because labeling something a disease makes it possible for insurance money to pay for services provided to addicts, does not necessarily mean that the disease model is valid, or that everybody in the addictions field agrees with it. It is valuable to clarify what those two models are, how they differ, and why it may be important to be aware of them.

The Disease Model

Firstly let us examine the disease model. The disease model basically says that the individual suffering from addiction is a helpless victim of forces beyond his or her control; a leaf in the wind, and that the condition is all due to internal biological vulnerabilities. When these vulnerability factors are operating, in the presence of the right substance, addiction develops. The object of the addiction does not have to be a substance, but can be anything that provides instant gratification. It could be sex, food, or the roulette wheel. Whatever it is, it is all set into motion by biological proclivity and the individual is powerless to do anything about it.

The second tenet in the disease model is that the goal of treatment is total abstinence. In this model, there is just no other way. The addict is either using and out of control or abstaining and living an addiction-free life. The treatment philosophy in the disease model essentially equates the person with the person's behavior – this is the interesting way that Marlatt and Gordon [1] describe it. A person is an addict, a compulsive gambler, a compulsive overeater, or a pedophile. That's it. He is his behavior. The approach to treatment is the medical disease approach; do what you have to in order to extinguish the behavior. The treatment procedures in the disease model involve confrontation and conversion; in effect saying, "You are an alcoholic, you are an addict, admit it. Once you've admitted it we can get you to change." Group support, like that available through Alcoholics Anonymous (AA) or Narcotics Anonymous (NA), is enormously important. These groups espouse a variety of simple dogmas; for example, one of the most famous ones of AA is, "The man takes a drink and then the drink takes the man." Aphorisms such as this are easy to understand and remember.

The general approach of the disease model until relatively recently has been that each addiction is unique. If you were an alcoholic, you would go to AA, if you were an incest survivor, you would be in a group for survivors of incest. If you were a compulsive gambler, you would go to Gamblers Anonymous. If you were a pedophile, you would go to special program for pedophiles, and so forth. The differences rather than the commonalities in the addiction process are emphasized, and again the stress is that addiction is based on physiological processes. In keeping with the conceptualization of addictions as diseases, treatments for addictions based on the disease model include hospital inpatient treatments, aversion treatments such as Antabuse (which is quite effective if a patient is willing to use it), and of course group support like AA and NA. It is sometimes confusing that the advocates of the disease model of addiction also use the phrase "relapse prevention" to describe their approach to maintaining recovery from addiction; an example of the disease model approach to relapse prevention is provided by T.T. Gorski [3].

The Self-Control Model

The self-control model that Marlatt and Gordon support is quite different. The construct underlying self-control is that of locus of control. An idea developed into a quantifiable quality by Rotter [4], it refers to generalized expectancies for internal versus external control of reinforcement. People with an internal locus of control believe that their own actions determine the rewards that they obtain, while those with an external locus of control believe that their own behavior doesn't matter much and that rewards in life are generally outside of their control. In the self-control paradigm, individuals are understood not as helpless victims of forces beyond their control, but rather as beings able to control their behavior. They may not know how to do this, but that is an entirely different matter that can be addressed through skills training. You have an automobile to drive and you don't drive it without taking lessons. You have an addiction problem, so you can't deal with it unless you are taught how to deal with it, but just as you can learn how to drive a car, you can learn how to deal with an addiction problem. Relapses are viewed as mistakes that mean better skills are needed to cope effectively with circumstances that increase the likelihood of substance abuse. Rather than signs of moral failures or weaknesses, relapses provide opportunities to learn new ways of coping.

TREATMENT GOALS IN RELAPSE PREVENTION

The treatment goals in the self-control model are also controversial, because abstinence is not the only option considered in this model; rather there is a choice between abstinence and moderation. The idea that there is a choice is based on the fact that the great majority of people in our society drink but, the great majority of people in our society are not alcoholics. The problem is not necessarily the consumption of alcohol. The problem is how to consume alcohol in the right way, at the right time, in the right manner so that there are no or minimal aversive consequences. The self-control model suggests that it is possible for people to learn how to behave like everybody else does – in ways that are not intrinsically self-destructive, in ways that are moderate. They don't necessarily have to abstain. Closely related to this idea and much more fashionably named these days is the whole concept of "harm reduction." The goal of harm reduction is not necessarily to get people to stop risky behavior, but to reduce the risk that the behavior they are engaging in is going to hurt themselves or anyone else. Instead of telling a teenager "Just say no," a proponent of harm reduction would counsel the youth about reducing risk. For example, instead of saying "Just don't have sex," you tell the teenager how to use a condom and how to have safer sex. The same approach holds with addiction.

Coping Skills and Cognitive Restructuring

The treatment approach is primarily teaching behavioral coping skills and using cognitive restructuring techniques. As previously noted, the general approach to addictions in the self-control model is to focus on the commonalities across all addictions. Thus, in this model, there are more commonalities between persons addicted to alcohol and those addicted to heroin than there are differences. This approach means that addiction is viewed as essentially the same phenomenon in terms of the psychological factors that need to be considered in order to establish or have a hope of establishing control. Addiction is conceptualized as based on maladaptive over-learned habits, which, like all over-learned habits, are resistant to change, but nonetheless can be changed. The types of therapy employed in the self-control model differ from those used in the disease model. They are basically outpatient cognitive behavioral therapies. There are self-control programs, such as SMART Recovery® (which has an extensive website at www.smartrecovery.org). There are also controlled drinking programs. While everyone is aware of AA and Rosner [5,6] has written elsewhere about 12-step facilitation, very few therapists have been trained in SMART Recovery facilitation, and controlled drinking programs are even less well known.

Determinants of Relapse

Intrapersonal High-Risk Situations

Marlatt and Gordon found, when they studied conditions leading to relapse, that there were two large clusters of situations in which relapse occurred. The first they labeled intra, meaning within the person. These include both negative emotional states – "I'm so blue" – and positive emotional states – "I just passed the test, let's go celebrate by go getting drunk!" Testing personal control is another relapse-inducing situation – a person thinks, "It may be said that the man takes the drink and then the drink takes the man, but let me find out for myself. Let me take that drink and see whether or not I can control myself." Then there are urges and temptations. While the sources of temptations may be external cues – such as being around other people who are drinking – the experiences themselves are intrapsychic.

Marlatt and Gordon found that negative emotional states were the major cause of relapsing in their initial studies. This cause and effect relationship is illustrated in the following case example.

Case Example

A young man's negative emotional state was precipitated by a breakup with his girlfriend. His assumption was that this girl must have perceived him for what he was really worth – nothing. Therefore no girl would ever like him, he would be alone for the rest of his life, he would be lonely for the rest of his life, and therefore his life was not worth living and he should kill himself.

A large-scale study funded by the National Institute on Alcohol Abuse and Alcoholism resulted in some modifications of Marlatt and Gordon's original classifications of high-risk situations, and found that the situations themselves had poor predictive validity, but confirmed the relationship between coping skills in high-risk situations and likelihood of relapse.

A large number of people seen because of their problems with addiction are extremely sensitive and over-reactive. In this respect they resemble people with borderline personality disorder. In fact some of the techniques of dialectical behavior therapy (DBT) [7] are being applied to people with addictive problems, and in some instances with reasonable levels of success [8].

Interpersonal Conflicts

The other large cluster of determinants for a relapse are interpersonal conflicts – "I can't stand my boss" – social pressure – "Come on have a drink, everybody else is having a drink, just one, come along" – or as an example of positive emotional states – "I just got married," "I'm feeling on top of the world, I may just as well get high."

You can actually label those high-risk situations and once you know what those high-risk situations are, you can share that knowledge with persons who are suffering with addictive problems and teach them how to identify those high-risk situations in advance, teach them coping skills to deal with those high-risk situations, and teach them ways in which they can have greater control over their behavior. The idea is that it is not mysterious.

Somebody is in a high-risk situation and one possibility is that the person has a coping response. The coping response is accompanied by an experience of increased self-efficacy. Self-efficacy is the interesting concept that basically deals with a type of reality-based sense of personal confidence and self-esteem [9]. The cognitions associated with self-efficacy are: "I've dealt with this before. I just dealt with it right now. The likelihood is that the next time it comes along, although I am not looking forward to it, I'll be able to deal with it then too." As a result of the positive outcome of the coping response, there is a decreased probability of relapse occurring.

The alternative outcome is that the high-risk situation comes along and the person does not have a coping response. These situations are analogous to being behind the wheel of a car, and told to drive, but having never had driving lessons. When people like this get in a high-risk situation, they don't know how to deal with it, because nobody taught them how to deal with it. The outcome of such an experience is a sense of decreased self-efficacy, manifested by thoughts like, "I have never been able to cope with this" "I can't cope with this right now" or "I'll never be able to cope with it."

Outcome Expectancies

Being in such a high-risk situation is often associated with what are referred to as positive outcome expectancies [10]: "I'll feel better if I take a drink" or "I'll feel better if I get high," and that is perhaps correct. In the vast majority of the cases, certainly in the beginning, what happens at first is positive. The negative outcome that follows is downplayed. "It's true I'll feel lousy some time after I feel better, but I'll probably feel better immediately after I take the heroin." But they don't focus on the "I'll feel lousy after I feel better" they focus on the "I'll feel better."

There have been some interesting studies of the way in which people who are suffering from addictive problems perceive long-term and short-term outcomes. They have a much greater capacity to discount the value of long-term outcomes than do people who are not suffering from substance abuse. So the person with an addiction reasons, "The fact that I'll feel good in 20 seconds outweighs the fact that I'm going to feel terrible in eight hours." This reasoning then leads to the use of a substance. This is accompanied by an interesting intrapsychic experience, which Marlatt and Gordon have termed the "abstinence violation

effect." The person erroneously thinks that any use whatsoever will make him or her become one of the bad guys who use, in accordance with the disease model that the world is compartmentalized into the good guys who abstain and the bad guys who use. If the world is viewed as being made up of the people who have the power to resist, and people who have no spine and no willpower at all and who succumb, the person who relapses is viewed as having no willpower, worthless, and without moral fiber. A drop in self-esteem follows, and people usually feel guilty because they fail to abstain. They have said a million times that they are going to; as Mark Twain said, "Quitting smoking is easy. I've done it hundreds of times." Of course, every time they succumb they feel poorly, and they feel that they are not in control of themselves so they have learned that "I can't control myself," and this mindset increases the probability that a relapse will occur. A high-risk situation usually occurs in the overall context of an imbalanced lifestyle or, in the language of DBT, a "life not worth living." In behavioral terms an imbalance exists between the demands being made upon an individual and the satisfaction that life provides for the individual. When the 'shoulds' – "You should do this," "You should get up in the morning and go to school," "You should get up and go to work" – outweigh the positive good of the satisfaction of your own wants and desires, your life is out of balance. According to Marlatt and Gordon that out-of-balance circumstance causes people to want to redress the balance. They want their wants to be satisfied and they often want what they want when they want it and there is a desire for immediate gratification. This is illustrated in the following exchange between a therapist and a patient: the therapist said "You really have a lot of trouble waiting to get your reward," and the patient replied, "Yes, I like my reward now and large." In response to that desire for immediate gratification, people may experience subjective urges and cravings and may seek immediate gratification through substances. They may also engage in rationalizations: "I deserve this," or "I earned this." They use denial: "I'm not really an alcoholic, once in a while I just drink too much," "Other people will get caught if they use illegal drugs; not me, I'm smart." They make what Marlatt and Gordon term "Apparently Irrelevant Decisions," or AIDs. For example, a teenager might say to himself, "Gee, I'm on my way home from a tough day at school. Why don't I walk this time instead of taking the bus," and the walk just happens to be through the neighborhood where the drug dealers are. So the apparently irrelevant decision leads to relapse. He didn't decide that he was going to use drugs; he decided that he would walk home. Part of relapse prevention therapy is teaching people to recognize that AIDs can lead to disastrous consequences. If you have a problem with addictions you can't be casual in these matters. A great deal of self-monitoring is required.

TECHNIQUES IN RELAPSE PREVENTION

Let's take a look at this cluster of specific intervention strategies. First, if there is an issue of being at risk for entering a high-risk situation, you have to help the person become aware of what his or her personal high-risk situation may be. For someone who is addicted to Belgian chocolate of at least 72% cocoa content, it is of no concern whatsoever if he takes a walk past a bar, and it doesn't hurt him in the slightest to walk through a neighborhood endemic with drug dealers. That's not high risk for him. He couldn't care less about that stuff. He has to be careful about not walking past the wrong sort of confectionery store. He has to know where every one of them is in his neighborhood and he has to avoid them like the plague.

One also has to teach people to engage in honest behavioral assessments. For example: "Gee, today I'm feeling hungry. Today I'm feeling angry. Today I'm feeling lonely. Today I'm feeling tired. I know that when that happens, my commitment to staying on the wagon is reduced. I have to be particularly careful today to do whatever I can to avoid high-risk situations because today is not a day when I am going to be at my best to resist them."

Then one has to work on the various relapse fantasies that people have. This means understanding what really happened as opposed to what one *thinks* happened. The therapist has to help the patient to understand the behavioral change that actually led up to the past relapses so he or she can be taught to avoid them.

Then, of course, for people who have no real coping skills, you've got to teach them coping skills. An important component of skills training is relapse rehearsal. What do you do if you actually slip? Carry a card with you with the name of your AA sponsor. Carry a card with you that tells you where to go and who to call. Have the name of three or four friends available whom you can contact. Get out of the place that you are in and go where the temptation is less. All of these are coping strategies to use to avoid slipping to begin with, as well as skills to employ if there is a slip. In addition, technical skills such as relaxation training and imagery can be used to enhance one's sense of self efficacy.

SLIPS VERSUS RELAPSES

When one does have a slip and one again has an experience of decreased self-efficacy (the abstinence violation effect and accompanying loss of self-esteem,

which have been mentioned above), relapse prevention teaches that a slip is a mistake, it is not a sin, and that a slip is not the same as a relapse. Once again skills training is involved and there is education again about the immediate and delayed effects of substances and helping people to think beyond the good feelings and become aware of the bad stuff around the corner awaiting them after the good feelings have passed.

People have to understand that to use once does not mean that it is inevitable that they will go on and use again. They have to be taught that it is not that either you are abstaining or you are out of control. You slipped, now regain control. When a baby slips when it's learning to walk, it doesn't say "I'll never learn to walk." It gets up and tries again. So if you slip you pick yourself up, dust yourself off, and start all over again on the right foot.

Finally, there is the overall issue of lifestyle imbalance, which increases vulnerability to slips and relapses. So you have to teach people how to have a balanced lifestyle and get them involved in positive addictions rather than negative addictions. Positive addictions are activities such as jogging, or meditation, or what Marlatt and Gordon call "body time," all ways of making oneself feel good. The clinician must help the patient to find indulgences that do not have negative side effects and that are adaptive rather than maladaptive. You have to teach patients how to deal with urges and cravings, how to deal with rationalization and denial, apparently irrelevant decisions, and how to deal with high-risk situations: how to avoid them if possible, or if unavoidable, how to cope with them.

DISCUSSION

There is, of course, a difference between knowing the concepts and actually doing the nuts and bolts. Do not assume that you can go out and immediately start working in this without doing much of the background reading and obtaining supervised "hands-on" experience. Fortunately there are some excellent books on how to deal with the nuts and bolts, one of which is actually free, and the other of which specifically addresses the adolescent population.

The United States Department of Health and Human Services through the Substance Abuse and Mental Health Services Administration and the Center for Substance Abuse Treatment has published a series of Technical Assistance Publications (TAP). One of these is the *Counselor's Manual for Relapse Prevention with Chemically Dependent Criminal Offenders* [11]. It is available free from the US government. The front part explains what a counselor needs to know to use this *Manual for Relapse Prevention*. The back part is the workbook that your patient follows.

The Adolescent Relapse Prevention Workbook: A Brief Strategic Approach [3] is a step-by-step approach designed specifically for teenagers. You go through it with the adolescent patient, who fills in the material. You then use the teen's own data and life experience to help him or her recognize what high-risk situations are, what the feelings, thoughts, and behaviors are that lead to use, and what strategies he or she can develop to cope.

There are a variety of helpful books that you can use to educate yourself about relapse prevention. In addition to Marlatt and Gordon's classic book on relapse prevention [1], there is an article summarizing their model on the NIH website [12]. Marlatt has been an author, co-author, or editor of 17 books. There is even an "Idiot's Guide" [13]. The second edition of the classic book on relapse prevention describes the application of the relapse prevention model in a variety of addictive disorders, and discusses the evidence base for the relapse prevention approach [2]. And finally, a fairly recent book contains several chapters that focus on adolescents [14].

This chapter has attempted to sketch out the rationale behind Marlatt and Gordon's approach to relapse prevention. It aims to encourage you to acquaint yourself further with relapse prevention and use it and expand the scope of your practice.

References

1. Marlatt GA, Gordon JR. *Relapse Prevention: Maintenance Strategies in the Treatment of Addictive Behaviors*. New York: Guilford, 1985.
2. Marlatt GA, Donovan DM. *Relapse Prevention: Maintenance Strategies in the Treatment of Addictive Behaviors*, 2nd edn. New York: Guilford Press, 2005.
3. Gorski TT. *The Adolescent Relapse Prevention Workbook: A Brief Strategic Approach*. Independence, MO: Herald Publishing House, 1996.
4. Rotter JB. Generalized expectancies for internal versus external control of reinforcement. *Psychol Monogr* 1966; **80**:1–28.
5. Rosner R. Anonymous encounters: Alcoholics Anonymous, Al-Anon, and Overeaters Anonymous. *Adolesc Psychiatry* 2011;**1**:138–139.
6. Rosner R. Saving adolescents. *Adolesc Psychiatry* 2008;**30**:35–46.
7. Linehan MM. *Cognitive Behavioral Treatment of Borderline Personality Disorder*. New York: Guilford Press, 1993.
8. Sher L. Behavioural therapy for the treatment of alcohol abuse and dependence. *Can J Psychiatry* 2002;**47**:586.
9. Bandura A. Self-efficacy: toward a unifying theory of behavioral change. *Psychol Rev* 1977;**84**:191–215.
10. Brown SA, Goldman MS, Inn A, Anderson LR. Expectations of reinforcement from alcohol: their domain and relation to drinking patterns. *J Consult Clin Psychol* 1980;**48**:419–426.
11. Center for Substance Abuse Treatment. *Counselor's Manual for Relapse Prevention with Chemically Dependent Criminal Offenders*. TAP 19 (1996) NCADI # BKD723. Rockville, MD: Department of Health and Human Services, Substance Abuse and Mental Health Services Administration, 1996.
12. Larimer ME, Palmer RS, Marlatt GA. Relapse prevention: an overview of Marlatt's cognitive-behavioral model. *Alcohol Res Health* 1999;**23**:151–160.
13. Marlatt GA, Romaine DS. *The Complete Idiot's Guide to Changing Old Habits for Good*. New York: Alpha Books, 2008.
14. Marlatt GA, Witkiewitz K. *Addictive Behaviors: New Readings on Etiology, Prevention, and Treatment*. Washington, DC: American Psychological Association, 2009.

29

Adolescent Intensive Outpatient Treatment

Tiffany Tsai

UCLA-Kern Department of Psychiatry, Bakersfield, CA, USA

INTRODUCTION

The growing numbers of adolescents with substance use disorders (SUD) necessitate increased availability, awareness, and options for treatment. The treatment of the adolescent versus the adult with SUD differs in many important aspects. A savvy clinician must continually keep the unique needs of the adolescent in mind when selecting an appropriate level and type of treatment. One method of treatment becoming better recognized and more utilized are intensive outpatient programs (IOPs). However, there exists a wide variety of IOPs and there is no current universal standard. This chapter seeks to further expand knowledge, understanding, and awareness of intensive outpatient programs. It will focus exclusively on intensive outpatient programs and not community outpatient care.

DEFINITION

Historically, over the last two decades there has been movement toward developing the least-cost and highest-efficacy treatments for SUD. This entailed development of the intensive outpatient treatment (IOT) model for substance abuse treatment [1]. There is not always a clear distinction in the definition of an intensive outpatient and a day or partial hospital program. Often, clinicians will confuse the terms and use them interchangeably. A certain amount of this ambiguity arose from the differences in defining an intensive outpatient program in the research literature. For example, in 1997 McKay *et al.* used the term "intensive outpatient" in reference to the Philadelphia VA day program consisting of 27 hours/week [1]. However, another study by

McLellan *et al.* in 1997 utilized a minimum criterion of 9 hours/week comprising three sessions per week as a definition of 10 intensive outpatient programs. This same study also differentiated IOPs from six "traditional" outpatient programs offering a maximum of two 2-hour sessions per week [1]. American Society of Addiction Medicine (ASAM) guidelines in 2001 called for 9 hours/week of planned programming for IOPs and 20 hours/week for partial hospital programs. Partial hospital programs, however, generally have more direct access to psychiatric and medical services [1]. Of note, the ASAM guidelines do not specify the duration of treatment in IOP. However, the definition of an IOP should encompass more than a tally of the number of patient contact hours per week, since there is a significant range from the minimum of 9 hours up to 70 hours per week [2]. Often, there is variation in the treatment intensity level and type of services provided by an IOP among different programs. State law and regulations may mandate certain requirements of an IOP.

LEVEL OF CARE

Matching of a patient's biopsychosocial needs to the appropriate level of care through a range of different levels and services is a major goal of effective treatment in SUD [1,3]. For adolescents, treatment occurs at one of many different levels of care across a variety of settings that reflect treatment intensity and level of supervision/restriction of movement [4]. Factors influencing the treatment setting decision include the following:

1. Provision of a safe environment and the capability of the adolescent for self-care.

Clinical Handbook of Adolescent Addiction, First Edition. Richard Rosner.
© 2013 John Wiley & Sons, Ltd. Published 2013 by John Wiley & Sons, Ltd.

2. Motivation and willingness of the adolescent and the family in treatment cooperation.
3. The adolescent's need for structure and limit-setting unachievable in a less restrictive environment.
4. The presence of medical or psychiatric conditions.
5. The availability of specific types of treatment settings designated for adolescents.
6. The preference of the adolescent and family for a particular treatment environment.
7. Less restrictive setting or level of care resulting in insufficient treatment success [4].

A commonly used and accepted guideline for level of care in SUDs is the American Society of Addiction Medicine Patient Placement Criteria for Treatment of Substance-Related Disorders (ASAM-PPC) [3,5,6]. The four levels of care are:

1. Level I – outpatient treatment.
2. Level II – intensive outpatient treatment.
3. Level III – medically monitored intensive inpatient treatment.
4. Level IV – medically managed intensive inpatient treatment.

The criteria describe intensive outpatient treatment, including partial hospitalization, as a planned and organized service where addiction professionals deliver several alcohol and other drug (AOD) treatment services to patients. Treatment comprises scheduled sessions totaling a minimum of 9 hours per week within an overall structured program. Flexibility exists in the timing of the programming, but patients universally live at home or in their customary environment [2]. IOPs were designed to bridge the gap between the high-intensity, medically monitored inpatient or residential treatment setting and the low-intensity, traditional outpatient treatment consisting of one weekly session of individual or group therapy [5].

SPECIFIC NEEDS OF ADOLESCENTS

Adolescents with SUDs are not just miniature versions of adults but require treatment tailored to their unique needs [7]. The ASAM-PPC delineates several distinguishing factors that differentiate SUD treatment in adolescents from adults, which include the following: (i) potential for intoxication and withdrawal; (ii) medical conditions and complications; (iii) behavioral, emotional, and cognitive state in conjunction with developmental stages; (iv) willingness for change; (v) potential for continued use, relapse, or problems; and (vi) recovery environment [6,8]. The reasons why adolescents use

drugs and alcohol stem from different sources than those of adults, and the future consequences are even less apparent to adolescents [9]. Therefore, treatment of the adolescents with SUD necessitates a tailored approach where the clients' distinctive developmental problems, differences in values and beliefs, and external environmental pressures are taken into consideration. A core component of treatment is the family and their active participation. By changing the manner in which adolescents interact with others and their environment, substance use may potentially impair the mental and emotional development from youth to adulthood [9]. Thus, treatment needs to be comprehensive and encompass the unique medical, social, and psychological needs of an adolescent. The adolescents best suited for IOPs are those experiencing difficulties resulting from recent, moderate-to-heavy use of legal or illegal substances with functional but ineffective coping skills, and who require a marginally structured setting without complete removal from their current living situation [10]. In addition, careful assessment of the adolescent and restraint in premature diagnosis of substance dependence is needed given that signs of dependence in adolescents present differently than adults [11].

PROGRAM COMPONENTS

The seven key parts of several adolescent substance abuse treatment programs, including IOPs, are the following:

- orientation;
- daily scheduled activities;
- peer monitoring;
- conflict resolution;
- client contracts;
- schooling; and
- vocational training [9].

Orientation is the first exposure to the program for the adolescent and sets the tone for treatment, delineating expectations and what substance abuse treatment comprises. Given that adolescents enter treatment through a multitude of difference avenues, such as parental coercion, school referral, and court mandate, they experience significant anxiety and ambivalence about treatment. A main objective of orientation is to calm the anxiety as well as to strengthen the motivation for treatment. Scheduling structured time for activities such as homework, school, and healthy recreational outlets allows adolescents to build a framework to maintain sobriety. Peer monitoring allows adolescents to learn to respond appropriately to the pressures of a peer group. Conflict resolution is essential to mediate friction between patients and staff as well as to manage a patient's resistance in meeting program expectations. Client contracts, consisting of behavioral contracts and substance-free contracts, are written between the adolescent and the primary counselor in order to lay the groundwork for treatment goals, expectations, consequences, and timelines. The schooling is an essential factor and requires a seamless integration into treatment of an adolescent. Some programs provide education on site as part of the IOP; however, the same IOP can work together with the adolescent's off-site school in addition. Vocational training in terms of career guidance, job search skills, and prevocational training gives adolescents the tools to support themselves so they are less likely to resort to illegal activites or relapse [9].

An effective IOP consists of different levels and types of service, ranging from core to optimal to enhancing components. Every IOP as part of its core services should provide screening, assessment, treatment planning, 24-hour crisis management, pharmacotherapy, individual and group therapy, education for patient and family, toxicology screen, and program outcome evaluation [12]. Adolescents in particular benefit from group therapy given their developmental stage and greater susceptibilty to influence, both positive and negative, of their peer group [13]. However, individual therapy is often needed to give adolescents privacy when they do not feel comfortable discussing things openly in a group setting. Optimal elements include family therapy, parenting skills training, leisure activities aimed at fostering drug-free recreation, transportation, aftercare, and alumni activities. Examples of enhancing elements that further amplify treatment include art therapy, meditation, biofeedback, acupuncture, and stress reduction techniques [12].

STAFFING CONSIDERATIONS

Thorough understanding of the development and unique treatment needs of adolescents is important for the IOP staff. They should maintain appropriate and distinct personal boundaries, yet remain warm and adaptable in engaging with adolescents. Sensitivity to family dynamics and a large fund of knowledge regarding the school system are essential. Given the high likelihood of conflict with authority in adolescents, program staff need to set definitive behavioral limits in a manner that is not perceived as judgmental or punishing. Current knowledge of the vernacular, types, and combinations of substances used by adolescents is key. A clinical coordinator trained in adolescent substance abuse treatment is needed among the roster of program staff [10]. The program staff credentials include a range and different

combinations of licensed marriage and family therapists (LMFT), doctorate of philosophy (PhD), doctor of psychology (PsyD), medical doctors (MD), licensed clinical social workers (LCSW), and certified alcohol and drug addiction counselor (CADAC) staff.

ADVANTAGES

There exist numerous advantages to an IOP. Financial benefits include providing a longer duration of treatment for a lower cost as compared to the traditional 28-day inpatient care, without loss of favorable clinical outcomes [14]. Patients are able to remain productive and continue their education and occupational and social obligations without major interruption. There are also future cost savings in terms of prevention of advancement of the SUD and comorbidity [12]. This is especially relevant to adolescents since early intervention and appropriate treatment may alter the trajectory of the SUD and may allow resumption of normal development of the adolescent. The patient also benefits from an IOP in terms of greater flexibility, the ability to individualize and tailor treatment, and improved confidentiality and convenience [12]. One major advantage of an IOP is the flexibility it gives adolescents by allowing them to continue to attend school while they are receiving treatment for their SUD. Most groups in an IOP are scheduled in the afternoons and evenings, with some programs also having an independent school program as an additional service provided by the IOP. Additional advantages of IOPs include allowing patients daily to practice their newly learned behaviors and coping skills in their native, unsheltered environments, and develop their recovery identity free from substances. The flexibility of the IOP means that it can quickly respond and react to changes in the clinical presentation of the patient, whether an improvement or deterioration. Relapse management support with an IOP is integral as it addresses triggers and issues that arise in the context of real-life situations, which facilitate positive learning experiences [12]. Retention rates are better in IOPs, a feature that has been associated with improved abstinence due to longer time spent in treatment [12]. Given the active participation inherent in an IOP, this shifts responsibility onto the patient and empowers them in their own treatment. Two other unique beneficial features of IOPs are the capacity for an enhanced therapeutic milieu that fosters relationships that often continue beyond treatment, and the acclimatization during treatment to the 12-Step group participation (e.g., with Alcoholics Anonymous and Narcotics Anonymous) [12]. However, despite these many advantages, there remain challenges and disadvantages with IOPs.

CHALLENGES

The same advantages discussed previously can also become a limitation or barrier in treatment depending on the patient and circumstance [12]. Two of the major challenges include retention of the patient and crisis management. Unlike adult patients, adolescents most likely are entering treatment for the first time, may have little knowledge of the treatment process, and need more orientation [10]. A more comprehensive approach to treatment and planning is required in adolescents given that they are part of several different, overlapping systems such as school, family, and peer groups. Therefore, information from multiple sources is necessary for a complete biopsychosocial treatment plan. Working with the family poses its own challenges; this is integral to recovery, but unhealthy family dynamics, resistance, or unwillingness to participate can hinder treatment progress. Additional clinical challenges include treatment non-compliance, continuation or relapse of substance abuse, arriving at sessions intoxicated, and affordability [14]. A significant challenge is motivation of the adolescent as most enter treatment not on self-referral, but rather due to external factors such as parents, court, school, or social welfare agencies [15]. Since there is no uniform, standard definition of an IOP in terms of its constitution, besides the minimum requirement of 9 hours per week, much of what defines an IOP is left to the discretion of individual IOPs. This leads to quite a variety in terms of intensity, duration, financial cost, services provided, and staffing credentialing. Therefore, finding the appropriate IOP for an adolescent can present difficulties, and good knowledge of the available local programs is needed.

THERAPEUTIC APPROACHES

A variety of different theories exist as regards therapeutic approaches to treatment in IOPs. Six of the most widely utilized and researched approaches include the 12-Step facilitation, cognitive behavorial, motivational enhancement, matrix model, therapeutic community, and contingency management and community reinforcement [16]. No one theoretical method is superior to another, and effective IOPs design treatment specific to the needs of the popluation served, in this case adolescents. Adolescents tend to respond better to the cognitive behavorial and motivational enhancement and interviewing techniques [10]. An integral component of treatment in adolescents involves engagement of the family and active participation of both the adolescent and parents. Often comprehensive treatment of the adolescent necessitates treatment of the parents and family, whose problems may be contributing to the adolescent's SUD.

LITERATURE

There exists a paucity of research studies on adolescent substance abuse IOPs. Part of the problem stems from the lack of a standard definition for what an intensive outpatient program entails. The literature tends not to make a clear distinction between day treatment programs, partial hospitalization programs, and intensive outpatient programs. In 2004, White *et al.* conducted a study looking at 59 marijuana-dependent adolescents receiving treatment in an IOP, and the possible predictors of relapse. They found that comorbid psychiatric disorders of depression and attention-deficit/hyperactivity disorder (ADHD) were associated with reduced likelihood of successful program completion and greater likelihood of relapse [17]. Current research literature specifically on IOPs is very limited and further research is needed to examine IOPs and understand how to help adolescents with SUDs.

SELECTED INTENSIVE OUTPATIENT PROGRAM EXAMPLES

There exist a number of adolescent IOPs across the United States. One of the best known is the Chestnut Health Systems – Bloomington Adolescent Outpatient and Intensive Outpatient Treatment Model. It was established in 1985 and is located in Bloomington, Illinois. This treatment model developed from a combination of four theoretical backgrounds (Rogerian, behavioral, cognitive, and reality) with emphasis on behavioral and emotional change. The treatment plan is tailored to the individual adolescent and includes both the family and the adolescent [18,19]. It is included in the National Registry of Evidence-Based Programs and Practices (NREPP) and has been used for many notable studies on adolescent substance abuse treatment, such as the Cannabis Youth Treatment (CYT) study. Skill-building and counseling groups form the two main treatment methods in this model [19]. Skill-building is conducted in a group environment with 14 different subjects covered each week including life skills, self-esteem, family issues, recovery lifestyle, and relapse prevention [19]. An individualized Master Treatment Plan (MTP) dictates which and how many skill-building groups an adolescent attends. There are 12 30–45-minute presentations in each group [19]. Counseling groups occur weekly and last 35–40 minutes. They allow adolescents to openly discuss how to cope with their problems with peer feedback [19]. To incorporate flexibility around school and work, these group sessions are conducted in both the morning and evening.

Another example of an adolescent substance abuse IOP is Insight Treatment Centers: A Program for Teens and their Families, located in Sherman Oaks and Pasadena, California. The program is an alternative to the adolescent residential treatment center and provides a higher intensity level than the traditional outpatient treatment. The target population comprises adolescents ranging in age from 13 to 18 years who are dealing with SUDs, comorbid mental health disorders, social and family issues, behavioral problems, and self-harming behaviors [20]. A key element of treatment is the fundamental approach of IOPs where the adolescent undergoing treatment remains in school and lives at home, which facilitates development of new coping skills and supportive drug-free peer groups in the safety of a highly structured treatment program [20]. This promotes growth and long-term change in family interactions, and there is a strong emphasis in the program on family therapy. However, many different modalities are used in treatment that is tailored to the individual adolescent. Some examples of the enhanced services provided include EEG biofeedback, art and music therapy, guided imagery, and meditation. The program begins with attendance on 4 days per week with structured weekend plans, integration with community 12-Step groups and counselors available on call for crisis 24 hours by phone.

There are additional groups in addition to the standard curriculum such as process groups, gender-specific groups, and multi-family groups. Individual and family therapy sessions and case management are done at a minimum of once per week [20]. Adolescents remain in their regular school environment during treatment, or attend independent schooling that is integrated into the IOP as a separate service. As adolescents achieve therapeutic goals in their treatment, there are progressive steps down in the number and days in treatment [20]. Insight IOP is just one example of the many different adolescent substance abuse IOPs available for adolescent substance abuse treatment.

SUMMARY

Intensive outpatient programs for adolescent substance use disorders remain an under-utilized community resource, due to many factors. However, awareness of this valuable modality of treatment can help promote successful treatment of the adolescent by providing a continuum and seamless transition between higher and lower levels of care. Multiple services can be provided by an IOP, and there is considerable variation among different programs in terms of intensity level, duration, program content, therapeutic modalities, and services provided. Numerous advantages and challenges exist and more research is needed to elucidate various aspects of IOPs and how they can best benefit adolescents struggling with SUDs.

References

1. Kaminer Y. Adolescent substance abuse. In: Galanter M, Kleber H (eds), *Textbook of Substance Abuse Treatment*, 4th edn. Arlington, VA: American Psychiatric Publishing, 2008; pp. 483–484.
2. Center for Substance Abuse Treatment (CSAT). Placement criteria and expected treatment outcomes. In: *Treatment Improvement Protocol (TIP) Series 8. Intensive Outpatient Treatment for Alcohol and Other Drug Abuse*. DHHS Publication No. (SMA) 94B2077. Rockville, MD: Substance Abuse and Mental Health Services Administration, 1994.
3. Jaffe SL, Solhkhah R. Substance abuse disorders. In: *Textbook of Child and Adolescent Psychiatry*, 3rd edn. Arlington, VA: American Psychiatric Publishing, 2004; pp. 800–805.
4. American Academy of Child and Adolescent Psychiatry (AACAP). Practice parameter for the assessment and treatment of children and adolescents with substance use disorders. *J Am Acad Child Adoles Psychiatry* 2005;**44**: 609–621.
5. Center for Substance Abuse Treatment. Introduction. In: *Treatment Improvement Protocol (TIP) Series 8. Intensive Outpatient Treatment for Alcohol and Other Drug Abuse*. DHHS Publication No. (SMA) 94B2077. Rockville, MD: Substance Abuse and Mental Health Services Administration, 1994.
6. American Society of Addiction Medicine (ASAM). *ASAM PPC-2R: ASAM Patient Placement Criteria for the Treatment of Substance-Related Disorders*, 2nd edn, revised. Chevy Chase, MD: American Society of Addiction Medicine, Inc. 2001.
7. Deas D, Riggs P, Langenbucher J, *et al.* Adolescents are not adults: Developmental considerations in alcohol users. *Alcohol Clin Exp Res* 2000;**24**:232–237.
8. Milin R, Walker S. Adolescent substance abuse. In: Ruiz P, Strain E (eds), *Lowinson and Ruiz's Substance Abuse: A Comprehensive Textbook*, 5th edn. Philadelphia, PA: Lippincott Williams & Wilkins, 2011; pp. 792–801.
9. Center for Substance Abuse Treatment (CSAT). Executive summary and recommendations. In: *Treatment Improvement Protocol (TIP) Series 32. Treatment of Adolescents with Substance Use Disorders*. DHHS Publication No. (SMA) 99-3283. Rockville, MD: Substance Abuse and Mental Health Services Administration, 1999.
10. Center for Substance Abuse Treatment (CSAT). Adapting intensive outpatient treatment for specific populations. In: *Treatment Improvement Protocol (TIP) Series 47. Substance Abuse: Clinical Issues in Intensive Outpatient Treatment*. DHHS Publication No. (SMA) 94B2077. Rockville, MD: Substance Abuse and Mental Health Services Administration, 1994.
11. Martin CS, Winters KC. Diagnosis and assessment of alcohol use disorders among adolescents. *Alcohol Health Res W* 1998;**22**:95–105.
12. Center for Substance Abuse Treatment. Components of an effective IOT program. In: *Treatment Improvement Protocol (TIP) Series 8. Intensive Outpatient Treatment for Alcohol and Other Drug Abuse*. DHHS Publication No. (SMA) 94B2077. Rockville, MD: Substance Abuse and Mental Health Services Administration, 1994.
13. Myers MG, Brown SA. The adolescent relapse coping questionnaire: psychometric validation. *J Stud Alcohol* 1996;**57**:40–46.

14. Fink EB, Longabaugh R, McCrady BM, *et al.* Effectiveness of alcoholism treatment in partial versus inpatient settings: twenty-four month outcomes. *Addict Behav* 1985;**10**:235–248.

15. Muck R, Zempolich KA, Titus JC, *et al.* An overview of the effectiveness of adolescent substance abuse treatment models. *Youth Soc* 2001;**33**:143–168.

16. Center for Substance Abuse Treatment (CSAT). Intensive outpatient treatment approaches. In: *Treatment Improvement Protocol (TIP) Series 47. Substance Abuse: Clinical Issues in Intensive Outpatient Treatment.* DHHS Publication No. (SMA) 94B2077. Rockville, MD: Substance Abuse and Mental Health Services Administration, 1994.

17. White AM, Jordan JD, Schroeder KM, *et al.* Predictors of relapse during treatment and treatment completion among marijuana-dependent adolescents in an intensive outpatient substance abuse program. *Subst Abuse* 2004;**25**:53–59.

18. Dembo R, Muck RD. Adolescent outpatient treatment. In: Leukefel CG, *et al.* (eds), *Adolescent Substance Abuse.* New York: Springer Science + Business Media LLC, 2009; pp. 97–117.

19. NREPP. Chestnut Health Systems – Bloomington Adolescent Outpatient (OP) and Intensive Outpatient (IOP) Treatment Model. NREPP, 2007. Available from: http://nrepp.samhsa.gov/ViewIntervention.aspx?id=140 on 6/6/2011.

20. Insight Treatment Programs. Website: www.insighttreatment.com.

30

Adolescent Behaviors Out of Control: An Introduction To Adolescent Residential Treatment

Reef Karim

The Control Center For Addictions, Beverly Hills, CA, USA

INTRODUCTION

Research and clinical experience reveal addiction to be a disease of our youth. The majority of adults with substance use disorders admit they began using in their adolescence. As such, the proper treatment of adolescent substance abuse with the inclusion of comprehensive family therapy is paramount to sustained recovery.

Approximately 90% of individuals who develop chronic substance dependence disorders with associated severe mental, psychiatric, and behavioral problems start using illicit substances while under the age of 18 years [1]. Drug and alcohol abuse and dependence are the most prevalent causes of adolescent morbidity and mortality in the United States. Consequences of adolescent substance abuse may include academic failure, social and familial disruption, overdose, automobile accidents, increased risk for sexually transmitted diseases, arrest, and incarceration [2].

Unintentional death involving prescription drugs in adolescence increased 150% between 2001 and 2009. In 2008, drug overdose exceeded highway fatalities as a leading cause of death among adolescents [3].

One size does not fit all. Residential substance abuse programs designed to treat adults often fail to meet the unique needs of adolescents. Compared to adults, adolescents have higher rates of dual diagnosis [4], different developmental needs [5], and higher rates of binge and opportunistic use [6]. The developmental period of adolescence is distinguished by a transition from the dependent, family-oriented state of childhood to the independent, peer-oriented state of adulthood [7]. In this transition, there is an alteration in emotional, cognitive, and social skills that often facilitates novelty-seeking, sensation-seeking, and exploratory behavior. These behavioral changes facilitate substance use and experimentation. The notion of enhanced reward-seeking combined with the relatively delayed maturation of cognitive control is a common model for understanding the peak onset of substance abuse in adolescence [8]. And the direct neurobiological effect of drugs of abuse on adolescent brains may have more severe consequences than in adults because of the additional effects on ongoing development.

The majority of adolescents with a substance use disorder are not in treatment. Only 10% of the estimated 1.4 million adolescents in the U.S., ages 12–17, with an illicit drug problem are receiving treatment compared with one in five adults [9]. There is very little data supporting the efficacy of inpatient adolescent treatment. Research on the effectiveness of treatment for adolescents is still a new field, with relatively few scientifically rigorous studies published to date [10].

ASSESSMENT AND ADOLESCENT PROBLEM BEHAVIOR

In assessing an adolescent for residential treatment, a multiple assessment approach is recommended as substance abuse will affect multiple areas of a youth's life.

Clinical Handbook of Adolescent Addiction, First Edition. Richard Rosner.
© 2013 John Wiley & Sons, Ltd. Published 2013 by John Wiley & Sons, Ltd.

A good adolescent assessment will include:

1. Substance use history – illicit drugs, prescription drugs, over-the-counter drugs, supplements, tobacco, inhalants, synthetic drugs (bath salts, spice, etc.).
2. Mental health impairment – depression, suicidal ideation or attempts, anxiety disorders, conduct disorders, autism, attention-deficit/hyperactivity disorder (ADHD), behavioral disorders, personality disorders, psychotic disorders, eating disorders, trauma, etc.
3. Family history – substance use by parents, guardians, or extended family; mental and physical health impairment and treatment.
4. School experience – academic and behavioral performance, learning disabilities, attendance.
5. Social history – peer relationships, romantic relationships, interpersonal skills, neighborhood environment, gang involvement.
6. Juvenile justice involvement.
7. Sexual history – sexual orientation, sexual activity, sexual abuse, sexually transmitted diseases, HIV status, risky behaviors.
8. Medical health status.
9. Strengths and resources – self-esteem, family, community supports, coping skills, motivation for treatment.

Assessments should include psychological testing measures and (with the adolescent's consent) the gathering of information from parents, other family members, and adults and peers who are important to the youth [11].

Understanding the motivation for adolescent substance use is obviously important. Lecca and Watts report three primary motivations for adolescent substance use: a coping motive; a drug experience motive, and a peer motive [12].

A thorough evaluation of potential risk factors for adolescent substance abuse is vital. Hawkins and Catalano provide a good overview of potential risk factors, as noted in Table 30.1 [13]. Further, families experiencing high levels of conflict are more likely to have low levels of parent-child involvement. These family conditions are related to poor parental monitoring and association with deviant peers 1 year later. Poor parental monitoring and associations with deviant peers are strong proximal predictors of engagement in an array of problem behaviors at a 2-year follow-up [14].

RESIDENTIAL TREATMENT PROGRAMS

There is a paucity of outcomes research for residential treatment programs in general. Some treatment centers

Table 30.1 Potential risk factors for adolescent substance abuse.

- Availability of drugs
- Laws and norms being favorable toward behavior
- Extreme economic deprivation
- Neighborhood disorganization
- Physiological factors
- Family history of alcohol and drug behavior and attitudes
- Poor and inconsistent family management practices
- Family conflict
- Low bonding to family
- Early and persistent problem behaviors
- Academic failure
- Low degree of commitment to school
- Peer rejection in elementary grades
- Association with drug-using peers
- Alienation and rebelliousness
- Attitudes favorable to drug use
- Early onset of drug use
- Comorbidities with mental health disorders

will boast an 85% "cure" or "still sober" rate which often means eighty-five percent of the alumni they got hold of reported continued sobriety a few months after discharge. But the research methodology for these "self-reported" studies is often flawed. Many residential treatment programs have no incentive to initiate outcome studies as marketing often trumps data and realistic numbers of former patients with continued sobriety may not be as impressive. When a family or individual is looking for an inpatient residential treatment program, many factors come to mind, including: location, quality and professionalism of the staff, cost, accreditation, admissions experience, a feeling of safety, quality of the accommodations, food, atmosphere of respect from clients and staff, customization of a therapeutic treatment plan, diversity of groups, specialization of treatment, other amenities, etc. The inclusion of objective data and diagnostic measures during the admissions stay (objective data measures pre-, during, and post stay) are often not collected. A successful stay and good patient care are often difficult to define objectively.

DATOS-A: NIDA's Ongoing Drug Abuse Treatment Outcome Studies for Adolescents

In the first large-scale study designed to evaluate drug abuse treatment outcomes among adolescents in age-specific treatment programs, National Institute on Drug Abuse (NIDA)-supported researchers found that longer stays in these treatment programs can effectively decrease drug and alcohol use and criminal activity as well as improve school performance and psychological adjustment. This study analyzed data from 23 community-based adolescent treatment programs that addressed peer relationships, educational concerns, and family issues such as parent-child relationships and parental substance abuse. The 418 adolescents in the residential treatment programs received education, individual and group counseling, and interventions to develop social responsibility [15]. Residential treatment for adolescents would be indicated if 24-hour supervision, a sober and safe environment, mental health treatment in an inpatient setting, or other clinical decision was deemed necessary for inpatient residential treatment.

With regards to overall outcomes, adolescents showed significant declines in the use of marijuana and alcohol when comparing the year before treatment to the year after treatment. Weekly or more frequent marijuana use dropped from 80% to 44%, and abstinence from any use of illicit drugs increased from 52% to 58%. Heavy drinking decreased from 34% to 20%, and criminal activity decreased from 76% to 53%. Adolescents also reported fewer thoughts of suicide, lower hostility, and higher self-esteem. In the year following treatment, more adolescents attended school and reported better than average grades.

Overall, previous research indicates that a minimum of 90 days of treatment for residential drug-free programs is predictive of positive outcomes for adults in treatment. Better treatment outcomes were reported among adolescents who met or exceeded this length of treatment as well. This study confirms that community-based drug treatment programs designed for adolescents can reduce substance abuse and have a positive impact on many other aspects of their life [15].

NATIONAL SURVEY STUDY: ADOLESCENT SUBSTANCE ABUSE PROGRAMS

Brannigan et al. published an article on the results of a systematic evaluation of the quality of highly regarded adolescent treatment programs in the United States to develop a guide that would define effective treatment [16]. Utilizing an advisory panel of 22 experts in the field, directors of 50 US states' alcohol and drug abuse agencies, national organizations, and federal agencies, their research team used written questionnaires followed by a structured, recorded telephone interview from each program and a follow-up interview 12 months later.

Program characteristics were measured and nine key elements of effective adolescent drug treatment were found [16]:

1. *Assessment and treatment matching:* Programs should conduct comprehensive assessments that cover psychiatric, psychological, and medical problems, learning disabilities, family functioning, and other aspects of the adolescent's life.
2. *Comprehensive, integrated treatment approach:* Program services should address all aspects of an adolescent's life.
3. *Family involvement in treatment:* Research shows that involving parents in the adolescent's drug treatment produces better outcomes.
4. *Developmentally appropriate program:* Activities and materials should reflect the developmental differences between adults and adolescents.
5. *Engaging and retaining teens in treatment:* Treatment programs should build a climate of trust between the adolescent and the therapist.
6. *Qualified staff:* Staff should be trained in adolescent development, co-occurring mental disorders, substance abuse, and addiction.
7. *Gender and cultural competence:* Programs should address the distinct needs of adolescent boys and girls as well as cultural differences among minorities.
8. *Continuing care:* Programs should include relapse prevention training, aftercare plans, referrals to community resources, and follow-up.
9. *Treatment outcomes:* Rigorous evaluation is required to measure success, target resources, and improve treatment services.

In ranking the 144 highly regarded adolescent-only substance abuse treatment programs in the survey, the top quartile programs were more likely to be 20 years old or more and were more likely to offer multi-dimensional family therapy and the therapeutic community approach. The elements with the poorest overall performance were assessment and treatment matching, engaging and retaining teens in treatment, gender and cultural competence, and treatment outcomes. Less than half of the programs (45%) reported using a standardized substance abuse instrument or a clinical interview [16].

For engaging and retaining teens in treatment, 39% of the programs reported an emphasis on building a therapeutic alliance between staff and clients; 41% reported utilizing motivational enhancement techniques, such as motivational interviewing, and 48% reported incorporating positive reinforcements to provide incentives for client participation. Regarding gender and cultural competence, 35% of programs reported providing content that differs for male and female patients; 24% of programs were designed to meet the needs of minorities, and 12% of programs in the survey were designed to meet the needs of gay and lesbian adolescents. For treatment outcomes, 44% of the programs reported not collecting any data related to client outcomes, and 35% reported analyzing their own internally gathered data [16].

SPECIALIZED ADOLESCENT TREATMENT STRATEGIES

Adolescents have little motivation to stop using drugs or participate in treatment. Many teens don't find their substance use to be a problem or they would rather make repeated attempts to stop using on their own than go to treatment.

Studies reveal that the use of motivational incentives can be effective with adolescents. Incentives can help adolescents decrease resistance to treatment. Even if they don't believe they have a substance use disorder, they will often actively participate in treatment to receive the incentives [17]. Once the decision is reached to participate in treatment, adolescents who receive incentives achieve greater abstinence, better school attendance, improved relationships with their parents, and less depression, compared to control groups [18].

By targeting the right reinforcer to the right target population with a clear identification of the desired target behavior, contingency management can be a powerful tool in adolescent treatment. Additionally, intermittent reinforcers have been found to work well, as has receiving the incentive soon after achieving the targeted behavior.

Additionally, the use of family-based treatment approaches for adolescent substance abuse has shown great promise. There is more data emerging on MDFT (multi-dimensional family therapy) in both outpatient and inpatient adolescent treatment settings. The MDFT model approaches the treatment of the multi-dimensional aspect of the teen's life, emphasizing the teen's internal world, their relationship with parents and peers, and the world of the parents themselves. Each aspect of the teen's life is addressed in a manner consistent with the motivational interviewing principle of "rolling with resistance." According to NIDA, MDFT for adolescent drug abuse offers broad and lasting benefits compared with cognitive-behavioral therapy (CBT). The therapeutic approach integrating individual, family, and community interventions of MDFT had a better one-year success rate with fewer drug-related problems and improved health compared to those treated with standard counseling based on CBT [19].

SUMMARY

Adolescent residential treatment programs need to be studied further. Clinical programs reveal difficulties in engaging and retaining teens in treatment as the primary challenge. Few adolescents seek treatment on their own, and denial about their drug use is high. Programs need to find creative techniques to engage and retain adolescents in treatment by making activities relevant to their concerns [16].

There are still relatively few substance use treatment programs designed specifically for adolescents, with very little research and evidence comparing the efficacy of different types of adolescent treatment strategies. Clinical experience and preliminary survey data show that sensitivity to sex and cultural differences helps develop a successful therapeutic alliance as well as a safe environment that can lead to behavioral change.

It is also critical that more adolescent substance abuse treatment programs adopt standardized assessment tools to ensure that adolescents are evaluated and matched properly [16].

In conclusion, effective treatment for adolescents with substance abuse disorders (and possible co-occurring disorders) requires key elements including: appropriate assessment specific to the world of the adolescent; family involvement throughout treatment; developmentally appropriate, gender-specific groups; a highly qualified and experienced staff; addressing co-occurring mental health disorders; and management strategies used to motivate teens to continue with treatment [19].

References

1. Dennis M, Barbor TF, Roebuck MC, Donaldson J. Changing the focus: the case for recognizing and treating marijuana use disorders. *Addiction* 2002;**97**:514–515.
2. Botvin GJ, Griffin KW. Life Skills Training: Theory: methods and effectiveness of a drug abuse prevention approach. In: Wagner E, Waldron H (eds), *Innovations in Adolescent Substance Abuse Interventions*. New York, NY: Elsevier Science, 2001; pp. 31–50.
3. Cermak T. *A Blueprint for Adolescent Addiction Treatment*. CSAM Review Council, 2009.
4. Brown SA, Myers MG, Mott MA, Vik PW. Correlates of success following treatment for adolescent substance abuse. *Appl Prev Psychol* 1994;**3**:61–73.
5. Winters KC. Treating adolescents with substance use disorders: an overview of practice issues and treatment outcome. *Subst Abuse* 1999;**20**:203–224.
6. Dennis ML. Treatment research on adolescent drug and alcohol abuse: despite progress many challenges remain. *Connection*. Washington, DC:Academy for Health Services Research and Health Policy, 2002.
7. Hardin MG., Ernst M. Functional brain imaging of development-related risk and vulnerability for substance use in adolescents. *J Addict Med* 2009;**3**(2):47–54.

8. Spear LP. The adolescent brain and age related behavioral manifestations. *Neurosci Biobehav Rev* 2000;**24**:417–463.

9. Office of Applied Studies. *Report From the 2001 National Household Study on Drug Abuse Volume 1: Summary of National Findings*. Rockville, MD: Substance Abuse and Mental Health Services Administration, 2002.

10. Williams RJ, Chang SY. A comprehensive and comparative review of adolescent substance abuse treatment outcome. *Clin Psychol-Sci Pr* 2000;**7**:138–166.

11. Center for Substance Abuse Treatment. *Screening and Assessing Adolescents for Substance Use Disorders*. Treatment Improvement Protocol (TIP) Series No. 31. Substance Abuse and Mental Health Services Administration, 2001.

12. Lecca LJ, Watts DT. Preschoolers and Substance Abuse; Strategies for prevention and intervention. *Journal of Abnormal Clinical Psychology* 1993;**21**:153–64.

13. Hawkins JD, Catalano RF, Miller JY. Risk and protective factors for alcohol and other drug problems in adolescence and early adulthood: Implications for substance abuse prevention. *Psychological Bulletin* 1992;**112**(1): 64–105.

14. Arv DV, Duncan TE, Duncan SC, Hops H. Adolescent problem behavior: the influence of parents and peers. *Behav Res Ther* 1999;**37**:217–230.

15. Hser Y-I, Grella CE, Hubbard RL. An evaluation of drug treatment for adolescents in four U.S. cities. *Arch Gen Psychiatry* 2001;**58**:689–695.

16. Brannigan R, Schackman B, Falco M, Millman R. The quality of highly regarded adolescent substance abuse treatment programs. results of an in-depth national survey. *Arch Pediatr Adolesc Med* 2004;**158**:904–909.

17. Petry N. A comprehensive guide to the application of contingency management procedures in clinical settings. *Drug Alcohol Depend* 2000;**58**:9–25.

18. Higgins S, Silverman K, Heil S (eds). *Contingency Management in Substance Abuse Treatment*. New York: Guilford Press, 2008.

19. Smith D, Nosal B. Integrating Multi-Dimensional Family Therapy (MDFT) with substance abusing adolescents in a residential treatment setting. *Counselor Magazine* June 2011; pp. 28–33.

31

Adolescent Group Treatments: Twelve-Step and Beyond

Jeremy Martinez

UCLA Addiction Medicine Clinic, Los Angeles, CA, USA

INTRODUCTION

Relatively brief residential or outpatient addiction treatment of 3–9 months' duration is often insufficient for sustained, life-long sobriety for the adolescent. Additional support comes in the form of mutual self-help groups, or group therapy. Mutual self-help groups, such as the twelve-step groups, Alcoholics Anonymous (AA) and Narcotics Anonymous (NA), provide extended support for the addicted adolescent. Facilitated recovery groups provide treatment, having a trained group leader or a licensed therapist to guide the process. This is the distinction between a "support group," which does not include a licensed facilitator, and a "treatment" or "therapy" group, which may be led by a licensed drug counselor, social worker, psychologist, psychiatrist, or other mental health professional. Common facilitated groups include cognitive-behavioral therapy (CBT), motivational enhancement therapy (MET), and twelve-step facilitated (TSF) groups.

The group process, whether as a *treatment (therapy) group* or *support group*, is helpful in the recovery from addiction in several ways. Dr Irvin D. Yalom [1] describes group psychotherapy as having 11 key elements (see Table 31.1). These curative parts of the group process are integral to mutual self-help groups as well as therapy groups. Specifically, there are several of these principles that are crucial in the process of recovery from drugs and alcohol. One of these is the *instillation of hope*, whereby members who have longer periods of sobriety may encourage newer members, while in facilitated groups the therapist can instill hope by maintaining a positive reference frame in the therapy. *Universality* is another important principle described

by Yalom. In recovery groups, addicts and alcoholics are able to identify with one another, having similar life struggles related to drug and alcohol use; this allows for some relief, or *catharsis* (another of Yalom's principles), when realizing that others are dealing with, and have overcome, similar problems. *Development of socialization* is another important principle in the recovery from drug and alcohol addiction. Addicts and alcoholics tend to use their substance of choice in a solitary manner as their disease progresses, and the ability to have quality relationships often suffers. Participation in group therapy or support provides new relationships with other sober adolescents. The other principles of group treatment are listed in Table 31.1.

HISTORY OF TWELVE-STEP GROUPS

Alcoholics Anonymous (AA) was started in 1935 as the brainchild of a New York stockbroker, Bill Wilson ("Bill W."), and a physician, Dr Robert Smith ("Dr Bob"). As alcoholics, they strived to create a program of mutual self-help, which had its origins in the Oxford Group, a non-denominational Christian movement [2]. AA, also known as "The Program," is based on the principles of the addict's powerlessness over drugs and alcohol, self-reflection, making amends for past wrongs, and helping others.

In addition to the Twelve Steps (see Table 31.2) are Twelve Traditions, which explain the rules of AA groups, such as protecting the anonymity of its members; the Twelve Traditions also explain the AA leadership structure [3]. AA has expanded to include over 100 other groups, including Narcotics Anonymous (NA),

Clinical Handbook of Adolescent Addiction, First Edition. Richard Rosner.
© 2013 John Wiley & Sons, Ltd. Published 2013 by John Wiley & Sons, Ltd.

Table 31.1 Yalom's eleven principles of group psychotherapy [1].

1. Instillation of hope
2. Universality
3. Imparting of information
4. Altruism
5. The corrective recapitulation of the primary family group
6. Development of socializing techniques
7. Imitative behavior
8. Interpersonal learning
9. Group cohesiveness
10. Catharsis
11. Existential factors

Cocaine Anonymous (CA), Marijuana Anonymous (MA), and Gamblers Anonymous (GA).

ADOLESCENTS AND THE TWELVE-STEPS

In the community, twelve-step groups are widely available, are free of charge, and the only requirement is to have a desire to stop using drugs and alcohol. Only 10% of the membership of AA is under age 30 [4]. Many adolescents feel uncomfortable in AA groups, feel they do not belong, or have difficulty identifying as an alcoholic or addict. Dr Steven Jaffe produced a workbook describing possible modifications of the steps of Alcoholics Anonymous for adolescents [5]. His recommendations include placing emphasis on *empowerment* through cessation of drugs and alcohol, rather than focusing on *powerlessness* in the first step. Exploring the additional activities the adolescent can perform when *sober* is one way to establish this empowerment. Other issues that Jaffe mentions include the difficulty of establishing a safe and consistent "higher power." Most adolescents have only known their parents as a higher power, and many of those with drug or alcohol problems have grown up in unstable home environments, experiencing abuse and neglect. Difficulty forming healthy attachments can be an obstacle when conceptualizing a higher power, whether it be God or the fellowship of an AA group. Consistent, nurturing relationships in the context of twelve-step participation can be a formative experience for adolescents working toward sobriety.

Each and every twelve-step meeting has its own demographics, and young people should be encouraged to explore multiple meeting locations to find an appropriate fit. Local meetings may be found by writing PO

Table 31.2 The 12 steps of Alcoholics Anonymous [2].

1. We admitted we were powerless over alcohol – that our lives had become unmanageable
2. Came to believe that a Power greater than ourselves could restore us to sanity
3. Made a decision to turn our will and our lives over to the care of God *as we understood Him*
4. Made a searching and fearless moral inventory of ourselves
5. Admitted to God, to ourselves, and to another human being the exact nature of our wrongs
6. Were entirely ready to have God remove all these defects of character
7. Humbly asked Him to remove our shortcomings
8. Made a list of all persons we had harmed, and became willing to make amends to them all
9. Made direct amends to such people wherever possible, except when to do so would injure them or others
10. Continued to take personal inventory and when we were wrong promptly admitted it
11. Sought through prayer and meditation to improve our conscious contact with God *as we understood Him*, praying only for knowledge of His will for us and the power to carry that out
12. Having had a spiritual awakening as the result of these steps, we tried to carry this message to alcoholics, and to practice these principles in all our affairs

Box 459, Grand Central Station, New York, NY, or online at http://www.aa.org.

EFFICACY AND SAFETY OF TWELVE-STEP MEETINGS

Several recent studies have investigated the efficacy of twelve-step meetings for alcoholism and drug addiction in adolescents. As has been found in adults, the adolescents who participate in twelve-step meetings in the community tend to be those with greater severity of addiction [2,6]. Adolescents who participate in AA/NA groups are nearly twice as likely to remain abstinent from drugs and alcohol at 6-month follow-up (based on percentage of days abstinent) compared to those who did not attend meetings [4]. In a review of 11 studies examining community involvement in twelve-step meetings, adolescents who participated in AA/NA were two to three times more likely to remain sober [3].

There have been some concerns about the safety of teens attending twelve-step meetings, and this has been examined [7]. Youths attending AA/NA meetings generally rate their feeling of safety as "high," with a mean of 8.6 on a scale of 1 being "not at all safe" and 10 being "very safe." Parents of these teens rated safety slightly lower, but still considered twelve-step meetings generally safe, with a mean of 7.6 out of 10. Over the course of AA/NA involvement, 21.9% of adolescents reported at least one instance of a negative experience: feeling threatened, intimidated, or sexually harassed. Complaints by teens included "people coming drunk to meetings and harassing others." Despite these negative experiences, none of the teens in this study discontinued AA/NA meetings due to safety concerns.

FACILITATED GROUP TREATMENT FOR ADOLESCENTS

Group treatment involves a licensed facilitator, such as a drugs counselor, social worker, psychologist, psychiatrist, or other mental health professional. Once again, these groups are considered *treatment* rather than *support* because of the presence of a licensed group leader, trained to facilitate the prescribed treatment. These treatment groups range from facilitated twelve-step groups, to MET and CBT-oriented groups; combinations of these treatment modalities may also be used. Some of the evidence-based treatment groups will be discussed here.

FACILITATED TWELVE-STEP GROUPS

Twelve-step groups are facilitated in a number of settings, most commonly as part of a residential (or *inpatient*) treatment program, day treatment (or *outpatient*) program, or intensive outpatient program (IOP). These details of these treatment formats are discussed in previous chapters. Twelve-Step Facilitation (TSF) has been investigated in adults, and its efficacy has been reviewed by several authors [8,9]. There has been limited study of this technique among adolescents, although this may be considered an evidence-based treatment for adults.

This type of treatment involves assisting patients in seven areas, which are addressed in AA/NA [10]. The first of these is *Acceptance*, whereby the clinician assists the patient in the understanding of addiction as a disease, realizing the chronic and relapsing nature of the disorder. The next is *Surrender*, where the patient recognizes the powerlessness of the addicted individual over drugs and/or alcohol. The *Cognitive* step helps the patient to understand the errors of one's thinking related

to substance use, including defense mechanisms such as denial. There may be *Emotional* difficulties, as well as unproductive *Behavioral* patterns that are involved in the drug or alcohol use, and the astute clinician will explore these with the patient. The *Social* environment of the addict or alcoholic can limit the patient's progress, and providing a new support network in AA/NA can be very helpful. Finally, the clinician may guide the patient through the development of *Spirituality*, finding assistance through a "Higher Power." This does not mean that the patient must believe in a Judeo-Christian God; a higher power may be general spirituality, a general belief in morality, or karma, or the fellowship of AA/NA. Facilitating involvement in AA/NA allows the patient to have a continued network of sober individuals, with a focus on personal development and service to others.

MOTIVATIONAL ENHANCEMENT THERAPY AND CBT

There is clinical evidence for the effectiveness of Motivational Enhancement (or Effectiveness) Therapy in adolescents [11–14]. Motivational interviewing is a technique formulated by William Miller and Steven Rollnick, which is patient-centered, explores ambivalence to change, focuses on patient strengths, and provides support for behavioral change [15]. This technique respects patient *autonomy,* which can be useful when engaging adolescents in treatment – treating the patient as an *individual*.

Motivational interviewing can be used to assist patients along the continuum of the *Stages of Change* (Table 31.3). Behavioral change begins with *Precontemplation*, the stage where an individual refuses to admit that a problem exists, or acknowledges the problem but refuses to make behavioral change. Next is *Contemplation*, the stage where the patient begins to realize the problem exists, yet continues to have ambivalence about treatment or behavioral change. When the patient acknowledges the problem and begins to take steps toward behavioral change, this is the phase of *Preparation*. This might include researching treatment facilities or patient care providers. The *Action* step involves engaging in treatment for behavioral change, which may include entering residential or outpatient treatment. For addicts and alcoholics, this is the stage when initial sobriety develops; this requires long-term investment of time in sobriety-related efforts, which is the *Maintenance* phase of behavioral change. These may take the form of involvement in twelve-step groups, participation in "aftercare" programs affiliated with

Table 31.3 Stages of change (based on Prochaska and Diclemente 1984 [16]).

Stage	Description
Precontemplation	In this stage, the patient does not believe, or refuses to admit, that he or she has an addiction. Alternatively, the individual may admit to a problem and this stage, but refuses to make changes in the behavior
Contemplation	The *contemplative* individual questions whether a problem exists, or recognizes the problem but has ambivalence about making changes
Preparation	At this stage, the patient recognizes the problem, and begins to take steps toward behavioral change
Action	In the *action* phase, the patient has begun taking steps toward change. For drug and alcohol-related problems, this might include entering residential or outpatient rehabilitation, or attending twelve-step meetings
Maintenance	*Maintenance* involves actively working to maintain behavioral change (or abstinence from drugs and alcohol). This may take the form of regular attendance at twelve-step meetings, attending "aftercare" programs through the attended rehabilitation facility, or participating in outpatient treatment with an addiction professional

their drug treatment program, or following-up in outpatient treatment with an addiction professional.

The stages of behavioral change are fluid, and may not progress in a linear fashion; the patient may switch from one stage to another, forward or reverse, at various times in the treatment process. Ambivalence is part of the psychology of addiction, so the clinician should not be discouraged by apparent backward progress along these stages of change. Many patients will continue to have doubts about proceeding with behavioral change as the treatment process progresses, which does not necessarily mean there is no overall improvement.

Motivational Effectiveness Therapy plus CBT (MET/CBT 5) is an evidence-based treatment for addiction that was proven to be successful for adolescents in the Cannabis Youth Treatment Trial [17]. MET/CBT 5 consists of two individual sessions of motivational interviewing or MET, followed by three group sessions of CBT. MET in this trial examined risks and benefits of continued marijuana use, and exploring the patient's goals for treatment according to their progress on the continuum of *Stages of Change*. Additional sessions were added in this trial, with an additional group of family treatments, including creating a "MET/CBT 12" group; however, it was found that MET/CBT 5 was just as efficacious as the other groups, and was more cost-effective [10].

SUMMARY

Maintaining abstinence from drugs and alcohol is difficult for adolescents, but group treatment and support can provide increased rates of maintained sobriety. Twelve-step groups such as AA/NA are mutual self-help groups that are generally safe and effective for adolescents. Drug or alcohol *treatment* involves a licensed provider, such as a drug counselor, psychiatrist, or other therapist. Facilitated twelve-step groups are a common part of treatment in drug and alcohol rehabilitation settings. CBT and MET can be administered in as few as five sessions, and may be a more cost-effective alternative to longer-term group therapies.

References

1. Yalom ID. *The Theory and Practice of Group Psychotherapy*. New York: Basic Books, 1970.
2. Alcoholics Anonymous. Timeline. Available at: http://aa.org/aatimeline.
3. Sussman S. A review of Alcoholics Anonymous/Narcotics Anonymous programs for teens. *Eval Health Prof* 2010;**33**:26–55.
4. The A.A. Grapevine, Inc. *Young People and A.A.* New York, NY:Alcoholics Anonymous World Services, Inc., 2007.
5. Jaffe SL. *Step Workbook for Adolescent Chemical Dependency Recovery: A Guide to the First Five Steps*. Washington, DC:American Psychiatric Press, 1990.
6. Kelly JF, Dow SJ, Yeterian JD, Kahler CW., Can 12-step group participation strengthen and extend the benefits of adolescent addiction treatment? A prospective analysis. *Drug Alcohol Depend* 2010;**110**:117–125.
7. Kelly JF, *et al. J Subst Abuse Treat* 2011;**40**:419–425.
8. Kelly JF, McCrady BS. Twelve step facilitation in non-specialty settings. *Recent Dev Alcohol* 2008;**18**:321–346.
9. Donovan DM, Floyd AS. Facilitating involvement in twelve step groups. *Recent Dev Alcohol* 2008;**18**:303–320.
10. Galanter M, Kleber HD. *The American Psychiatric Publishing Textbook of Substance Abuse Treatment*. Arlington, VA:American Psychiatric Publishing, 2008; pp. 376–380.

11. Riley KJ, Rieckmann T, McCarty D., Implementation of MET/CBT5 for adolescents. *J Behav Health Serv Res* 2008;**35**:304–314.

12. Cornelius JR, Douaihy A, Bukstein OG, Daley DC, Wood SD, Kelly TM, Salloum IM. Evaluation of cognitive behavioral therapy/motivational enhancement therapy (CBT/MET) in a treatment trial of comorbid MDD/ AUD adolescents. *Addict Behav* 2011;**36**:843–848.

13. Ramchand R, Griffin BA, Suttorp M, Harris KM, Morral A. Using a cross-study design to assess the efficacy of motivational enhancement therapy-cognitive behavioral therapy 5 (MET/CBT5) in treating adolescents with cannabis-related disorders. *J Stud Alcohol Drugs* 2011; **72**:380–389.

14. Miller WR, Rollnick S. *Preparing People to Change Addictive Behavior*. New York:Guilford Press, 1991.

15. Levonius, Arnaout B. *Handbook of Motivation and Change: A Practical Guide for Clinicians*. Washington, DC: American Psychiatric Publishing, Inc., 2010; pp. 12–14.

16. Prochaska JO, DiClemente CC. Self change processes, self efficacy and decisional balance across five stages of smoking cessation. *Prog Clin Biol Res*. 1984;**156**: 131–40.

17. Dennis M, Godley SH, Diamond G, Tims FM, Babor T, Donaldson J, et al. The Cannabis Youth Treatment (CYT) Study: main findings from two randomized trials. *J Subst Abuse* 2004;**27**:197–213.

32

Psychopharmacology for the Addicted Adolescent

Timothy W. Fong

Semel Institute for Neuroscience and Human Behavior at UCLA; UCLA Addiction Psychiatry Fellowship; UCLA Addiction Medicine Clinic, Los Angeles, CA, USA

INTRODUCTION

The use of medications for the management of addictive disorders has seen increased attention and effort since the mid-1990s. Currently, the US Food and Drug Administration (FDA) has approved several medications for opioid, alcohol, and nicotine dependence. Ongoing research continues to investigate the use of vaccines, genetic profiling, and injectable medications as means of offering a variety of treatment options [1]. In adults, the use of medications for addictive disorders has produced mixed results in the office-based setting. For experienced addiction specialists, the addition of medications to the available treatment toolbox has allowed a greater range of patients to be treated. For non-addiction specialists, there remain questions on how most effectively to use these medications.

To date, none of the FDA-approved medications for addictive disorders is approved for use in children and adolescents. Significant questions remain about how effective and safe these medications are with an adolescent population. Further questions about the role of medications in addictive disorders are raised by recent reviews, which suggest that medications for treatment of depression in adolescents are not significantly better than placebo [2].

There are other explanations about why the field has been so limited. First, there is a general bias against the use of medications for the treatment of addictive disorders [3]. This comes from treatment providers, families, and patients themselves. Recovery groups for a long time stressed that any medication prescribed meant that "you are not sober." For an adolescent population, these attitudes can have a profound impact on readiness to accept medications. Secondly, obtaining funding for adolescent clinical trials focusing on medications is difficult, especially without industry support and with growing concerns about psychoactive medications in children and adolescents. With the recent controversy over antidepressant use in children and adolescents, pharmaceutical companies have been reluctant to fund studies in this population [4]. Thirdly, there is the hope that adolescents will "mature out" of addictive behaviors naturally, as the frontal lobe develops. This belief comes out of optimism that natural recovery and time will restore behavioral controls and that adding psychotropic medication may in fact be more damaging than helpful to recovery [5].

Some researchers believe that one of the challenges to developing effective pharmacological treatments for addicted adolescents is because the adolescent brain is "a changing organ" [5]. The brain's developmental growth processes may result in a drug affecting adolescents differently than adults –both intended and unintended – depending on their individual stage of maturation. Thus, research on adults may identify promising pharmacological treatments but claims that they are effective with adolescents must be met with doubt. Definitive medication recommendations for substance-abusing adolescents will need the completion of well-designed, controlled, clinical trials.

Still, the possibility that medications can help the addicted adolescent is a compelling one. Given that addiction is a brain disease with biological, psychological, and social origins, it makes sense that any early intervention with an effective medication may limit the

Clinical Handbook of Adolescent Addiction, First Edition. Richard Rosner.
© 2013 John Wiley & Sons, Ltd. Published 2013 by John Wiley & Sons, Ltd.

development of symptoms that will lead to full-blown expression of the disease.

One of the clear-cut tasks is to figure out which adolescents will respond to medications. Examples of the types of adult subtypes that do respond to medications are those with a strong family history for addiction and an early age (12–14 years) of onset [6]. Medications should always be considered as adjuncts to proven psychosocial interventions for adolescents with addictive disorders.

MEDICATION APPROACHES

Pharmacotherapy for addictive disorders in adults targets the symptoms of substance dependence, such as withdrawal symptoms, and reducing urges and cravings to use [7].

Substitution therapy utilizes medications that act on the same receptors as the drug of abuse. They are used to treat withdrawal because they mimic the effects of the abused drug and then they can eliminate drug craving, and, in some instances, block the euphoric effects of the abusable drug. Examples of substitution medications include methadone maintenance for opioid dependence, and nicotine replacement therapy [8].

Aversive interventions, such as disulfiram (Antabuse) create an aversive consequence of using, which will lead to avoidance of the drug of abuse. Aversive approaches are considered different from targeting the core pathophysiology of addictive disorders because they are not addressing fundamental changes or targeting regions of the brain known to be affected by drugs of abuse [9].

Anti-craving agents are intended to reduce the urges and cravings felt toward using substances of abuse. This is a relatively newer approach because it is targeting signs and symptoms of the addictive disorder that are automatic and compulsive, and when experienced can quickly lead to relapse. Acamprosate and naltrexone are examples of medications that aim to blunt or reduce cravings [7].

Another pharmacological approach is to treat co-occurring disorders. The premise is that reducing symptoms of psychiatric conditions will reduce the frequency and intensity of drug and alcohol use. Although there are limited data on pharmacological treatment for adolescents with addictive disorders, the use of pharmacotherapy is very prevalent, reaching 55% of adolescents seen in addictive disorders treatment [10]. The bulk of these prescriptions are used to treat co-occurring psychiatric disorders, such as depression, generalized anxiety disorder, and attention-deficit/hyperactivity disorder (ADHD).

There have been only a limited number of controlled trials of pharmacological interventions targeting the treatment of substance use in adolescents. Geller and colleagues conducted a double-blind, placebo-controlled study of lithium in adolescents (12–18 years old) with bipolar disorder and secondary addictive disorders [11]. Subjects ($n = 25$) were randomly assigned to 6 weeks of treatment with either lithium or placebo. Random weekly collection of serum for lithium levels and of urine for drug assays were performed. At study's end there were no significant group differences in outcome on the substance dependence items from the *Diagnostic and Statistical Manual of Mental Disorders* (DSM). Those in the lithium group had fewer positive urine drug tests after 3 weeks of treatment.

ALCOHOL USE DISORDERS

Advances in the understanding of the pathophysiology involved with alcohol use disorders has led to the discovery, testing, and release of several medications specifically for the treatment of alcohol use disorders. Three medications (disulfiram, naltrexone, and acamprosate) are currently approved by the FDA for patients over 18 years of age [10].

Disulfiram (Antabuse)

Disulfiram (Antabuse) is a medication that inhibits alcohol metabolism by blocking the activity of aldehyde dehydrogenase. The result is an accumulation of acetaldehyde, which triggers severe nausea, vomiting, and flushing when a person drinks alcohol. Awareness that this unpleasant reaction will occur instills the motivation (and fear) that will allow the patient to refrain from drinking. This medication has been available for more than 45 years and it appears to be most effective for adult patients who are highly motivated and/or under directly observed conditions [12].

In adolescents, Niederhofer conducted a placebo-controlled study of disulfiram and reported that the 13 adolescents receiving medication had more days of abstinence during the 90-day trial than did the 13 adolescents on placebo. The results were limited by a high drop-out rate of participants who were not included in the follow-up assessment [13].

Clinical barriers with disulfiram are primarily compliance. For adolescents, directly observed treatment with disulfiram may provide for relief in the knowledge that medications have been taken. The other barrier is determining how long patients should remain on disulfiram. Long-term side effects of the medication include hepatitis, neuropathy, and, rarely, psychosis and mood disturbances.

Naltrexone (ReVia)

Naltrexone (ReVia) has been shown to be effective in decreasing heavy drinking days in patients with alcohol dependence [14,15]. It "curbs your consumption" of alcohol and reduces overall intake. Naltrexone is an opioid antagonist that purportedly blocks the urges and cravings for alcohol. In theory, patients who take naltrexone and then drink do not report the positive reinforcement experience of alcohol. Patients who respond well to naltrexone describe a muted impact of alcohol, less preoccupation about alcohol, and an easier time of "walking away from drinks" [9].

Although no randomized, double-blind, placebo-controlled studies of naltrexone in an adolescent population have been published, it is important to note that a small open-label trial with adolescents has been reported. Deas and colleagues found reductions in both craving and alcohol consumption (an average reduction of 7.6 standard drinks over a 6-week period), and that naltrexone was well tolerated and safe when dosage levels were reduced [16,17].

Naltrexone is available as an oral tablet and as an injectable, long-acting depot preparation. The injectable version was approved in 2006 and has a 30-day duration of effectiveness. The availability of an injectable medication greatly improves medication adherence (provided the patient shows up), one of the main criticisms with medications for alcohol use disorders. No known studies have been published examining injectable naltrexone in an adolescent population.

Recently, a functional allele of the gene for the opioid receptor (OPRM) has been associated with a good response to naltrexone treatment among alcoholics [18]. This serves as an example of the potential of patient profiling and matching based on genetic portfolios. Office tests for this genetic marker (OPRM1) are currently available for use by clinicians.

Acamprosate (Campral)

Acamprosate (Campral) has been used in Europe since the 1990s. Acamprosate is a competitive inhibitor of the N-methyl-D-aspartate (NMDA)-type glutamate receptor. The drug appears to normalize the dysregulated neurotransmission associated with chronic ethanol intake and thereby to attenuate one of the mechanisms that lead to relapse [19].

A number of controlled studies, done in Europe, have found acamprosate to reduce drinking relapse and to increase days of abstinence for alcohol-dependent adults [19]. Acamprosate is a derivative of taurine, a non-essential amino acid, and is purported to reduce the negative reinforcement aspects of drinking. The medication was FDA-approved for alcohol dependence in 2004 but since its inception it has failed to take a significant market share. Questionable efficacy in the real-world setting, likely due to a combination of poor compliance and lack of an effective profile, seem to limit its impact in the addiction field. Limitations with acamprosate include its three-times-a-day dosing, which in an adolescent population would be especially challenging.

Recent studies for an adolescent population have not been as promising. Two well-designed studies were negative, whereas another study by Nierderhoffer did find a mild beneficial effect [13,20]. In this study, acamprosate and placebo groups were examined in a small sample of adolescent alcohol-dependent subjects. ($n = 13$). At the end of the 3-month trial period, results showed increased rates of abstinence in the acamprosate group compared to the placebo group [13].

Potential Medications for Alcohol Use Disorders

Ondansetron

Serotonin has been implicated as playing a significant role in alcohol use disorders. Ondansetron is a serotonin receptor (5-HT$_3$) antagonist, principally used for intractable nausea, that decreases alcohol consumption in adults, especially those with early-onset alcohol dependence. In adolescents, there has been recent preliminary work with a small, open-label study that showed significant within-group decreases in self-reported alcohol consumption in adolescents with alcohol use disorders who took ondansetron [21,22]. The mechanism of the drug's anti-craving properties is not fully understood but it may center around attenuating the reward effects of alcohol and associated cues. Further controlled studies have not been conducted.

Selective Serotonin Reuptake Inhibitors (SSRIs)

Several double-blind, placebo-controlled trials examining selective serotonin reuptake inhibitors (SSRIs) (e.g., citalopram and fluoxetine) have been conducted in adults with alcohol use disorders with the intention of impacting alcohol use, but the results are mixed. The premise centers around the idea that restoring serotonergic tone will help to diminish symptoms of alcoholism.

In the adolescent population, a small open-label study of 13 adolescent participants who had both depression and an alcohol use disorder indicated that fluoxetine 20 mg/day may decrease drinking [23]. In another study, Deas and colleagues conducted a pilot study using 10 outpatient adolescents with concurrent depression and alcohol dependence [17]. Participants enrolled into a 12-week, double-blind, placebo-controlled study in which they were randomly assigned to receive sertraline or placebo. In addition, all subjects received cognitive-behavioral group therapy. The outcome measures were Hamilton Depression (HAM-D) total score, percentage of days drinking, and drinks per drinking day. Results failed to show a statistical separation between groups, suggesting that sertraline was no different than placebo.

Topiramate

Medications that antagonize glutaminergic neurotransmission, or facilitate GABAergic function, or both, have been shown to be effective in the treatment of adult alcohol dependence, according to Dawes and Johnson. Examples include acamprosate, topiramate, and gamma-hydroxybutyrate. In a recent study by Johnson *et al.*, topiramate was shown to be effective in adults for reducing cravings and heavy drinking [24]. Both acamprosate and topiramate hold promise as adjuncts to psychosocial treatments for adolescent alcohol use disorders.

MEDICATIONS FOR NICOTINE DEPENDENCE

Smoking prevalence rates for adults have decreased from approximately 50% of the general population in the mid-1960s to around 21% in 2010, primarily due to a shift in public health policies and a change in culture around smoking. For adolescents, nicotine use continues to serve as an early introduction into drug use and abuse, yet smoking cessation programs geared specifically for adolescents are infrequent [25].

As an example, tobacco use commonly present in adolescents with addictive disorders and/or psychiatric disorders, but screening and brief interventions with smoking cessation techniques are not routine. Even fewer who are in residential adolescent treatment are offered smoking cessation treatment [26].

Nicotine replacement therapy (NRT; transdermal patch, gum, inhaler, and lozenge), varenicline, and bupropion sustained-release (SR) are currently approved by the FDA for smoking cessation in adults [27]. In adolescents, NRT and bupropion SR provide the most empirical data.

Nicotine Replacement Therapy (NRT)

The efficacy of the transdermal nicotine patch has been modest among adolescents, with resulting abstinence rates ranging from 5% to 18% [28]. Efficacy rates for adults are not significantly higher (approximately 21%), and there are some clear reasons why success is low. First, compliance is an issue as effective NRT protocols take time and require care in tapering, with the need to stay disciplined and not to take more than intended. Secondly, adolescent motivation to quit smoking is not usually driven by fears of medical problems, job loss, or pressure from spouses, leading to a greater likelihood of return to smoking. Finally, approximately one-quarter of all adolescent smokers will develop adult nicotine dependence, suggesting that a significant percentage of adolescent smokers do not meet nicotine dependence criteria as they are currently defined [29].

Comparisons with placebo treatment show large benefits of nicotine replacement at 6 weeks, but the effect diminishes over time. The nicotine patch produces a steady blood level and offers better patient compliance than observed with nicotine gum. The necessary goal of complete abstinence contributes to the poor success rate; when ex-smokers "slip" and begin smoking a little, they usually relapse quickly to their prior level of tobacco use.

Further evidence clouds the picture of NRT's role with adolescent smokers. In one study, to help adolescents quit smoking, researchers randomized 100 13–19-year-olds to one-on-one cognitive treatment sessions and the nicotine patch or placebo patch. At the end of the 13-week intervention, there was no difference between groups [30]. These studies demonstrate that NRT is safe, and without serious side effects in adolescents. However, only short-term effects have been evaluated.

As a result, the use of nicotine replacement therapy (NRT) among adolescents remains controversial [31]. In the United States, the FDA labels NRTs for use by individuals at least 18 years old. Current clinical practice guidelines for treating tobacco use and dependence suggest that NRT be a first-line treatment for adults [30]. These same guidelines suggest that physicians consider the use of NRT in adolescents with obvious nicotine dependence who want to quit smoking.

Various NRT options, because they are available over the counter or online, are easily accessible by minors without proof of age and are often tried by adolescents before presentation to the clinician [30].

Bupropion (Zyban)

A sustained-release (SR) preparation of the antidepressant bupropion improves abstinence rates among smokers and remains a useful option for smoking cessation. Bupropion, an aminoketone inhibitor antidepressant, is an effective treatment for smoking cessation in adults and has been FDA approved for more than 10 years [32].

For adolescents, the effectiveness has not held up. In one published study, 211 adolescent smokers were randomized to receive nicotine patch and bupropion SR 150 mg/day versus nicotine patch plus placebo. Continuous abstinence rates (not a single puff of cigarettes) were measured at weeks 10 and 26 [33]. These rates were 23% (NRT + bupropion) versus 28% (NRT + placebo). This study used half the usual adult dose of bupropion in the treatment arm and failed to show a difference between groups. Although this study shows decreased cigarette consumption across both groups, there was no separation or added benefit of bupropion for smoking cessation in adolescents.

Results from another study suggest that bupropion SR with counseling may help teens quit smoking, regardless of whether or not they have ADHD [34]. Participants were titrated over 1 week to bupropion SR 150 mg twice a day and maintained at this dosage for 6 weeks. They were seen for weekly outpatient visits and also received two 30-minute smoking cessation counseling sessions based on American Cancer Society brochures involving psychoeducation, coping and craving, and identification of triggers for smoking and how to avoid them. Nine participants received at least 4 weeks of medication. There was a significant decrease in the average number of cigarettes smoked and in carbon monoxide (CO) levels over the course of treatment. Intent-to-treat analysis showed that 31.25% of the adolescents were completely abstinent (5/16) after 4 weeks of taking bupropion SR. Participants' weight did not change significantly during the study, and there was no significant change in ADHD symptoms during the study. The authors conclude that bupropion SR along with brief counseling may be safe and potentially efficacious for adolescents with nicotine dependence with and without ADHD.

Varenicline (Chantix)

Varenicline is a partial nicotinic agonist at the α4β2 receptor, found primarily in the nucleus accumbens. It was approved in 2006 and represented a novel mechanism of action in addressing nicotine dependence. Varenicline partially stimulates nicotinic receptors, thereby reducing craving and preventing most withdrawal symptoms [35]. It has high receptor affinity, thus blocking access to nicotine. Patients who take varencline who then smoke describe a blunted effect from the cigarette and less urges/cravings for cigarettes throughout the day. In one recent clinical trial with adults, the abstinence rate for varenicline at 1 year was 36.7% versus 7.9% for placebo [36].

Despite an impressive achieved outcome, varenicline received a black box warning from the FDA because of post-marketing reports of suicidal ideation, nightmares, and behavioral changes (hostility). Given the black box warning and the experience of antidepressants in adolescents, it would not be surprising for physicians to hesitate at the idea of prescribing varenicline.

However, a recent study demonstrated that varenicline does have a treatment effect in adolescent smokers. In this trial, treatment-seeking older adolescent smokers (ages 15–20) were randomized (double-blind) to varenicline ($n = 15$) or bupropion XL ($n = 14$), with 1-week titration and active treatment for 7 weeks [37]. Over the course of treatment, participants receiving varenicline reduced from 14 cigarettes per day to 2, while those on bupropion XL reduced from 16 to 3.

MEDICATIONS FOR OPIOID DEPENDENCE

Withdrawal and Maintenance

The first step in medication use for opioid dependence is addressing withdrawal symptoms. Opioid withdrawal symptoms are not life-threatening but at their peak they can be debilitating and incapacitating. One of the primary reasons why opioid users do not attempt to stop is fear of going through opioid withdrawal. Currently, the FDA has approved methadone and buprenorphine for the treatment of opioid withdrawal.

Once the detoxification period is completed, maintenance on these medications is considered important to minimize relapse. Additionally, naltrexone, both oral and injectable, is approved for maintenance treatment of opioid dependence.

If patients are simply discharged from the hospital or other treatment setting after withdrawal from opioids, there is a high probability of a quick return to compulsive opioid use. One factor is that the withdrawal syndrome does not end in 5–7 days. There are subclinical signs and symptoms, often called the protracted withdrawal syndrome, that can persist for up to 6 months. This is where staying on methadone or buprenorphine for an extended period can be essential to retaining patients in treatment [38].

Methadone

Methadone remains the most effective treatment for opioid dependence and consists of stabilization and dispensing in accordance with state and federal regulations. The dose of methadone must be sufficient to prevent withdrawal symptoms for at least 24 hours. Combined with behavioral therapies or counseling and other supportive services, methadone enables patients to stop using heroin (and other opiates) and return to more stable and productive lives. Methadone has also been shown to reduce addiction-related death, criminal recidivism, and the spread of HIV [39].

For adolescents aged 16–18 years, accessing methadone clinics is similar to adults (18 years and older). Patients under the age of 16 can access methadone detoxification but staying in a methadone maintenance program may require special approval from state or federal regulators.

Detoxification and subsequent maintenance of opiate dependence with methadone is specifically limited to accredited opioid treatment programs (OTPs) and is regulated by Federal Opioid Treatment Standards. Physicians who prescribe methadone in the office setting for opioid dependence (withdrawal or maintenance) are violating state and federal rules, which can result in loss of medical license and/or criminal prosecution.

No formal data on methadone treatment in opioid-dependent adolescents are currently available. Clinically, methadone maintenance is the treatment of choice for pregnant adolescents given known risks and benefits to the fetus [40].

Buprenorphine (Suboxone, Subutex)

Methadone was FDA-approved for the treatment of opioid dependence in 1957 and although there are numerous facilities to access care, treatment barriers such as stigma, rigid program policies, and daily attendance requirements exist. The approval of buprenorphine in 2002 heralded a new era of opioid treatment that could be done from the office, thereby prompting the hope that many new patients would seek treatment services.

The Drug Abuse Treatment Act 2000 (DATA 2000) permits qualified physicians to obtain a waiver from the separate registration requirements of the Narcotic Addict Treatment Act to treat opioid addiction with Schedule III, IV, and V opioid medications or combinations of such medications that have been specifically approved by the FDA for that indication. Such medications may be prescribed and dispensed [41].

Buprenorphine is a partial opioid agonist that creates a ceiling effect of opioids, making overdose theoretically less likely. The combination of buprenorphine with naloxone (opiate antagonist) decreases the likelihood of diversion through intravenous routes because the naloxone counteracts any such effort. Naloxone blocks the opiate receptors and hence no euphoric effects of buprenorphine are experienced.

Buprenorphine has been shown to be safe and effective in improving abstinence from opioids in two controlled clinical trials for adolescent populations [41]. In a recent double-blind, double-dummy trial of buprenorphine versus clonidine detoxification in a 28-day outpatient clinic with 36 adolescents with opiate dependence, buprenorphine had almost double the retention and half the number of positive urine tests for opiates compared to clonidine [42]. More research is needed in several clinically relevant areas: appropriate duration of agonist treatment; ways to enhance medication adherence; the value of integrated treatments for co-occurring conditions; and the role of opioid antagonists in opioid-dependent youths.

In order to prescribe buprenorphine for opioid dependence, providers must first take an 8-hour training course (available through the American Academy of Addiction Psychiatry or the American Psychiatric Association) and then submit a form to the Drug Enforcement Administration (DEA) to receive a unique DEA number. Since its inception in 2002, well over 10 000 physicians have taken this training, but fewer than 10% of those trained actually prescribe buprenorphine regularly. There are ample training tools and strategies on how to prescribe it correctly to minimize side effects, complications, and provider and patient anxiety, but it has remained a medication for addiction specialists. Diversion of buprenorphine product into the street has become a significant problem in some parts of the country, but this can be mitigated through careful prescribing practices and routine monitoring. Buprenorphine has a unique formulation in that it comes in both sublingual tablets that dissolve in 5–10 minutes or as a sublingual film strip that is absorbed much quicker.

For adult patients, buprenorphine has proven to be a consistently effective product, opening up many more treatment slots for addiction. However, for adolescent patients, these data are not yet proven and there is a degree of controversy among those in recovery. Since it is an opioid product, some members of the recovery community do not view it as true sobriety. There is also the critical question of how long someone should remain on the product.

The long-term impact of buprenorphine in adolescent brains has not been established, although some studies implicate less of a lasting impact on mood, attention, and learning skills than seen with long-term use of methadone.

Naltrexone

Naltrexone, as an opioid antagonist, is used for the maintenance treatment of opioid dependence. It is not routinely used for opioid detoxification although some practitioners use the intravenous form of naloxone in "ultra-rapid detoxifications." Naltrexone for opioid dependence blocks urges/craving while also blocking the effects of any exogenous opioids used. Currently, the FDA has approved both the oral formulation and, recently, the long-term injectable version for opioid dependence in adults.

In the adolescent population, there have been only case reports recently published. In one study, 16 cases of adolescents were openly prescribed naltrexone for opioid dependence; 10 of 16 (63%) were retained in treatment for at least 4 months, and 9 of 16 (56%) substantially decreased opioid use and showed an improvement in at least one psychosocial domain [42].

STIMULANTS

Since cocaine and methamphetamine withdrawal is generally self-limited, and not known to create significant medical consequences, treatment of withdrawal symptoms is usually with supportive meds such as low-dose benzodiazepines and rest.

The main treatment issue is not detoxification but helping the patient to resist the urge to resume compulsive drug use. Numerous medications have been tried in placebo-controlled clinical trials with stimulant dependence, but no medication has emerged that will clearly surpass treatment effects seen by evidenced-based behavior treatments.

Animal models suggest that enhancing GABAergic inhibition can reduce reinstatement of cocaine self-administration, and a controlled clinical trial of topiramate showed a significant reduction in cocaine use [19]. Baclofen, a $GABA_B$ agonist, was found in a single-site trial to reduce relapse in cocaine addicts, but was not effective in a multisite trial [43]. A different approach was taken using modafinil, a medication that increases alertness and is approved for the treatment of narcolepsy. This medication was found to reduce the euphoria produced by cocaine and to relieve cocaine withdrawal symptoms. Modafinil is currently being tested in clinical trials of cocaine, methamphetamine, alcohol, and other substance abuse disorders.

A novel approach to cocaine addiction employs a vaccine that produces cocaine-binding antibodies. Preliminary studies showed some success in reducing cocaine use [19,44].

No systemic or controlled trials for stimulant dependence have been conducted on an adolescent population. In one case report, desipramine was administered to an adolescent cocaine-dependent patient and showed continued abstinence and improvements in life domains 6 months later [45].

SEDATIVE-HYPNOTICS

For adolescent patients who have been taking benzodiazepines for more than 4 weeks, the primary method of stopping is through gradual dose reduction. This may take several days, weeks, or months depending on the subjective complaints of the patient. If anxiety symptoms return, a non-benzodiazepine such as buspirone or gabapentin may be prescribed, but such agents usually are less effective than benzodiazepines for treatment of anxiety in these patients. It is also an untested approach, although commonly used by clinicians and inpatient settings.

Some authorities recommend transferring the patient to a long-half-life benzodiazepine, such as diazepam, during detoxification, while others recommend the anticonvulsants carbamazepine and phenobarbital. Controlled studies comparing different treatment regimens are lacking.

The specific benzodiazepine receptor antagonist flumazenil has been found useful in the treatment of overdose and in reversing the effects of long-acting benzodiazepines used in anesthesia. It has been used experimentally in the treatment of persistent withdrawal symptoms after cessation of long-term benzodiazepine treatment [46].

Deliberate abusers of high doses of benzodiazepines will require inpatient detoxification. Frequently, benzodiazepine abuse is part of a combined dependence involving alcohol, opioids, and cocaine.

After detoxification, the prevention of relapse requires a long-term outpatient rehabilitation program similar to the treatment of alcoholism. No specific medications have been found to be useful in the rehabilitation of sedative abusers at this time.

Medication approaches to address this issue in adolescent populations have not been addressed.

MARIJUANA

Marijuana dependence does not have any FDA-approved medications for adults. The effects of marijuana withdrawal, now scientifically proven to exist, are usually time limited and may require symptomatic relief only. The CB_1 receptor antagonist rimonabant has been reported to block the acute effects of smoked marijuana, but development of this drug has been halted due to safety concerns, namely suicidal ideation [47]. Other researchers have investigated a variety of medications including topiramate, antipsychotics, and mood stabilizers without much traction [48]. Psychopharmacological trials for adolescent marijuana smokers have not been conducted at this time. One 5-week, open-label trial of divalproex in eight adolescent marijuana-use-disordered participants showed reductions in marijuana use, as measured by self-report [48]. This has not been replicated or conducted on a controlled basis.

NON-SUBSTANCE-RELATED DISORDERS

Non-substance-related disorders, otherwise known as behavioral addictions, impulse-control disorders, or process addictions, comprise pathological gambling, hypersexual disorders, compulsive shopping, video game addiction, and kleptomania. To date, no FDA-approved medication is available for adults for any of the above disorders. Collectively, these disorders are often insidious and hidden, but they can have enormous and profound consequences. For adults, studies have suggested that naltrexone may have an impact on reducing the urges, cravings, and preoccupations in pathological gamblers, kleptomaniacs and compulsive sexual behaviors [5]. Clinicians who prescribed medications for these conditions are urged to monitor treatment effects closely by checking the patient's clinical status frequently.

In an adolescent population, these conditions have been known to begin and fully express themselves at an early age, signaling the importance for early intervention and treatments. Pharmacological interventions in this population have not been studied extensively, and the potential for effectiveness remains; however, too little is understood about the biological and psychological targets that are present.

CLINICAL GUIDELINES FOR PRESCRIBING MEDICATIONS

Given the paucity of evidence-based strategies for medication management of addictive disorders for adolescents, addiction physicians have come to rely on trial-and-error methods. In general, specific clinical knowledge, skills, and attitudes should be employed by general practitioners when prescribing medications for addiction. These practice principles are taken from a combination of the National Institute on Drug Addiction (NIDA) principles on treatment of addiction, the American Psychiatric Association (APA) guideline for treatment of substance use disorders, and Substance Abuse and Mental Health Services Administration (SAMHSA) treatment improvement protocols and clinical experience.

1. *Ensure diagnosis is correct:* Addicted adolescents may minimize or exaggerate amounts of drug use and the physiological effects of drugs. Given the wide availability of information, many patients can come "armed" with information about the correct thing to say to get the physician to prescribe something. To counter these possibilities, employ collateral information, urine drug screens, and rating scales, and actively listen for inconsistencies in clinical history.
2. *Inform patients about treatment choices:* Since there are no FDA-approved medications for addictive disorders for adolescents, these patients must be informed about this prior to prescribing any medication. This requires informed consent for discussing off-label use of medications, even if they are approved for adults.
3. *Manage expectations:* When prescribing medications, providers are encouraged to educate patients about what the impact of the medications will be on their disease of addiction. For instance, none of the approved medications should be thought of as a panacea, or something that will manage all symptoms forever. Providers are encouraged to target symptoms for which medications are known to work, such as reducing urges/cravings and/or diminishing positive or negative reinforcements. Medications that are being targeted for mood or anxiety symptoms should be considered separately.
4. *Monitor for treatment compliance:* The number one reason why medications do not work for substance use disorders is because patients do not take them. This can be partially avoided by using an injectable formulation such as naltrexone. Directly observed therapy is possible in structured settings but this technique may not increase the motivation of the patient and can be seen as punitive. Monitoring techniques, such as random urine testing for the presence of buprenorphine, is an alternative strategy to enhance/document compliance. The key element in any urine testing program is that it is random. Providers should also be very aware of prescription practices; for instance, if a refill for an antidepressant or mood stabilizer is due but no timely appointment has been made, consider that a sign of possible non-compliance.
5. *Monitor for side effects:* Because the symptoms of psychiatric conditions, substance abuse, and side effects from medications (e.g. anxiety, nausea, insomnia) are often similar and coexist, it can be very difficult for providers to sort out which symptoms are which. To manage this, consider using a very clear medication log, tracking side effects over time and concentrating on documenting the somatic complaints during the initial assessment period. For instance, if a patient has insomnia identified at the start of treatment this will help to identify what is iatrogenic and what is secondary to psychiatric illness.
6. *Always consider length of time in treatment:* Clinicians and patients often wonder how long to maintain medication management for patients with addictive disorders. In general, consideration for tapering or reducing medications is made after one full year of sobriety and significant reductions of psychiatric symptoms. Because addiction is a chronic, relapsing disease, those who need to be considered for longer-term therapies typically have multiple relapse histories, strong genetic components, significant co-occurring illnesses, and poor social support and structure.
7. *Medications lay the groundwork for recovery:* One helpful way of conceptualizing the role of medications is that they can be used to reduce the

symptoms of substance dependence thus enabling the user to pay attention in therapy and recovery groups. This is especially true for adolescent substance abusers, who may already have difficulty with attention, concentration, and the ability to listen. Medications that can reduce urges/cravings and allow patients to be more present will increase the likelihood of them being able to remain in treatment.

8. *What is the impact on brain development?* In choosing medications for use in adolescents, practitioners should be aware of the biological and behavioral changes that occur during adolescence. Clinicians should carefully determine if the medications selected might affect brain or body growth and development. Dosage and duration of treatment should be chosen with the developmental issues of teenagers in mind.

CONCLUSIONS

There is a paucity of evidence-based research and a complete lack of treatment guidelines for the use of medications to treat addictive disorders in the adolescent population. In reality though, clinicians are likely to try to prescribe medications that are approved in adults, but they should be wary that the same results and effectiveness may or may not hold true for an adolescent population. As more pharmaceutical products become available for use, there will be more treatment options for clinicians. Until then, clinicians are urged to practice practical pharmacology with an emphasis on informed consent, setting an appropriate expectation of treatment, and monitoring signs and symptoms very closely. As more research is done in this area, clinicians can expect to see refinements in patient–medication matching, optimal dosing, and, perhaps, genotyping.

Acknowledgements

Time to work on this chapter was facilitated by a NIDA K23 Career Developmental Award.

References

1. Rahman S. Drug addiction and brain targets: from preclinical research to pharmacotherapy. *CNS Neurol Disord-Dr* 2008;**7**:391–392.
2. Bridge JA, Birmaher B, Iyengar S, Barbe RP, Brent DA. Placebo response in randomized controlled trials of antidepressants for pediatric major depressive disorder. *Am J Psychiatry* 2009;**166**:42–49.
3. Livingston JD, Milne T, Fang ML, Amari E. The effectiveness of interventions for reducing stigma related to substance use disorders: a systematic review. *Addiction* 2012;**107**:39–50.
4. Taurines R, Gerlach M, Warnke A, Thome J, Wewetzer C. Pharmacotherapy in depressed children and adolescents. *World J Biol Psychiatry* 2011;**12**(Suppl. 1):11–15.
5. Grant JE, Potenza MN. Pharmacological treatment of adolescent pathological gambling. *Int J Adolesc Med Health* 2010;**22**:129–138.
6. Oliva EM, Maisel NC, Gordon AJ, Harris AH. Barriers to use of pharmacotherapy for addiction disorders and how to overcome them. *Curr Psychiatry Rep* 2011;**13**:374–381.
7. Edens E, Massa A, Petrakis I. Novel pharmacological approaches to drug abuse treatment. *Curr Top Behav Neurosci* 2010;**3**:343–386.
8. Montoya ID, Vocci F. Novel medications to treat addictive disorders. *Curr Psychiatry Rep* 2008;**10**:392–398.
9. Ross S, Peselow E. Pharmacotherapy of addictive disorders. *Clin Neuropharmacol* 2009;**32**:277–289.
10. Clark DB, Wood DS, Cornelius JR, Bukstein OG, Martin CS. Clinical practices in the pharmacological treatment of comorbid psychopathology in adolescents with alcohol use disorders. *J Subst Abuse Treat* 2003;**25**:293–295.
11. Geller B, Cooper TB, Sun K, *et al.* Double-blind and placebo-controlled study of lithium for adolescent bipolar disorders with secondary substance dependency. *J Am Acad Child Adolesc Psychiatry* 1998;**37**:171–178.
12. Sofuoglu M, Kosten TR. Pharmacologic management of relapse prevention in addictive disorders. *Psychiatr Clin N Am* 2004;**27**:627–648.
13. Niederhofer H, Staffen W. Acamprosate and its efficacy in treating alcohol dependent adolescents. *Eur Child Adolesc Psychiatry* 2003;**12**:144–148.
14. Mannelli P, Peindl K, Masand PS, Patkar AA. Long-acting injectable naltrexone for the treatment of alcohol dependence. *Expert Rev Neurother* 2007;**7**:1265–1277.
15. McGeary JE, Monti PM, Rohsenow DJ, Tidey J, Swift R, Miranda RJr., Genetic moderators of naltrexone's effects on alcohol cue reactivity. *Alcohol Clin Exp Res* 2006;**30**:1288–1296.
16. Lifrak PD, Alterman AI, O'Brien CP, Volpicelli JR. Naltrexone for alcoholic adolescents. *Am J Psychiatry* 1997;**154**:439–441.
17. Deas D, May MP, Randall C, Johnson N, Anton R. Naltrexone treatment of adolescent alcoholics: an open-label pilot study. *J Child Adolesc Psychopharmacol* 2005;**15**:723–728.
18. Sturgess JE, George TP, Kennedy JL, Heinz A, Muller DJ. Pharmacogenetics of alcohol, nicotine and drug addiction treatments. *Addiction Biol* 2011;**16**:357–376.
19. Olive MF, Cleva RM, Kalivas PW, Malcolm RJ. Glutamatergic medications for the treatment of drug and behavioral addictions. *Pharmacol Biochem Behav* 2012;**100**:801–810.
20. De Wildt WA, Schippers GM, Van Den Brink W, Potgieter AS, Deckers F, Bets D. Does psychosocial treatment enhance the efficacy of acamprosate in patients with alcohol problems? *Alcohol Alcoholism* 2002;**37**:375–382.
21. Dawes MA, Johnson BA, Ma JZ, Ait-Daoud N, Thomas SE, CorneliusJR. Reductions in and relations between "craving" and drinking in a prospective, open-label trial of ondansetron in adolescents with alcohol dependence. *Addict Behav* 2005;**30**:1630–1637.
22. Dawes MA, Johnson BA, Ait-Daoud N, Ma JZ, CorneliusJR. A prospective, open-label trial of ondansetron in adolescents with alcohol dependence. *Addict Behav* 2005;**30**:1077–1085.

23. Cornelius JR, Bukstein OG, Birmaher B, *et al.* Fluoxetine in adolescents with major depression and an alcohol use disorder: an open-label trial. *Addict Behav* 2001;**26**:735–739.

24. Johnson BA, Ait-Daoud N, Bowden CL, *et al.* Oral topiramate for treatment of alcohol dependence: a randomised controlled trial. *Lancet* 2003;**361**:1677–1685.

25. Colby SM, Gwaltney CJ. Pharmacotherapy for adolescent smoking cessation. *JAMA* 2007;**298**:2182–2184.

26. Upadhyaya HP, Deas D, Brady KT, Kruesi M. Cigarette smoking and psychiatric comorbidity in children and adolescents. *J Am Acad Child Adolesc Psychiatry* 2002;**41**:1294–1305.

27. Mitrouska I, Bouloukaki I, Siafakas NM. Pharmacological approaches to smoking cessation. *Pulm Pharmacol Ther* 2007;**20**:220–232.

28. Moolchan ET, Robinson ML, Ernst M, *et al.* Safety and efficacy of the nicotine patch and gum for the treatment of adolescent tobacco addiction. *Pediatrics* 2005;**115**:e407–414.

29. Miyata H, Kono J, Ushijima S, Yanagita T, Miyasato K, Fukui K. Clinical features of nicotine dependence compared with those of alcohol, methamphetamine, and inhalant dependence. *Ann N Y Acad Sci* 2004;**1025**:481–488.

30. Grimshaw GM, Stanton A. Smoking cessation services for young people. *Brit Med J* 2008;**337**:a1394.

31. Grimshaw GM, Stanton A. Tobacco cessation interventions for young people. *Cochrane Database Syst Rev* 2006 (4): CD003289.

32. Aubin HJ, Karila L, Reynaud M. Pharmacotherapy for smoking cessation: present and future. *Curr Pharm Des* 2011;**17**:1343–1350.

33. Killen JD, Robinson TN, Ammerman S, *et al.* Randomized clinical trial of the efficacy of bupropion combined with nicotine patch in the treatment of adolescent smokers. *J Consult Clin Psychol* 2004;**72**:729–735.

34. Upadhyaya HP, Brady KT, Wang W. Bupropion SR in adolescents with comorbid ADHD and nicotine dependence: a pilot study. *J Am Acad Child Adolesc Psychiatry* 2004;**43**:199–205.

35. Faessel HM, Obach RS, Rollema H, Ravva P, Williams KE, Burstein AH. A review of the clinical pharmacokinetics and pharmacodynamics of varenicline for smoking cessation. *Clin Pharmacokinet* 2010;**49**:799–816.

36. Williams KE, Reeves KR, Billing CBJr, Pennington AM, Gong J. A double-blind study evaluating the long-term safety of varenicline for smoking cessation. *Curr Med Res Opin* 2007;**23**:793–801.

37. Gray KM, Carpenter MJ, Lewis AL, Klintworth EM, Upadhyaya HP. Varenicline versus bupropion XL for smoking cessation in older adolescents: a randomized, double-blind pilot trial. *Nicotine Tob Res* 2011; doi: 10.1093/ntr/ntr130.

38. Ebner R, Schreiber W, Zierer C. [Buprenorphine or methadone for detoxification of young opioid addicts?] *Psychiatrische Praxis* 2004;**31**(Suppl. 1):S108–110.

39. Vlahov D, O'Driscoll P, Mehta SH, *et al.* Risk factors for methadone outside treatment programs: implications for HIV treatment among injection drug users. *Addiction* 2007;**102**:771–777.

40. Kraus ML, Alford DP, Kotz MM, *et al.* Statement of the American Society of Addiction Medicine Consensus Panel on the use of buprenorphine in office-based treatment of opioid addiction. *J Addict Med* 2011;**5**:254–263.

41. Woody GE, Poole SA, Subramaniam G, *et al.* Extended vs short-term buprenorphine-naloxone for treatment of opioid-addicted youth: a randomized trial. *JAMA* 2008;**300**: 2003–2011.

42. Marsch LA, Bickel WK, Badger GJ, *et al.* Comparison of pharmacological treatments for opioid-dependent adolescents: a randomized controlled trial. *Arch Gen Psychiatry* 2005;**62**:1157–1164.

43. Somaini L, Donnini C, Raggi MA, *et al.* Promising medications for cocaine dependence treatment. *Recent Pat CNS Drug Discov* 2011;**6**:146–160.

44. De La Garza R2nd, Zorick T, London ED, Newton TF. Evaluation of modafinil effects on cardiovascular, subjective, and reinforcing effects of methamphetamine in methamphetamine-dependent volunteers. *Drug Alcohol Depend* 2010;**106**:173–180.

45. Kaminer Y. Desipramine facilitation of cocaine abstinence in an adolescent. *J Am Acad Child Adolesc Psychiatry* 1992;**31**:312–317.

46. Mintzer MZ, Griffiths RR. Flumazenil-precipitated withdrawal in healthy volunteers following repeated diazepam exposure. *Psychopharmacology* 2005;**178**: 259–267.

47. Gorelick DA, Heishman SJ, Preston KL, Nelson RA, Moolchan ET, Huestis MA. The cannabinoid CB1 receptor antagonist rimonabant attenuates the hypotensive effect of smoked marijuana in male smokers. *Am Heart J* 2006;**151**:754 e1–e5.

48. Donovan SJ, Nunes EV. Treatment of comorbid affective and substance use disorders. Therapeutic potential of anticonvulsants. *Am J Addictions* 1998;**7**:210–220.

33

What's Old is New: Motivational Interviewing for Adolescents[1]

Lois T. Flaherty

University of Maryland School of Medicine, Baltimore, MD, USA

INTRODUCTION

Two groups of alcoholics received either one counseling session or several months of in- and outpatient treatment. One year later there were no significant differences in outcome between the two groups.

Edwards *et al.* [1], p. 1004.

Foremost in my mind is how it works at all . . . How could it possibly be, then, that a session or two of asking clients to verbalize their own suffering and reasons for change would unstuck a behavior pattern that has been so persistent.

Miller [2], p. 840.

Motivational interviewing (MI) involves five basic skills:

1. open-ended questions;
2. reflective listening;
3. eliciting self-motivational statements;
4. supportive and affirming statements; and
5. summary statements.

Examples of each of these are appended to this chapter.

According to its developer, William Miller, motivational interviewing was discovered by accident; Miller found, when studying an intervention for problem drinkers in the 1970s, that control groups did as well as treatment groups [2]. In the process of unraveling what

was going on in the control groups, who received an initial assessment, encouragement, and advice, he was able to tease out what seemed to be the ingredients in the apparently minimal interventions they received that resulted in their changing their behavior. Not all of the controls improved, but those who did had counselors who were empathetic, non-confrontational, and gave helpful information. The kind of information that seemed to be most useful was the creating of a discrepancy between the client's stated goal and their current behavior. There was no urging the client to make changes, but rather an emphasis that the decision about whether to change was up to the client, and that they could do so whenever they were ready.

From that beginning, MI was developed into protocols and tested in a variety of situations. Books and journal articles appeared, although it remained largely unknown outside the psychiatric literature. Perhaps it was deemed too simple, or perhaps because it was developed in the addictions field, which has historically developed independently of psychiatry, it did not make it into the mainstream. But a brief intervention that appeared to work for a variety of problems with diverse patients and required little formal training was bound to spread. In a 1990 report the Institute of Medicine recommended brief intervention, namely MI, for all patients with alcohol problems [3].

A therapeutic approach that respected patients' autonomy and decision-making capacity, and was encouraging and supportive, while at the same time providing feedback about the person's current situation with respect to where he or she wants to be eventually, would appear to be a natural fit for adolescents. This in fact proved to be the case. By mid-2011, 74 articles on MI

---

[1] What's Old is New: Motivational Interviewing for Adolescents. Reprinted with kind permission from Adolescent Psychiatry, Vol 30, pages 117–127. © Francis and Taylor, 2008.

with adolescents in various contexts had appeared in English language peer-reviewed journals indexed in PubMed. The settings reported on range from adolescent inpatient units to internet chat rooms [3,4]. While most of these articles describe pilot studies, their number indicates a growing popularity of MI in a variety of psychiatric and non-psychiatric situations.

CONDITIONS IN WHICH MI HAS BEEN STUDIED

Motivational interviewing was originally developed to treat alcohol use disorders, and has been extensively studied in this context first in adults [1], and more recently in adolescents [5–13]. MI has been used for marijuana use and dependence [14], as well as for addictions to heroin and other drugs [14–21]. Extension of the early work on substance abuse led to trials of MI with other kinds of behavior viewed as having an addictive or habitual component, including smoking [22] and obesity [23]. Other situations not characterized by compulsive behavior in which MI has been tested are adherence to antiretroviral treatment [24], dietary adherence [25], diabetes and other long-term medical care [26,27], and avoidance of dental care in older adolescents [28] – evidently a significant problem.

WHAT DO WE KNOW ABOUT MI?

Miller observed that a confrontational stance on the part of the therapist increased the client's resistance. Challenging the patient's assertions, disbelieving, criticizing, or arguing were all counterproductive, decreasing the likelihood that a patient would want to change. These observations led him to reframe "resistance" and "denial" as arising from interpersonal interactions, rather than qualities that resided inherently in patients. His reframing led to a conceptualization of motivation also as a dynamic interpersonal process resulting from the relationship.

Miller noted that in contrast to the negative, resistance-increasing actions on the part of ineffective therapists, successful therapists behaved in an empathetic, supportive way, engaging in reflective listening and offering positive feedback. For example, they offered advice about community resources, and discussed ways to change. They monitored readiness to change and did not push clients to change before they were ready. In psychological parlance, they enhanced self-efficacy and elicited motivational statements from their clients. Finally, they fostered an awareness of the difference between current reality and the person's own stated goals for him or herself. This awareness of difference, termed cognitive dissonance, has been suggested as the crucial active ingredient in MI [29]. In sum, what the

therapists provided was a combination of modes of interaction (the supportive, non-judgmental stance) and techniques (the advice and creation of cognitive dissonance).

THE TRANSTHEORETICAL MODEL OF CHANGE

Motivational interviewing is closely tied to the transtheoretical model of change (TMC), which was in fact developed simultaneously with MI by Prochaska and DiClemente [30] based on their review of many types of therapy and their empirical observations of smokers who were able to stop by themselves; see Rosner [31] for a more complete discussion of TMC. The idea here is that it is possible to categorize stages in the process by which individuals (and even institutions) undergo change and that these stages apply to all change and occur regardless of what method or theory is invoked to explain the change. MI can be used at any stage, but its appropriate use depends on an awareness of a person's current stage with respect to change.

MODERATORS OF MI

Prior conditions have an effect on the outcome of MI. These include pre-treatment substance abuse history, school adjustment, and emotional abuse history. Lack of prior treatment and only mild to moderate dependence are also factors, as is a view of alcohol use as a bad habit rather than a disease. The fact that this is the case suggests that comorbidity is important to consider. As we know, comorbidity is the rule with adolescent substance abuse, raising questions about how effective an intervention MI might be with the typical adolescent seen in a psychiatric setting. Nonetheless, Battjes and colleagues [14], using a manual-guided, group therapy format, found MI to be effective in reducing marijuana use in a large sample of adolescent outpatients, although neither substance abuse nor criminal behavior decreased in this group. Only modest effects were found in reducing smoking in adolescent psychiatric inpatients [22]. On a more positive note, a small group (13 subjects) of inpatients aged 18–35 and with comorbid non-opioid drug abuse and psychosis reduced their drug use and maintained their gains over a 12-month period [16].

HARM REDUCTION ASPECTS OF MI

Harm reduction is one of the more interesting aspects of MI. The concept has to do with accepting a partial change in high-risk behavior, with the idea that something is better than nothing. Harm reduction tends to be controversial, as for example, in the case of needle-exchange programs for addicts. Promoting condom use among adolescents is another example – critics are convinced these measures lead to more of the behavior that is undesirable in the first place. Advocates of harm reduction argue that the behavior is going to occur anyway, so we are better off making it safer. Harm reduction is used in MI as a way of encouraging patients involved in high-risk behavior who might despair of being able to change the behavior completely, to realize that more modest goals are within their reach.

Typical harm reduction strategies with alcohol use include setting limits on alcohol consumption, and increasing awareness of safe driving levels and of the effects of alcohol abuse [6]. Harm reduction may be a particularly salient approach for adolescents – as much adolescent high-risk behavior is time limited and phase-specific anyway. The rationale is that if one can help the adolescent get through the teen years without serious harm he or she is likely to discontinue the behaviors as an adult. Obviously this is not the case for all adolescents who engage in high-risk behavior, and harm reduction has attracted much criticism from those who see it as encouraging the behavior it is designed to modify.

PARAMETERS OF MI

Motivational interviewing is usually administered in a single session. The duration of interviews averages about $1\frac{1}{2}$ hours in research settings. Training in reported studies has varied from 2 hours to 31 hours. Most studies use relatively untrained therapists. An online continuing medical education (CME) course is available [3,4,32]. A baseline evaluation can be done using the Readiness to Change Questionnaire [33], a 12-item questionnaire based on Prochaska and DiClemente's stages of change model [30].

MI seems to be effective as a stand-alone intervention – for some people. For others whose impairment and duration of problem behavior is such that they need inpatient or residential treatment, detoxification, or other services besides counseling or therapy, MI has been considered a type of treatment induction. That is, it gets the interviewee thinking about what he or she needs to do and creates receptivity for further intervention.

MI can be considered a type of planned single-session psychotherapy, an intervention for whose efficacy there is considerable empirical support [34,35]. Bloom identified the essential features of this approach as:

1. the identification of and focus on one issue;
2. an active stance on the part of the therapist (who should ask questions and listen but not lecture or exhort);
3. the imparting of relevant information;
4. assessing the patient's current level of self-awareness.

He advised commenting on affect and making sure that whatever interpretations were offered were acceptable to the patient. The goal at the end of the session is that the patient and therapist have identified some aspect of the patient's cognitive or affective life that is below his or her awareness and is creating problems, and that a template is created for making changes. Single-session or other short-term psychotherapy is facilitated by the presence of a crisis, which serves to increase motivation to change. Slaff [35] gave several clinical examples in which patients did not return for a second session but made dramatic improvements, and reviewed the literature on successful single-session interventions, which emphasized the importance of the readiness of the patient to make changes.

In Bloom's model, a follow-up is done by telephone to ascertain what changes have occurred as a result of the session. If patients say they did not act on the recommendations, they are told that they can always do so later when they are ready. One can see parallels with aspects of MI, such as the focus on a single issue, the use of reflective listening, and monitoring of readiness to change.

MI has been embraced as a technique that can be incorporated into primary healthcare settings. Given the fact that 20–30% of adults seen in these settings have problems with alcohol, MI would, if successful, indeed be a cost-effective primary or secondary prevention strategy. A high proportion of adolescents seen in hospital emergency departments have drug- and/or alcohol-related medical problems, especially those seen after automobile accidents, so this is another site where a brief intervention makes sense [9,11,36–41]. Another venue where it has been tried is college campuses, where binge drinking and alcohol-related problems are a major concern [5,8,42,43].

Interventions in such non-substance abuse treatment settings are termed opportunistic interventions. That is, a patient may come into the office (or clinic or emergency room) with an unrelated (at least ostensibly) presenting problem, but is discovered to have an alcohol use problem, and can be given a brief intervention for this. There is a counterpart for this with psychiatric practice, where comorbid alcohol and substance abuse are estimated to occur in upwards of 50% of patients seen in mental health settings [44].

As with any intervention studied in research settings, transferability to real-world settings is always a question. If in fact MI is most useful as an opportunistic intervention, research settings are not places where people are seen who just happen to have the targeted problem, rather they are selected for it. And, of course, the therapists are research staff and not real-world clinicians.

CONCLUSION

Adolescents who present to primary care settings, or who come to the attention of school personnel or emergency rooms, are seldom in the end-stage throes of addiction, making them ideal candidates for brief interventions. This is also true of those adolescents seen in outpatient psychotherapy whose substance abuse or other health-endangering behavior is not impairing them enough for them to need more intensive forms of treatment. Finally, for those adolescents seen in psychiatric settings who have problems that are not the primary reason for their mental health treatment, such as smoking or being overweight, MI offers the possibility for opportunistic interventions, which, if successful, could have a long-term impact on health and quality of life.

MI is intriguing from a variety of standpoints. First, despite its apparent simplicity, it defies explanation. It gives addicts, who view themselves as helpless in the face of their addiction, a new way of seeing themselves, as being capable of change. Together with its companion, TMC, it stands in contrast to the many highly specific treatment modalities that have been developed in recent years. Yet, like cognitive-behavioral therapy, interpersonal psychotherapy, and others, it has a good evidence base. It is a relatively "old" modality, harking back to the pioneering work of such early theorists as Carl Rogers. Information is presented to a patient by a non-judgmental therapist who listens to the patient's point of view and conveys hope and optimism. It seems to revolve around the interpersonal relationship that is the core of the therapeutic process. And let's not forget the importance of empathy, long recognized as a crucial ingredient to all effective therapy. That sounds uncomplicated. Yet, it is also mysterious; perhaps it is because it speaks to the essence of human freedom, which is essentially unknowable, and human choice, which is essentially unpredictable. Isn't this always the case with good psychotherapy?

APPENDIX 33.1: MOTIVATIONAL INTERVIEWING TECHNIQUES[2]

- Use open-ended questions.
  "Tell me about your drinking."
  "What concerns do you have about your drinking?"
  "How can I help you with your drinking?"

- Use reflective listening.
  "I hear you."
  "I'm accepting, not judging you."
  "Please say more."
- Use affirmative assessments
  "You are very courageous to be so revealing about this."
  "You've accomplished a lot in a short time."
  "I can understand why drinking feels good to you."
- Use summary statements.
  "What you said is important. Let's talk about it . . . "
- Elicit self-motivational statements – these statements fall into four categories.
  1. Problem recognition – "I never realized how much I am drinking." "Maybe I have been taking foolish risks."
  2. Expression of concern – "I am really worried about my grades and how alcohol may be affecting them."
  3. Intention to change – "I don't know how, but I want to try."
  4. Theme about optimism – "I think I can do it. I am going to overcome this problem."

Additional Points About Motivational Interviewing

1. The primary goal of MI is to resolve ambivalence and resistance and to move patients into a commitment to change their behavior.

Example
From: "I am not interested in reducing my alcohol use. I drink less than my friends." "I see no reason to change how much I drink. It is part of the college experience. I am not having problems so why should I cut down?"

To: "If I stop drinking I will feel better and maybe do better in school. However I am not sure what my friends will think. I am not sure how I can party and have fun if I don't drink so much."

To: "Maybe I do drink too much. I am willing to try to cut down. How much do you think it is safe for me to drink?"

2. Motivation to change is elicited from the student from within. It is not imposed from without. MI does not involve the use of external threats.

Provider statements not based on MI:
"If you don't stop drinking, you will be expelled."
"If you don't stop drinking, you will lose your job."
"If you don't stop drinking, you will never get into graduate school."
"If you don't stop drinking now, you will turn into an alcoholic."

---

[2] Adapted from the: National Institute on Alcohol Abuse and Alcoholism *College Drinking Prevention*. Accessed May 17, 2006, at http://www.collegedrinkingprevention.gov/NIAAACollegeMaterials/trainingmanual/module_4.aspx.

3. In MI, the clinicians are not passive agents or mirrors. They direct and facilitate change with a number of methods. Clinicians utilize empathy, summarization, reflective listening, and other techniques. MI is not 100% clinician-directed or 100% client-centered but, rather, someplace in between. It is meant to be interactive, with both sides giving and taking. In this way, it is similar to developing a relationship based on mutual respect, trust, and acceptance.

4. MI avoids arguments, coercion, and labels. While a therapist who is using MI techniques may not agree with a student, he/she respects the student's perspective. A counselor can disagree. For example:

   Student: "Doc, I don't think I have a problem or need to cut down."

   Provider: "John, I have to respectfully disagree. You had a serious accident after you were drinking. You are not doing well in your classes. Your girlfriend left you. I am not sure how serious things are, but I think you should consider how alcohol is contributing to these problems."

5. MI does not use negative comments.

ACKNOWLEDGEMENT

This chapter originally appeared in *Adolescent Psychiatry* 2008;**30**:117–127. Reprinted with permission of The Analytic Press, New York.

References

1. Edwards G, Orford J, Egert S, *et al.* Alcoholism: a controlled trial of "treatment" and "advice". *J Stud Alcohol* 1977;**38**:1004–1031.
2. Miller WR. Motivational interviewing: Research, practice, and puzzles. *Addict Behav* 1996;**21**:835–842.
3. Institute of Medicine Division of Mental Health and Behavioral Medicine. *Broadening the Base of Treatment for Alcohol Problems.* Washington, DC: National Academy Press, 1990.
4. Woodruff SI, Edwards CC, Conway TL, Elliott SP. Pilot test of an Internet virtual world chat room for rural teen smokers. *J Adolesc Health* 2001;**29**:239–243.
5. Baer JS, Kivlahan DR, Blume AW, McKnight P, Marlatt GA. Brief intervention for heavy-drinking college students: 4-year follow-up and natural history. *Am J Public Health* 2001;**91**:1310–1316.
6. Bailey KA, Baker AL, Webster RA, Lewin TJ. Pilot randomized controlled trial of a brief alcohol intervention group for adolescents. *Drug Alcohol Rev* 2004;**23**:157–166.
7. Boekeloo BO, Jerry J, Lee-Ougo WI, *et al.* Randomized trial of brief office-based interventions to reduce adolescent alcohol use. *Arch Pediatr Adolesc Med* 2004;**158**:635–642.
8. Collins SE, Carey KB, Sliwinski MJ. Mailed personalized normative feedback as a brief intervention for at-risk college drinkers. *J Stud Alcohol* 2002;**63**:559–567.
9. Gregor MA, Shope JT, Blow FC, Maio RF, Weber JE, Nypaver MM. Feasibility of using an interactive laptop program in the emergency department to prevent alcohol misuse among adolescents. *Ann Emerg Med* 2003;**42**:276–284.
10. Hungerford DW, Williams JM, Furbee PM, *et al.* Feasibility of screening and intervention for alcohol problems among young adults in the ED. *Am J Emerg Med* 2003;**21**:14–22.
11. Kelly TM, Donovan JE, Chung T, Cook RL, Delbridge TR. Alcohol use disorders among emergency department-treated older adolescents: a new brief screen (RUFT-Cut) using the AUDIT, CAGE, CRAFFT, and RAPS-QF. *Alcohol Clin Exp Res* 2004;**28**:746–753.
12. Larimer ME, Turner AP, Anderson BK, *et al.* Evaluating a brief alcohol intervention with fraternities. *J Stud Alcohol* 2001;**62**:370–380.
13. Stewart SH, Conrod PJ, Marlatt GA, Comeau MN, Thush C, Krank M. New developments in prevention and early intervention for alcohol abuse in youths. *Alcohol Clin Exp Res* 2005;**29**:278–286.
14. Battjes RJ, Gordon MS, O'Grady KE, Kinlock TW, Katz EC, Sears EA. Evaluation of a group-based substance abuse treatment program for adolescents. *J Subst Abuse Treat* 2004;**27**:123–134.
15. Breslin C, Li S, Sdao-Jarvie K, Tupker E, Ittig-Deland V. Brief treatment for young substance abusers: a pilot study in an addiction treatment setting. *Psychol Addict Behav* 2002;**16**:10–16.
16. Kavanagh DJ, Young R, White A, *et al.* A brief motivational intervention for substance misuse in recent-onset psychosis. *Drug Alcohol Rev* 2004;**23**:151–155.
17. Levy S, Vaughan BL, Knight JR. Office-based intervention for adolescent substance abuse. *Pediatr Clin N Am* 2002;**49**:329–343.
18. Spoth RL, Redmond C, Shin C. Randomized trial of brief family interventions for general populations: adolescent substance use outcomes 4years following baseline. *J Consult Clin Psychol* 2001;**69**:627–642.
19. Tait RJ, Hulse GK. A systematic review of the effectiveness of brief interventions with substance using adolescents by type of drug. *Drug Alcohol Rev* 2003;**22**:337–346.
20. Tait RJ, Hulse GK. Adolescent substance use and hospital presentations: a record linkage assessment of 12-month outcomes. *Drug Alcohol Depend* 2005;**79**:365–371.
21. Tevyaw TO, Monti PM. Motivational enhancement and other brief interventions for adolescent substance abuse: foundations, applications and evaluations. *Addiction* 2004;**99**(Suppl. 2):63–75.
22. Brown RA, Ramsey SE, Strong DR, *et al.* Effects of motivational interviewing on smoking cessation in adolescents with psychiatric disorders. *Tob Control* 2003;**12**(Suppl. 4):IV3–10.
23. Kirk S, Scott BJ, Daniels SR. Pediatric obesity epidemic: treatment options. *J Am Diet Assoc* 2005;**105**(5 Suppl. 1): S44–S51.
24. DiIorio C, Resnicow K, McDonnell M, Soet J, McCarty F, Yeager K. Using motivational interviewing to promote adherence to antiretroviral medications: a pilot study. *J Assoc Nurses AIDS Care* 2003;**14**:52–62.
25. Berg-Smith SM, Stevens VJ, Brown KM, *et al.* A brief motivational intervention to improve dietary adherence in adolescents. The Dietary Intervention Study in Children (DISC) Research Group. *Health Educ Res* 1999;**14**:399–410.

26. Channon S, Smith VJ, Gregory JW. A pilot study of motivational interviewing in adolescents with diabetes. *Arch Dis Child* 2003;**88**:680–683.

27. Aliotta SL, Vlasnik JJ, Delor B. Enhancing adherence to long-term medical therapy: a new approach to assessing and treating patients. *Adv Ther* 2004;**21**:214–231.

28. Skaret E, Weinstein P, Kvale G, Raadal M. An intervention program to reduce dental avoidance behaviour among adolescents: A pilot study. *Eur J Paediatr Dent* 2003;**4**: 191–196.

29. Draycott S, Dabbs A. Cognitive dissonance. 2: A theoretical grounding of motivational interviewing. *Br J Clin Psychol* 1998;**37**:355–364.

30. Prochaska JO, DiClemente CC. Transtheoretical therapy: Toward a more integrative model of change. *Psychother-Theor Res* 1982;**19**:276–287.

31. Rosner R. The scourge of addiction: What the adolescent psychiatrist needs to know. *Adolesc Psychiatry* 2005;**29**: 19–31.

32. Etheridge RM, Sullivan E, Tanner TB. *Brief Interventions for Alcohol Use Problems*. Clinical Tools, Inc., 2003.

33. Rollnick S, Heather N, Gold R, Hall W. Development of a short 'readiness to change' questionnaire for use in brief, opportunistic interventions among excessive drinkers. *Br J Addict* 1992;**87**:743–754.

34. Bloom BL. *Planned Short-term Psychotherapy*. Boston: Allyn & Bacon, 1992.

35. Slaff B. Thoughts on short-term and single-session therapy. *Adolesc Psychiatry* 1995;**20**:299–306.

36. Burke PJ, O'Sullivan J, Vaughan BL. Adolescent substance use: brief interventions by emergency care providers. *Pediatr Emerg Care* 2005;**21**:770–776.

37. Johnston BD, Rivara FP, Droesch RM, Dunn C, Copass MK. Behavior change counseling in the emergency department to reduce injury risk: a randomized, controlled trial. *Pediatrics* 2002;**110**:267–274.

38. Maio RF, Shope JT, Blow FC, *et al.* Adolescent injury in the emergency department: opportunity for alcohol interventions? *Ann Emerg Med* 2000;**35**:252–257.

39. Maio RF, Shope JT, Blow FC, *et al.* A randomized controlled trial of an emergency department-based interactive computer program to prevent alcohol misuse among injured adolescents. *Ann Emerg Med* 2005;**45**: 420–429.

40. Monti PM, Colby SM, Barnett NP, *et al.* Brief intervention for harm reduction with alcohol-positive older adolescents in a hospital emergency department. *J Consult Clin Psychol* 1999;**67**:989–994.

41. Spirito A, Monti PM, Barnett NP, *et al.* A randomized clinical trial of a brief motivational intervention for alcohol-positive adolescents treated in an emergency department. *J Pediatr* 2004;**145**:396–402.

42. Borsari B, Carey KB. Effects of a brief motivational intervention with college student drinkers. *J Consult Clin Psychol* 2000;**68**:728–733.

43. Marlatt GA, Baer JS, Kivlahan DR, *et al.* Screening and brief intervention for high-risk college student drinkers: results from a 2-year follow-up assessment. *J Consult Clin Psychol* 1998;**66**:604–615.

44. Grilo CM, Becker DF, Walker ML, Levy KN, Edell WS, McGlashan TH. Psychiatric comorbidity in adolescent inpatients with substance use disorders. *J Am Acad Child Adolesc Psychiatry* 1995;**34**:1085–1091.

Section Six

Special Issues in Adolescent Addiction

Edited by Stephen Bates Billick and Dean De Crisce

34

Substance Abuse Impact on Adolescent Brain Development

Adam Raff

New York University Medical Center, New York, NY, USA

INTRODUCTION

Adolescence is a crucial phase of development that is widely understood to be characterized by significant changes in an individual's neurobiology and related maturational processes. While the time frame defining adolescence has its sociocultural variations, the onset of puberty typically marks this critical period of transition from childhood, characterized by a surge in hormonal production and the emergence of secondary sexual characteristics. In addition to an array of unique biological changes that lay the foundations for adult functioning, adolescence is also a phase when sensation-seeking and impulsive behaviors tend to be much more prevalent. Developmentally, these behaviors potentially fuel the adolescent's development of an independent and autonomous identity by promoting the necessary social skills and peer interactions. With their social, as well as neurobiological roots, these reward-seeking behaviors are also, unfortunately, associated with their maladaptive consequences such as motor vehicle accidents and teenage pregnancy. Specifically, these risky behaviors have become increasingly implicated as one of several factors for increased risk for alcohol and substance abuse.

With growing evidence that more adolescents are being exposed to substance abuse at even younger ages, the unique quality of adolescent brain development and its vulnerability have become a greater focus of national attention. Alcohol is the most commonly consumed substance within the adolescent population, and one-third of all high-school seniors have used alcohol to intoxication within the previous month. Statistics measuring the consumption and frequency of alcohol use by adolescents are cause for alarm given the studies linking early alcohol use with the heightened risk for subsequent abuse, dependence, and alcohol-related medical problems in adulthood [1]. A 2006 report from the National Survey on Drug Use and Health noted that a majority of adolescents ranging in age from 12 to 20 years had used alcohol at least once in their lifetime, with the same age group representing 11.2% of all national alcohol consumption in a given month. An Office of Applied Studies Report from the Substance Abuse and Mental Health Services Administration (SAMHSA) indicated that in 2006 one-third of all adolescents ranging in age from 12 to 17 used alcohol in the prior year and approximately 20% had used an illicit substance in the same time frame. Of related concern, studies have also revealed that underage drinkers tend to use more alcohol on a given occasion compared with those individuals above the legal limit of 21 [2,3].

It is well established that normal adolescent brain development is characterized by considerable neurobiological changes with correlated behavioral expressions such as greater impulsivity and lower frustration tolerance. In addition to and because of the continuing maturation of brain structures, adolescence represents a period of significant changes in neuroplasticity and neurotransmission. Of concern, therefore, is that such a developmentally vulnerable brain is a sensitive substrate to the neurotoxicity of addictive substances. In a proposed vicious cycle, the resulting exposure to addictive substances lowers the already compromised threshold of inhibition for impulsivity, thereby disrupting any emerging developmental processes that would otherwise regulate risk-taking behaviors. This phenomenon has

Clinical Handbook of Adolescent Addiction, First Edition. Richard Rosner.
© 2013 John Wiley & Sons, Ltd. Published 2013 by John Wiley & Sons, Ltd.

been repeatedly illustrated in growing trends of earlier and heavier abuse of substances as well as rising rates of substance dependency in the adolescent population.

Understanding the relationship between substance abuse and its effect on the developing brain is complicated by several issues, including the adolescent brain's premorbid vulnerabilities and the role of the brain's regulatory mechanisms in behavioral, emotional, and cognitive responses to such exposures. The underlying brain structures responsible for regulation of those responses, both influence and are influenced by exposure to intoxicating substances. The neurobiology is such that substance-abusing adolescents, including those with comorbid psychiatric disorders, are then predisposed to further addiction and associated neuronal damage. As a result, scientific studies aimed at explaining the direct effect of substance abuse on the developing brain must be understood to be limited by a host of biopsychosocial variables such as mental illness, socioeconomic distress, trauma, and genetics. Adolescent brain development is marked by a series of multi-system neurobiological changes, ranging from molecular to macrostructural, that interface with both environmental and genetic forces. This period of significant brain remodeling is increasingly thought to represent a significant juncture of neurodevelopment that is highly vulnerable to the effects of toxic substances [4].

Studies of neurobiological and cellular effects of addictive substances on the adolescent brain are limited and composed of both prospective and retrospective research. Advances in imaging techniques such as functional magnetic resonance imaging (fMRI) processing in recent years have yielded a more richly differentiated understanding of the arch of neuroanatomical and microstructural development once considered to be essentially complete at puberty. This modality allows researchers to avoid exposing the brain to ionizing radiation compared with prior imaging methods; it also affords an invaluable tool in the study of the brain's function in real time.

In studying the effects of toxic substances on the brain, another useful measurement of structural change is white matter volume. In contrast to the non-linear changes in gray matter growth, white matter structural organization increases uniformly throughout childhood and adolescence in all four brain lobes. Neurodevelopment of white matter occurring into an individual's twenties, is associated with increase in white matter volume and integrity of fiber connections. Studies comparing white matter volume measurement using diffusion tensor imaging (DTI) have yielded results that suggest the latter may more sensitively detect white matter tissue distortions and potentially play a greater role in the evaluation of the brain with substance-related

exposure. Specifically, DTI is an enhanced magnetic resonance imaging technique that can measure both the magnitude and directionality of white matter tissue water diffusion in three directions. Using fractional anisotropy (FA) and radial diffusivity (RD), researchers can empirically determine microstructural growth and organization of tissue.

In contrast to the vast amount of imaging and research devoted to the effects of substance abuse on the adult brain, studies of brain development in substance-abusing adolescents have more recently emerged to address this phase-specific relationship. With late neuromaturation of the higher executive functioning areas within the adolescent brain, such as the prefrontal cortex, findings from the adult literature should not be generalized to the adolescent population.

ADOLESCENT BRAIN DEVELOPMENT

Before embarking upon a review of the impact of substance abuse on the adolescent brain, a more focused discussion of normal neurodevelopment is given to provide an appropriate context. The normal neural constructs underlying the adolescent's patterns of heightened impulsivity, risk-taking, and poor frustration tolerance may be the substrate upon which correlating behavioral patterns of adolescent substance abuse emerge. Research into the neurobiological underpinnings of these adolescent behaviors points in particular to the unique and crucial interrelationship between the prefrontal cortex, limbic system, and their differential rates of maturation. The neural maturation of the limbic system is relatively early when compared with that of the prefrontal cortex. The limbic system, with precortical and subcortical structures in its make-up, plays a central role in the motivational behaviors of risk and reward, while the prefrontal cortex, the seat of behavioral and inhibitory control, is the last of the major brain structures to reach its final development. Interestingly, it is in children and adults, where, simultaneously, both poles of this opposing neural circuitry are either wholly immature or mature, respectively. In contrast, the adolescent brain undergoes an important and unique transition, both in the emergence from childhood and the entrance into adulthood, which brackets a period of delicate imbalance between these two interrelated functional structures [4].

Studies of neuroanatomical data used to map the adolescent brain and its regional maturational changes have been based on the imaging of several cohorts of healthy adolescent volunteers. While an individual's brain size is noted to be 90% of its final volume by the age of 6 years, the subsystems of brain architecture undergo enormous differentiation in their neurodevelopment throughout adolescence and even into young adulthood. While the infant and child's brain is characterized by the tremendous growth in the total number of neurons, there is a tectonic shift during adolescent brain development to greater systemic efficiency between and within its neuronal circuitry. Neuroanatomical development proceeds in a differentiated manner within different areas of the cortex. Those brain divisions dedicated to more primal and homeostatic functions, mature first. In contrast areas responsible for higher executive functioning, such as the prefrontal cortex and the association cortices, complete their maturation last. Although both regions differ in their rates of neuromaturation, their connections remain highly interdependent and in delicate balance of one another [5].

During adolescent development, the brain's surface gray matter adopts an inverted "U" shape in growth, with volumetric increase at variable stages before an overall decline in size. It is thought that the changes in gray matter are related to changes in the cell neuron structure and their axonal apparatus and not a proliferation of tissue cells. The two cellular processes that characterize the asynchronous development of neural structures in adolescent brain are the myelination of axons and the cycle of overproduction (synaptogenesis or "arborization") followed by their eventual reduction ("pruning").

The neuromaturation of myelination usually begins in the first several years of life with the formation of axonal myelin sheaths persisting until late in adolescence. From ages 7 to 16, approximately half of all synapses are pruned with most synaptic pruning taking place in the neural inputs of the glutaminergic system. The differential stages of myelination in early adolescence occur across a spatial and temporal axis, with the brainstem and cerebellum myelinating first and cortical hemispheres and frontal lobes developing last. Progressively, neural connectivity and speed between the frontal cortex and other brain regions are consolidated throughout adolescence. The second process that occurs in the prefrontal cortex during adolescence is an increase in synaptic density followed by a period of synaptic pruning. Thus there is a non-linear pattern of development in the cortex, with frontal gray matter volume increasing until early adolescence and then decreasing between adolescence and adulthood [5].

The etiology of such neurodevelopment is unclear to investigators but an evolutionary based "use it or lose it" theory has been proposed by some researchers, the implications of which are particularly significant for an active adolescent brain. Research has demonstrated progressive gray matter pruning starting in the major sensorimotor areas with concluding maturation in associated areas of higher executive functioning such as the dorsolateral prefrontal cortex. The latter structure and its maturation – considered to be

responsible for a vast range of growing inhibitory functions including impulse control, assessment of judgment and consequences, and formation of future planning – appear to be consistent with the unregulated behavioral expressions commonly associated with early adolescence [6].

Cortical and subcortical structures have demonstrated significant development during adolescence, including the basal ganglia, amygdala, and hippocampus, which are of particular interest due to their prominent roles in memory formation, memory retrieval of state-specific emotional responses, affect regulation, and language synthesis. Another area undergoing significant maturation is the corpus callosum, the prominent bundle of commissural axons that links sections of the left and right hemispheres. Given its vast regulatory activity of motor output, sensory field integration, memory formation, and higher level executive functioning, the corpus callosum's functional role of integrating critical interhemispheric tasks is of paramount importance in the maturation of the adolescent brain. Imaging studies have revealed that, like the prefrontal cortex, posterior portions of the corpus callosum demonstrate prolonged development into the mid-twenties [5].

Normal cortical and subcortical structural development is predicated upon various underlying neurotransmitter systems, including dopamine, gamma-aminobutyric acid /termDefinition> (GABA), and glutamate. These neurotransmitter systems undergo radical reorganization in the prefrontal cortex with increases in cortical neurotransmitter concentration, densities of neurotransmitter afferents, and in the activity of COMT, the dopamine eliminating enzyme, catechol-O-methyl transferase. Other cellular changes, including the synthesis and reorganization of biogenic amine pathways, have been shown to have dramatic changes, both pre- and postnatally in human and animal studies. In contrast to the input of the excitatory glutamatergic system, which is reduced in the prefrontal cortex during adolescence, dopamine and serotonin as well as their receptor-binding capacity, have peak levels of synthesis and transmission during adolescence.

Understood to have a central role in the cycles of euphoria and reward, enhanced levels of dopamine may be particularly important in explaining the elated behaviors characterized by adolescence. Specifically, receptor levels of D1 and D2 are 30–50% higher in the caudate nucleus and putamen of adolescents compared to those in adults. The cortico-mesolimbic dopamine system undergoes significant reorganization, with D1 and D2 receptors showing amplified growth before the onset of the normal pruning process. In contrast to the overall decrease in dopaminergic production in the prefrontal cortex, several subcortical structures signal increased turnover and production of dopamine synthesis including projections to the nucleus accumbens, ventral tegmental area, and amygdala.

Finally, parallel to regional brain changes during adolescent brain growth, major neurological and psychological processes have also been found to undergo developmental changes and differential stages of maturation, including processing speed, response inhibition, and spatial working memory. Studies indicate that given specific cognitive tasks, and despite similar measures of performance, adolescents demonstrated immature patterns of brain activation and alternate neural circuitry when compared with adults. Variations in regional neuromaturation are also noted in studies of differential gender development. Some neuroanatomical studies indicate that females tend to demonstrate earlier peaking of gray matter volume compared with males but possess smaller overall brain volumes. Such gender differences in brain development are postulated to confer varying levels of neurotoxic vulnerability during substance exposure.

STUDIES OF THE IMPACT OF SUBSTANCE USE

In addition to the direct neurotoxic effect of substances on the growing brain, research has increasingly studied their unique neurobiological interactions, such as the reinforcing properties that propagate their dependence. Commonly used neurotoxic substances are thought to distort neurotransmission in the mesolimbic dopaminergic tract while overactivating the dopaminergic-rich ventral striatum projecting to the frontal lobe. The ventral striatum, an already highly activated structure in adolescence, is thought to be further enhanced by the substance exposure resulting in a cementing of the substance's reinforcement properties. Thus toxic substance exposure is thought simultaneously to disrupt the brain's emerging regulatory mechanisms and to overstimulate its reward centers, compromising the delicate balance between the competing forces of higher cortical inhibitory functions and lower subcortical structures linked to reward and motivation [4].

ANIMAL STUDIES

In an effort to approximate the impact of substance abuse on the adolescent brain and due to ethical constraints on human experiments, research has relied on the parallels of neurobiology and physiology in animal studies, particularly rodents. The dramatic biological changes and related behavioral changes that typify adolescent human development, such as increases in socialization, impulsivity, risk-taking, and novelty-seeking, are also evident in a host of other species, particularly the adolescent rat. Conventionally marked by enhanced neurogenesis, adolescence in the rat typically begins between postnatal days 28 to 42, characterized by significant growth changes, hormonal spurts, and behavioral expressions of socially extroverted group behaviors. As in humans, glutamate and N-methyl-D-aspartate (NMDA) glutamate receptor densities in rat brains have also been demonstrated to be markers presaging the neural pruning process. In adolescent rats, too, glutamate and glutamate-NMDA receptors have shown increases in density growth compared with adult rats.

Monti et al. investigated the effects of binge drinking on both the adolescent and adult rat brain. While both populations revealed signs of alcohol-induced neuronal damage, the adolescent rat brain demonstrated specific neuroanatomical deficits in the forebrain corresponding to the orbital-frontal and temporal areas of the human brain, areas responsible for working memory and learning. An increasing number of studies have also demonstrated that binge drinking can be differentiated from other levels of alcohol intake by its association with lasting neurotoxic effects. Such investigations of the effects of binge drinking are of particular importance because a large segment of the national adolescent population binge drinks to a significant degree [7].

One emerging hypothesis of binge drinking stems from studies of alcohol-preferring rats, which have been associated with increased binge-induced brain damage and decreased levels of phospho-mitogen-activated protein kinase, compared with controls. It is widely observed that both adolescent alcohol-preferring rats and adolescent humans are noted to be resistant to the sedative effects of alcohol, which may be caused by a disruption in cellular signaling mechanisms, thereby lowering regulatory mechanisms and enhancing the propensity to continue drinking alcohol. In fact, normal adolescent neurogenesis has been found to be inhibited by alcohol binge drinking, with associated pathogenic effects on cellular signaling and neurotransmission pathways [8].

Monti et al. also studied the effects of alcohol binge drinking on the distribution of serotonin transporters in the adolescent rat brain using citalopram-binding capacity. Compared to controls, rats with exposure to binge drinking in adolescence demonstrated increased levels of serotonin transporter density and citalopram binding as adults. Such alterations in serotonergic innervation are thought to decrease synaptic serotonin concentration leading to changes in sleep patterns, impulsivity, satiation, and other serotonin-mediated behaviors. In other rodent studies, significant alcohol exposure in adolescents compared with adults demonstrated various molecular and neuropsychological effects including greater impairment in spatial memory, alcohol-induced neurodegeneration, and alcohol-induced inhibition of neurogenesis. In adolescent rats, disturbances in NMDA-mediated synaptic transmission have been associated with increased dendritic spine size, which has been hypothesized to represent cellular manifestations of neuroadaptive mechanisms involved in the establishment of addictive behaviors and resulting cognitive impairments. The aforementioned studies support the growing research implicating heavy alcohol exposure in forebrain damage during adolescence, when this area is itself undergoing significant neuromaturation. Neuronal loss and increased levels of local inflammatory cells are thought to result, causing further disruption of forebrain functioning and neurotransmission [7].

Both human and rodent studies have indicated a range of sequelae resulting from the brain's exposure to alcohol. An analysis of differentiating variables for exposure includes the stage of brain development, blood alcohol concentrations, and pattern of exposure. With increasing empirical evidence demonstrating alcohol's toxic effects on the growing brain after binge-like exposure, studies have attempted to explore the effects of chronic alcohol exposure and the degree to which the brain can compensate for such exposure. In animal studies, researchers chronically exposed adolescent rat brains to 6 weeks of alcohol inhalation followed by a 10-week period of abstinence. The initial morphological effects of the chronic exposure, measured by immuno-histochemical assay, included expected changes in the serotonergic system, astrocytes, and cystoskeleton. In addition, the study revealed that despite a longer period of abstinence, molecular and cell-related damage was only partially recovered, compared to a baseline state of development [8].

ALCOHOL

A significant body of research exploring the differential effects of alcohol on human adolescent brains compared to adult brains lends empirical support to the often observed phenomenon that adolescents appear more immune to the sedating effects of alcohol and its withdrawal effects than their adult counterparts. Such age-dependent resilience to alcohol's depressive effects – sometimes a negative reinforcement for further exposure in adults – raises concerns that adolescents are biologically predisposed for continued abuse compounded by the influence of social pressures.

With 10% of late adolescents meeting criteria for alcohol use disorder (AUD), individuals with a family history of AUD have an increased risk for developing AUD compared to individuals without such a positive

family history. Individuals with a positive family history have demonstrated cognitive deficits as well as neuro-anatomical differences compared with such controls groups. In healthy populations, the hippocampus evidences a natural asymmetry of right greater than left lobes, with increases in volume throughout adolescence. Given the particular vulnerability of the hippocampus to the effects of alcohol and the continued neuromaturation of adolescence, a limited number of studies have explored the role of an AUD history on hippocampal volume development in adolescents. The significance of such hippocampal changes may provide information regarding future risk factors for these populations.

Although not uniformly consistent, various findings in adolescents with AUD histories suggest both overall decreased hippocampal volume in right and left lobes and increased asymmetry of left and right hippocampus without concomitant volume decreases in other major brain structures. Research involving the comparisons of adolescent populations exposed to heavy alcohol use, alone or in combination with marijuana, with controls, has consistently demonstrated either smaller hippocampal volumes or greater degrees of asymmetry directly correlated to age of onset and duration of AUD. In contrast, other studies, involving both alcohol and marijuana, have reported actual increases in hippocampal volumes suggesting a complexity of interactions with multiple forms of substance exposure and the developing brain [9–11].

In one of the earlier neuroimaging studies of its kind, DeBellis et al. (2000) compared the hippocampal volumes of adolescents and young adults having a history of adolescent-onset AUD with healthy matched controls. Given the age-related relationship between the neurotoxic effects of alcohol and significant brain pathology in adults, it was hypothesized that the two groups would not significantly differ in their respective hippocampal development. Instead, the MRI measurements of 12 subjects with AUDs compared to 24 control subjects revealed that both left and right hippocampal volumes were smaller in the former. Significantly, these hippocampal volumes correlated positively with the age at onset of alcohol use and negatively with the duration of the alcohol use disorder [9–11].

Researchers suggest several possible mechanisms for the findings including the direct neurotoxic effects of alcohol on the hippocampal development through the NMDA receptors as well as the possibility that the smaller hippocampus may itself be a risk factor for subsequent alcohol abuse. Regarding the former, in animal studies, chronic alcohol exposure is associated with upregulation of NMDA receptors and resulting neuronal damage secondary to its heightened excitatory process. Thus, hippocampal development during adolescence may be exquisitely sensitive to the effects of alcohol through NMDA-mediated neurotoxicity [9].

More extensive studies in adult alcohol-dependent individuals previously demonstrated hypometabolism in the medial frontal region of the cerebral cortex, as well as decreased volumes in various subcortical and cerebellar regions. While significant cognitive deficits have been studied in adolescent alcohol use, it was also noted that offspring of adult alcoholics independently performed poorly on cognitive function measures. In order to explore the notion that pre-existing structural vulnerabilities may increase the risk of AUD, DeBellis et al. [12] compared structures in the prefrontal-thalamic-cerebellar tract in adolescents having AUDs and their healthy controls, hypothesizing smaller volumes in the former.

Results indicate that adolescents with AUDs had smaller prefrontal cortex and prefrontal cortex white matter volumes compared with control subjects, with no significant difference in some subcortical and cerebellar structures. In a study of the effect of gender, results showed that males with AUDs compared with control males had smaller cerebellar volumes, while the two female groups demonstrated no differences in cerebellar volumes. Finally, the study concluded that prefrontal cortex volumes significantly correlated with measures of alcohol consumption. These findings underscore the association between a smaller prefrontal cortex and early-onset drinking [12].

The effects of alcohol abuse on the prefrontal cortex are of special significance given its late maturation and its centrality to executive functioning and decision-making. Traditionally, imaging studies of adults with heavy alcohol usage have consistently reflected an array of neural deteriorations at both macro- and micro-structural levels of the prefrontal cortex. More recently, imaging techniques have localized these microstructural changes to interconnecting white matter tracts of the frontal and parietal cortices. Studies have compared prefrontal cortex total volume and white matter volume in individuals with adolescent-onset AUDs, with their controls. The results revealed smaller volumes of pre-frontal cortex associated with early-onset drinking in comparison with healthy controls. Smaller cerebellar volumes in AUD males were also reported, whereas no significant differences were noted between female cohorts. Significantly these volumetric findings correlated positively with measures of alcohol consumption [12].

Research by Medina et al. [13] sought to examine the relationship between AUD and the effects on prefrontal cortex volume in adolescents without comorbid psychiatric disorders. Fourteen adolescents with AUD were compared with 17 healthy controls, excluding any history of psychiatric or neurological disorder other than AUD and conduct disorder. The results showed that alcohol exposure during adolescence was associated with prefrontal cortex (PFC) volume abnormalities as well as PFC white matter differences. Notably, there were marked gender-related differences: males with AUD demonstrated overall larger PFC volumes than girls with AUD, and each study group had increased volumes compared with their controls. Paralleling the adult literature, the findings suggest that gender may regulate the relationship between alcohol use and PFC volume in response to cognitive tasks.

These findings may be relevant to a better under-standing of adolescent neurodevelopment, considering that boys typically exhibit a delayed pruning process in brain development compared with girls. Researchers have postulated that early exposure to heavy alcohol consumption in males may inhibit this maturational process, resulting in larger volumes. A potential explanation is that the brain of male adolescents is less vulnerable than female adolescents to the neurotoxic effects of alcohol and thus myelination and overall growth continue to advance [13].

However, similar investigations have yielded some contradictory results, including smaller volumes of PFC and white matter for both boys and girls with AUD histories. In addition to an older population of adolescents, another factor explaining the differences in volumes may be that comorbid Axis I psychiatric disorders (e.g. attention-deficit/hyperactivity disorder, conduct disorder, major depressive disorder-recurrent, and post-traumatic stress disorder) are also associated with structural abnormalities, only furthering the complexity of these interacting variables. Nonetheless, Medina's research supports previous studies indicating smaller PFC total and white matter volumes in adolescent AUD females compared to female controls. Underlying processes of programmed cell loss (e.g. neuronal cell death or atrophy) or proliferation of inflammatory mediators have both been proposed as mechanisms for reduced volumes. The PFC is highly dense with exci-tatory amino acid pathways; during adolescence these may be exquisitely vulnerable to the neurotoxic effects of alcohol, yielding further cell reduction and pruning.

Research has attempted to explore further the relationship between brain structure and psychiatric disturbances in populations of adolescent substance abusers. Although there is a substantial body of neuroimaging research in adult populations linking morphological changes in the brain and psychiatric conditions, it is difficult to extrapolate such effects to child and adolescent development given the dramatic changes of neuro-maturation. The complexity of these variables is borne out by studies measuring various structural or volumetric abnormalities, which have yielded results without uniform findings. Also, various substances, such as marijuana, with its high prevalence of use in adolescents, are independently associated with a risk of depressive syndrome, especially among heavy and earlier onset users.

MARIJUANA

Marijuana is the most commonly used illicit substance among adolescents in the United States [3]. Recent statistics indicate that nearly 45% of senior high-school students have tried marijuana, and 5% have reported daily use. Historically, marijuana has been considered a gateway drug, although this continues to be debatable. Of significance, there is growing concern that early marijuana abuse may be directly related to the development or acceleration of underlying psychiatric disturbances. Studies examining the effects of long-term marijuana abuse in adult populations seem to suggest a relatively higher risk of psychological deficits when developing brains are exposed to marijuana, with some studies demonstrating greater propensity to depressive symptoms in marijuana-using adolescents.

Medina et al. [14] sought to examine the relationship between white matter and hippocampal volumes and depressive symptoms in marijuana-using adolescents. Sixteen marijuana-using adolescents with no past or current history of depressive symptoms were compared with healthy controls. Using MRI, the Beck Depression Inventory, and Hamilton Depression Rating Scale, among other tools, these researchers demonstrated that smaller white matter volumes among adolescent marijuana users predicted greater depressive symptoms than the controls [14].

Studies of the general population and the effects of chronic marijuana exposure have revealed diminished cognitive functioning in terms of working memory and learning. In adolescents, studies using neuropsychological functioning and fMRI validate the deleterious effects of cannabis exposure in the adolescent brain, including deficits in working memory and attentional and overall cognitive performance [15]. Studies of gray matter changes in adults who initiated marijuana use in early adolescence reveal volume reductions in various cortical and subcortical areas including the hippocampus, cingulate cortex, and amygdala. These reductions were found to be inversely related to chronicity of marijuana exposure. There is limited DTI research on the effects of chronic cannabis exposure on white matter integrity, even in the adult population. Results have varied due to small sample sizes, heterogeneity of cannabis abuse, and differing methods of image analysis. Findings have ranged from no changes

in white matter volume to reduced white matter volumes in the left parietal lobe.

Ashtari et al. [16] hypothesized that DTI would demonstrate white matter tissue deficits and microstructural changes in key brain regions undergoing developmental maturation during adolescence as well as in brain areas where cannabinoid receptors have also been found to influence neurodevelopment during adolescence. Cannabinoid receptors are considered to be most densely located in the frontal cortex, hippocampus, basal ganglia, cerebellum, amygdala, and striatum. In these regions, increased marijuana use is known to be associated with increased local metabolism on fMRI and decreased gray matter density. Hypothesized findings were to be measured by decreased fractional anisotropy (FA) and increased mean and radial diffusivity (MRD), using a more comprehensive whole brain analysis of data.

In the Ashtari study, 14 male adolescents with histories of heavy cannabis use (HCU), residing in a residential drug treatment center, were compared with healthy subjects matched on various demographic and socioeconomic markers. The marijuana user group, other than drug-related charges, had no history of violent crimes, was drug-free for at least 3 months, and was monitored by routine urine toxicology tests to ensure their diagnosis of cannabis dependence. Participants were reported to have used marijuana daily for 1 year prior to treatment, but subjects with a lifetime history of greater than 10 uses of illicit substances other than marijuana were excluded from the study. Finally, while individuals with psychiatric disorders including major depressive disorder, bipolar disorder, and psychotic disorders were also excluded, a history of past alcohol abuse, due to its high rate of association with marijuana use, was not viewed as an exclusionary variable.

Resulting analyses confirmed the hypothesis of white matter disruption in the HUC population, as evidenced by four neuroanatomical clusters with decreased FA in the internal capsule, thalamic radiation, left middle temporal gyrus, and right superior temporal gyrus – areas considered to undergo significant structural development in adolescence. Other positive findings such as increased MRD, in combination with decreased FA values, also reflect the likelihood of decreased myelination or its disruption of normal development during adolescence. A second set of analyses focusing on specific white matter tracts, the right and left arcuate fiber tracts (brain areas thought to be populated with cannabinoid system receptors and highly susceptible to insults during neuromaturation), were also found to have similar patterns of deficits, with decreased FA. Cannabinoid receptors have been shown to be present in white matter tissue in early developmental stages of growth, indicating their potentially influential role in white matter differentiation, migration, and maturation. Thus, chronic exposure to marijuana of the cannabinoid receptor system may likely interfere with the generation and functioning of oligodendrocytes [16].

While volumetric and structural studies of brain tissues in adult cannabis users have demonstrated variable results, there is evidence to suggest that the sub-population of early marijuana users may reveal significant patterns of tissue alteration during neuro-development. Along these lines, there is continuing research exploring the link between early-age marijuana use and heightened risk of psychosis in individuals with associated genetic diathesis. On a cellular level, marijuana abuse has been hypothesized to lead to the down-regulation of CB1 receptors as well as to suppress oligodendrocyte genesis and functioning, thereby disrupting optimal neural transmission in the myelin tissue. Such pervasive white matter damage would presumably account for a host of sensory deficits characteristic of psychosis. In support of this hypothesis, Grigorenko et al. demonstrated decreased expression of myelin-related genes in association with long-term cannabis exposure [17].

Bossong et al. [18] reviewed the growing body of scientific research to support the implicated role of marijuana's neurotoxic effects in precipitating a psychotic illness. Specific risk factors for the development of psychosis in the context of marijuana use include the timing of exposure with respect to the neurodevelopment of the adolescent and the frequency of use. Despite its controversy, research investigators have sought to explore the relationship between marijuana exposure and its role preceding new-onset psychotic episodes. A mounting foundation of data has encouraged further research into this relationship. Clear explanations of neurobiological mechanisms underlying this link have historically been absent but marijuana's neurotoxicity is borne out in some pilot animal research. Animal studies indicate that adolescent rats, when compared to adult rats, sustain greater structural brain deficits with associated functional disturbances when exposed to chronic levels of delta-7-tetrahydrocannabinol (THC). These animal studies suggest that the structural brain changes are mediated by excessive exposure to CB1 receptors.

In their work, Bossong et al. [18] suggest a toxicological model implicating THC, the intoxicating agent in marijuana, as having direct and irreversible effects on brain tissue with resulting microstructural and functional aberrations. Specifically, exposure to THC disrupts neural circuitry in the PFC that is most vulnerable during adolescent brain development. The CB1 receptor and endogenous cannabinoids are found in developing white matter in the PFC. During normal brain development, the binding of the CB1 receptor and endogenous cannabinoids plays a crucial role in the regulation of glutamate and gamma-aminobutyric acid (GABA) release. Glutamate is a neurotransmitter with functional properties central to the pruning and final differentiation of synaptic development during key phases of neuro-maturation. It has been proposed that THC exposure negatively affects CB1 receptors, which then dysregulate glutamate release, potentially disturbing emerging structural development and neural circuitry in the PFC. Distortions in the PFC and related neural connections to subcortical structures are thought to promote the aberrant neurotransmitter synthesis of dopamine and GABA, which are historically implicated in the etiology of schizophrenia [18].

COMBINED USE OF ALCOHOL AND MARIJUANA

National statistics on adolescent substance use indicate that adolescents most frequently use both alcohol and cannabis in combination. This poses significant challenges in attempting to assess the complexity of inter-active effects on the development of brain structure and central nervous system functioning during a period of continued neuromaturation. With evidence of cannabinoid receptor distribution in myelin cell formation and data already implicating the toxic effects of alcohol on white matter development, work by Bava et al. [19] explored the impact of heavy alcohol and marijuana use combined on microstructural white matter development.

Using DTI, this study involved the assessment of white matter development in 36 marijuana- and alcohol-using adolescents, aged 16–19, compared to 36 non-using controls. The substance-using adolescents demonstrated significantly decreased FA compared with controls in multiple regions including left superior longitudinal fasciculus and fronto-temporal white matter tracts. Simultaneously, increased FA in right occipital and superior longitudinal fasciculus regions was noted. The findings suggest that perhaps as a result of the neurotoxic effects on the adolescent's fronto-parietal circuitry and resulting distortions in axonal and myelin development, there are enhanced or compensatory cognitive processes in alternate brain regions.

In studying similar populations of dual substance users, researchers have demonstrated neurocognitive deficits in attention, visuo-spatial functioning, and verbal and non-verbal encoding learning, as well as changes in related brain morphology, anisotropic differences in white matter development, and evidence of alternate neural pathway formation. Using DTI, Bava *et al.* [20] studied the relationship between brain regions of both decreased and increased FA in order to determine if there were correlating and enduring neurocognitive manifestations stemming from changes in white matter microstructure. Specifically it was hypothesized that decreased FA and decreased white matter integrity would be associated with poorer performance on neurocognitive measures, and that increased FA would be associated with improved performance due to compensatory processes. Measured scores of attention, working memory, and speed processing were, in fact, discovered to be lower in those brain areas of decreased FA. In contrast, regions of increased FA activation, including the right occipital area, correlated with enhanced measures of visuo-motor performance that appear to support the anticipated compensatory process [19,20].

NEUROPSYCHOLOGICAL EFFECTS OF SUBSTANCE USE

Related adult literature and rodent studies have repeatedly shown the direct neurotoxic effects of alcohol as well as the resultant effects on working memory, attention, and learning. Nonetheless, in the past, the limited number of retrospective studies examining the effects of substance use on neuropsychological functioning in the adolescent population did not reveal significant deficits. By the late 1990s, reports increasingly found poorer performance scores in a range of cognitive tasks including visuo-spatial functioning, inhibitory control, and language and attention skills. Nonetheless, the full impact of alcohol's effects on adolescent neurocognitive functioning is yet to be determined due to the frequent cross-sectional nature of much research.

Tapert *et al.* [21] prospectively studied neuropsychological functioning associated with adolescent substance abuse and withdrawal over a period of 8 years. The authors followed a previously studied cohort from ages 16 to 24 with neuropsychological testing and substance abuse monitoring. The results indicated that protracted substance use differentially influenced neurocognitive functioning and that heavy use is specifically associated with learning, attention, and retention deficits. While language functioning did not appear to be adversely effected, attentional deficits were found to be most sensitive to the commonly used substances, alcohol, marijuana, and stimulants. Both prolonged marijuana and stimulant use modestly predicted poor attention and dysregulated psychomotor processing speeds in the final year of the study. Finally, visuospatial functioning correlated with substance use and withdrawal over the study's duration. This and other

similar studies underscore the subtle but conclusively damaging effects of prolonged substance abuse and, particularly withdrawal states, on neurocognitive abilities [21].

Using fMRI techniques and measured neural activity via blood oxygen levels in response to specific cognitive tasks, Tapert *et al.* [22] attempted to measure the spatial working memory of adolescents with heavy alcohol use compared with adolescents with light alcohol use. Their results revealed that, although both groups performed similarly on the respective cognitive tasks, the parietal lobes of the heavy drinkers demonstrated increased activation in a blood oxygen-level-dependent signal and decreased activation in the occipital lobe and cerebellum. Related investigations in adolescents with even longer histories of heavy alcohol use resulted in greater deficiencies in similar spatial working memory tasks. This and other supportive work suggest that while heavy alcohol use of 1–2 years can potentially distort neural activity in response to spatial working memory tasks, extended periods of heavy alcohol use overwhelm and compromise the brain's capacity to compensate during the execution of such neurocognitive tasks [22].

Research into the role of post-drinking effects such as hangover and withdrawal has further supported the risk of lasting brain changes. Some studies have suggested that the actual quantity of alcohol causing withdrawal is less damaging to neurocognitive functioning during adolescence than the effects of the withdrawal syndrome itself. Squeglia *et al.* [23] examined neurocognition in adolescents prior to the onset of any heavy drinking and then prospectively studied cognitive functioning at follow-up in those transitioning into moderately heavy alcohol use. The differential effect of alcohol on gender was also evaluated. Results indicated that for girls, more drinking days in the year before the follow-up of neurocognitive assessment predicted worsening visuo-spatial functioning. For boys, greater hangover symptoms in the year before the follow-up were linked to relative worsening in sustained attention [23].

NICOTINE

Cigarette smoking remains the most common cause of preventable death in the United States (Centers for Disease Control and Prevention [CDC], [24]). Epidemiological studies indicate that earlier use of nicotine, compared with individuals over 20, is associated with more extended periods of subsequent smoking as an adult and greater difficulty with attempts at cessation. Research has recently suggested that exposure to smoking in early adolescence may foster a cycle of increased neurotoxicity, impaired cognitive functioning, and heightened impulsivity that contributes to hardened smoking patterns and nicotine dependency. One theory suggests that tobacco-induced neurotoxicity of adolescent cognitive development points to nicotine-induced damage in the prefrontal cortex and its neuronal connections during the brain's most vulnerable state of development [25].

Full maturation of the cholinergic system is typically attained in the PFC during the course of adolescence, with acetylcholine playing several critical regulatory functions. Acetylcholine has been shown to be crucial to the mechanism of neuronal proliferation and differentiation, as well as modulating axonogenesis and synaptogenesis. Cholinergic activity is significant for its role in shaping the foundations for neural architecture and has also been studied in regard to learning and memory of early adolescence.

Significant biochemical differences exist between acetylcholine and nicotine. Acetylcholine is released in amounts exponentially smaller than nicotine, and acts on neuronal acetylcholine receptors before being rapidly metabolized by acetylcholinesterase. Compared with acetylcholine, exogenous nicotine from a cigarette perfuses the brain in a higher concentration, at a more gradual rate, and remains unmetabolized for longer periods of time outside the central nervous system. In a nicotine-stimulated cholinergic system, a desensitization and upregulation of neuronal acetylcholine receptors results, leading to disturbances in synaptic activity, functioning, and neurotransmission.

In rodent studies of exposure to heightened levels of nicotine, adolescent rats, when compared to adults, demonstrated a neurotoxic overproduction of neuronal acetylcholine receptors and a more prolonged suppression of cholinergic activity after nicotine withdrawal. These neurochemical changes in the adolescent rat brain are associated with enduring cognitive impairments in the adult [26].

The theory of tobacco-induced neurotoxicity and its deleterious effect on the adolescent PFC represents another explanation for a neurotoxic substance to enhance the cycle of its overuse by compromising executive functioning and lowering the threshold for impulse control. Impulsivity in smokers has been studied and particular areas of the PFC, such as the orbitofrontal cortex, have been implicated. Imaging studies have demonstrated smaller prefrontal cortical volumes and densities in smokers than non-smokers, and pack-year smoking history was noted to be inversely correlated with PFC volume. Given that multiple studies have shown nicotine's effect on enhancing cognitive performance and attention, the plight of the adolescent smoker with poor executive functioning is more readily understood. Whether or not the adolescent smoker's poor executive functioning was initially induced by nicotine's deleterious effects, a vicious cycle of cognitive reward and further neurotoxicity is propagated [27].

References

1. National Survey on Drug Use and Health. *Trends in Substance Abuse, Dependence or Abuse, and Treatment among Adolescents: 2002 to 2007*. Washington, DC:Office of Applied Studies, Substance Abuse and Mental Health Services Administration, 2008.
2. National Survey on Drug Use and Health. *Quantity and Frequency of Alcohol Use among Underage Drinkers*. Washington, DC:Office of Applied Studies, Substance Abuse and Mental Health Services Administration, 2008.
3. National Survey on Drug Use and Health. *A Day in the Life of American Adolescents: Substance Use Facts*. Washington, DC:Office of Applied Studies, Substance Abuse and Mental Health Services Administration, 2007.
4. Casey BJ. Neurobiology of the adolescent brain and behavior: implications for substance use disorders. *J Am Acad Child Adolesc Psychiatry* 2010;**49**:1189–1201.
5. Giedd J. Adolescent brain development: vulnerabilities and opportunities. *Ann N Y Acad Sci* 2004;**1021**:77–85.
6. Spear LP, Varlinskaya EI. Sensitivity to ethanol and other hedonic stimuli in an animal model of adolescence: implications for prevention science? *Dev Psychobiol* 2010;**52**:236–243.
7. Monti P, Miranda R Jr, Nixon K, *et al.* Adolescence: booze, brains and behavior. *Alcohol Clin Exp Res* 2005;**29**:207–220.
8. Evrard SG, Duhalde-Vega M, Tagliaferro P, Mirochnic S, Caltana LR, Brusco A. A low chronic ethanol exposure induces morphological changes in the adolescent rat brain that are not fully recovered even after a long abstinence: An immuno-histochemical study. *Exp Neurol* 2006;**200**:438–459.
9. DeBellis MD, Clark DB, Beers SR, *et al.* Hippocampal volume in adolescent onset alcohol use disorder. *Am J Psychiatry* 2000;**157**:737–744.
10. Nagel BJ, Schweinsburg AD, Phan V, Tapert SF. Reduced hippocampal volume among adolescents with alcohol use disorders without psychiatric co-morbidity. *Psychiatry Res* 2005;**139**:181–190.
11. Medina KL, Schweinsburg AD, Cohen-Zion M, Nagel BJ, Tapert SF. Effects of alcohol and combined marijuana and alcohol use during adolescence on hippocampal volume and asymmetry. *Neurotoxicol Teratol* 2007;**29**:141–152.
12. DeBellis MD, Narasimhan A, Thatcher DL, Keshavan MS, Soloff P, Clark DB. Prefrontal cortex, thalamus, and cerebellar volumes in adolescents and young adults with adolescent-onset alcohol use disorders and comorbid mental disorders. *Alcohol Clin Exp Res* 2005;**29**:1590–1600.
13. Medina, KL, McQueeny T, Nagel BJ, Hanson KL, Schweinsburg AD, Tapert SF. Prefrontal cortex volumes in adolescents with alcohol use disorders: unique gender effects. *Alcohol Clin Exp Res* 2008;**32**:386–394.
14. Medina KL, Nagel BJ, Park A, McQueeny T, Tapert SF. Depressive symptoms in adolescents: associations with white matter volume and marijuana use. *J Child Psychol Psychiatry* 2007;**48**:592–600.

15. Medina KL, Hanson KL, Schweinsburg AD, Cohen-Zion M., Nagel BJ, Tapert SF. Neuropsychological functioning in adolescent marijuana users: subtle deficits detectable after a month of abstinence. *J Int Neuropsychol Soc* 2007;**13**:807–820.

16. Ashtari M. Diffusion abnormalities in adolescents. *J Psychiatric Responsibilities* 2009;**43**:189–204.

17. Grigorenko E, Kittler J, Clayton C, *et al.* Assessment of cannabinoid induced gene changes: tolerance and neuro-protection. *Chem Phys Lipids* 2002;**121**:257–266.

18. Bossong MG, Niesink RJ. Adolescent brain maturation, the endogenous cannabinoid system and the neurobiology of cannabis-induced schizophrenia. *Progr Neurobiol* 2010;**92**: 370–385.

19. Bava S, Frank LR, McQueeny T, Schweinsburg BC, Schweinsburg AD, Tapert SF. Altered white matter micro-structure in adolescent substance users. *Psychiatry Res* 2009;**173**:228–237.

20. Bava S, Jacobus J, Mahmood O, Yang TT, Tapert SF. Neurocognitive correlates of white matter quality in adoles-cent substance users. *Brain Cognition* 2010;**72**:347–354.

21. Tapert S, Granholm E, Leedy NG, Brown SA. Substance use and withdrawal: neuropsychological functioning over 8 years in youth. *J Int Psychol Soc* 2002;**8**:873–883.

22. Tapert S, Schweinsburg AD, Bartlett VC, *et al.* Blood oxygen level dependent response and spatial working memory in adolescents with alcohol use disorders. *Alcohol Clin Exp Res* 2004;**28**:1577–1586.

23. Squeglia L, Spadoni AD, Infante MA, Myers MG, Tapert SF. Initiating moderate to heavy alcohol use predicts changes in neuropsychological functioning for adolescent girls and boys. *Psychol Addict Behav* 2009;**23**:715–722.

24. Prevalence of Current Cigarette Smoking Among Adults and Changes in Prevalence of Current and Some Day Smoking—United States, 1996–2001. Centers For Disease Control and Prevention. April 11, 2003, Vol. 52, No. 14.

25. DeBry SC, Tiffany ST. Tobacco-induced neurotoxicity of adolescent cognitive development (TINACD): A proposed model for the development of impulsivity in nicotine dependence. *Nicotine Tob Res* 2008;**10**:11–25.

26. Slotkin T. Nicotine and the adolescent brain: insight from an animal model. *Neurotoxicol Teratol* 2002;**24**: 369–384.

27. Jacobsen LK, Krystal JH, Mencl WE, Westerveld M, Frost SJ, Pugh KR. Effects of smoking and smoking abstinence on cognition in adolescent tobacco smokers. *Biol Psychiat* 2005;**57**:56–66.

35

Neuropsychological Effects of Substance Abuse in Adolescents

Diane Scheiner,[1] Ari Kalechstein,[2] and Wilfred G. van Gorp[3]

[1]*Department of Psychology, Fordham University, New York, NY, USA*
[2]*Baylor College of Medicine, The Menninger Department of Psychiatry, Houston, TX, USA*
[3]*Columbia University College of Physicians & Surgeons, Department of Psychiatry, New York, NY, USA*

Adolescent substance abuse is an international public health concern. While only a minority of youths eventually develop substance use disorders, recreational drug abuse represents a major social policy challenge worldwide [1,2]. Recent surveys of middle- and high-school students reveal that the overwhelming majority of adolescents have used alcohol by the time they complete high school, and nearly half have experimented with illicit substances [1,2]. Despite declines in the use of some illicit drugs in the United States over the past two decades [3], abuse of alcohol and other substances; including over-the-counter (OTC) medications, prescription medications, and chemical inhalants; remains high in a substantial portion of young people.

The concerns raised by these epidemiological studies cannot be overstated, given that adolescence marks a critical stage in neurodevelopment (i.e., when the brain is particularly vulnerable to the neurotoxic effects of psychoactive substances) [4]. Disruptions to normal brain development may have far-reaching implications for functioning in adulthood. Early-adolescent-onset substance use, for example, is associated with greater probability of later substance dependency [5–7], highlighting the potential long-term risk associated with substance use during this critical developmental period.

Because adolescents experiment with various substances that modulate central nervous system (CNS) function, it is important that clinicians treating adolescent patients are knowledgeable about how acute intoxication and protracted use of recreational drugs affect cognition. The effects of adolescent substance use on the brain are complicated by the fact that a subset of adolescents have pre-existing neuropsychological deficits, particularly frontal/executive deficits, as a result of a learning disability and/or attention-deficit/hyperactivity disorder (ADHD), and these conditions are risk factors for onset of substance abuse themselves [8–10]. Long-term adolescent substance use is associated with changes in brain physiology and structure, as well as related deficits in a number of neuropsychological functions, including attention, learning and memory, and visuo-spatial skills [11–14].

Studies of adolescents have for the most part focused on the effects of protracted substance use. Thus, many of the findings reviewed in this chapter describe the neuropsychological implications of chronic substance abuse in adolescents-either during periods of continued use or following periods of abstinence-as opposed to the acute effects of intoxication.

NEUROPSYCHOLOGICAL SEQUELAE OF SUBSTANCE ABUSE IN YOUTH

Alcohol

The literature on substance abuse and neuropsychological functioning in adolescence has primarily focused on alcohol. Early studies of adolescent drinking reported lower intellectual functioning in alcohol-abusing youths, as well as poorer language skills [15,16], though findings were inconsistent [15]. More recent studies, however, have employed sophisticated brain

Clinical Handbook of Adolescent Addiction, First Edition. Richard Rosner.

imaging techniques, refined methodologies (e.g., longitudinal study designs,) and more focused neuro-psychological batteries. As a result of these technological advances, greater consistency in study findings has been observed regarding the cognitive deficits associated with adolescent alcohol abuse.

Animal models of the effects of alcohol use on the still-developing brain find associated physiological and cellular abnormalities in hippocampal tissue [17,18]. Corresponding declines in maze-learning behavior are observed in ethanol-exposed adolescent mice [19]. Human adolescent studies employing *in vivo* structural imaging techniques identified volumetric decreases in the hippocampus, a structure that is critical for learning and memory [20–22]. Deficits in verbal and non-verbal information encoding and retention are also found in human adolescents with histories of heavy drinking [23,24]. Specific learning and memory deficits, as indexed by performance on the California Verbal Learning Test – Children's Version [25] and the Visual Reproduction subtests of the Wechsler Memory Scale – Revised [26], were reported in some of the early longitudinal studies that tracked adolescents with alcohol use disorders (AUDs) into early adulthood [12,13]. Deficits in learning and memory were particularly marked in youths reporting higher levels of alcohol withdrawal symptoms.

Most youths investigated in early studies of the effects of heavy drinking also met criteria for polysubstance abuse/dependence, which is not surprising given the high rate of comorbid abuse of other substances among those with alcohol abuse or dependence diagnoses [12,27]. This complication potentially confounded the results of many longitudinal studies. In an effort to resolve this sampling issue, more recent studies have recruited adolescents who primarily use alcohol with no other clinical levels of abuse/dependence of other substances ("AUD-pure"). Consistent with the findings of earlier studies, AUD-pure adolescents demonstrated verbal memory deficits, as indexed by poorer performance on immediate and delayed recall of the thematic units on the Verbal Story Memory subtest from the Children's Memory Scale [28]. Another recent study used functional magnetic resonance imaging (fMRI) to examine verbal learning and memory in a small sample of "binge-drinking" adolescents, (where binging was defined as episodes of consuming five or more drinks in a row) in comparison to demographically matched non-drinkers [29]. Encoding deficits were observed in a word-pair association task, along with reduced hippocampal activation and increased fronto-parietal activity [29]. These findings suggest altered neural processing of novel verbal information in adolescent heavy (binge) drinkers; that is, they may be recruiting different brain regions in order to complete these tasks, perhaps to compensate for deficiencies in medial temporal lobe/hippocampal function.

Working memory abnormalities, particularly in spatial working memory (SWM), are documented in adolescent heavy drinkers. fMRI studies consistently find evidence of altered brain activity in alcohol-abusing youths during visuo-spatial information-processing tasks. Specifically, the brains of heavy drinking adolescents have been found to recruit additional network resources to accomplish these tasks, which suggests that the brains of these adolescents work less efficiently and that more resources are recruited as a compensatory mechanism. One such study of heavy-drinking adolescents aged 15–17 years found that, while they obtained similar test scores as demographically matched light drinkers on an experimental SWM task and on other neuropsychological measures, heavy drinkers exhibited increased parietal lobe activation and decreased occipital and cerebellar activity [30]. Adolescents reporting greater frequency of hangover and/or withdrawal symptoms evidenced the highest degree of abnormal brain activation during the SWM task, despite otherwise adequate (non-impaired) performance compared to controls. Similarly, adequate SWM task performance accompanied by abnormal brain activity is reported in AUD-diagnosed adolescents and in binge-drinking college students [31,32], with evidence pointing toward greater abnormality in the brains of young female heavy drinkers [31].

Other frontal lobe functions are detrimentally impacted by heavy drinking. A trend toward smaller prefrontal cortical volumes in AUD-diagnosed adolescents, measured using structural MRI, is reported [33]. In a study of AUD-pure adolescents aged 13–15 years [28], deficits in self-monitoring/inhibition as measured by the interference effect on the Stroop Color-Word Test [34] were observed. Inhibitory processing abnormalities in adolescent binge-drinkers, indexed using a go/no-go inhibition task and blood-oxygen level-dependent (BOLD) fMRI response, are also reported [35].

Deficits in prospective memory (ProM), as measured by the Prospective and Retrospective Memory Questionnaire (PRMQ) [36] and objective performance on a Prospective Remembering Video Procedure, were found in teenage binge drinkers when compared to light drinker controls [37]. Described as "remembering to remember" stored intentions [38], ProM is subserved by a combination of executive (planning, behavioral initiation, monitoring) and memory (recall) functions [39], both of which have been found to be detrimentally impacted in heavy-drinking youths [11].

Reductions in the white matter integrity of adolescent heavy drinkers [11], and in comorbid alcohol and marijuana adolescent heavy users [40,41], were found using advanced imaging techniques such as diffusion tensor imaging. This finding correlated with poorer performance on tasks of attention, working memory, and processing speed. Psychomotor speed and coordination deficits in active and abstinent adolescent heavy drinkers are described elsewhere as well [16,28,42]. A general trend in motor slowing has been observed, though it is interesting to note that in animal models, adolescents appear to be less affected by the sedating effects of immediate alcohol intoxication commonly seen in adults [43,44].

In summary, heavy alcohol use during adolescence is associated with poorer performance on measures of learning and memory, attention, processing speed, visuo-spatial information processing, and aspects of executive functioning. Abnormal brain response patterns during tasks involving spatial working memory and executive functioning have also been observed in the context of adequate task performance. Adolescent alcohol use may affect male and female brains differently, with females appearing somewhat more vulnerable to the deleterious effects of heavy use during this period. Deficits across all domains of neuropsychological function are most pronounced in youths reporting a greater number of withdrawal symptoms after episodes of heavy drinking, although heavy drinking in general is associated with poorer cognitive functioning and failure to attain age-level expectations [12,13]. More research is necessary to determine whether deficits persist into adulthood.

Cannabis

Marijuana is the most commonly abused illicit substance among adolescents [2,3]. Studies of adolescent marijuana use and its impact on cognition are less conclusive than those examining the effects of alcohol, but available research has generally shown a deficit pattern similar to that reported in the adult literature. Specifically, studies of adult marijuana users reveal greatest deficits in attention, learning and memory, processing speed, and executive functions during the initial phases of abstinence [45,46]. There is debate, however, as to whether deficits persist after periods of sustained abstinence [47].

Poorer performance on measures of memory, attention/working memory, psychomotor speed, and planning and sequencing abilities has been documented in marijuana-abusing adolescents after 1 month of abstinence [48,49]. A consistent finding of attentional difficulties in adolescent marijuana abusers has been observed, both after recent (12-hour [50]) and more protracted (3-week [51]) abstinence periods. Abstinent

adolescent marijuana users also evidence abnormal fMRI activity when conducting a SWM task [52], suggesting the potential for altered neurodevelopment in the context of heavy cannabis exposure during youth. A recent study of young adult current marijuana users aged 19 to 21 years replicated these findings [53]. Using available longitudinal data on participants (which included prior cognitive performance data, data on prenatal drug exposure, and current/past other drug use history), this study found unique effects of current marijuana use on SWM function. Recruitment of brain regions not typically associated with visuo-spatial working memory was observed, although the marijuana users appeared to perform as well as controls on the cognitive task, suggesting once again that additional brain regions were being recruited to maintain cognitive competency. The extent to which such alterations may impact real-world functioning remains to be investigated.

Given that adolescence encompasses a period of rapid neurodevelopmental change, more longitudinal research on illicit substance use in adolescent users is clearly needed. From the young adult literature, a study examining the consequences of earlier, as opposed to later, age-of-onset regular marijuana usage found poorer general verbal ability, verbal fluency, and verbal memory performance in individuals who began using marijuana before age 17 [54]. Because there were no data regarding premorbid function, a causal relationship for these findings could not be determined. Another study examined the effects of current and past regular marijuana use on current neuropsychological functioning in a sample of 17–21-year olds, where cognitive data, "pre-marijuana use," had been collected when participants were 9–12 years of age [55]. Accounting for premorbid cognitive function, the investigators found that heavy current users performed significantly worse on measures of general IQ, processing speed, and memory compared to non-using controls, whereas former (not current) heavy marijuana users did not evidence such impairments. The latter finding suggests that a recovery of cognitive function occurs after cessation of regular use. This, of course, is encouraging as it preliminarily indicates that heavy marijuana use is not associated with permanent, adverse effects upon cognition after prolonged cessation.

Taken together, it can be concluded that current use of marijuana during adolescence negatively impacts attention, as well as learning, memory, and processing speed, similar to findings in the adult literature. During the initial stages of abstinence, adolescents may continue to evidence these deficits, but these do not appear to persist beyond 1–3 months. Mixed but generally encouraging results suggest the potential for remediation of marijuana-induced effects with sustained abstinence.

Nicotine

In the United States, the good news is that adolescent use of nicotine products has been steadily declining [56]. Nonetheless, despite efforts to curtail the tobacco industry's aggressive advertising campaigns aimed at minors, nicotine remains one of most frequently used substances by US high-school students [1]. The harmful effects of cigarette smoking on cardiovascular and lung health are well established, but less is known about the effects of nicotine on the developing brain.

Review of the adult literature suggests that chronic cigarette smoking can adversely impact some neuropsychological functions [57], but acute nicotine exposure actually *improves* sustained attention, suggesting a short-term beneficial effect of the drug's stimulant properties [58]. In adolescent regular smokers, deficits in working (selected and divided attention tasks) and verbal memory were found after smoking cessation, with greater deficits exhibited in those who began smoking at younger ages [59]. A longitudinal study of young adult smokers aged 18–21 years with neuropsychological data available from young adolescence (pre-smoking initiation) [60] found that current smokers exhibited select verbally mediated skill deficits (receptive/expressive vocabulary and auditory memory) compared to non-smokers, with greater deficits corresponding to heavier current use and greater lifetime smoking duration. Former smokers exhibited only slight deficits on an auditory working memory task compared to non-smokers, suggesting that the negative cognitive consequences of heavy, long-term smoking are reversible with prolonged cessation.

Hallucinogens

MDMA (methylene dioxymethamphetamine, or "ecstasy") is an amphetamine derivative with both hallucinogenic and stimulant properties that has gained popularity in the adolescent demographic. Studies in adults find that heavy use can lead to poorer performance on measures of executive function/self-control, sustained attention, and verbal and visual learning and memory that correlate with serotonin depletion in the brain [61,62]. One study of adolescent MDMA users found associated difficulties on a divided attention task, as well as abnormal hippocampal activity [63]. The long-term effects of MDMA use beginning in adolescence have not been documented, though studies finding protracted behavioral and neuropsychiatric deficits in

adults, despite sustained abstinence from the drug, are concerning because of their potentially negative implications for the adolescent brain as well.

Inhalants

Inhalants have become a particularly important category of psychoactive drug among adolescent substance abusers; when including volatile substances within the larger definition of illicit drugs, over a quarter of US teenagers report using drugs by 13–14 years of age [1]. Inexpensive and easily accessible, inhalants are often an adolescent's first recreational drug experience, preceding even experimentation with cigarettes or alcohol. US prevalence statistics reflect higher levels of volatile substance abuse among younger teenagers in comparison to older teens [1], underscoring the need for better understanding of inhalant abuse on early brain development.

As a category, inhalants encompass a number of chemical substances that affect the brain in different ways. In general, any chemical solvent that vaporizes at room temperature can be considered an inhalant [64]. Common household products such as paint, nail polish remover, aerosol hairspray, glues, propellants, and cleaning supplies contain compounds that can induce feelings of euphoria when inhaled. Abuse can result in immediate death from acute intoxication, or cause more protracted damage to the heart, lungs, kidney, liver, and central and peripheral nervous systems [65]. A discussion of these effects is beyond the scope of this chapter, but they are important to consider as damage to peripheral organ systems can potentially and indirectly modulate neurocognition.

Inhalants may be more toxic to the developing brain than other substances of abuse. The high lipid solubility of organic solvents affords them a particular affinity for the CNS [66], given their ability to easily cross the blood–brain barrier. In a study of chronic adult inhalant abusers compared to cocaine abusers (which may allow some generalization to adolescents) greater structural abnormalities were found in the chronic inhalant abusers [67]. In general, inhalant abuse has been associated with coordination disturbances related to cerebellar dysfunction [65], and impairment in a number of cognitive functions [68] including impaired attention, speed of information processing, psychomotor coordination, learning and memory, and executive functions (see refs [65,69] for review). Protracted use has also been associated with decreases in IQ and symptoms akin to subcortical dementia, with profound impairments seen in attention and psychomotor functions [68]. However, the extent to which solvent abusers' cognitive performance is influenced by premorbid impairment, comorbid psychopathology, or socioeconomic variables is often unaddressed [65], as a case study of the neuro-psychological presentation of two inhalant-abusing adolescents recently demonstrated [70].

Another recent study examined children and adolescents aged 10–17 years who were occupationally exposed to a variety of solvents (including benzene, toluene, xylene, methyl ethyl ketone, styrene, and n-hexane), while controlling for the influential factors described above [71]. A dose–response relationship between level of solvent exposure and cognitive impairment was found. That is, those with higher levels of exposure had greater deficits in reaction time, significantly shorter digit spans, more variable responses on the NES2 Continuous Performance Test (CPT) [72], and impairment on Grooved Pegboard [73] performance.

The specific deleterious effects of toluene inhalation have been documented extensively in the substance abuse literature. Commonly found in household products such as adhesive glue and paint thinner, toluene toxicity has been linked to cerebellar white matter morbidity and associated ataxic symptoms [74]. Abuse of substances containing toluene may be particularly damaging to the CNS, with long-term abuse reported to be associated with development of dementia-like symptoms [75,76]. A small study of protracted toluene abusers (mean length of abuse 2.3 years) among Turkish adolescents [77] showed higher rates of impaired cognitive function in toluene abusers on a brief mental status examination when compared to controls. Other volatile substances including n-hexane, methyl-n-butyl ketone, and methyl isobutyl ketone are also found in glues and paints, and have been associated with development of peripheral neuropathy [64,78].

In contrast to toluene and related toxins, the neurological and neuropsychological effects of gasoline (petrol) inhalation, characterized by impaired learning, recognition memory, and attention, have been found to improve with abstinence [79]. Nitrous oxide is reported to cause mild euphoric and dissociative sensations in abusers [80] and has been associated with short-term memory impairment, though effects appear to reverse with cessation of abuse [68]. Similarly, sustained abuse of alkyl nitrates (e.g., "poppers") has not been associated with long-term cognitive impairment [68].

FUNCTIONAL OUTCOMES IN ADOLESCENT SUBSTANCE ABUSE

From the research findings discussed in the previous section, it is clear that neuropsychological instruments serve as a reliable and valid proxy for measuring the manner in which adolescent substance use modulates various cognitive functions, such as general intellectual functioning, attention, information processing speed, language, visuo-spatial function, learning and memory for verbal and visual information, and executive/frontal lobe function. As the field of neuropsychology has matured, research has amassed evidence that neuropsychological test data are related to many aspects of "real-world" functioning. Deficits in neuropsychological functioning are, for example, correlated with inability to perform basic activities of daily living, as documented in adults diagnosed with schizophrenia (e.g., ref. [81]), HIV infection (e.g., refs [82,83]), epilepsy (e.g., ref. [84]), and traumatic brain injury (e.g., ref. [85]).

Within the last few years, an emergent body of literature has examined the association between neuropsychological functioning and functional outcomes in adult substance abusers. For example, cocaine addicts who demonstrate executive function deficits tend to relapse more frequently than those with more intact neuropsychological functioning [86]. Moreover, in a sample of polysubstance users, neuropsychological impairment was associated with reduced likelihood of completing treatment [87]. In samples of alcohol abusers, impairment in executive function was also associated with poorer vocational outcome [88]. In another study, poorer neuropsychological functioning was associated with subsequent poorer treatment outcomes [89].

Another compelling study examined the choices that cocaine-dependent adult individuals make following exposure to cocaine [90]. In that study, participants were given either actual cocaine or a placebo, then asked if they preferred cocaine or, instead, cash. Following exposure to cocaine, the addicts always asked for cocaine over cash, regardless of the amount of money offered; in contrast, following exposure to placebo, they always took cash rather than the placebo. These findings illustrate the reinforcement value of cocaine and the difficulty in maintaining permanent abstinence. The relationship between neuropsychological functioning and real-world outcomes was succinctly described by Bates and colleagues [91], who stated in regard to their research with alcohol abusers: "cognitive abilities are necessary components of a number of the skills used in treatments for addictive behaviors, including initiation and planning of activities, complex problem solving, impulse control, and abstract reasoning. Heavy users of alcohol thus may lack the very skills they need to stop drinking."

To date, only a limited number of studies have examined the relationship between neuropsychological profile, substance use, and functional outcomes in adolescent samples. Those that have were primarily interested in alcohol, cannabis, and nicotine effects. To our knowledge, few studies have focused on the effects of stimulants (cocaine, methamphetamine), hallucinogens (MDMA), or prescription medications (benzodiazepines, pain medications). Furthermore, relative to studies of adult samples, the range of outcome measures examined is limited. In terms of outcome variables relevant to adolescents, our review will focus on academic achievement, aggressive behavior, and interpersonal functioning, primarily in relation to alcohol consumption.

With regard to academic functioning, in a group of Chinese adolescent students, poorer performance on a measure of working memory was associated with poorer academic performance after controlling for age, education level, and school type [92]. However, alcohol consumption profile was not associated with academic functioning or performance on the working memory task. In terms of interpersonal functioning, studies by Tarter and colleagues showed that cognitive disinhibition is associated with increased alcohol and drug use frequency [93]. Increased frequency of drug administration and neurobehavioral disinhibition were independently associated with social maladjustment, which was partially defined as social incompetence, school-related difficulties, and problems with peer social relationships. Another study showed that adolescents demonstrating relatively poor performance on a series of executive/frontal lobe measures also exhibited poorer performance on measures of social competence, increased likelihood of conduct disorder diagnosis, and reduced capacity to learn information about strategies to minimize use of alcohol and other drugs [94]. In that same study, substance use was independently associated with increased likelihood for aggressive behavior. A related experimental study showed that younger individuals with baseline executive/frontal lobe deficits were more likely to respond in an aggressive manner when given alcohol [95].

We also identified one study that examined the relationship between cognition and future alcohol use [96]. In that study, poorer performance on a measure of working memory was associated with greater levels of historic alcohol use, greater levels of alcohol consumption, a shorter interval since the last drink prior to study completion, and greater craving for alcohol. Moreover, the authors observed that adolescents characterized as relatively heavy drinkers demonstrated impulsive decision-making and an attentional bias toward alcohol-related cues.

In summary, the data from the studies reviewed here preliminarily show that substance use modulates neuropsychological function. Moreover, these changes in neurocognition are associated with poorer functional outcomes, such as increased aggression and poorer social competence. Nonetheless, from our perspective, it was surprising that, given the prevalence of adolescent substance abuse, only a handful of studies have endeavored to link adolescent alcohol and drug use to changes in cognitive function *and* changes in day-to-day functioning. Because this association is well established in studies of adult substance use psychopathology, it is reasonable to infer that a similar association will be observed in adolescents as well.

CONSIDERATIONS FOR NEUROPSYCHOLOGICAL ASSESSMENT IN SUBSTANCE-ABUSING ADOLESCENTS

The first consideration in any neuropsychological assessment of adolescents is to ask, in starkly neutral terms during the clinical interview, about substance use behavior. The unique aspect of this situation, of course, is that the interviewee will be a minor and hence, in most circumstances, the parent will hold the privilege. The adolescent may ask if the parent has to be informed of their answers– before they give them – and the response will usually depend upon state law in that jurisdiction. Once these issues are raised, if at all, and addressed, the examination can proceed. The interviewer should ask about substance use in non-judgmental terms, such as "Can you tell me a bit about your use of alcohol?" versus "You don't drink alcohol, do you?"

The second consideration of the neuropsychological examination of an adolescent with a known substance abuse history is whether the adolescent has used substances acutely, and if so, to what extent the substances may be affecting his or her current test performance. We have, on several occasions, examined adolescents who later confessed to drinking alcohol during the examination (one in a "Big Gulp" paper cup from a convenience store) and another who bought two beers from a nearby store during a testing break. Under unusual circumstances, and with parental consent, a breathalyzer or urine stick can be utilized to assure the examiner that the adolescent has not recently used alcohol or other substances.

The third consideration regards which test instruments to utilize. This, of course, will depend upon the referral question, but certain cognitive domains are especially relevant to adolescents with a history of substance abuse. As has been discussed above, working memory is affected in the acute phase of substance use and withdrawal; more importantly, this construct has been shown to relate to outcome and risk for relapse. Therefore, measures of working memory (such as from the Wechsler Intelligence Scale for Children – Fourth Edition (WISC-IV) or Wechsler Adult Intelligence Scale – Fourth Edition (WAIS-IV) [97,98], continuous performance tasks, and the Auditory Consonant Trigrams [99]) will be particularly important to examine in these adolescents.

Multiple measures of memory are also important, as memory relates to "real-world" functioning and the sequelae of long-term substance abuse. Useful measures include the Wide Range Assessment of Memory and Learning – Second Edition (WRAML2) [100], California Verbal Learning Test [25,101] (child or adult version, as appropriate for the age of the adolescent), and in persons age 16 and over, the Wechsler Memory Scale-IV (WMS-IV) [102].

As discussed, cognitive disinhibition has been shown to be related to potential for relapse. Inclusion of the Stroop Color-Word Interference Test [99] and/or battery measures such as the Delis–Kaplan Executive Functioning Scale (D–KEFS) [103], which highlight disinhibition, should be used with adolescents to assess for signs of executive dysfunction that are excessive for the examinee's age.

Beyond these three key domains to assess in adolescent substance abusers, additional domains will be included based upon the referral questions. If one issue is neurodevelopment, other measures with age-appropriate norms such as the test of Visual Motor Integration (Beery VMI) [104] should be included. US adolescents who exhibit stigmata of either long-term substance abuse or such conditions as fetal alcohol syndrome may be candidates for accommodations in school, based upon the Americans with Disabilities Act. In such cases, measures of academic achievement such as the Wechsler Individual Achievement Test – Third Edition (WIAT-III) [105] or the Woodcock–Johnson Tests of Achievement – Third Edition (WJ-III) [106] should be included, in addition to measures of speed of reading (e.g., Nelson-Denny Test of Reading Comprehension [107]), writing (Test of Written Language – Fourth Edition; TOWL-4 [108]), Trail Making Test (child or adult versions, depending of course, on age) [99], and other timed measures of functioning.

Finally, adolescents with current or past use and abuse of substances may have psychological or emotional features that either put them at risk for further substance abuse (e.g., impulsivity) or are a result of abuse (e.g., depression). Assessment of emotional state using measures such as the Minnesota Multiphasic Personality Inventory-Adolescent version (MMPI-A) [109] and child behavior checklists completed by parents and/or teachers (as appropriate for the examinee's age) will be important. Indeed, cognitive slowing, inattention, and even poor performance on measures of effortful learning/memory and executive functions can result from depression and other emotional factors.

CONCLUSION

Neuropsychological effects of substance abuse and dependence represent a complex issue, dependent on both the recency and extent of substance use. Working memory, episodic memory, and disinhibition represent key domains that are affected by substance abuse that can put the adolescent at risk for relapse and for poorer outcome in their "real-world" functioning. Assessment that focuses on these domains, as well as emotional factors, will be necessary to examine the effects of past substance abuse, and determine success in remaining abstinent as the adolescent enters adulthood.

References

1. Johnston LD, O'Malley PM, Bachman JG, Schulenberg JE. *Monitoring the Future National Results on Adolescent Drug Use: Overview of Key Findings, 2008*. Bethesda, MD: National Institute on Drug Abuse, 2009.
2. Hibell B, Guttormsson U, Ahlström S, *et al. The 2007 ESPAD Report – Substance Use Among Students in 35 European Countries*. Stockholm: The Swedish Council for Information on Alcohol and Other Drugs, 2009.
3. Johnston LD, O'Malley PM, Bachman JG, Schulenberg JE. National press release: Teen marijuana use tilts up, while some drugs decline in use. Ann Arbor, MI: University of Michigan News Service, 14 Dec 2009.
4. Crews F, He J, Hodge C. Adolescent cortical development: a critical period of vulnerability for addiction. *Pharmacol Biochem Behav* 2007;**86**:189–199.
5. Chen CY, Storr CL, Anthony JC. Early-onset drug use and risk for drug dependence problems. *Addict Behav* 2009;**34**:319–322.
6. Grant BF, Dawson DA. Age of onset of drug use and its association with DSM-IV drug abuse and dependence: results from the National Longitudinal Alcohol Epidemiologic Survey. *J Subst Abuse* 1998;**10**:163–173.
7. King KM, Chassin L. A prospective study of the effects of age of initiation of alcohol and drug use on young adult substance dependence. *J Stud Alcohol Drugs* 2007;**68**: 256–265.
8. Ernst M, Grant SJ, London ED, *et al.* Decision making in adolescents with behavior disorders and adults with substance abuse. *Am J Psychiatry* 2003;**160**:33–40.
9. Nigg JT, Glass JM, Wong MM, *et al.* Neuropsychological executive functioning in children at elevated risk for alcoholism: findings in early adolescence. *J Abnorm Psychol* 2004;**113**:302–314.
10. Schweinsburg AD, Paulus MP, Barlett VC, *et al.* An fMRI study of response inhibition in youths with a family history of alcoholism. *Ann N Y Acad Sci* 2004;**1021**:391–394.
11. Squeglia LM, Jacobus J, Tapert SF. The influence of substance use on adolescent brain development. *Clin Electroencephal Neurosci* 2009;**40**:31–38.

12. Tapert SF, Brown SA. Neuropsychological correlates of adolescent substance abuse: four-year outcomes. *J Int Neuropsychol Soc* 1999;**5**:481–493.

13. Tapert SF, Granholm E, Leedy NG, Brown SA. Substance use and withdrawal: neuropsychological functioning over 8 years in youth. *J Int Neuropsychol Soc* 2002;**8**: 873–883.

14. Zeigler DW, Wang CC, Yoast RA, et al. The neuro-cognitive effects of alcohol on adolescents and college students. *Prev Med* 2005;**40**:23–32.

15. Moss HB, Kirisci L, Gordon HW, Tarter RE. A neuro-psychologic profile of adolescent alcoholics. *Alcohol Clin Exp Res* 1994;**18**:159–163.

16. Tarter RE. Genetics and primary prevention of drug and alcohol abuse. *Int J Addict* 1995;**30**:1479–1484.

17. Oliveira-da-Silva A, Vieira FB, Cristina-Rodrigues F, et al. Increased apoptosis and reduced neuronal and glial densities in the hippocampus due to nicotine and ethanol exposure in adolescent mice. *Int J Dev Neurosci* 2009;**27**:539–548.

18. Pyapali GK, Turner DA, Wilson WA, Swartzwelder HS. Age and dose-dependent effects of ethanol on the induc-tion of hippocampal long-term potentiation. *Alcohol* 1999;**19**:107–111.

19. Markwiese BJ, Acheson SK, Levin ED, Wilson WA, Swartzwelder HS. Differential effects of ethanol on memory in adolescent and adult rats. *Alcohol Clin Exp Res* 1998;**22**:416–421.

20. DeBellis MD, Clark DB, Beers SR, et al. Hippocampal volume in adolescent-onset alcohol use disorders. *Am J Psychiatry* 2000;**157**:737–744.

21. Medina KL, Schweinsburg AD, Cohen-Zion M, Nagel BJ, Tapert SF. Effects of alcohol and combined marijuana and alcohol use during adolescence on hippocampal volume and asymmetry. *Neurotoxicol Teratol* 2007;**29**: 141–152.

22. Nagel BJ, Schweinsburg AD, Phan V, Tapert SF. Reduced hippocampal volume among adolescents with alcohol use disorders without psychiatric comorbidity. *Psychiatry Res* 2005;**139**:181–190.

23. Brown SA, Tapert SF, Granholm E, Delis DC. Neuro-cognitive functioning of adolescents: effects of protracted alcohol use. *Alcohol Clin Exp Res* 2000;**24**:164–171.

24. Schweinsburg A, McQueeny T, Nagel B, Eyler L, Tapert SF. A preliminary study of functional magnetic resonance imaging response during verbal encoding among adoles-cent binge drinkers. *Alcohol* 2010;**44**:111–117.

25. Delis DC, Kramer JH, Kaplan E, Ober BA. *Manual for the California Verbal Learning Test Manual – Children's Version*. San Antonio, TX: The Psychological Corpora-tion, 1994.

26. Wechsler D. *Manual for the Wechsler Memory Scale – Revised*. San Antonio, TX: The Psychological Corpora-tion, 1987.

27. Substance Abuse and Mental Health Services Adminis-tration. *Results from the 2006 National Survey on Drug Use and Health: National Findings*. NSDUH Series H-32, DHHS Publication No. SMA 07-4293. Rockville, MD: Office of Applied Studies, 2007.

28. Ferrett HL, Carey PD, Thomas KG, Tapert SF, Fein G. Neuropsychological performance of South African treat-ment-naive adolescents with alcohol dependence. *Drug Alcohol Depend* 2010;**110**:8–14.

29. Schweinsburg AD, McQueeny T, Nagel BJ, Eyler LT, Tapert SF. A preliminary study of functional magnetic resonance imaging response during verbal encoding among adolescent binge drinkers. *Alcohol* 2010;**44**: 111–117.

30. Tapert SF, Schweinsburg AD, Barlett VC, et al. Blood oxygen level dependent response and spatial working memory in adolescents with alcohol use disorders. *Alco-hol Clin Exp Res* 2004;**28**:1577–1586.

31. Caldwell LC, Schweinsburg AD, Nagel BJ, et al. Gender and adolescent alcohol use disorders on BOLD (blood oxygen level dependent) response to spatial working memory. *Alcohol Alcoholism* 2005;**40**:194–200.

32. Crego A, Rodriguez-Holguin S, Parada M, et al. Reduced anterior prefrontal cortex activation in young binge drink-ers during a visual working memory task. *Drug Alcohol Depend* 2010;**109**:45–56.

33. Medina KL, McQueeny T, Nagel BJ, et al. Prefrontal cortex volumes in adolescents with alcohol use disorders: unique gender effects. *Alcohol Clin Exp Res* 2008;**32**: 386–394.

34. Golden CJ, Freshwater SM. *Stroop Color and Word Test: A Manual for Clinical and Experimental Uses*. Los Angeles, CA: Stoelting Company, 2002.

35. Schweinsburg AD, Paulus MP, Barlett VC, et al. An fMRI study of response inhibition in youths with a family history of alcoholism. *Ann N Y Acad Sci* 2004;**1021**: 391–394.

36. Crawford JR, Smith G, Maylor EA, Della Sala S, Logie RH. The Prospective and Retrospective Memory Ques-tionnaire (PRMQ): normative data and latent structure in a large non-clinical sample. *Memory* 2003;**11**:261–275.

37. Heffernan T, Clark R, Bartholomew J, Ling J, Stephens S. Does binge drinking in teenagers affect their everyday prospective memory? *Drug Alcohol Depend* 2010;**109**: 73–78.

38. Winograd E. Some observations on prospective remem-bering. In: Gruneberg MM, Morris PE, Sykes RN (eds), *Practical Aspects of Memory: Current Research and Issues*. Chichester: John Wiley & Sons, Ltd, 1988; pp. 348–353.

39. McDaniel MA, Einstein GO. *Prospective Memory: an Overview and Synthesis of an Emerging Field*. Los Angeles, CA: Sage, 2007.

40. Bava S, Frank LR, McQueeny T, et al. Altered white matter microstructure in adolescent substance users. *Psy-chiatry Res* 2009;**173**:228–237.

41. Bava S, Jacobus J, Mahmood O, Yang TT, Tapert SF. Neurocognitive correlates of white matter quality in adolescent substance users. *Brain Cognition* 2010;**72**: 347–354.

42. Tapert SF, Brown SA. Substance dependence, family history of alcohol dependence and neuropsychological functioning in adolescence. *Addiction* 2000;**95**:1043–1053.

43. Silveri MM, Spear LP. Decreased sensitivity to the hypnotic effects of ethanol early in ontogeny. *Alcohol Clin Exp Res* 1998;**22**:670–676.

44. Swartzwelder HS, Richardson RC, Markwiese-Foerch B, Wilson WA, Little PJ. Developmental differences in the acquisition of tolerance to ethanol. *Alcohol* 1998;**15**:311–314.

45. Bolla KI, Brown K, Eldreth D, Tate K, Cadet JL. Dose-related neurocognitive effects of marijuana use. *Neurol-ogy* 2002;**59**:1337–1343.

46. Grant I, Gonzalez R, Carey CL, Natarajan L, Wolfson T. Non-acute (residual) neurocognitive effects of cannabis use: a meta-analytic study. *J Int Neuropsychol Soc* 2003;**9**:679–689.

47. Pope HGJr, Gruber AJ, Hudson JI, Huestis MA, Yurge-lun-Todd D. Neuropsychological performance in long-term cannabis users. *Arch Gen Psychiatry* 2001;**58**: 909–915.

48. Jacobus J, Bava S, Cohen-Zion M, Mahmood O, Tapert SF. Functional consequences of marijuana use in adolescents. *Pharmacol Biochem Behav* 2009;**92**: 559–565.

49. Medina KL, Hanson KL, Schweinsburg AD, *et al.* Neuropsychological functioning in adolescent marijuana users: subtle deficits detectable after a month of absti-nence. *J Int Neuropsychol Soc* 2007;**13**:807–820.

50. Harvey MA, Sellman JD, Porter RJ, Frampton CM. The relationship between non-acute adolescent cannabis use and cognition. *Drug Alcohol Rev* 2007;**26**:309–319.

51. Hanson KL, Winward JL, Schweinsburg AD, *et al.* Longitudinal study of cognition among adolescent mari-juana users over three weeks of abstinence. *Addict Behav* 2010;**35**:970–976.

52. Schweinsburg AD, Nagel BJ, Schweinsburg BC, *et al.* Abstinent adolescent marijuana users show altered fMRI response during spatial working memory. *Psychiatry Res* 2008;**163**:40–51.

53. Smith AM, Longo CA, Fried PA, Hogan MJ, Cameron I. Effects of marijuana on visuospatial working memory: an fMRI study in young adults. *Psychopharmacology* 2010;**210**:429–438.

54. Pope HGJr, Gruber AJ, Hudson JI, *et al.* Early-onset cannabis use and cognitive deficits: what is the nature of the association? *Drug Alcohol Depend* 2003;**69**:303–310.

55. Fried PA, Watkinson B, Gray R. Neurocognitive conse-quences of marihuana: a comparison with pre-drug per-formance. *Neurotoxicol Teratol* 2005;**27**:231–239.

56. Johnston LD, O'Malley PM, Bachman JG, Schulenberg JE. National press release: More good news on teen smoking: rates at or near record lows. Ann Arbor, MI: University of Michigan News Service, 11 Dec 2008.

57. Durazzo TC, Gazdzinski S, Meyerhoff DJ. The neuro-biological and neurocognitive consequences of chronic cigarette smoking in alcohol use disorders. *Alcohol Alco-holism* 2007;**42**:174–185.

58. Sacco KA, Bannon KL, George TP. Nicotinic receptor mechanisms and cognition in normal states and neuro-psychiatric disorders. *J Psychopharmacol* 2004;**18**: 457–474.

59. Jacobsen LK, Krystal JH, Mencl WE, *et al.* Effects of smoking and smoking abstinence on cognition in adoles-cent tobacco smokers. *Biol Psychiatry* 2005;**57**:56–66.

60. Fried PA, Watkinson B, Gray R. Neurocognitive conse-quences of cigarette smoking in young adults: a compari-son with pre-drug performance. *Neurotoxicol Teratol* 2006;**28**:517–525.

61. Bolla KI, McCann UD, Ricaurte GA. Memory impair-ment in abstinent MDMA ("Ecstasy") users. *Neurology* 1998;**51**:1532–1537.

62. Morgan MJ, Impallomeni LC, Pirona A, Rogers RD. Elevated impulsivity and impaired decision-making in abstinent Ecstasy (MDMA) users compared to polydrug and drug-naive controls. *Neuropsychopharmacology* 2006;**31**:1562–1573.

63. Jacobsen LK, Mencl WE, Pugh KR, Skudlarski P, Krystal JH. Preliminary evidence of hippocampal dysfunction in adolescent MDMA ("ecstasy") users: possible relationship to neurotoxic effects. *Psychopharmacology* 2004;**173**: 383–390.

64. National Institute on Drug Abuse. *NIDA InfoFacts: Inhal-ants*. NIDA, 2010. Available from: http://www.drugabuse.gov/publications/infofacts/inhalants.

65. Williams JF, Storck M. Inhalant abuse. *Pediatrics* 2010;**119**:1009–1017.

66. Lubman DI, Yucel M, Lawrence AJ. Inhalant abuse among adolescents: neurobiological considerations. *Brit J Pharmacol* 2008;**154**:316–326.

67. Rosenberg NL, Grigsby J, Dreisbach J, Busenbark D, Grigsby P. Neuropsychologic impairment and MRI abnormalities associated with chronic solvent abuse. *J Toxicol Clin Toxicol* 2002;**40**:21–34.

68. Brouette T, Anton R. Clinical review of inhalants. *Am J Addict* 2001;**10**:79–94.

69. Chadwick OF, Anderson HR. Neuropsychological con-sequences of volatile substance abuse: a review. *Hum Toxicol* 1989;**8**:307–312.

70. Takagi MJ, Lubman DI, Yucel M. Interpreting neuro-psychological impairment among adolescent inhalant users: two case reports. *Acta Neuropsychiatrica* 2008;**20**: 41–43.

71. Saddik B, Williamson A, Black D, Nuwayhid I. Neuro-behavioral impairment in children occupationally exposed to mixed organic solvents. *Neurotoxicology* 2009;**30**:1166–1171.

72. Letz R, Baker EL. *NES2: Neurobehavioral Evaluation System Manual*, 4th edn. Winchester, MA: Neurobeha-vioral Systems, Inc, 1988.

73. Lafayette Instruments. *Grooved Pegboard Test User Instructions Manual*. Lafayette, IN: Lafayette Instrument Company, 2002.

74. Yamanouchi N, Okada S, Kodama K, *et al.* White matter changes caused by chronic solvent abuse. *Am J Neuro-radiol* 1995;**16**:1643–1649.

75. Filley CM, Heaton RK, Rosenberg NL. White matter dementia in chronic toluene abuse. *Neurology* 1990;**40**: 532–534.

76. Fornazzari L, Wilkinson DA, Kapur BM, Carlen PL. Cerebellar, cortical and functional impairment in toluene abusers. *Acta Neurol Scand* 1983;**67**:319–329.

77. Uzun N, Kendirli Y. Clinical, socio-demographic, neuro-physiological and neuropsychiatric evaluation of children with volatile substance addiction. *Child Care Hlth Dev* 2005;**31**:425–432.

78. Lolin Y. Chronic neurological toxicity associated with exposure to volatile substances. *Hum Toxicol* 1989;**8**: 293–300.

79. Cairney S, Maruff P, Burns C, Currie B. The neuro-behavioural consequences of petrol (gasoline) sniffing. *Neurosci Biobehav Rev* 2002;**26**:81–89.

80. Beckman NJ, Zacny JP, Walker DJ. Within-subject com-parison of the subjective and psychomotor effects of a gaseous anesthetic and two volatile anesthetics in healthy volunteers. *Drug Alcohol Depend* 2006;**81**:89–95.

81. Green MF. What are the functional consequences of neuro-cognitive deficits in schizophrenia? *Am J Psychiatry* 1996;**153**:321–330.

82. Heaton RK, Velin RA, McCutchan JA, *et al.* Neuro-psychological impairment in human immunodeficiency virus-infection: implications for employment. HNRC Group. HIV Neurobehavioral Research Center. *Psychosom Med* 1994;**56**:8–17.

83. vanGorp WG, Baerwald JP, Ferrando SJ, McElhiney MC, Rabkin JG. The relationship between employment and neuropsychological impairment in HIV infection. *J Int Neuropsychol Soc* 1999;**5**:534–539.

84. Dikmen S, Morgan SF. Neuropsychological factors related to employability and occupational status in persons with epilepsy. *J Nerv Ment Dis* 1980;**168**:236–240.

85. Schwab K, Grafman J, Salazar AM, Kraft J. Residual impairments and work status 15 years after penetrating head injury: report from the Vietnam Head Injury Study. *Neurology* 1993;**43**:95–103.

86. Aharonovich E, Nunes E, Hasin D. Cognitive impairment, retention and abstinence among cocaine abusers in cognitive-behavioral treatment. *Drug Alcohol Depend* 2003;**71**:207–211.

87. Teichner G, Horner MD, Roitzsch JC, Herron J, Thevos A. Substance abuse treatment outcomes for cognitively impaired and intact outpatients. *Addict Behav* 2002;**27**: 751–763.

88. Moriyama Y, Mimura M, Kato M, *et al.* Executive dysfunction and clinical outcome in chronic alcoholics. *Alcohol Clin Exp Res* 2002;**26**:1239–1244.

89. Allsop S, Saunders B, Phillips M. The process of relapse in severely dependent male problem drinkers. *Addiction* 2000;**95**:95–106.

90. Donny EC, Bigelow GE, Walsh SL. Choosing to take cocaine in the human laboratory: effects of cocaine dose, inter-choice interval, and magnitude of alternative reinforcement. *Drug Alcohol Depend* 2003;**69**:289–301.

91. Bates ME, Bowden SC, Barry D. Neurocognitive impairment associated with alcohol use disorders: implications for treatment. *Exp Clin Psychopharmacol* 2002;**10**: 193–212.

92. Johnson CA, Xiao L, Palmer P, *et al.* Affective decision-making deficits, linked to a dysfunctional ventromedial prefrontal cortex, revealed in 10th grade Chinese adolescent binge drinkers. *Neuropsychologia* 2008;**46**:714–726.

93. Tarter RE, Kirisci L, Habeych M, Reynolds M, Vanyukov M. Neurobehavior disinhibition in childhood predisposes boys to substance use disorder by young adulthood: direct and mediated etiologic pathways. *Drug Alcohol Depend* 2004;**73**:121–132.

94. Fishbein DH, Hyde C, Eldreth D, *et al.* Neurocognitive skills moderate urban male adolescents' responses to preventive intervention materials. *Drug Alcohol Depend* 2006;**82**:47–60.

95. Wiers RW, Beckers L, Houben K, Hofmann W. A short fuse after alcohol: implicit power associations predict aggressiveness after alcohol consumption in young heavy drinkers with limited executive control. *Pharmacol Biochem Behav* 2009;**93**:300–305.

96. Field M, Christiansen P, Cole J, Goudie A. Delay discounting and the alcohol Stroop in heavy drinking adolescents. *Addiction* 2007;**102**:579–586.

97. Wechsler D. *Wechsler Intelligence Scale for Children – Fourth Edition*. San Antonio, TX: Pearson Education, Inc., 2003.

98. Wechsler D. *Wechsler Adult Intelligence Scale – Fourth Edition*. San Antonio, TX: Pearson Education, Inc., 2008.

99. Mitrushina MN, Boone KB, Razan J, D'Elia LF. *Handbook of Normative Data for Neuropsychological Assessment*. New York: Oxford University Press, 2005.

100. Sheslow D, Adams W. *Wide Range Assessment of Memory and Learning, Second Edition*. Lutz, FL: PAR Inc., 2003.

101. Delis DC, Kramer JH, Kaplan E, Ober BA. *California Verbal Learning Test – Second Edition*. San Antonio, TX: The Psychological Corporation, 2000.

102. Wechsler D. *Wechsler Memory Scale – Fourth Edition*. San Antonio, TX: Pearson Education, Inc., 2009.

103. Delis DC, Kaplan E, Kramer JH. *Delis–Kaplan Executive Function System*. San Antonio, TX: Pearson Education, Inc., 2001.

104. Beery KE, Buktenica NA, Beery NA. *Beery VMI – Sixth Edition*. San Antonio, TX: Pearson Education, Inc., 2010.

105. Wechsler D. *Wechsler Individual Achievement Test – Third Edition*. San Antonio, TX: Pearson Education, Inc., 2009.

106. Woodcock R, McGrew K, Mather N. *Woodcock–Johnson III: Tests of Achievement*. Itasca, IL: Riverside Publishing, 2001.

107. Brown JI, Fishco VV, Hanna GS. *Nelson–Denny Reading Test*. Itasca, IL: Riverside Publishing, 1993.

108. Hammill DD, Larsen SC. *Test of Written Language – Intermediate, Fourth Edition*. San Antonio, TX: Pearson Education, Inc., 2009.

109. Butcher JN, Williams CL, Graham JR, *et al. Minnesota Multiphasic Personality Inventory – Adolescent*. San Antonio, TX: The Psychological Corporation, 2006.

36

Trauma and Adolescent Addiction

Michal Kunz

Kirby Forensic Psychiatric Center; New York University School of Medicine, New York, NY, USA

Trauma, both physical and psychological, has long been recognized as a causative factor in emotional disorders. Although initially the deleterious effect of trauma gained recognition in military combat veterans, trauma-related disorders are now also recognized in victims of various peace-time traumas as well. Sexual and physical assault can give rise to trauma-related disorders, as can less serious insults, such as being a witness to a violent event, or even listening to a traumatic narrative. While many psychiatric conditions may have trauma as a predisposing or precipitating factor, it is post-traumatic stress disorder (PTSD) that explicitly defines trauma as one of the condition's necessary diagnostic criteria.

The diagnostic criteria for PTSD in adult patients, as defined by the *Diagnostic and Statistical Manual of Mental Disorders, Fourth Edition, Text Revision* (DSM-IV-TR) [1], include:

1. history of a traumatic event;
2. symptoms reflecting the re-experience of the traumatic event;
3. avoidance of stimuli associated with the traumatic event and/or emotional numbing; and
4. hypervigilance.

The symptoms have to last for more than 1 month and cause significant distress or impaired functioning.

Since PTSD was introduced as a formal diagnosis in the DSM-III [2], youth post-traumatic symptoms have been evaluated using criteria designed for adults. However, within the field of pediatric trauma, debate continues about the uniqueness of youth post-traumatic symptoms and whether distinct criteria should be established. Although research suggests that youths may manifest these symptoms differently (see below),

few qualifiers for symptoms have been introduced. The DSM-III-R [3] included alternative criteria for children within cluster B "re-experiencing" criterion 1 (repetitive play) and cluster C "avoidance/numbing" criterion 4 (loss of recently acquired developmental skills). DSM-IV [4] introduced additional child criteria for cluster A "exposure" criterion 2 (disorganized or agitated behavior) and cluster B criterion 2 (frightening dreams) and criterion 3 (trauma-specific re-enactment). However, the child qualifier in cluster C criterion 4 was removed from the 1987 edition. These criteria are consistent with those within DSM-IV-TR [1].

PREVALENCE OF TRAUMA AND TRAUMA-RELATED DISORDERS AMONG ADOLESCENTS

The lifetime prevalence of PTSD among adults was found to be 1%, according to the Epidemiological Catchment Area (ECA) [5] study. A study by Breslau *et al.* [6] found that the lifetime prevalence of PTSD among young adults enrolled in a Detroit health maintenance organization was 9.2%, or nine times that found in the ECA.

The exposure to trauma in children and adolescents can be gauged by reviewing the data collected by child protective agencies. Child protection services in the United States receive approximately 3 million referrals each year, representing 5.5 million children [7]. Those figures may only represent a portion of the child maltreatment cases that occur; researchers estimate that two-thirds of maltreatment cases are unreported. Of those cases referred, about 30% are substantiated and occur in the following frequencies [7]: 65% neglect; 18% physical abuse; 10% sexual abuse, and 7%

Clinical Handbook of Adolescent Addiction, First Edition. Richard Rosner.
© 2013 John Wiley & Sons, Ltd. Published 2013 by John Wiley & Sons, Ltd.

psychological abuse. In addition, anywhere from 3 to 10 million children are exposed to domestic violence each year [8], 40–60% of which cases also involve child physical abuse [9].

Studies of the general population have examined rates of exposure and PTSD in children and adolescents. Results from these studies indicate that 15–43% of girls and 14–43% of boys experience at least one traumatic event. Of those children and adolescents who have experienced a trauma, 3–15% of girls and 1–6% of boys could be diagnosed with PTSD.

Rates of PTSD are much higher in children and adolescents recruited from at-risk samples. The rates of PTSD in these at-risk children and adolescents vary from 3% to 100%. For example, studies have shown that as many as 100% of children who witness a parental homicide or sexual assault develop PTSD. Similarly, 90% of sexually abused children, 77% of children exposed to a school shooting, and 35% of urban youths exposed to community violence develop PTSD.

With the exception of combat trauma, adolescents are at risk for all types of traumas required for a diagnosis of PTSD, including rape, physical assault, seeing someone hurt or killed, natural disasters, threat of injury or harm, narrow escape, sudden injury or accident, receiving news about the sudden death of someone close, and learning that any of these events happened to a close friend or relative [10]. Giaconia *et al.* [11] reported that 43% of their adolescent sample had experienced at least one DSM-III-R trauma, and 6.3% overall (or 14.5% of those exposed to traumas) subsequently developed PTSD. Cuffe *et al.* [12] determined that 16% of their sample of adolescents and young adults aged 16–22 years experienced a lifetime DSM-IV trauma, and 12.4% of those exposed to traumas met criteria for a current (past-year) diagnosis of PTSD. According to the US National Comorbidity Survey, 8% of adolescents aged 15–24 years met lifetime DSM-III-R criteria for PTSD [13].

Adolescents are particularly vulnerable to experiencing traumas involving interpersonal violence, such as assault, rape, and robbery [14], types of traumas that are most frequently linked to PTSD in both adolescents and adults [10–13]. Among participants in the National Survey of Adolescents (NSA), an epidemiological study that examined a nationally representative sample of 4023 American youths who were 12 to 17 years of age, approximately 50% had experienced at least one form of interpersonal violence [15]. Substantially higher rates among young adolescents in an inner-city neighborhood were reported [16]; 93% had been exposed to at least one violent event in the past year, and 6.4% manifested clinically significant levels of PTSD symptoms.

PRESENTATION OF PTSD IN CHILDREN AND ADOLESCENTS

Researchers and clinicians have recognized that PTSD may not present itself in children the same way it does in adults. As noted above, criteria for PTSD now include age-specific features for some symptoms.

Elementary School-Aged Children

Clinical reports suggest that elementary school-aged children may not experience visual flashbacks or amnesia for aspects of the trauma. However, they do experience "time skew" and "omen formation," which are not typically seen in adults. Time skew refers to a child mis-sequencing trauma-related events when recalling the memory. Omen formation is a belief that there were warning signs that predicted the trauma. As a result, children often believe that if they are alert enough, they will recognize warning signs and avoid future traumas.

School-aged children also reportedly exhibit post-traumatic play or re-enactment of the trauma in play, drawings, or verbalizations. Post-traumatic play is different from re-enactment in that post-traumatic play is a literal representation of the trauma, involves compulsively repeating some aspect of the trauma, and does not tend to relieve anxiety. An example of post-traumatic play is an increase in shooting games after exposure to a school shooting. Post-traumatic re-enactment, on the other hand, is more flexible and involves behaviorally recreating aspects of the trauma (e.g., carrying a weapon after exposure to violence).

Adolescents and Teens

Post-traumatic stress disorder in adolescents may begin to more closely resemble PTSD in adults. However, there are a few features that have been shown to differ. As discussed above, children may engage in traumatic play following a trauma. Adolescents are more likely to engage in traumatic re-enactment, in which they incorporate aspects of the trauma into their daily lives. In addition, adolescents are more likely than younger children or adults to exhibit impulsive and aggressive behaviors.

ASSESSMENT OF PTSD IN CHILDREN AND ADOLESCENTS

Numerous formal evaluative instruments have been developed to assess the symptoms of PTSD in adults. Historically, these measures and interviews designed for adults have been adapted for youths by simplifying language and concepts. Discussion continues on whether separate criteria should be created for young populations because of unique differences with interpretation of trauma, manifestation of post-traumatic stress symptoms (PSS), and expression of affect [17]. Youths' understanding and memory of trauma and subsequent reactions may differ tremendously depending on developmental stage. Symptoms can include typical stress responses such as nightmares, fear, and general distress reactions [18]; however, symptoms can also be unique to youth, such as re-enactment of the event, regressed behavior, separation anxiety, and specific forms of behavior, academic, and somatic problems [19–21].

Studies have suggested that children experience the full range of PSS, but with different symptom manifestation than adults [22]. Scheeringa *et al.* [23] note that in the DSM-IV, eight criteria require verbal descriptions of experiences and emotional states. The lack of developmental modifications may result in the under-diagnosis of PTSD. Evidence suggests that children may experience disabling PSS that warrant treatment, but not meet criteria for PTSD [24].

Although many youth and parent interviews and youth self-report PTSD/PSS measures exist, there is not yet a "gold standard" [19]. McNally [25] reviewed measures of PTSD developed for youths, but existing measures were criticized for lack of synchronicity with DSM-III-R criteria, limited or non-existent establishment of psychometric properties, or for being incompletely tailored to developmental stage. Lonigan *et al.* [26] found that despite the availability of increasing numbers of sophisticated measures for assessing PTSD among children, it is not yet clear how best to use diagnostic techniques to advance knowledge of this disorder and assess treatment effects. Currently, few well-validated, DSM-IV-based standardized measures exist.

Clinicians and researchers increasingly use a multimodal, multi-informant approach for assessment and diagnosis of psychiatric disorders in young people; however, debate remains continues about how child and/or parent report of symptoms should inform a diagnosis of PTSD [19,27]. Despite low levels of agreement between parent and child reports of diagnostic conditions, both informants provide valuable information [27]. Evidence suggests that parents may not correctly report levels of PSS in their children as compared to child reports [28]. Parents may also be experiencing PSS from exposure to the trauma experienced by their child, such as cancer [29], or may be victims of trauma themselves [30]. Child/adolescent self-report measures are not problem-free. The veracity of youth self-report depends on many factors, including the child's developmental level, questions posed, the manner in which questions are asked, and factors about the event itself.

However, after trauma, children provide more reliable information on their own internal states than others [31].

MEASURES

Child Interview with Companion Parent Interview

Diagnostic Interview for Children and Adolescents – Revised

The Diagnostic Interview for Children and Adolescents (DICA) [32] was developed in 1969 primarily for clinical and epidemiological research and has since received many revisions. The DICA-R, the most recent version, is a semi-structured interview designed to assess present and lifetime diagnoses. The PTSD portion of the interview is based on an event the child identifies as traumatic. Lay interviewers, who receive 2–4 weeks of training, can administer the DICA-R. A diagnosis can be based on either parent or child/adolescent interview, but a thorough assessment should consider information from both sources. The DICA-R PTSD module consists of 17 questions and is 1 of 18 diagnostic scales. The DICA-R or earlier versions were used in 8/65 studies reviewed [38]. The studies primarily included non-US populations (4/8); fewer studies involved multi-ethnic youths (2/8). Both parent and youth interviews were utilized in 3/8 studies.

Kiddie Schedule for Affective Disorders and Schizophrenia for School-Age Children – Present and Lifetime Version

The original Kiddie Schedule for Affective Disorders and Schizophrenia for School-Age Children (K-SADS) [33] was designed as a comprehensive instrument to assess psychopathology in children. This semi-structured interview assesses full and partial diagnosis, including present and lifetime diagnosis of PTSD. Intensive training is recommended to administer the instrument because of the importance of diagnostic classification and differential diagnosis. The clinician integrates the parents' report of observable behavior and the child's self-report when formulating a diagnosis. In the PTSD module, the scale initially assesses whether any of a variety of traumatic events occurred recently or in the past, then assesses PTSD diagnostic criteria for one specific event. The PTSD module is one of 32 scales and varies in length depending on the number of endorsed items. The K-SADS Present and Lifetime Version (K-SADS-PL) or other versions were used in 8/65 studies reviewed [38]. The studies primarily included multi-ethnic youths (5/8) and fewer studies involved non-US populations (2/8). Both parent and youth interviews were utilized in one study.

Child/Adolescent Interview Only

Clinician-Administered PTSD Scale for Children and Adolescents

The Clinician-Administered PTSD Scale for Children and Adolescents (CAPS-CA) [34] is a semi-structured clinical interview designed to assess PTSD symptoms and associated symptoms in children and adolescents. This is a developmentally modified version of the Clinician-Administered PTSD Scale [35]. The CAPS-CA evaluates current and lifetime diagnosis, frequency and intensity of symptoms as well as social, developmental, and scholastic functioning. The CAPS-CA consists of 36 questions based on a specific event the child identifies as most distressing. A diagnosis also incorporates clinical judgment, regarding the type of trauma and impact on functioning. The CAPS-CA was used in 5/65 studies reviewed [38]. The studies were used primarily with US populations and multi-ethnic youths (3/5).

Child/Adolescent Self-Report

Impact of Events Scale – Revised

The Impact of Events Scale – Revised (IES-R) [36] is an adaptation of the Impact of Events Scale (IES), a self-report measure that assessed adults' intrusive and avoidant reactions associated with a particular event [37]. The IES-R was designed to also include items that assess the domain of hyperarousal. The IES-R was neither designed nor validated with children, but is probably comprehensible for children at approximately the formal operations level [38]. The author notes that any results from this scale with youths should be considered preliminary. The IES-R was not intended for use as a diagnostic tool and consists of 22 items composing three scales: hyperarousal, intrusion, and avoidance. The IES-R or IES were used in 11/65 studies reviewed [38]. The studies primarily included non-Hispanic white youths (5/11) and non-US groups (3/11).

Child Post-Traumatic Stress Disorder Reaction Index

The Child Post-Traumatic Stress Disorder Reaction Index (CPTSD-RI) [39] was originally intended for use as an interview, but is most often used as a self-report measure. The CPTSD-RI only assesses reactions to a specific traumatic event and was not designed as a diagnostic tool. The CPTSD-RI consists of 20 items composing three factors: intrusiveness/numbing/avoidance, fear/anxiety, and disturbances in sleep and concentration. The CPTSD-RI was the measure most frequently used overall (33/65) [38] and with non-US groups. The studies primarily included non-Hispanic white youths (15/33), with

fewer studies involving multi-ethnic youths (7/33) or non-US populations (7/33). Both parent and youth self-reports were utilized in 4/33 studies. Researchers at the University of California, Los Angeles (UCLA) have developed a series of self-report measures to assess trauma symptoms in children and adolescents [40]. The UCLA PTSD Reaction Index includes child, adolescent, and parent versions to provide preliminary PTSD diagnoses using DSM-IV criteria. All measures are based upon the CPTSD-RI and contain approximately 20 questions. The validity and reliability of these measures have been described [41].

PTSD Symptom Scale

The PTSD Symptom Scale (PSS) [42] was developed to assess the presence and severity of PTSD symptoms in adults, with a known trauma history, as a semi-structured interview or self-report questionnaire. Although the PSS has been used with many youth populations, it has not been validated with these groups. The PSS measures symptom severity for a specific traumatic event and consists of 17 items composing three scales: re-experiencing, avoidance, and arousal. The PSS was used in 5/65 studies reviewed [38] and primarily included non-US populations (3/5). Foa and colleagues have recently published a revised measure for children, called the Child PTSD Symptom Scale (CPSS) [43]. The CPSS is a self-report measure designed to diagnose and assess the severity of PTSD, as outlined in DSM-IV, in children and adolescents. This measure shows strong preliminary psychometric properties.

Trauma Symptom Checklist for Children

The Trauma Symptom Checklist for Children (TSCC) [44] is a self-report measure developed to assess a wide range of symptoms in children. Although the TSCC was not designed for use as a diagnostic tool, it assesses exposure to a variety of trauma, including sexual trauma, and PSS related to the events. The administration of the TSCC does not require specialized training, but the interpretation of scores does. The complete version contains 54 items and the post-traumatic stress scale is one of six clinical scales. The TSCC or a previous version were used in 7/65 studies reviewed and included multi-ethnic youths (4/7) [38].

TREATMENT OF PTSD IN CHILDREN AND ADOLESCENTS

The American Academy of Child and Adolescent Psychiatry has developed practice parameters for the treatment of PTSD. The primary interventions include psychoeducation, individual therapy – mostly cognitive-behavioral therapy (CBT) – family therapy, group therapy, and psychopharmacology [19]. Since the practice parameters were published in 1998, new studies in PTSD and trauma treatment have been completed.

Psychotherapy

Psychotherapy can involve teaching the patient stress management techniques. These include progressive muscle relaxation, thought stopping, positive imagery, and deep breathing. These techniques are taught to children to help them master their anxiety. They are then ready for direct exploration, which involves retelling their story to help them work through the trauma. Trowell et al. [45] randomly assigned 71 girls (6–14 years old) with PTSD to individual psychotherapy or group therapy. Both groups improved. However, the individual psychotherapy group had a slightly greater reduction in PTSD re-experiencing and avoidance symptoms up to 1 year after study completion [45].

Cognitive-Behavioral Therapy (CBT)

Cognitive-behavioral therapy is a popular and effective treatment option for children with PTSD symptoms. It addresses the core features of PTSD (i.e., re-experiencing, avoidance, and arousal). Psychoeducation provides the basis for CBT intervention. Avoidance is addressed through graded exposure to the trauma. A hierarchy of feared aspects of the trauma is developed so that the child or adolescent can confront and overcome each aspect of the event in stages [46]. Cognitive processing can also help patients to correct misconceptions they may have. For example, traumatized children often blame themselves for the trauma. In CBT, an accurate account of the event is created and consequently distorted to relieve the child and to allow him or her to develop alternate cognitions. This is done by identifying the sources for his or her beliefs about blame, responsibility, and shame regarding the event. These cognitions are then critically assessed to effect change [46]. Several studies have pointed out CBT's effectiveness in children and adolescents with PTSD. The largest and most recent study, by Cohen et al. [47], assessed sexually abused children aged 8 to 14 years. These children and their primary caretakers were randomly assigned to trauma-focused CBT or child-centered therapy. At treatment follow-up, the CBT group had significantly fewer children who fulfilled diagnostic criteria for PTSD. Furthermore, they showed fewer symptoms of depression, behavior problems, and shame- and abuse-related attributions.

CBT may also be an effective treatment for preschool-aged children with PTSD symptoms. Deblinger et al. [48] randomly assigned sexually abused children, aged 2 to 8 years, and their mothers to group CBT or supportive therapy. CBT allowed children to discuss their feelings about the traumatic event, educated children regarding personal safety skills and coping mechanisms, and helped children to learn about appropriate touching with adults. The parents discussed their feelings about their child's abuse and were taught how to deal with their child's behavioral outbursts and to facilitate communication with their child regarding the experience. Therapy included 11 2-hour sessions. Each session concluded with a 15-minute joint activity that included the children and their parents. The supportive therapy group had therapy sessions for the parents and children similar to those of the CBT group. However, no joint activity took place at the end. During follow-up assessment, mothers in the CBT group reported reductions in intrusive thoughts and negative emotional reactions to the abuse, and children had a greater knowledge about personal safety [48].

Eye Movement Desensitization and Reprocessing (EMDR)

EMDR is a more recent treatment. In one study [49], 32 children, aged 6 to 12 years, who had not responded to CBT treatment of PTSD symptoms that developed after a hurricane were treated with EMDR. A randomized, lagged group design was used. PTSD symptoms were reduced and the symptom reduction maintained at 6-month follow-up [49]. The relative effectiveness of CBT and EMDR was compared in a group of sexually abused girls, 12 to 13 years old, randomly assigned to a maximum 12-session intervention for each treatment. Both interventions focused on exposure to traumatic memories. However, the CBT group received a greater emphasis on symptom management skills training. Both groups had an improvement in general behavior and an overall reduction in PTSD symptoms. However, EMDR worked slightly better in less time than CBT [46,50]. Suggested PTSD symptoms may be reduced in a shorter period with EMDR compared with standard CBT intervention.

Psychopharmacology

Psychopharmacological treatment of PTSD usually focuses on specific symptoms and comorbid conditions. Selective serotonin reuptake inhibitors (SSRIs) are typically used to treat comorbid depression and anxiety. Clonidine is used to treat hyperarousal. Lithium and anticonvulsants are often used for the mood lability and poor affect regulation associated with trauma exposure [51]. Antipsychotics are used to target aggression and auditory hallucinations related to the trauma. However, a better understanding of the psychobiology of PTSD is needed to determine which psychopharmacological agents are most helpful in treating different symptom clusters of PTSD. Van der Kolk [52] recently reviewed the psychobiology and psychopharmacology of PTSD. Unfortunately, the data on psychopharmacological treatment of PTSD in children and adolescents are very limited. To date, double-blind, placebo-controlled studies are lacking. A PubMed review yielded only four open-label pharmacology trials in this age group. The first trial used citalopram, 20–40 mg, to treat PTSD symptoms in 24 children and adolescents (10 to 18 years old) and in 14 adults (19 years old or older). In this study, children and adolescents had significant reductions in mean Clinician-Administered Post-traumatic Stress Disorder Scale (CAPS) total scores and Clinical Global Impression scores at endpoint (8 weeks). Symptoms of hyperarousal improved, but re-experiencing and avoidance symptoms did not [53]. Another trial by Seedat *et al.* [54] included eight adolescents, 12 to 18 years old. This was a 12-week open trial of a fixed dose of citalopram (20 mg). CAPS (child and adolescent version) was the main outcome measure. PTSD symptom improvement was evidenced by a 38% reduction in the CAPS total score. However, depression did not improve. Thus, the authors suggested that improvement was not due to lessening of depression but rather to improvement of PTSD [54]. The third trial involved seven preschool children, 3 to 6 years old, with PTSD who were treated with clonidine, 0.05–0.20 mg (total dose), after failing all psychotherapy modalities. Aggression, hyperarousal, and sleep difficulties were reduced [55]. Famularo *et al.* [56] reported that propranolol improved hyperarousal and agitation in 11 children with PTSD. In this study, children manifested fewer PTSD symptoms when they were on propranolol than when they were not [56]. Finally, one case report showed improvement of PTSD symptoms with clonidine [57].

COMBORBIDITY OF TRAUMA AND ADDICTIVE DISORDERS IN ADOLESCENTS

In adult populations, comorbidity of PTSD with addictive disorders leads to poorer treatment outcomes as compared to addictive disorders alone; patients with the comorbidity tend to have longer duration of substance use and more symptoms of substance dependence, undergo more episodes of substance abuse treatment, and demonstrate less improvement during treatment than patients with an addictive disorder alone.

Prevalence of Addiction Among Adolescents

The use of drugs and alcohol by adolescents is an ongoing public health problem in the United States [58]. The prevalence of drinking increases quickly among children between 10 and 13 years of age, with more than 50% having begun to drink by age 13 [59]. According to data gathered in the 1999 Monitoring the Future study [60], which surveyed more than 45 000 adolescents in 433 schools across the nation, 52% of 8th-grade students reported having consumed alcohol in their lifetime and 25% reported having been drunk. Early onset of alcohol use in youths has been found to be strongly associated with use of other illegal drugs, as well as subsequent alcohol abuse and related problem behaviors in later adolescence, including injuries, drinking and driving, and absenteeism from school or work [61]. Substance use accounts for the largest number of years of potential life lost [62]. Thus, the negative outcomes associated with adolescent substance use are numerous and costly.

Comorbidity of Addictive and Trauma-Related Disorders

There is a large body of research with adult populations concerning prevalence, onset, course, sequelae, and treatment of comorbidity between addictive disorders and trauma-related disorders. There is substantially less corresponding research about such comorbidity in adolescents. Furthermore, few studies are available that adequately appraise the impact of the comorbidity between addictive disorders and trauma-related disorders on psychosocial functioning during adolescence, a distinct and critical developmental period when youths are still acquiring the social, educational, and occupational skills they will need throughout adulthood.

In a study of adolescents with alcohol dependence [63], it was reported that 59% of these adolescents (aged 14–18 years) experienced one or more DSM-III-R traumas, and 13% met DSM-III-R lifetime criteria for PTSD. Van Hasselt *et al.* [64] explored the history of maltreatment in a population of 150 hospitalized dually diagnosed substance-abusing adolescents. Their results indicated that 61% of the sample experienced or had a history that warranted suspicion of past and/or current maltreatment. Physical abuse was the most frequent form of maltreatment, followed by sexual abuse and neglect.

Perron *et al.* [65] found a high level of victimization in a group of 259 African-Americans receiving substance-abuse treatment in an inner city program. Fifty-four percent reported a lifetime history of victimization, mostly by being threatened with a weapon. PTSD contributed to teen and young adult cannabis use disorders [66].

In a study of 18-year-olds in a predominantly white, working-class community, Giaconia et al. [67] found that 18.5% of these adolescents met DSM-III-R criteria for lifetime addictive disorders and had experienced at least one qualifying trauma; 3.6% of the total sample (or 8.5% of those exposed to traumas) met all DSM-III-R lifetime criteria for both addictive disorders and PTSD. An even higher prevalence of PTSD was found in a group of 297 chemically dependent adolescents [10]. The lifetime prevalence of PTSD was 29.6% overall ($n = 88$), 24.3% for the males ($n = 54$) and 45.3% for the females ($n = 34$). The current prevalence, defined as within the past 4 weeks, was 19.2% ($n = 57$), 12.2% for the males ($n = 27$) and 40.0% for the females ($n = 30$). For the entire group overall and for the females specifically, PTSD was the most common diagnosis in terms of both lifetime and current prevalence, taking precedence over major depression, dysthymia, simple phobia, and bulimia. Among the males, PTSD ranked as the second most common disorder, preceded only by simple phobia. Overall, trauma was reported by 222 (74.7%) of the subjects. The females were somewhat more likely than the males to have experienced a trauma (80.0% vs 73%). Rape, seeing someone hurt or killed, physical assault, and threat of injury were the most common traumas for females. Among males, seeing someone hurt or killed, threat of injury, and sudden injury or accident were the most frequent traumatic events. Deykin and Buka [10] further explored the temporal sequence of the first episode of PTSD and the beginning of chemical dependence (either alcohol or other drugs). The onsets of chemical dependence and PTSD were intertwined. More of the females (58.8%, 20 of 34) than males (27.8%, 15 of 54) had experienced PTSD before chemical dependence. The average age of onset of chemical dependence was 12.7 years for the males (SD = 1.8) and 13.4 years for females (SD = 1.3). The mean age of onset of PTSD was 11.5 years (SD = 4.2) for the females and 13.5 years (SD = 4.4) for the males. The sample consisted of treated chemically dependent individuals. The rates of PTSD might be lower in untreated populations.

Conversely, the rates of addictive disorders in populations of adolescents with PTSD have also been substantial. Data from a community study of 14 to 24-year-olds [68] indicate that 34.7% of participants who had experienced DSM-IV traumas had a lifetime DSM-IV substance-related disorder. Among those with diagnosis of PTSD, 5.3% had a comorbid substance-related disorder. Although declines in specific types of adolescent substance use were observed recently, these declines were less pronounced in cigarette smokers and alcohol users with a history of PTSD [69] as compared with cigarette smokers and alcohol users without a history of PTSD.

As for the temporal relationship between the onset of the addictive disorder (AD) and the onset of PTSD, there are the following three possibilities: (i) AD precedes trauma/PTSD; (ii) AD and trauma/PTSD occur at the same time; or (iii) AD follows the onset of trauma/PTSD. Studies have found no overall sequencing of onset that characterizes this comorbidity. There seem to be diverse and multiple pathways leading to the comorbity of AD and trauma/PTSD during adolescence.

When substance use problems precede trauma exposure and PTSD symptoms, researchers argue that substance use interferes with adaptation. Specifically, substance use is viewed as a coping strategy that fosters escape or avoidance of the stressor and associated emotional distress, which may interfere with more adaptive efforts at processing the event and problem-solving, leading to an increase in maladaptive outcomes such as PTSD symptoms [70–72].

However, ample research with adults [69,73] and adolescents [74,75] has documented increased substance use following trauma exposure. Most researchers interpret this increased use as self-medication, an attempt to reduce the distress associated with the immediate and ongoing effects of the trauma and symptoms of PTSD [10,72]. Giaconia et al. [67] argue that rather than a single sequence of onset, substance use problems likely play multiple roles in the onset and maintenance of PTSD. Namely, Giaconia et al. [67] found that for about half (56.3%) of the adolescents in their sample the onset of AD preceded that of the earliest trauma, for 18.3% both occurred during the same year, and for 25.4% the AD emerged later than the trauma. The relationship between the onset of an AD and the onset of PTSD was similarly varied: For 50% of adolescents with comorbid AD-PTSD, the onset of AD preceded that of PTSD; for 35.7% AD and PTSD developed during the same year; and for 14.3% the AD developed more than 1 year later than the PTSD. The patterns of onset may depend on the type of AD: for drug disorders the AD preceded the PTSD in 75%, whereas for alcohol disorders the AD preceded PTSD for 55.5% of the participants [68].

The interplay between trauma, PTSD, and substance use is further complicated by the presence of secondary stressors [76].

Severity of PTSD was a significant predictor of negative situational drug use, and emotion-focused coping was found to mediate this relationship [77]. A higher number of experienced potentially traumatic events was associated with incremental risk for PTSD and PTSD associated with a substance abuse disorder [78].

The addictive behaviors often occur in the context of other high-risk behaviors, such as delinquent behavior, risky sexual behaviors, and self-injurious behaviors. Adolescence is a period of life when there is, in any case, an increased risk for these types of behaviors. Research has shown that victimization experiences and high-risk behaviors frequently co-occur in at-risk adolescents.

TREATMENT OF COMORBID ADDICTIVE AND TRAUMA-RELATED DISORDERS

Many treatment approaches that separately address addictive disorders and trauma-related disorders have been implemented and will not be reviewed here. However, little is known about the effect of the comorbidity on the success of these treatments. One longitudinal study could be found utilizing traumatic stress as a predictor of substance abuse treatment. Jaycox et al. [79] examined longitudinal data among 212 adolescents in long-term residential substance abuse treatment, where 29% of the sample indicated a PTSD diagnosis. At baseline, the authors found that PTSD was associated with internalizing behaviors (e.g., anxiety, depression), but not externalizing behaviors. Dividing the sample into three groups (no trauma, trauma but no PTSD, trauma and PTSD), the authors examined treatment retention at 6 months and found that although youths with PTSD did not differ from the other groups on retention, youths with trauma without PTSD dropped out of treatment significantly faster than youths never experiencing trauma. The authors concluded that these youths may have been particularly resilient and no longer felt the need for treatment. However, it is also possible that these youths were exhibiting the avoidant behaviors related to PTSD and that youths with some trauma may be difficult to retain in substance abuse treatment.

Williams et al. [80] examined 108 youths (ages 11–17) looking at how youths who enter outpatient substance abuse treatment with high traumatic stress (HTS) compared to youths who enter treatment without such HTS, at intake and at 3 and 6 months following intake on substance abuse treatment outcomes. HTS was defined as a score of 5 and higher on the GAIN'S Traumatic Stress Scale. Despite having significantly higher rates of co-occurring mental health disorders, emotional abuse, sexual abuse, and use of other drugs, the HTS group showed equal or greater improvement on substance abuse treatment outcomes over time compared to their counterparts. The authors point out that early steps in substance abuse treatment generally appear to mirror recommended early steps of trauma treatment, and this may have accounted for the success of treatment in

the youths with HTS. Alternatively, treatment provided the youths with HTS with alternative ways of coping with the trauma thus lessening their motivation to "self-medicate" with substances. The authors proposed that this might indicate a subgroup of substance-abusing youths, whose use of substances is temporary and contingent on the experience of traumatic sequelae.

There is a need for integrated interventions that target high-risk behaviors, such as substance abuse, in adolescents who have experienced interpersonal violence in order to incorporate into treatment potential victimization-related memories, distress, or other symptoms that are unique to victims and may be related to the expression of the high-risk behaviors. Unfortunately, empirical data on the efficacy or effectiveness of these integrative approaches are very limited. Several integrated interventions involving victimized youth populations have begun to be developed and tested, including "Seeking Safety," trauma systems therapy, and risk reduction through family therapy.

Seeking Safety [81] is a treatment for individuals with comorbid PTSD and substance use problems that has been well evaluated in various adult populations. It consists of 24 sessions and includes cognitive, behavioral, and interpersonal components, with each component addressing a safety coping skill relevant to both PTSD and substance abuse. Treatment is based on five key principles:

1. Safety as the priority of the first stage of treatment.
2. Integrated treatment of PTSD and substance abuse.
3. Focus on ideals with the title of topics framed positively to combat pathology (e.g., honesty to combat denial, lying, and false self).
4. Four content areas: cognitive, behavioral, interpersonal and case management (the interpersonal aspect helps the patient maximize the presence of supportive people and let go of destructive people).
5. Attention to therapist processes.

Although the results of Seeking Safety have been promising with adult populations, no efficacy studies to date have been published on this intervention with adolescents.

Trauma Systems Therapy (TST), developed at the Center for Medical and Refugee Trauma at Boston Medical Center [82], is currently being adapted to address the complex treatment needs of adolescents experiencing traumatic stress and abusing substances, through work being done at the Adolescent Traumatic Stress and Substance Abuse Treatment Center at Boston University. Interventions in TST are designed to work in two dimensions: strategies that operate through and in the social environment to promote change, and strategies that enhance the individual's capacity to self-regulate. The implementation of TST begins with an assessment of an individual's level of emotional regulation as well as the degree of environmental stability in the adolescent's world. Within the TST framework, youths are considered to be at the most acute levels of emotional dysregulation when, in addition to experiencing emotional distress (e.g., anxiety, depression, and PTSD symptoms), they are also displaying behaviors that are harmful to themselves and others (e.g., substance use, self-injury, bingeing and purging, delinquency). In addition, contextual information is taken into consideration to evaluate whether the environment is stable, distressed, or threatening.

The TST model involves choosing a series of interventions that correspond to the fit between the traumatized youth's own emotional regulation capacities and the ability of the child's social environment and system-of-care to help manage emotions or offer protection from threat. TST is implemented using a modular approach in which interventions are selected based on the level of need. These interventions include home and community-based care, psychopharmacology, services advocacy, emotional regulation skills training, trauma processing, and meaning making skills training.

Preliminary data from an open trial of TST in a sample of traumatized youths ($n = 110$; mean age = 11.21, SD = 3.6) demonstrated a significant reduction of trauma symptoms, improvements in emotional and behavioral regulation, as well as a more stable social environment after 3 months of treatment [83]. TST contributed significantly to transitioning from more intensive to less intensive phases of treatment. In addition, gains in psychiatric symptoms and environmental stability were correlated with the clinician's assessment of children's improvements in functioning after 3 months. Further, the substance-abuse adaptation of TST for adolescents who have experienced traumatic events (TST-SA) is currently being piloted at the Center for Anxiety and Related Disorders at Boston University.

Risk Reduction through family Therapy (RRFT) [84] is an intervention developed to reduce the risk of substance abuse and other high-risk behaviors, revictimization, and trauma-related psychopathology in adolescents who have been sexually assaulted. RRFT integrates several existing empirically supported treatments, such as trauma-focused cognitive-behavioral therapy (TF-CBT), Multisystemic Therapy (MST), and other risk-reduction programs for revictimization and risky sexual behaviors. Adolescents participating in this treatment can be heterogeneous with regard to symptom expression, thus a clinical pathways approach is taken in the RRFT manual. The manual consists of six primary treatment components: (i) psychoeducation;

(ii) coping; (iii) substance abuse; (iv) PTSD; (v) sexual education and decision-making; and (vi) sexual revictimization risk reduction. Results of a pilot trial of RRFT showed reductions in multiple areas of clinical concern, including substance use and related risk factors, PTSD, and depression symptoms, which were maintained through a 6-month follow-up [84].

SUMMARY

Comorbidity of trauma and PTSD with addictive disorders is common in adolescents. The interrelationship between the two conditions is complex, with addictive behaviors following the trauma, as well as preceding it. While there are established treatments for each of the conditions separately, few treatments addressing the comorbidity have been developed and tested. Little is known about the impact of the comorbid addictive disorders and trauma-related disorders on the adolescent developmental trajectory – the ability of the adolescent to acquire crucial psychosocial skills in the face of these twin disorders. In view of the adolescent tendency not to self-disclose, proactive screening for trauma in the population of addicted adolescents, as well as screening for substance abuse in those who have experienced trauma, is highly indicated.

References

1. American Psychiatric Association (APA). *Diagnostic and Statistical Manual of Mental Disorders, 4th edn, Text Revision* (DSM-IV-TR) Washington, DC: APA, 2000.
2. American Psychiatric Association (APA). *Diagnostic and Statistical Manual of Mental Disorders, 3rd edn* (DSM-III) Washington, DC: APA, 1980.
3. American Psychiatric Association (APA). *Diagnostic and Statistical Manual of Mental Disorders, 3rd edn, Revised* (DSM-III-R) Washington, DC: APA, 1987.
4. American Psychiatric Association (APA). *Diagnostic and Statistical Manual of Mental Disorders, 4th edn* (DSM-IV) Washington, DC: APA, 1994.
5. US Department of Health and Human Services, National Institute of Mental Health. Epidemiologic Catchment Area Study, 1980–1985. Rockville, MD: US Department of Health and Human Services, National Institute of Mental Health [producer], 1992. Ann Arbor, MI: Interuniversity Consortium for Political and Social Research [distributor], 1994. doi:10.3886/ICPSR06153.v1.
6. Breslau N, Davis CG, Andeski P, Peterson E. Traumatic events and posttraumatic stress disorder in an urban population of young adults. *Arch Gen Psychiatry* 1991;**48**: 216–222.
7. US Department of Health and Human Services, Administration on Children, Youth and Families. Child Maltreatment 2006. Washington, DC: US Government Printing Office, 2008. Available from: http://www.acf.hhs.gov/programs/cb/pubs/cm06/cm06.pdf.
8. Jouriles E, McDonald R, Norwood W, Ezell E. Issues and controversies in documenting the prevalence of children's

exposure to domestic violence. In: Graham-Bermann SA, Edelson JL (eds), *Domestic Violence in the Lives of Children: The Future of Research, Intervention, and Social Policy*. Washington: American Psychological Association, 2001; pp. 13–34.

9. Edelson JL. Studying the co-occurrence of child maltreatment and domestic violence in families. In: Graham-Bermann SA, Edelson JL (eds), *Domestic Violence in the Lives of Children: The Future of Research, Intervention, and Social Policy*. Washington: American Psychological Association, 2001; pp. 91–110.

10. Deykin EY, Buka SL. Prevalence and risk factors for posttraumatic stress disorder among chemically dependent adolescents. *Am J Psychiatry* 1997;**154**:752–757.

11. Giaconia RM, Reinherz HZ, Paradis AD, Stashwick CK. Comorbidity of substance use disorders and posttraumatic stress disorder in adolescents. In: Ouimette P, Brown PJ (eds), *Trauma and Substance Abuse*. Washington, DC: American Psychological Association, 2003; pp. 227–242.

12. Cuffe SP, Addy CL, Farrison CZ, *et al.* Prevalence of PTSD in a community sample of older adolescents. *J Am Acad Child Adolesc Psychiatry* 1998;**37**:147–154.

13. Kessler RC, Sonnega A, Bromet E, Hughers M, Nelson CB. Posttraumatic stress disorder in the National Comorbidity Survey. *Arch Gen Psychiatry* 1995;**52**:1048–1060.

14. Centers for Disease Control and Prevention (CDC). Youth Risk Behavior Surveillance – United States, 2005. *Morb Mortal Wkly Rep* 2006;**55**(SS-5):1–112 (www.cdc.gov/mmwr/PDF/SS/SS5505.pdf).

15. Kilpatrick DG, Acierno R, Saunders B, *et al.* Risk factors for adolescent substance abuse and dependence: Data from a national sample. *J Consult Clin Psychol* 2000;**68**:19–30.

16. Mazza JJ, Reynolds WM. Exposure to violence in young inner-city adolescents: relationships with suicidal ideation, depression, and PTSD symptomatology. *J Abnorm Child Psychol* 1999;**27**:203–213.

17. Scheeringa MS, Zeanah CH, Myers L, Putman FW. New findings on alternative criteria for PTSD in preschool children. *J Am Acad Child Adolesc Psychiatry* 2003;**42**:561–570.

18. Silverman WK, La Greca AM. Children experiencing disasters: Definitions, reactions, and predictors of outcomes. In: La Greca AM, Silverman WK, Vernberg EM, Roberts MC (eds), *Helping Children Cope with Disasters and Terrorism*. Washington, DC: American Psychological Association, 2002; pp. 11–33.

19. AACAP Official Action: Practice Parameters. Practice parameters for the assessment and treatment of children and adolescents with posttraumatic stress disorder. *J Am Acad Child Adolesc Psychiatry* 1998;**37**:4S–26S.

20. Drake EB, Bush SF, van Gorp WG. Evaluation and assessment of PTSD in children and adolescents. In: Spencer E (ed.), *PTSD in Children and Adolescents*. Washington, DC: American Psychiatric Publishing, Inc., 2001; pp. 1–31.

21. Pfefferbaum B. Posttraumatic stress disorder in children: A review of the past 10 years. *J Am Acad Child Adolesc Psychiatry* 1997;**36**:1503–1511.

22. Pynoos RS, Steinberg AM, Goenjian A. Traumatic stress in childhood and adolescence: Recent developments and current controversies. In: van der Kolk BA, McFarlane AC (eds), *Traumatic Stress: The Effects of Overwhelming Experience on Mind, Body, and Society*. New York: Guilford Press, 1996; pp. 331–358.

23. Scheeringa MS, Zeanah CH, Drell MJ, Larrius JA. Two approaches to diagnosing posttraumatic stress disorder in infancy and early childhood. *J Am Acad Child Adolesc Psychiatry* 1995;**34**:191–200.

24. Carrion VG, Weems CF, Ray RD, Glaser B, Hessl D, Reiss AL. Diurnal salivary cortisol in pediatric posttraumatic stress disorder. *Biol Psychiatry* 2002;**51**:575–582.

25. McNally RJ. Assessment of posttraumatic stress disorder in children and adolescents. *J School Psychol* 1996;**34**:147–161.

26. Lonigan CJ, Phillips BM, Richey JA. Posttraumatic stress disorder in children: Diagnosis, assessment, and associated features. *Child Adolesc Psychiatr Clin N Am* 2003;**12**:171–194.

27. Jensen PS, Rubio-Stipec M, Canino G, *et al.* Parent and child contributions to diagnosis of mental disorder: Are both informants always necessary? *J Am Acad Child Adolesc Psychiatry* 1999;**38**:1569–1579.

28. Korol M, Green BL, Gleser GC. Children's responses to a nuclear waste disaster: PTSD symptoms and outcome prediction. *J Am Acad Child Adolesc Psychiatry* 1999;**38**:368–375.

29. Brown RT, Madan-Swain A, Lambert R. Posttraumatic stress symptoms in adolescent survivors of childhood cancer and their mothers. *J Trauma Stress* 2003;**16**:309–318.

30. De Bellis MD, Broussard ER, Herring DJ, Wexler S, Moritz G, Benitez JG. Psychiatric co-morbidity in caregivers and children involved in maltreatment: A pilot research study with policy implications. *Child Abuse Neglect* 2001;**25**: 923–944.

31. Vogel JM, Vernberg EM. Children's psychological responses to disasters. *J Clin Child Psychol* 1993;**22**: 464–484.

32. Reich W, Leacock N, Shanfield C. *Diagnostic Interview for Children and Adolescents – Revised (DICA-R)*. St Louis, MO: Washington University, 1994.

33. Kaufman J, Birmaher B, Brent D, *et al.* Schedule for Affective Disorder and Schizophrenia for School-age Children – Present and Lifetime version (K-SADS-PL): Initial reliability and validity data. *J Am Acad Child Adolesc Psychiatry* 1997;**36**:980–988.

34. Newman E, Weathers FW, Nader K, *et al. Clinician-Administered PTSD Scale for Children and Adolescents (CAPS-CA)* Los Angeles: Western Psychological Services, 2004.

35. Blake DD, Weathers FW, Nagy LM, *et al.* A clinician rating scale for assessing current and lifetime PTSD. The CAPS-1. *Behav Therapist* 1990;**13**:187–188.

36. Weiss DS, Marmar CR. The Impact of Events Scale – Revised. In: Wilson JP, Keane TM (eds), *Assessing Psychological Trauma and PTSD*. New York: Guilford Press, 1997; pp. 399–411.

37. Horowitz MJ, Wilner N, Alvarez W. Impact of events scale: A measure of subjective stress. *Psychosom Med* 1979;**41**:209–218.

38. Hawkins SS, Radcliffe J. Current measures of PTSD for children and adolescents. *J Pediatric Psychol* 2006;**31**: 420–430.

39. Pynoos RS, Frederick C, Nader K, *et al.* Life threat and posttraumatic stress in school-age children. *Arch Gen Psychiatry* 1987;**44**:1057–1063.

40. Rodriguez N, Steinberg A, Pynoos RS. *ULCA PTSD Index for DSM-IV Instrument Information: Child Version, Parent Version, Adolescent Version*. Los Angeles, CA: UCLA Trauma Psychiatry Service, 1999.

41. Steinberg AM, Brymer MJ, Decker KB, Pynoos RS. The University of California at Los Angeles Post-Traumatic

Stress Disorder Reaction Index. *Curr Psychiatry Rep* 2004;**6**:96–100.

42. Foa EB, Riggs DS, Dancu DV, Rothbaum BO. Reliability and validity of a brief instrument for assessing post-traumatic stress disorder. *J Trauma Stress* 1993;**6**:459–473.

43. Foa EB, Johnson KM, Feeny NC, Treadwell KRH. The child PTSD symptom scale: A preliminary examination of its psychometric properties. *J Clin Child Psychol* 2001;**30**: 376–384.

44. Briere J. *Trauma Symptom Checklist for Children (TSCC)*. Odessa, FL: Psychological Assessment Resources, 1996.

45. Trowell J, Kolvin I, Weeramanthri H, *et al.* Psychotherapy for sexually abused girls: psychopathological outcome findings and patterns of change. *Br J Psychiatry* 2002;**180**: 234–247.

46. Stallard P. Psychological interventions for post-traumatic reactions in children and young people: a review of randomized controlled trials. *Clin Psychol Rev* 2006;**26**: 895–911.

47. Cohen JA, Deblinger E, Mannarino AP, Steer RA. A multisite randomized controlled trial for children with sexual abuse related PTSD symptoms. *J Am Acad Child Adolesc Psychiatry* 2004;**43**:393–402.

48. Deblinger E, Stauffer LB, Steer RA. Comparative efficacies of supportive and cognitive behavioral group therapies for young children who have been sexually abused and their nonoffending mothers. *Child Maltreat* 2001;**6**:332–343.

49. Chemtob CM, Nakashima J, Carlson JG. Brief treatment for elementary school children with disaster-related post-traumatic stress disorder: a field study. *J Clin Psychol* 2002;**58**:99–112.

50. Jaberghaderi N, Greenwald T, Rubin A, *et al.* A comparison of CBT and EMDR for sexually abused Iranian girls. *Clin Psychol Psychother* 2004;**11**:358–368.

51. Donnelly CL. Pharmacologic treatment approaches for children and adolescents with posttraumatic stress disorder. *Child Adolesc Psychiatr Clin N Am* 2003;**12**:251–269.

52. Van der Kolk BA. The psychobiology and psychopharmacology of PTSD. *Hum Psychopharmacol* 2001;**16**: S49–S64.

53. Seedat S, Stein DJ, Ziervogel C, *et al.* Comparison of response to a selective serotonin reuptake inhibitor in children, adolescents, and adults with posttraumatic stress disorder. *J Child Adolesc Psychopharmacol* 2002;**12**:37–46.

54. Seedat S, Lockhat R, Kaminer D, *et al.* Open trial of citalopram for adolescents with PTSD. *Int Clin Psychopharmacol* 2001;**16**:21–26.

55. Harmon RJ, Riggs PD. Clonidine for posttraumatic stress disorder in preschool children. *J Am Acad Child Adolesc Psychiatry* 1996;**35**:1247–1249.

56. Famularo R, Kinscherff R, Fenton T. Propranolol treatment for childhood posttraumatic stress disorder, acute type. A pilot study. *Am J Dis Child* 1988;**142**:1244–1247.

57. Porter DM, Bell CC. The use of clonidine in post-traumatic stress disorder. *J Natl Med Assoc* 1999;**91**:475–477.

58. Substance Abuse and Mental Health Services Administration (SAMHSA). *National Household Survey on Drug Abuse: Main Findings 1996*. DHHS Pub. No. (SMA) 98-3200. Rockville, MD: SAMHSA, 1998.

59. Komro KA, Toomey TL. Strategies to prevent underage drinking. *Alcohol Res Health* 2002;**26**:5–14.

60. Johnston LD, O'Malley PM, Bachman JG. The Monitoring the Future National Survey results on adolescent drug use:

Overview of key findings 1999. NIH Pub. No. 00-4690. Rockville MD: National Institute on Drug Abuse, 2000.

61. Gruber E, DiClemente RJ, Anderson MM, *et al.* Early drinking onset and its association with alcohol use and problem behavior in late adolescence. *Prev Med* 1996;**25**: 293–300.

62. US, Department of Justice, National Drug Intelligence Center. *The Economic Impact of Illicit Drug Use on American Society*. Washington, DC: United States Department of Justice, 2011. Available from: http://www.justice.gov/ndic/pubs44/44731/44731p.pdf.

63. Clark DB, Lesnick L, Hegedus A. Trauma and other stressors in adolescent alcohol dependence and abuse. *J Am Acad Child Adolesc Psychiatry* 1997;**36**:1744–1751.

64. Van Hasselt VB, Ammerman RT, Glancy LJ, Bukstein OG. Maltreatment in psychiatrically hospitalized dually diagnosed adolescent substance abusers. *J Am Acad Child Adolesc Psychiatry* 1992;**31**:868–874.

65. Perron BE, Gotham HJ, Cho D. Victimization among African-American adolescents in substance abuse treatment. *J Psychoactive Drugs* 2008;**40**:67–75.

66. Cornelius JR, Kirisci L, Reynolds M, *et al.* PTSD contributes to teen and young adult cannabis use disorders. *Addict Behav* 2010;**35**:91–94.

67. Giaconia RM, Reinherz HZ, Hauf AC, Paradis AD, Wasserman MS, Langhammer DM. Comorbidity of substance use and posttraumatic stress disorder in a community sample of adolescents. *Am J Orthopsychiatry* 2000;**70**: 253–262.

68. Perkonigg A. Kessler RC. Storz S, Wittchen HU. Traumatic events and post-traumatic stress disorder in the community: prevalence, risk factors and comorbidity. *Acta Psychiatr Scand* 2000;**101**:46–59.

69. McCart MR, Zajac K, Danielson CK, *et al.* Interpersonal victimization, posttraumatic stress disorder, and change in adolescent substance use prevalence over a ten-year period. *J Clin Child Adolesc Psychol* 2011;**40**:136–143.

70. Adams R, Boscarino J, Galea S. Alcohol use, mental health status, and psychological well-being 2 years after the World Trade Center attacks in New York City. *Am J Drug Alcohol Abuse* 2006;**32**:203–224.

71. Cooper M, Frone M, Russell M, *et al.* Drinking to regulate positive and negative emotions: a motivational model of alcohol use. *J Pers Soc Psychol* 1995;**69**:990–1005.

72. Windle M. Paternal, sibling, and peer influences on adolescent substance use and alcohol problems. *Appl Dev Psychol* 2000;**4**:98–100.

73. Vetter S, Rossegger A, Rossler W, *et al.* Exposure to tsunami disaster, PTSD symptoms and increased substance abuse – an internet based survey of male and female residents of Switzerland. *BMC Public Health* 2008;**8**:1–6.

74. Reijneveld SA, Crone MR, Verhulst FC, Verloove-Vanhorick SP. The effect of a severe disaster on the mental health of adolescents: A controlled study. *Lancet* 2003;**362**: 691–696.

75. Wu P, Duarte CS, Mandell DJ, *et al.* Exposure to the World Trade Center attack and the use of cigarettes and alcohol among New York City public high school students. *Am J Public Health* 2006;**96**:804–807.

76. Overstreet S, Salloum A, Badour C. A school-based assessment of secondary stressors and adolescent mental health 18 months post-Katrina. *J School Psychol* 2010;**48**: 413–431.

77. Staiger PK, Melville F, Hides L, *et al.* Can emotion-focused coping help explain the link between post-traumatic stress disorder severity and triggers for substance

use in young adults? *J Subst Abuse Treat* 2009;**36**:220–226.

78. Macdonald A, Danielson CK, Resnick HS, *et al.* PTSD and comorbid disorders in a representative sample of adolescents: the risk associated with multiple exposures to potentially traumatic events. *Child Abuse Neglect* 2010;**34**:773–783.

79. Jaycox LH, Ebener P, Damesek L, Becker K. Trauma exposure and retention in adolescent substance abuse treatment. *J Trauma Stress* 2004;**17**:113–121.

80. Williams JK, Smith DC, Gotman N, *et al.* Traumatized youth and substance abuse treatment outcomes: a longitudinal study. *J Trauma Stress* 2008;**21**:100–108.

81. Najavits LM, Weiss RD, Shaw SR, *et al.* "Seeking safety": Outcome of a new cognitive-behavioral psychotherapy for women with posttraumatic stress disorder and substance dependence. *J Trauma Stress* 1998;**11**:437–456.

82. Saxe GN, Ellis BH, Kaplow JB. *Collaborative Treatment of Traumatized Children and Teens: The Trauma Systems Therapy Approach.* New York: Guilford Press, 2007.

83. Saxe GN, Ellis B, Fogler J, *et al.* Comprehensive care for traumatized children. *Psychiatr Ann* 2005;**29**:443–448.

84. Danielson CK. *Risk Reduction Through Family Therapy Treatment Manual.* Charleston, SC: National Crime Victims Research & Treatment Center, 2006.

37

Sexual Addiction and Hypersexual Behaviors in Adolescents

Dean De Crisce

New York University School of Medicine, Brooklyn, NY, USA

INTRODUCTION

Adolescence is a monumental period of global change characterized by rapid emotional, moral, social, cognitive, psychological, and physical lines of development, all of which occur independently. Adolescence is typically accompanied by the successful navigation of individuation, peer identification, and risk-taking behavior. The ability to predict the outcome of actions, as a function of cognitive development, may be preceded by behaviors that have a significant probability to cause harm. Such risky behaviors may include sexual experimentation, substance use, reckless driving, and other types of potentially problematic behaviors.

Problematic sexual behaviors are a potential concern to any clinician treating adolescents. Identification of those behaviors that deviate from "normal," and that may represent deviant or compulsive sexuality, will be helpful to the clinician. Sexual behavior is complex, and the literature is scant in regards to hypersexual disorder or sexual addiction in teenagers. Sexual behaviors, perhaps more so than any other high-risk behaviors, are set in a fragile and sociologically relative framework.

Addiction may be roughly defined as the compulsive pursuance of pleasure-producing substances and behaviors, despite significant problems, and associated with craving and impairment of control. According to the American Society of Addiction Medicine in a recent policy statement, "Addiction is a primary, chronic disease of brain reward, motivation, memory and related circuitry. Dysfunction in these circuits leads to characteristic biological, psychological, social and spiritual manifestations. This is reflected in an individual pathologically pursuing reward and/or relief by substance use

and other behaviors. Addiction is characterized by inability to consistently abstain, impairment in behavioral control, craving, diminished recognition of significant problems with one's behaviors and interpersonal relationships, and a dysfunctional emotional response. Like other chronic diseases, addiction often involves cycles of relapse and remission. Without treatment or engagement in recovery activities, addiction is progressive and can result in disability or premature death" [1].

Out of control sexual behavior has been considered and classified along with impulse control disorders, sexual disorders, addictive disorders, and as a result of mood disorders, obsessive-compulsive disorder, or even psychodynamic processes [2]. There is reasonable evidence for considering some problematic sexual behaviors as comprising a behavioral addictive disorder, given the strong similarities with substance use disorders in presentation, neuroadaptive responses, treatment approaches, and other features.

A primary feature of all addictive processes is an inability to control a compulsive, perceived pleasurable behavior that ultimately causes significant problems. Many addictive disorders begin in adolescence and represent chronic behavioral patterns that persist throughout adulthood. Initially producing a pleasurable "high," the behaviors often later become more motivated by an attempt to avoid dysphoria in their absence, and are associated with a decrease in the pleasure received over time. This leads to a need to increase intensity of the behavior to maintain the pleasurable state [3].

Similarities may be drawn between behavioral addictive disorders and substance abuse in terms of neuroadaptive responses, characterological traits, and psychiatric comorbidity. For example, neurotransmitters

Clinical Handbook of Adolescent Addiction, First Edition. Richard Rosner.

involved in memory, learning, and reward have been implicated in both behavioral addictive disorders and substance use disorders. Those with behavioral addictions have been shown to report high levels of impulsivity, sensation seeking, and compulsivity, similar to addicted substance users. Behavioral addictions likewise have been reported to be highly comorbid with major depressive disorder, bipolar disorder, obsessive-compulsive disorder, and attention-deficit/hyperactivity disorder [3,4].

There are valid arguments against defining disorders based on specific problematic behaviors. One could imagine the absurd extent to which that process might be applied. However, supportive arguments have been considered sufficiently salient to influence one proposal of a new diagnostic classification, "Addiction and Related Disorders," which would include both behavioral addictions and substance use disorders to be included in the future *Diagnostic and Statistical Manual of Mental Disorders, Fifth Edition* (DSM-5) [3,4]. A similar proposal suggests including compulsive sexual behaviors with gambling and other "behavioral addictions" in a category to be termed "Volitional Disorders, Not Elsewhere Classified" until it is determined whether they represent "addictive" processes, disorders of impulse control, or even if such a classification is appropriate [5].

The general concept of sexual addiction as a "behavioral addiction," or as a diagnostic entity is controversial. Theoretical justifications for the consideration of problematic sexual behavior as an addictive disorder have their merits and deficits. Its application in adolescence is even more problematic given the typical behavior that is the hallmark of adolescent development. Nevertheless, the construct has a practical utility in the clinical approach to the categorization, intervention, and treatment of compulsive sexually problematic behaviors in youth.

NORMATIVE ADOLESCENT SEXUAL BEHAVIOR

Sexuality and sexual behaviors rank among the most complex of human interactions. Aspects from every area of human existence, ranging from physiology to philosophy, contribute to the establishment of "normative sexual behavior." The definition of such a standard, if indeed one can be determined, is established by cultural, sociological, generational, individual, familial, biological, cognitive, psychological, and psychiatric factors. Sexual behaviors, like other human behaviors and experiences, occur on a continuum.

Prior to adolescence, many US and, presumably, other Western children engage in curiosity-driven childhood sexual play in an attempt to explore gender roles and

sexual biology. Such sexual play typically occurs alone or with same-aged, mixed gendered, non-sibling peers, and is not generally associated with significant feelings of shame or fear. These behaviors might include minor self-stimulation, kissing, hugging, peeking, touching, and exposure [6,7].

During early and middle adolescence, the development of secondary sexual characteristics and hormonal changes fixes sexuality as a prominent force. Most early adolescents are aware of sexual attraction, develop a sexual identity, and are engaged in sexual joking and conversation with peers, sexual fantasy, and self-stimulation. Actual interactive sexual behaviors with peers may involve open mouth kissing, mutual touching, and even simulated intercourse [8]. In late adolescence, the sexual behaviors of many approach those of adults, typified by appropriate peer-aged consensual sexual interaction, including oral sex and intercourse.

Subcultural values differ regarding opinions of the appropriateness of sexual behaviors in youth. An examination of data from various studies gives an indication of the actual, self-reported frequency of such behaviors. This may be reasonably considered to be *de facto* normative behaviors in the United States and other similar cultures. However, as self-report of these behaviors may be associated with shame in certain groups, it is likely that these self-reports underestimate masturbatory and other sexual practices.

Masturbation is the most common sexual behavior in youth. One 2011 survey of US teens between the ages of 14 and 17 years, reported increasing masturbatory activity, based on age, over that age range. For example, approximately 68% of 17-year-old males reported masturbation in the prior month, compared with 43% of 14-year-old males. More male teens reported masturbation (74%) than female teens (48%) [9]. In one Australian study, approximately 38% of high-school males, and 9% of high-school females reported masturbating three or more times per week [10].

Solitary sexual activities are followed by interactive sexual behaviors prior to the initiation of intercourse. Such behaviors in high-school-aged students include, in order of frequency, masturbation of a partner, receiving masturbation by a partner, cunnilingus, and fellatio. Males generally initiate such activity earlier than females, and report partners of the same age, or up to three years older. Adolescent females report a majority of partners within 2 years of their age, with one-quarter reporting partners older, by 4 years or more [11].

Oral sexual activity is common. According to data from the Centers for Disease Control and Prevention, approximately 30% of 15-year-olds have engaged in oral sex. In 19-year-olds, this proportion increases substantially, with approximately 80% having participated in oral sexual activity [12].

The age of initiation of intercourse depends upon a number of sociocultural and familial factors. Higher socioeconomic status, greater parental supervision, "moral or religious emphasis," and two-parent families have been associated with delayed sexual initiation. Of adolescents surveyed, 10% to 20% reported engaging in intercourse before the age of 15; however, intercourse in adolescent girls younger than 13 is most frequently involuntary. Age of onset of sexual activity has been reported earlier in urban populations, when compared to the general population. Approximately 30% of urban minority males and 8% of urban minority females report engaging in intercourse by the 7th grade (approximately 13 years of age). These numbers increased to 66% of males and 52% of females by the 10th grade (approximately 16 years of age) [11,13].

The US National Survey of Family Growth, a project compiled by the Centers for Disease Control between 2006 and 2010, surveyed approximately 22 682 individuals in order to provide US national estimates of sexual activity, contraceptive use, and other information among youths aged 15 to 19 years. According to those results, less than 50% of unmarried teens aged 15 to 19 had engaged in sexual intercourse at least once; that percentage declined slightly from mid-1980s surveys [13]. Approximately 25% of adolescents surveyed had engaged in intercourse within a month prior to the survey, and approximately 40% within the prior year. Most teenagers had their first experience of intercourse with someone with whom they were "going steady," but a sizable proportion had their first intercourse with someone they had just met or whom they considered to be "just friends." The actual proportion varied among ethnic groups [13]. Sexual activity among Canadian and European teens was reported at similar rates [14,15].

In the 2006–2010 US National Survey of Family Growth, approximately 25% of teenagers had engaged in intercourse with only one partner. Slightly fewer males reported a single partner when compared with females. Younger teens had less report of multiple partners in the prior 12 months when compared with older teens; the majority of respondents still reported intercourse with only one partner. For example, only 16% of females between the ages of 18 and 19 reported having two or three partners in the prior year, and 6.9% of males between the ages of 18 and 19 reported having four or more partners [13].

For sexually experienced teenagers, approximately 33% reported only one lifetime sexual partner, 16% had two partners, another 33% had between three and five partners, and a final 16% reported six or more partners. This was similarly reported by both males and females, although males were more likely to report more partners. The overwhelming majority reported use of contraception [13].

Among the more than 50% of teens surveyed who reported not having had intercourse, the most frequent reason reported was religious or moral values, along with concern about sexually transmitted diseases, a desire to avoid pregnancy, and "waiting for the right time" [13,16].

The medium of the internet has now become an additional forum for sexual behaviors in adolescents and adults. "Sexting" refers to the sending of sexually explicit messages or photographs via cell phone or the internet. Approximately 25% of over 600 adolescent girls surveyed in 2008 reported having engaged in "sexting" [17].

Establishment of normative sexual behaviors must be considered within the adolescent's gender, sociological, and developmental context. The United States has been noted to be more sexually conservative than European countries such as Germany, Sweden, and The Netherlands, and more sexually liberal than Asian and Islamic countries such as Japan, the Philippines, Morocco, and Bangladesh [18]. Such cultural factors and even subcultural factors must be explored when assessing for non-normative behaviors.

An illustrative, particular case demonstrating such factors concerns a 15-year-old immigrant Dominican girl ordered to undergo an emergent psychiatric evaluation by child protective services in a large US metropolitan area, after having been noted to be in a relationship with a 22-year-old Dominican male. In the process of performing the evaluation, both families presented to the interview. They were aware of, consented to, and even encouraged the relationship, which they hoped would lead to marriage. Both families explained that such an age discrepancy was not unusual in their culture, and they did not appear to be aware that such a relationship was a potentially indictable offense in that jurisdiction. There did not appear to be any evidence of harmful or unusual sexual behavior, or trauma, despite the fact that the behavior was considered to be illegal by the "greater US culture."

Ryan, in a 10-year study of childhood sexuality on behalf of the Kempe Children's Center, categorized adolescent sexual behaviors into four categories:

1. normal adolescent sexual behavior;
2. behavior requiring an adult response;
3. behavior requiring correction; and
4. illegal behaviors requiring immediate intervention.

Sexual behaviors that might be a cause of concern include the following [19]:

- Preoccupation with sexual themes that impair social and scholastic functioning.

- Degradation/humiliation of self or others.
- Single occurrences of voyeuristic, frotteuristic, or exposure activities.
- Coercive sexual behaviors.
- Sexual touching without consent.
- Compulsive masturbation, causing impairment in daily functioning.
- Sexual behaviors that cause injury to self or others.
- Sexual behaviors that create significant shame and fear.
- Sexual behaviors that place one in a position of significant vulnerability and morbidity.
- Unusual interest or preoccupation with pornography.
- Indiscriminate promiscuity with multiple partners.
- Significant discrepancy in age, developmental level, or supervisory status (e.g., babysitting).
- Significantly unusual sexual behaviors.
- Sexual harassment or repeated obscene phone calls.

SEXUAL ADDICTION AND HYPERSEXUAL DISORDER

Much of adolescent sexual behavior considered "problematic" in the media and literature includes relatively normative activities that specifically place teens at risk for pregnancy, sexually transmitted diseases, and other morbidity. While this is of concern in the treatment of all adolescent patients, it must be understood that most high-risk sexual activity does not comprise a compulsive, hypersexual, or addictive sexual disorder.

Problematic sexual behaviors in youth may be considered in various categories. Nomenclature in the literature is not standardized, resulting in the use of different criteria and terminology throughout various studies, confounding an already limited research base on hypersexual behaviors. At least one contributor to these disagreements involves differing theoretical assumptions [2]. Additionally, studies focusing on compulsive sexual behaviors in adolescents are almost non-existent. Therefore the clinician must apply literature regarding adult populations to the adolescent patient, understanding the unique physiology and developmental considerations of adolescence.

Problematic excessive sexual behaviors have been considered to be sexual disorders, addictive disorders, impulse control disorders, and expressions of obsessive-compulsive disorders [2]. The various terms used to designate compulsive sexual behaviors, including hypersexual disorders, problematic sexual behaviors, and sexual addiction, will be used interchangeably throughout the remainder of this chapter.

The view of compulsive sexual behaviors as "behavioral addictions" similar to substance-based addictions, subject to peer self-help group treatment, was presented by Carnes et al. approximately 25 years ago [20]. The Diagnostic and Statistical Manual of Mental Disorders, Fourth Edition, Text Revision (DSM-IV-TR) has not focused on the categorization of compulsive, non-paraphilic, sexual behaviors, although "sexual addiction" was given as an example of Sexual Disorder Not Otherwise Specified in a 1987 version (DSM-III-R) [21]. More recently, Kafka has proposed "Hypersexual Disorder" for inclusion in the upcoming DSM-V [22]. Those views that categorize compulsive sexual behavior as an addictive disorder utilize the general criteria of substance use disorders to define the addictive sexual disorder. Similarly, views that categorize compulsive sexual behaviors as non-paraphilic sexual disorders utilize the basic structure of diagnostic criteria for paraphilia as defining characteristics.

Stein, in 2008, proposed an A-B-C model when considering problematic sexual behaviors. This view avoids a singular classification based on theoretical assumptions, and encourages exploration of phenomenological and psychobiological components. Key components of the model include:

A   affective dysregulation,
B   behavioral addiction, and
C   cognitive dyscontrol [2].

Typical high-risk adolescent sexual behavior, as previously described, generally denotes relatively normative behaviors that place adolescents at risk for pregnancy and sexually transmitted diseases such as unprotected sex and sex with multiple partners. In contrast, compulsive sexual, or hypersexual, disorders indicate sexual behaviors that while mostly normative in nature, are engaged in excessively and compulsively, causing distress or impairment [23]. Subcategories of these behaviors have been described as non-coercive versus coercive, non-deviant versus deviant, and non-paraphilic versus paraphilic.

A basic definition of a behavioral addiction, which may be applied to certain patterns of sexual behavior, has been given as an obsessive and excessive engagement in a perceived pleasurable behavior, despite adverse consequences, in which the person experiences a perceived compulsion to continue the behavior. The disorder is also associated with a loss of insight with regards to the difficulty the behavior is causing. There may also be an experience of "tolerance," in which the person increases the frequency or intensity of the behavior to achieve a prior or pleasurable response, and the experience of a "withdrawal" syndrome if the behavior is ceased [24].

Using the categorization of compulsive sexual behaviors as a behavioral addiction similar to other substance-related addictions, Goodman (in 1993) proposed criteria for the diagnosis of Sexual Addiction, below [25]. Carnes (in 2001) established similar criteria [20].

Sexual Addiction:

A. Recurrent failure to resist impulses to engage in a specified sexual behavior.
B. Increasing sense of tension immediately prior to initiating the sexual behavior.
C. Pleasure or relief at the time of engaging in sexual behavior.
D. At least five of the following criteria:
    1. Frequent preoccupations with sexual behavior or with activity that is preparatory to the sexual behavior.
    2. Frequent involvement in sexual behavior to a greater extent or over a longer period than intended.
    3. Repeated efforts to reduce, control, or stop sexual behavior.
    4. A great amount of time spent in activities necessary for engaging in sexual behavior, or for recovering from its effects.
    5. Frequent involvement in sexual behavior when the subject is expected to fulfill occupational, academic, domestic, or social obligations.
    6. Important social, occupational, or recreational activities given up or reduced because of the behavior.
    7. Continuation of the behavior despite knowledge of having a persistent or recurrent social, financial, psychological, or physical problem that is caused or exacerbated by the sexual behavior.
    8. Need to increase the intensity or frequency of the sexual behavior in order to achieve the desired effect, or diminished effects obtained with sexual behavior of the same intensity.
    9. Restlessness or irritability if unable to engage in the sexual behavior.
E. Symptoms have persisted for at least 1 month, or have occurred repeatedly over a longer period of time [25].

Kafka proposed the following criteria for Hypersexual Disorder for inclusion in DSM-V:

A. Over a period of at least 6 months, recurrent and intense sexual fantasies, sexual urges, or sexual behaviors in association with three or more of the following five criteria:
    1. Time consumed by sexual fantasies, urges, or behaviors repetitively interferes with other important goals, activities, and obligations.
    2. Repetitively engaging in sexual fantasies, urges, or behaviors in response to dysphoric mood states.
    3. Repetitively engaging in sexual fantasies, urges, or behaviors in response to stressful life events.
    4. Repetitive but unsuccessful efforts to control or significantly reduce these sexual fantasies, urges, or behaviors.
    5. Repetitively engaging in sexual behaviors while disregarding the risk for physical or emotional harm to self or others.
B. There is clinically significant personal distress or impairment in social, occupational, or other important areas of functioning associated with the frequency and intensity of these sexual fantasies, urges, or behaviors.
C. These sexual fantasies, urges, or behaviors are not due to the direct physiological effects of an exogenous substance.

Specify if: Masturbation, Pornography, Sexual Behavior with Consenting Adults, Cybersex, Telephone Sex, Strip Clubs, Other [22].

In the criteria for the proposed DSM-V Hypersexual Disorder, Kafka synthesizes varying theoretical perspectives. In this view, compulsive sexual behaviors are considered as non-paraphilic sexual disorders. Notably, the diagnostic criteria incorporate the typical structure used in the diagnosis of other sexual disorders, but account for an "addictive process" in that the behavior serves to mitigate emotional states, and is repeatedly performed despite attempts to refrain from the behavior, and despite problematic outcomes [21,22]. Hypersexual disorder is viewed as a disorder of sexual desire, characterized by increased frequency and intensity of sexual fantasies and urges, associated with impulsive behaviors that carry adverse consequences. The behaviors may be associated with a response to ameliorate dysphoric states along with, possibly, progressive risk-taking or sensation seeking [22]. Similar to the criteria for established substance use disorders and sexual disorders, special consideration or criteria for adolescents have not been proposed.

Paraphilic disorders refer to deviant sexual arousal and practices, and are generally classified and discussed separately from sexual addiction or hypersexual disorders. One significant reason to separate the two classes of disorders, although there may be overlap, is that paraphilias generally involve behaviors that are illegal and harmful to others, whereas sexual addiction involves legal behaviors that are generally harmful to the individual, not unlike other typical addictions such as substance use disorders and gambling. Another general distinction is that paraphilias indicate deviant sexual attraction toward a socially unacceptable behavior or object, and sexual addiction or hypersexual disorder generally indicates more normative sexual arousal, with an excessive drive or persistent disinhibition [23,26]. An additional ethical consideration in classifying paraphilias as separate disorders involves the real concern that viewing an illegal behavior as an "addiction" might lead to an extreme legal argument that most criminals are not responsible for their behaviors because they are acting on impulses which they cannot control.

A paraphilia is generally defined by the DSM-IV-TR as:

A. Over a period of at least 6 months, recurrent, intense sexually arousing fantasies, sexual urges or behaviors generally involving (i) non-human objects, (ii) the suffering or humiliation of oneself or one's partner, or (iii) children or other non-consenting persons.

B. The person has acted on these sexual urges, or the sexual urges or fantasies cause marked or clinically significant distress, interpersonal difficulty, or impairment in social, occupational, or other important areas of functioning [27].

Various specifiers are given, based upon the specific paraphilic diagnosis. Typical paraphilic diagnoses include exhibitionism, fetishism, frotteurism, pedophilia, sexual sadism, voyeurism, and paraphilia, not otherwise specified. The paraphilia, not otherwise specified category refers to a multitude of paraphilic behaviors that are not elucidated individually. They include telephone scatalogia (obscene phone calls), zoophilia (bestiality), erotic asphyxiation, necrophilia, and many others. Special qualification is given when considering the diagnosis of pedophilia in adolescents, in that the person must be "at least 16 years and at least five years older than the child or children." It is also noted "not to include an individual in late adolescence involved in an ongoing sexual relationship with a 12 or 13 year old." No age consideration is given for other sexual disorders or substance use disorders [27,28].

DIAGNOSTIC CONSIDERATIONS

Sexual addiction and most other sexual disorders are diagnoses of exclusion. Hypersexuality can result from a number of psychiatric disturbances, medical disorders, intoxicants, and social processes, which must be explored prior to making a sexual diagnosis. Sexuality is a complex phenomenon, and hypersexual behaviors are best viewed in a multifactorial setting that includes neurobiological, psychological, social, and psychiatric components. Various contributors to hypersexual behavior are considered below.

Sexual interest, sexual activity, and androgen levels generally decline with age. Adolescents are physiologically "hypersexual" by comparison with later adulthood [29]. Testosterone surges during the pubertal period generally peak between the ages of 15 and 25 [30]. This age range generally, and additionally, corresponds to periods of greater recklessness and aggressiveness, as displayed by higher rates of property crime and violent crime in this age group, as indicated in US Federal Bureau of Investigation (FBI) arrest data [31].

Hypersexual behaviors are associated with a number of neurological disorders. Examples of such disorders that might be seen in adolescence include Tourette's syndrome, temporal lobe epilepsy, movement disorders, brain injury, or processes that increase intracranial pressure [32]. Similarly, hypersexuality might be seen in various endocrinological disturbances such as Klinefelter's syndrome, and adrenal and testicular tumors.

Psychiatric comorbidity has been considered to be common in individuals with compulsive sexual behaviors. Hypersexual behaviors may be frequently associated with mood disorders, substance use disorders, disruptive behavioral disorders, anxiety disorders, impulse control disorders, and cluster B personality traits and disorders [33].

Hypersexual behaviors may be frequently found in adolescents with bipolar disorder as a symptom of mania or hypomania. Mania may be accompanied by impulsivity and sensation-seeking, in the presence of impaired judgment. Therefore, a thorough assessment of mood disorders is essential in the exploration of hypersexual behaviors, keeping in mind that adolescents often present with more atypical mood symptoms than are classically seen in adults. Treatment would then be geared toward managing the sexual behaviors within the context of other high-risk and impulsive behaviors associated with the mood disorder [17].

Hypersexual behaviors are frequently comorbid with substance use disorders. Specific substances of abuse have been reported to be associated with increased libido, primarily stimulants such as cocaine and methamphetamine. Various substances may also be used to enhance sexual performance and pleasure (e.g., amyl nitrate, methylene dioxymethamphetamine (MDMA), gamma-hydroxybutyrate (GHB)), to decrease inhibitions (alcohol), or to overcome the resistance of a potential victim (benzodiazepines) [24].

Psychological factors associated with hypersexuality include poor impulse control, sensation-seeking, and poor self-esteem. Adolescent girls with poor self-esteem are more likely to engage in sexual activity as a coping mechanism, and to gain validation [17].

Social contributors to hypersexual behaviors include parental modeling, peer group affiliation, sociocultural identification, and media influence. For example, greater exposure to sexuality in media is correlated with early onset of sexual behaviors in some adolescent groups [17].

PRESENTATION

Significant epidemiological studies regarding the prevalence of compulsive sexual disorders have not been carried out. It is estimated to affect 3–6% of the US population, one-third of whom are female, although the symptom qualification for that specific estimate is unclear [32]. Marshall and Briken reported estimates of sexually addictive behaviors in up to 17% of an impoverished urban community, based upon self-reported items in an administered sexual addiction screening instrument [21]. At least one difficulty in performing such studies is disagreement on diagnostic classification. In addition, no such estimates exist for adolescents, as data available on the frequency and types of sexual behaviors in adolescents focus either on typical high-risk behavior associated with pregnancy and sexually transmitted diseases, or on criminal juvenile sexual offending behavior. These data sets are not directly applicable to non-paraphilic, non-criminal, compulsive sexual behaviors.

Techniques to assess the prevalence of non-criminal hypersexual behaviors rely almost exclusively on self-report. Reliability of self-report is variable and dependent upon presenting circumstances. Sexual offenders are known to under-report sexual symptoms and behaviors. It is assumed that most adolescents would tend to minimize problematic sexual behaviors, as they do with other problems.

Compulsive sexual behaviors often have their onset in adolescence, with paraphilic behaviors occurring earlier than non-paraphilic behaviors. Bradford reported that the average age of onset for transvestism is 13.6, for fetishism is 16, voyeurism is 17.4, non-incestuous homosexual pedophilia is 18.2, sadism is 19.4, and non-incestuous heterosexual pedophilia is 21.1, although the onset of the paraphilic fantasies and urges occurs significantly prior to victimization having occurred [34].

Most individuals who suffer from compulsive sexual behaviors neither have a deviant arousal pattern nor engage in criminally harmful sexual behaviors. The concept of sexual addiction or hypersexual disorder only partially overlaps with paraphilic disorders. If there is any correlation with non-criminal compulsive sexual

behaviors, the overwhelming majority of adolescent sexual offenders do not become adult sexual offenders. However, up to 50% of adult sexual offenders report the onset of their behaviors in adolescence [35].

The course of sexual addiction in adults, as in substance use disorders, is considered to be chronic and progressive. Most sufferers have reported that their thoughts and behaviors lead to tension relief and a sense of gratification; however, approximately one-third described the thoughts as intrusive, and up to two-thirds described attempts to resist thoughts and urges [33].

Various models conceptualizing hypersexual behaviors have been proposed and applied. Carnes described a cycle, consisting of "preoccupation," "ritualization," "compulsive sexual behavior," and "despair" to characterize addictive sexual behaviors [36]. A 12-step model of addiction includes phases in which use of the substance (in this case, initiation of the behavior) leads to craving and a resultant binge, followed by remorse and a resolution not to repeat the behavior, with continued buildup of discontentment leading again to use of the substance to provide relief [37]. A relapse prevention model of sexual offending described by Freeman-Longo and Bays proposes a cycle comprised of phases such as "buildup," "acting out," "justification," and "pretend normal" [38]. Again, conceptualization of the dynamic process is based on theoretical formulation.

Increasing levels of addiction have been proposed, in order of concern. Level 1 includes normative behaviors that could be problematic if compulsive, such as masturbation, serial relationships, pornography, strip clubs, and prostitution. Level 2 includes more intrusive behavior such as exhibitionism, voyeurism, and obscene phone calls. Level 3 includes the highest level of sexual victimization such as child molestation, rape, and violence [36]. This type of categorization may be helpful in determining level of treatment required.

Sexual addicts are often involved in multiple different sexual compulsivities. Males tend to engage in activities that allow for emotional detachment, such as voyeurism, anonymous sex, prostitution, internet pornography, and exploitative sex. Women are more likely to engage in sexual activities involving sexual conquest, pain exchange, or internet chat rooms. Sexual addiction is often also associated with substance use disorders [24]. It is similarly known that paraphilias frequently occur comorbidly with other paraphilias [23,34].

Compulsive sexual behaviors can take various specific forms. One proposed categorization includes:

- preoccupation with sexual fantasy and masturbation;
- focus on seductive "conquest" behavior;
- anonymous sexual activity;

- compulsive use of prostitution, phone, or internet sexual material;
- traditional paraphilic interests such as voyeurism, exhibitionism, frotteurism, bestiality, sadomasochism, and exploitative sex [24].

Based on clinical samples, Kafka categorizes specific hypersexual behaviors in general order of prevalence reported in evaluated males with sexual disorders [22]. A discussion of each category follows.

- compulsive masturbation
- pornography dependence
- telephone sex dependence
- cybersex dependence
- protracted promiscuity
- frequent use of "strip clubs."

Compulsive Masturbation

Compulsive masturbation was the most common hypersexual behavior reported in males. Although definitions of compulsive masturbation differ, reports of high-school and undergraduate students note an average report of masturbation occurring approximately three times a week, with much lower percentages reporting consistent daily masturbation [22].

Pornography Dependence

Compulsive pornography use was also reported to be fairly common and associated with compulsive masturbation and telephone sex. Pornography included internet images and videos, as well as written text-based sexual materials [22]. Internet-related pornography is easily accessible, and in many cases may be normative for most adolescent males with internet access (discussed separately below).

Telephone Sex Dependence

Telephone sex refers to sexually explicit conversations with others, often concurrent with masturbation, and is typically associated with phone and credit card charges. Although a common form of hypersexual behavior in adults, it is expected to be a less likely significant activity for most adolescents because of financial access, and the availability of internet resources.

Cybersex Dependence

Cybersex refers to internet pornography use and chat room participation. Although studies have primarily examined the phenomenon in adult populations, this relatively new sexual format is seen to be specifically relevant to adolescents and young adults, because of the easily accessed, unrestricted sexual content that might otherwise be limited. The anonymous format of the internet may allow engagement in sexual behaviors and interests that the individual would not pursue offline [18]. This may serve to replace normative social interaction, obscure the typical social restraint to sexual pursuits, and foster the reinforcement of unusual or deviant interests.

Internet exchange may lead to real-life sexual encounters, be accompanied by masturbation, or enable illegal behaviors such as distribution of illegal materials or "cyberstalking." Engagement in the internet sexual world from a solitary position at home might alter the perception of safety, decrease normal inhibitory thresholds to behavior, and foster a lack of consequences for the behavior [18]. Adolescent use of sexually related chat rooms may lead to vulnerability to predation.

Internet sexual use comprises both passive and active activities. Passive activities may be termed "cybersexual consumption," and include downloading or viewing sexually explicit images, videos, or text-based stories. Active activities may be termed "cybersexual interaction," and include chat-based exchange, real-time video exchange, or involvement in distribution or exchange of sexually explicit emails, texts, and multimedia messaging [18].

Males and females who identified themselves as having compulsive cybersexual activity engaged in online activity at least 1–2 hours per day [22]. Males were more likely to use internet pornography, followed by chat room use, and real-time online sexual interaction. Females were more likely to engage in chat room use, followed by real-time online sexual interaction, with only a small proportion using pornography. Women were also more likely to use the internet to lead to live sexual interaction than men. In those with self-identified excessive sexual internet use, the online sexual activity led to significant interpersonal problems, and decreases in work performance and self-esteem [38,39].

Promiscuity and Strip Club Use

Definitions of promiscuity are problematic as there is no single standard for acceptable levels of consensual sex. However, most adolescents reported having three or fewer sexual partners in the prior year, according to the US National Survey of Family Growth studies cited above, with very few reporting four or more sexual partners [13]. Promiscuity may involve heterosexual, bisexual, or homosexual activities. The choice of partners associated with the promiscuous behavior may not be consistent with the claimed sexual orientation of the individual. Typical promiscuous behaviors reported by adults include repetitive brief, casual sexual encounters, serial sexual affairs, and use of prostitutes, massage parlors, and "pickup bars" [22]. Most adolescents with these types of behaviors would be more likely to have repetitive sexual partners, casual sexual encounters, and engage in an anonymous sexual activity in clubs (e.g., raves), rather than the adult use of prostitutes and massage parlors, because of financial and access considerations. Similarly, only older adolescents and college-age adults could be expected to attend strip clubs frequently enough to cause adverse consequences.

In adult studies, males represent a substantial majority of those seeking treatment for sexually compulsive behaviors. In smaller samples of female participants, promiscuity, compulsive masturbation, and cybersex use were reported by those seeking treatment [22].

Negative outcomes associated with hypersexual behaviors include loss of interest in other activities, failure to meet obligations, harm to relationships, transmission of sexually transmitted diseases, unintentional pregnancy, and dysphoric states such as depression, anxiety, and shame [22].

ASSESSMENT

Adolescents rarely self-refer for treatment of behavioral or psychiatric disorders. A clinician presented with an adolescent referred for perceived out-of-control sexual behavior, is advised to take a comprehensive approach to evaluation. Referrals may involve behaviors along the entire spectrum of sexual activity, some problematic and some normative. Referring sources can include caretakers, school officials, child protective services workers, court and other legal officials, mental health professionals, pediatricians, and childcare service agencies concerned with the adolescent's behavior. Consider the following range of referral examples, along with a brief summary of the concerning circumstances.

Zachariah

Zachariah, a 15-year-old boy from a conservative religious community, is brought in by his parents for a mental health evaluation after being found masturbating to commercially available adult pornographic magazines. His parents strongly believe that masturbation is both morally unacceptable and dangerous. They conclude that he must have a mental illness to engage in such behavior after extensive religious education. The teen has otherwise had no significant history of psychiatric or other behavioral disturbance. He is well-liked by

his peers, and reportedly is functioning well in his religious school environment.

Tina

Tina, a 14-year-old girl, is brought in to the emergency room by her single mother, after a suspicion that she might be pregnant. During the emergency room evaluation, it is determined that she is indeed in early pregnancy. The teen reports to the pediatrician that she engaged in a one time, consensual, unprotected sexual exchange with an 18-year-old boy. In further discussion with the pediatric social worker, the girl admitted to having had repeated sexual contact with multiple boys and young men in her neighborhood, ranging in age from 15 to perhaps 25 or older. Her urine toxicology screening is positive for cocaine. An emergency psychiatric consult is placed.

Joe

Joe is a 17-year-old adolescent, referred for "psychiatric clearance" to return to school after it was determined that he had sent sexual pictures of his 16-year-old ex-girlfriend to other peers in school. He has been suspended until that clearance is obtained. Joe has a history of multiple problematic behaviors in school, such as truancy and class disruption, for which he has been suspended. The referral was requested by a school social worker, and Joe's parents located the psychiatrist through their insurance company. The social worker mentioned that there is a possibility that legal charges will be pursued by the police for possession and distribution of child pornography.

Adam

Adam is an 18-year-old freshman at a local university. Although described as relatively anxious by his successful parents, he has always performed exceptionally well in academics. He has a few close friends, and has enjoyed moving to student housing to attend a prestigious university where he resides in his own dormitory room. Adam tells his parents that he is having some difficulty with his class load, and is not performing as he would wish. On one weekend, his parents came to visit him at the dormitory; after a long discussion it became clear that Adam had withdrawn from the semester after he had failed a number of mid-term examinations. He denied any traumatic events, or substance abuse, and his parents were bewildered by his behavior. The father asked Adam to use his desktop computer to respond to a work-related email that he had received on his phone. Adam told his father that his computer was not working, and when the father went to investigate the computer problem, both parents became aware of multiple open screens of internet pornography, and folders containing hundreds of pornographic downloads. Adam yelled uncharacteristically, "You are always trying to control me," and began crying. He would no longer speak to his parents about the issue, and an appointment with a psychiatrist was made.

Jerome

A call is made to child protective services from a foster care mother after observing her 16-year-old foster child, Jerome, in a room with her 6-year-old biological son. Jerome was found kneeling in front of the young boy, whose pants had been lowered to his knees. Jerome stated that he was checking the boy after he told him that his "pee pee hurt." The young boy later told his mother privately that Jerome had touched him on a number of occasions over the prior 6 months, and had touched some of his friends. The mother recalled that Jerome had been unusually close with her son, frequently giving him toys and other gifts. The child protective services agency notified the police and initiated an investigation. Jerome was placed in a youth shelter facility pending the results of the investigation. No formal charges had yet been brought. The child protective services caseworker requested a psychiatric evaluation to determine if a psychiatric disturbance was present, and what treatment and placement recommendation were needed.

Clarification of the role that the clinician is serving is important in establishing the extent, duration, and type of assessment required. Mental health clinicians might be involved in a variety of roles. These include initial detection, intervention, recommendations for treatment, aftercare, and specialty consultation [40].

A primary goal of the average clinician is, in addition to role clarification, to surmise the general nature and scope of the disturbance, the urgency of the behaviors, and to provide for the initial clinical course of treatment. As sexual disorders are not commonly treated by most clinicians, a realistic consideration is whether more extensive evaluation or treatment is within the scope of expertise of the clinician. For example, evaluations of youths involved in legal proceedings might be best completed by those with specialized forensic training in answering specific legal questions involving risk, competency, and culpability that can withstand the scrutiny of court testimony. Non-forensic, general psychiatric evaluations that either knowingly or unknowingly infer opinions regarding those issues, might be utilized in the legal process and have a substantial influence on the legal outcome. Accordingly, clinicians should be aware of those potential pitfalls.

In establishing the nature of the disturbance and assessing the urgency of the behaviors, an appropriate evaluation will substantially regard collateral information, as adolescents tend to minimize symptoms and problems, especially in situations in which the outcome may be expected to be punitive. All available data should be reviewed including the clinical interview, caretaker reports, social service records, school records, prior mental health treatment records, medical records, and arrest reports, if applicable. Particular attention should be paid toward developmental considerations, family and school functioning, psychiatric history, relevant medical history, and other known sexual, criminal, or disruptive behaviors.

Traditional psychiatric assessment components should focus on determining the presence of commonly associated comorbid psychiatric disorders such as anxiety, substance use disorders, attention-deficit/hyperactivity disorder, other disruptive behavior disorders, major depression, dysthymia, impulse control disorders, bipolar disorder, or obsessive-compulsive disorder [22]. Evidence for traditional psychiatric symptoms, such as mood changes, recent impulsive behaviors, obsessive thoughts, substance abuse, or bizarre beliefs will of necessity precipitate more in-depth examination in those areas.

Underlying medical contributors to hypersexual behaviors should be considered, such as neurological disorders, endocrinological disorders, substance use, or medication reactions. Evidence for such disorders should be addressed and treated accordingly. Hypersexual behaviors reported in several cases of temporal lobe epilepsy, responded successfully to antiepileptic treatment. Similarly, neuroleptic treatment of Tourette's syndrome was successful in controlling hypersexual behaviors. Medication to reduce compulsive or aggressive sexual behaviors in adolescents with substantial developmental disabilities warrants consideration [32].

The clinical interview, while gathering information in the above-mentioned traditional categories, will also focus on the presenting sexual behaviors, exploring them so as to determine if they are associated with illegal behaviors, abusive relationships, physical or emotional harm, substantial fear or shame, or bizarre sexual behaviors, as a safety priority. Behaviors or symptoms that lead to an immediate concern for safety might warrant emergent hospitalization, or removal from the home, until a more thorough evaluation and intervention can be completed. Often, the clinician must attempt to strike a balance between rapport building and the need to ensure safety with hospitalization and/or the involvement of authorities.

Various instruments have been proposed to screen for, and assist in the detection of, hypersexual or addictive sexual disorders. The Sexual Addiction Screening Test (SAST), Hypersexual Behavior Inventory (HBI), Compulsive Sexual Behavior Inventory (CSBI), Internet Sex Screening Test (ISST), and the Sexual Compulsivity Scale (SCS) are examples of such instruments [21]. None of these scales has been primarily designed to be used with adolescents, and their usefulness in that population is unknown.

The Sexual Addiction Screening Test (SAST), one of the most widely used general assessments, now exists in a revised form of 45 items as of 2010. A recent attempt to provide a more concise screening method that might be used in general clinical settings was proposed by Carnes *et al.* in 2012. The PATHOS Questionnaire is a brief screener comprised of six items taken from the SAST, and utilizes as a theoretical foundation the consideration of hypersexual behaviors as a sexual addiction [20].

The PATHOS data published in the *Journal of Addiction Medicine* cite two study samples of approximately 2800 total individuals taken from patients treated at a residential inpatient treatment center for sex addiction, outpatients receiving treatment for sex addiction, and healthy volunteers from a university setting as a comparison group. Approximately 43% of the total participants were female; however, over 75% of the patient participants were male, reflective of the fact that males are more likely to seek treatment for sexual addiction than females. The age of all participants ranged from 18 to 79 years. In one study, approximately 60% of the student/healthy sample was Caucasian, 37% African American, and 3% Hispanic, Asian and "other." Demographic information on the patient participants in the first study was not collected for confidentiality reasons. In the second study, the patient/target population comprised approximately 73% Caucasian, 15% Hispanic, 4% African American, and 6% Asian and "other" [20].

The PATHOS Questionnaire was designed to be a rapid tool, to be used by general clinicians in screening for potential addictive sexual disorders, similar to the usefulness of the CAGE Questionnaire in screening for substance use disorders. The name represents a mnemonic of questions to be used when evaluating patients. The summarized items include [20]:

1. Do you find yourself **P**reoccupied with sexual thoughts?
2. Do you hide some of your sexual behavior from others? Are you **A**shamed about your sexual behaviors?
3. Have you ever sought help (**T**reatment) for sexual behavior you did not like?
4. Has anyone been **H**urt emotionally because of your sexual behavior?

5. You feel controlled by your sexual desire? Do you feel **O**ut of control?
6. When you have sex, do you feel depressed (**S**ad) afterwards?

Using a cutoff score of 3, the PATHOS Questionnaire was found to correctly identify approximately 80% or more of the male patient population (sensitivity) when compared to results reported in the revised SAST. The Questionnaire was also able to correctly identify approximately 80% or more of the healthy male sample (specificity). Results were slightly less accurate for female participants [20].

Preliminary evidence suggests that the PATHOS Questionnaire may be a useful tool in rapidly screening for and identifying individuals who might benefit from a referral for more extensive assessment. More validation studies are necessary, including perhaps alteration of the items for use in adolescents. It nevertheless serves as a potential guideline for questions to be addressed in an assessment.

In instances in which imminent safety issues do not appear to be present, and there does not appear to be a causative acute psychiatric or medical condition, further exploration may be carried out with the teenager to gain a more comprehensive sexual history. This might include questions regarding the history of sexual experiences, sexual knowledge, sexual self-perception, sexual orientation and identity, and the presence of genital anomalies [41]. A focus on the problematic behaviors themselves will attempt to ascertain their precipitants, duration, frequency, variety, and associated outcomes. Forensic evaluations, although not the focus of this particular chapter, will emphasize assessment of the known contributors to risk for the particular class of deviant behaviors, if they exist.

The PATHOS Questionnaire was designed to assist in rapid screening for sexual problems, as described above. Although a review of the various, more extensive assessments is outside the scope of this chapter, one additional helpful and relevant screener is the Internet Sex Screening Test (ISST), given the likelihood of this type of problematic behavior in adolescents and young adults. The ISST, developed by Delmonico in 1999, is a 34-item self-report questionnaire, with scores greater than 9 indicating "at risk" behaviors. The instrument has limited validation and was developed primarily for adults. It is available in the public domain, and may be helpful in evaluating for problematic online sexual behavior in youths [42,43].

Initial assessments will have at least made a number of preliminary conclusions. Acute safety issues associated with the sexual behaviors will require primary intervention, as will acute medical or psychiatric decompensation. A general formulation as to the nature of the sexual disorder should be made, with consideration for various differential diagnoses that require further workup. At this point, concurrent with the role or expertise of the clinician, recommendations or referrals can be made if appropriate to a pediatrician, endocrinologist, neurologist, sexual disorder specialist, or forensic specialist. Evaluating clinicians may wish to continue working with the adolescent for education, psychiatric treatment, or sexual disorder treatment, if the clinician has such expertise.

TREATMENT

It is generally accepted that sexual behaviors and arousal in adolescence are not fixed. Sexual behavior becomes decreasingly fluid as adolescence progresses into adulthood. Deviant arousal patterns, if present, are generally established in early adulthood [44]. Early clinical intervention and treatment may have a substantial impact in the course of compulsive sexual behaviors or potential deviant behaviors.

There is no single standard approach to treatment of compulsive sexual behaviors, for many of the same reasons that there is no single accepted approach to substance use disorders. Treatment may include psychosocial treatment, pharmacological treatment, and participation in peer self-help support groups. There is little in the literature regarding treatment of adolescents with non-criminal compulsive sexual behaviors.

Ultimate treatment goals for compulsive sexual behavior include development of healthy sexuality, refraining from engagement in problematic behaviors, addressing psychological contributors such as low self-esteem and social skills deficits, and increasing quality of life. This assumes that safety has been assured, primary psychiatric and medical disorders treated, and substance use disorders addressed. The process may be lengthy, as in the treatment of any habitual, compulsive behavior, and recurrence of the problematic behavior might be reasonably expected.

Whereas a "relapse" into compulsive sexual behaviors may cause impairment to the individual, a "relapse" into criminal paraphilic behaviors can cause substantial harm to others. Therefore, the goals for the treatment of criminal paraphilic behaviors differ, understandably, in approach and expectations from non-criminal sexual behaviors.

Psychosocial Interventions

Adolescents with non-criminal compulsive sexual behaviors may be treated in a manner similar to other chemical dependency treatment models, with addiction and sex education, group and individual therapy, and family involvement. This may additionally involve attendance in 12-step programs addressing sexual addictions [24]. The strongest evidence supports a multidisciplinary approach to problematic sexual behaviors that utilizes education, crisis intervention, relapse prevention treatment, psychiatric treatment, substance abuse treatment, monitoring, and family involvement for youths [36,40].

First steps in addressing the sexual behaviors might involve immediate actions to halt the behaviors, such as limiting access to various websites, other sexual material, or victims. Later strategies might involve assisting the individual in learning behavioral and cognitive techniques to self-regulate sexual urges and prevent relapse [45].

Family therapy is known to be a highly effective method of treatment for adolescents with substance use disorders, and may be useful in addressing hypersexual behaviors. The process redefines the addictive behavior as a dynamic family problem, addresses dysfunctional family processes, and establishes contracts with contingent reinforcers [46]. Involvement of family members in a program of education and confrontation is helpful when treating those with impulsive sexual behaviors [24].

Relapse prevention is a cognitive-behavioral therapy technique used in substance abuse treatment, and has been adapted for use in the treatment of paraphilias and sexual addiction. The therapy seeks to help individuals identify triggers for the problematic behaviors, potential interventions to prevent the recurrence of those behaviors, and address cognitive distortions [44].

Various 12-step programs based upon Alcoholics Anonymous and other organizations, have been created to address sexual addictions. These groups include the National Council on Sexual Addiction and Compulsivity (now called the Society for the Advancement of Sexual Health), Sexaholics Anonymous, Sex Addicts Anonymous, Sex and Love Addicts Anonymous, and Cybersex Chat Addicts Anonymous [36]. Associated with these groups are support groups for families of sex addicts, similar to Alanon [24]. The groups vary somewhat in their definitions of abstinence and basic tenets, but all are based on 12-step, spiritually based concepts, or view compulsive sexual behaviors as an addiction.

Twelve-step programs may be somewhat problematic for adolescents, yet they are a widely available resource that might be helpful. Twelve-step programs generally cater to those who have "hit bottom," have a heavy emphasis on spirituality, and view the self as the "source of the problem," which might not be directly applicable to adolescents [47,48]. There are generally fewer adolescent members in any given program compared to the numbers of adult members, providing fewer avenues for identification and less resources for teens. Additionally, the various sexually based 12-step programs differ in their definition of abstinence, which may not give a realistic therapeutic goal for the adolescent. For example, Sexaholics Anonymous defines "sobriety" as refraining from all sexual activity outside of a relationship with one's marital partner [40]. Finally, there is some realistic concern that without adequate supervision, an adolescent might be vulnerable to relapse, or predation at a primarily adult-based meeting of self-reported sexual addicts. Substantial literature regarding the usefulness of these programs for compulsive sexual behaviors in adolescents (and others) is unknown.

Psychotherapy can be useful to address issues of shame, trauma, and distorted thoughts about sexual activity and behavioral consequences [24]. Attention may be given to the functionality of the sexual behaviors, self-esteem, and interpersonal issues [45].

Comprehensive inpatient and outpatient treatment programs for sexual disorders may be available, and provide structured, formalized treatment by experienced professionals. This might be an appropriate clinical course of action for those with substantial impairment as the result of the sexually problematic behaviors, as well as for those adolescents displaying intrusive, victimizing, or harmful sexual behaviors. Various models exist, geared to specific types of problematic behaviors. A primary distinction is between treatment for sex offenders and those suffering from non-criminal problematic sexual behaviors. Programs do exist that either accept adolescents, or are designed for juvenile offenders.

Typical addiction-based programs that focus on treatment for non-criminal sexual behaviors are structured similar to those available for substance use and eating disorders. These programs can vary between 1 and 5 months in duration, or more. Sexual addiction programs focus on "recovery," which involves the attainment and maintenance of a healthy sexuality and lifestyle when coping with life's problems. Successful recovery is based upon the restructuring of the individual's core beliefs, expansion of problem-solving skills, honesty, and the utilization of support networks [40].

Pharmacological Treatment

Pharmacological treatment for sexual disorders has focused on paraphilias. Medication treatment of paraphilias has included off-label use of gonadotropin-releasing hormone agonists, gonadotropin-releasing inhibitors, and other medications that reduce sexual drive. Non-paraphilic, compulsive sexual behaviors have been additionally treated with selective serotonin reuptake inhibitors, lithium, atypical antipsychotics, naltrexone, bupropion, valproic acid, and tricyclic antidepressants in various case reports [45,49]. Similar to the situation regarding use of medication for substance use disorders, little work has been done focusing on medication treatment of compulsive sexual behaviors in adolescent populations.

In one case report, Fong et al. described the successful treatment with topiramate of an adult male compulsive user of strip clubs and massage parlors, after failure of a 12-session course of cognitive-behavioral therapy and fluoxetine at 80 mg/day. Topiramate was titrated to a dose of 200 mg/day, which proved successful in enabling the patient to control the problematic sexual behaviors after the sixth week of treatment, along with individual therapy and 12-step program attendance. The medication was stopped because of side effects, and then restarted successfully, after the return of urges and problematic behaviors. The group described that topiramate may have been successful as a result of enhanced inhibitory control function [49].

In another case report, naltrexone was explored as a medication for hypersexual behaviors. The rationale for that choice involved targeting dopaminergic activity in the ventral tegmental area, implicated in naltrexone's effectiveness in alcoholism treatment. In theory, naltrexone would be expected to block the capacity of endogenous opioids to trigger dopaminergic release, thereby interfering with reward mechanisms. Bostwick and Bucci described treating with naltrexone a 24-year-old male who presented to a psychiatrist with a complaint of escalating preoccupation with internet pornography, up to 8 hours each day, and depressive symptoms. This behavior interfered with the patient's marriage, and led to the loss of several jobs as a result of poor productivity [50].

In this case, the young man had not been successful with antidepressants, nor with group and individual psychotherapy, nor with 12-step programs. Along with sertraline 100 mg/day, oral naltrexone at 50 mg/day was added to the regimen, leading to a self-reported substantially decreased urge to continue the behavior after only a week of treatment. The naltrexone was increased to 150 mg/day, and the patient reported complete control over his impulses. Bostwick and Bucci reported that the patient had continued in nearly complete remission for both depressive symptoms and compulsive internet use while continuing on the sertraline and naltrexone for over 3 years. There have been other studies examining naltrexone's efficacy in reducing sexual offending behavior in adolescents, with participants describing decreases in fantasies, arousal and masturbation, along with increased control over sexual urges [50].

Larger scale studies have demonstrated the effectiveness of a gonadotropin-releasing inhibitor (triptorelin) in adult males with non-paraphilic compulsive sexual behaviors [44]. Other antiandrogenic medications used in the treatment of non-paraphilic sexual behaviors have included medroxyprogesterone acetate, leuprolide acetate, and cyproterone acetate, which may be given orally or by depot injection. Antiandrogen treatment in adolescents could only be justified in the most refractory cases where there exists a substantial risk of sexual violence. It should only be used after puberty and the attainment of bone maturation [51].

Various resources are available for clinicians seeking referrals for their patients suffering from sexual disorders. Referrals for both inpatient and outpatient treatment programs may be obtained from academic medical centers, individual private treatment programs specializing in the treatment of problematic sexual behaviors, and various organizations such as the American Board of Sexology, the American College of Sexologists, the Association for the Treatment of Sexual Abusers (www.atsa.com), and the Safer Society Foundation (www.safersociety.org) [52]. Although the focus of these last two organizations is primarily on sexual offenders, they might also be helpful in locating treatment resources for those with non-criminal, sexually problematic behaviors. Clinicians wishing to be helpful should expect to investigate the various resources available and their applicability to the specific adolescent.

A review of the available information presented in this chapter makes clear the need for more substantial research of hypersexual disorder in adolescents.

References

1. American Society of Addiction Medicine. Public policy statement: Short definition of addiction, adopted by the ASAM Board of Directors 4 December 2011. Available from: http://www.asam.org/for-the-public/definition-of-addiction.
2. Stein DJ. Classifying hypersexual disorder: compulsive, impulsive, and addictive models. *Psych Clin N Am* 2008;**31**:587–591.
3. Grant JE, Potenza MN, Weinstein A, Gorelick DA. Introduction to behavioral addictions. *Am J Drug Alcohol Abuse* 2010;**36**:233–241.
4. Martin PR, Petry NM. Are non-substance-related addictions really addictions? *Am J Addict* 2005;**14**:1–7.
5. Fontenelle LF, Mendlowicz MV, Versiani M. Volitional disorders: A proposal for DSM-V. *World J Bio Psych* 2009;**10**:1016–1029.
6. Johnson TC. Understanding the sexuality of children. *Child and Youth Care Workers* 2001;**30**:1–6.
7. Friedrich WN, Fisher J, Broughton D, Houston M, Shafran CR. Normative sexual behavior in children: A contemporary sample. *Pediatrics* 1997;**101**:1–8.
8. Simon W, Gagnon J. Psychosexual development. *Society* 1998;**35**:60–68.
9. Robbins CL, Schick V, Reece M, *et al.* Prevalence, frequency, and associations of masturbation with partnered sexual behaviors among US adolescents. *Arch Pediatric Adolesc Med* 2011;**165**:1087–1093.
10. Smith AM, Rosenthal DA, Reichler H. High schoolers masturbatory practices: Their relationship to sexual intercourse and personal characteristics. *Psychol Rep* 1996;**79**: 499–509.
11. Feldman J, Middleman AB. Adolescent sexuality and sexual behavior. *Curr Opin Obstet Gynecol* 2002;**14**: 489–493.
12. Centers for Disease Control and Prevention. Sexual behavior and selected health measures: Men and women 15 to 44 years of age, United States, 2002. *Vital Health Stat* 2005;**362**: 1–56.
13. Martinez G, Copen CE, Abma JC, National Center for Health Statistics. Teenagers in the United States: Sexual activity, contraceptive use, and childbearing, 2006–2010. National Survey of Family Growth. *Vital Health Stat* 2011;**23** (31):1–44.
14. Poulin C, Graham L. The association between substance use, unplanned sexual intercourse and other sexual behaviours among adolescent students. *Addiction* 2001;**96**:607–621.
15. Santelli J, Sandfort T, Orr M. Transnational comparisons of adolescent contraceptive use: What can we learn from these comparisons? *Arch Pediatr Adolesc Med* 2008;**162**: 92–94.
16. Martinez G, Copen CE, Abma JC. Teenagers in the United States: Sexual activity, contraceptive use, and childbearing, 2006–2008. National Survey of Family Growth. *Vital Health Stat* 2010;**23** (30):1–57.
17. Ramirez Basco M, Celis-de-Hoyos CE. Biopsychosocial model of hypersexuality in adolescent girls with bipolar disorder: Strategies for intervention. *J Child Adolesc Psych Nur* 2012;**25**:42–50.
18. Griffiths MD. Internet sex addiction. *Addict Res Theory* 2012;**20**:111–124.
19. Ryan G. Childhood sexuality: A decade of study. Part I – Research and curriculum development. *Child Abuse Neglect* 2000;**24**:33–48.
20. Carnes PJ, Green BA, Merlo LJ, Polles A, Carnes S, Gold MS. PATHOS: A brief screening application for assessing sexual addiction. *J Addict Med* 2012;**6**:29–34.
21. Marshall LE, Briken P. Assessment, diagnosis, and management of hypersexual disorders. *Curr Opin Psychiatry* 2010;**23**:570–573.
22. Kafka MP. Hypersexual disorder: A proposed diagnosis for DSM-V. *Arch Sex Behav* 2010;**39**:377–400.
23. Krueger RB, Kaplan MS. The paraphilic and hypersexual disorders: An overview. *J Psych Practice* 2001;**7**:391–403.
24. Schneider JP, Irons RR. Assessment and treatment of addictive sexual disorders: Relevance for chemical dependency relapse. *Subs Use Misuse* 2001;**36**:1795–1820.
25. Goodman A. Sexual addiction: designation and treatment. *J Sex Marital Ther* 1993;**18**:303–314.
26. Kafka MP, Hennan J. A DSM-IV Axis I comorbidity study of males (n=120) with paraphilias and paraphilia-related disorders. *Sexual Abuse* 2002;**14**:349–366.
27. American Psychiatric Association. *Diagnostic and Statistical Manual of Mental Disorders, Fourth Edition, Text Revision.* Washington, DC:American Psychiatric Association, 2000.

28. Kafka MP. The DSM diagnostic criteria for paraphilia not otherwise specified. *Arch Sex Behav* 2010;**39**:373–376.

29. Davidson JM, Chen JJ, Crapo L, Gray GD, Greenleaf WJ, Catania JA. Hormonal changes and sexual function in aging men. *J Clin Endocrinol Metab* 1983;**57**: 71–77.

30. Ewing LL, Davis JC, Zirkin BR. Regulation of testicular function: A spatial and temporal view. *Int Rev Physiol* 1980;**22**:41–115.

31. Snyder HN. Juvenile arrests 1999. *Juvenile Justice Bulletin*. Office of Juvenile Justice and Delinquency Prevention, December 2000; pp. 1–10.

32. Kreuger RB, Kaplan MS. Disorders of sexual impulse control in neuropsychiatric conditions. *Semin Clin Neuropsych* 2000;**5**:266–274.

33. Kuzma JM, Black DW. Epidemiology, prevalence and natural history of compulsive sexual behavior. *Psych Clin N Am* 2008;**31**:603–611.

34. Bradford JM. The paraphilias, obsessive compulsive spectrum disorder, and the treatment of sexually deviant behaviors. *Psych Quart* 1999;**70**:1–6.

35. Butler SM, Seto MC. Distinguishing two types of adolescent sex offenders. *J Am Acad Child Adolesc Psychol* 2002;**41**:83–90.

36. Plant M, Plant M. Sex addiction: A comparison with dependence on psychoactive drugs. *J Subst Use* 2003;**8**:260–266.

37. Anon. *Alcoholics Anonymous*, 4th edn. New York: Alcoholics Anonymous World Services, 2001.

38. Freeman-Longo R, Bays L. *Why Did I Do it Again? Understanding My Cycle of Problem Behaviors (Offender Guided Workbook, Part Two)*. Brandon, VT:Safer Society Press, 1988.

39. Schneider JP. A qualitative study of cybersex addiction on the family: Results of a survey. *Sex Addiction Compuls* 2000;**7**:249–278.

40. Manley G. Treatment and recovery for sexual addicts. *Nurs Pract* 1990;**15**:34–41.

41. Ryan G, Leversee TF, Lane S. *Juvenile Sexual Offending: Cause, Consequences, and Correction*. San Francisco: Jossey-Bass Publications, 1997.

42. Delmonico DL, Miller JA. The Internet sex screening test: A comparison of sexual compulsives versus nonsexual compulsives. *Sex Reln Ther* 2003;**18**:261–276.

43. Internet Sex Screening Test (ISST). InternetBehavior.com. Available from http://www.Internetbehavior.com/pdf/isst.pdf.

44. Veneziano C, Veneziano L. Adolescent sex offenders, a review of the literature. *Trauma Violence Abuse* 2002;**3**: 247–260.

45. Kaplan MS, Kreuger RB. Diagnosis, assessment and treatment of hypersexuality. *J Sex Res* 2010;**47**:181–198.

46. Azrin N, Donohue B, Besale V. Youth drug abuse treatment: A controlled outcome study. *J Child Adolesc Subst Abuse* 1994;**3**:1–16.

47. Chapple JN. Long term recovery from alcoholism. *Psych Clin N Am* 1993;**1**:177–187.

48. Chapple JN, DuPont RL. Twelve step and mutual help programs for addictive disorders. *Psych Clin N Am* 1999;**2**:425–447.

49. Fong TW, De LaGarza R, Newton TF. A case report of topiramate in the treatment of non-paraphilic sexual addiction. *J Clin Psychopharm* 2005;**24**:512–513.

50. Bostwick JM, Bucci JA. Internet sex addiction treated with naltrexone. *Mayo Clin Proc* 2008;**83**:226–230.

51. Garcia FD, Thibaut F. Sexual addictions. *Am J Drug Alcohol Abuse* 2010;**36**:254–260.

52. Kreuger RB, Kaplan MS. Treatment resources for the paraphilic and hypersexual disorders. *J Psych Pract* 2002;**8**:59–60.

38

Sexting, Cybersex, and Internet Use: the Relationship Between Adolescent Sexual Behavior and Electronic Technologies

Abigail M. Judge[1] and Fabian M. Saleh[2]

[1]*Harvard Medical School, Massachusetts Avenue, Cambridge, MA, USA*
[2]*Harvard Medical School; Sexual Violence Prevention & Risk Management Program (SVP&RMP), Beth Israel Deaconess Medical Center, Boston, MA, USA*

In 2007, Phillip Alpert of Florida was 18 years old when he argued with his former girlfriend and impulsively distributed her naked picture to dozens of her friends and family. This same ex-girlfriend had sent him this picture via electronic mail earlier in their almost 2-year relationship. Alpert explained, "It was a stupid thing I did because I was upset and tired and it was the middle of the night and I was an immature kid" [1]. As a result, Alpert was arrested, charged and convicted with a felony (child pornography distribution), and sentenced to 5 years' probation. He was also required by Florida law to register as a sex offender, which he is mandated to do for the next 25 years. Alpert complained to *The Orlando Sentinel* that following his arrest, peers teased him; he developed symptoms of depression, and neighbors and fellow students harassed him after he was discovered on the sex offender registry [2].

The popular press has featured cases of "sexting" like Alpert's over the last few years [3–6]. Defined as the creation, sharing, or forwarding of sexually suggestive (nude or nearly nude) images by minor teens via cell phone or computer, the practice may include text messaging only (although it most often refers to the transmission of images) [7]. Alpert's case is particularly compelling because it captures the range of possible uses of sexting: an amorous communication turned impulsive retaliation. Although the definition of sexting lacks a motivational component, it is popularly described as a form of flirtation, seduction, and sexual communication [8]. This has since evolved to include

potentially malicious acts that some consider a form of cyber-bullying [9]. Indeed, the suicide of 13-year-old Hope Witsell in 2009 followed relentless bullying after she sent a picture of her breasts to her boyfriend, which a female peer then distributed to friends at six other schools [10]. Of course, the circumstances surrounding the suicide of any adolescent cannot be reduced to a single factor. Nevertheless, the prominence of sexting in popular narratives about Witsell's death is striking, and it reflects the unease as well as curiosity that youth-produced sexual images can engender.

These cases raise important questions about the interface between adolescent sexual behavior and emerging technologies. These questions arise as the use of electronic communication devices (e.g., the computer, cell phone) among teens is nearly universal. Online activity is reported by more than 90% of US youths (ages 12 to 18) [11,12], and instant messaging (IM) is the most popular mode of online communication among teens [13]. Twenty-five percent of MySpace's 200 million profiles belong to those under the age of 18 years [13], suggesting the influence of social networking sites on youth interaction and identity development. Unfortunately, little is known about the effects of these phenomena on adolescent development and vice versa. Given the emerging nature of technology and the corresponding generation gap between youths and adults regarding online activities, the developmental significance of adolescent online activity needs to be better understood.

The concept of problematic internet use first appeared in psychological literature in the 1990s and has been based primarily on clinical observations of adults. The phenomenon is described in many ways: compulsive internet use [14–16], problematic internet use [17,18], and most controversially, internet addiction [19]. Internet addiction has been framed as "a genuine diagnosis, a new symptom manifestation of underlying disorders, or psychosocial problems in adjusting to a new medium" [20]. Subtypes of internet addiction have been proposed based on literature review and clinical observation (e.g., excessive gaming, sexual preoccupations, and email/text messages [19,21].

However, the validity of internet addiction remains controversial largely due to methodological weaknesses of recent research (e.g., varying definitions of internet addiction; reliance on instruments with limited psychometric validity; the overuse of non-representative samples and self-report data; and exploratory rather than confirmatory analytic techniques) (for a meta-analysis, see ref. [22]). These limitations contribute to an equivocal evidence base about the concept, even as it is increasingly applied to adolescent populations. Prevalence rates of so-called internet addiction among teens are highly variable (i.e., 0.9% to 38%) due in large part to the absence of standardized measures or established criteria [23]. Of note, research on internet addiction among adolescents has emerged only in the last few years, with much of it based on non-US samples (i.e., Chinese, Taiwanese, Korean) internet where overuse, particularly online gaming, is over-represented [24,25]. The more widespread use of internet cafes in Asian countries has also made data collection more accessible as compared with the primarily home based nature of internet use in the U.S. The South Korean government labeled the problem a major public health concern following 10 cardiopulmonary-related deaths in internet cafes and a game-related murder [21].

Given the dearth of data and the importance of understanding the internet to adolescents in developmentally appropriate terms, some have proposed whether the concept of internet addiction is at this point best understood as an analogy [26,27]. Turkle [28] has written extensively on how individuals subjectively experience computers and new technology. She cautioned that the concept of internet addiction may obscure other ways of understanding how adolescents derive meaning from online activity:

> People are tethered to the gratifications offered by their online selves. These include the promise of affection, conversation, a sense of new beginnings . . . Powerful evocative objects for adults,

they are even more intense and compelling for adolescents, at that point in development when identity play is at the center of life.

> S. Turkle (2008) [28]

The concept of addiction contrasts from Turkle's view, and these differences suggest important tensions in how problematic internet use is understood among adolescents in particular. Accordingly, this chapter offers a critical review of the empirical research on internet use in adolescents with a particular focus on the interplay between emerging technologies and adolescent sexual behavior. We hope to bear in mind Turkle's invitation to consider the range of "identity play" these behaviors may express, including but not limited to a critical evaluation of whether internet misuse may be an addiction and if so, for whom. Regardless of the diagnostic conceptualization, some youths who use the internet have a more complicated development; this review aims to consider lines of evidence that may help to characterize vulnerable youths and to suggest promising areas of future inquiry.

INTERNET USE AND PSYCHOSOCIAL RISK AMONG ADOLESCENTS: WEIGHING THE EVIDENCE

Since the 1990s, research has considered the effects of internet use on a range of psychosocial outcomes among adolescents. A seminal 2-year prospective study on the consequences of adolescent internet use (i.e., the HomeNet study) found that greater adolescent internet use was associated with declines in measures of psychological well-being (e.g., decreased communication with family members, declines in the size of social circles, increased depression and loneliness) [29]. The authors described this as the "internet paradox," since participants used the internet heavily for communication, which in general has positive psychosocial effects. Interestingly, those who reported loneliness or depression prior to internet use were not more attracted to the internet, suggesting that internet use in itself was related to decreases in well-being. The authors speculated that adolescents' usage of the internet for online communication resulted in compromised offline social relationships with friends and family, which could have resulted in observed declines in well-being. A 3-year follow-up study among the same sample showed that all of the negative effects on well-being dissipated over time, except for an increase in stress [30].

A second longitudinal study revisited the internet paradox and also addressed the original study's methodological limitations [30]; results were mixed. Greater internet use was associated with positive outcomes across a range of dependent measures of social involvement and psychological well-being. However, internet use was again associated with increased stress, decline in local knowledge, and diminished commitment to one's local area. This study also identified moderators of the association between internet use and well-being: online communication is related to a decrease in psychological well-being among introverts and those with low levels of social support. In contrast, the psychological well-being of extroverts and those with more social support tended to benefit from online communication [30] (referred to as the *rich-get-richer model*). Unfortunately, age was dichotomized (i.e., adult if age 18 years or older, or teen), with no within-group analyses of youth, and a smaller proportion of adolescent participants in this second study. Overall, results suggest that individuals who are already socially engaged may leverage internet use to healthier ends than those who struggle in social domains.

A more recent longitudinal study of Dutch youths aged 12 to 15 years in The Netherlands evaluated this pathway [31], and found that online communication (rather than other internet applications) was related to future compulsive internet use at 6-month follow-up. Compulsive internet use was defined using a validated measure that evaluated preoccupation or salience, loss of control, and continued internet use despite the intention to stop [32]. Instant online communication (i.e., instant messaging applications such as g-chat; IM) evoked the greatest compulsive tendencies among participants, and was positively associated with depression 6 months later. According to path analysis (i.e., a technique that provides estimates of the magnitude and significance of hypothesized causal connections between variables), IM affected compulsive internet use and depression rather than computer use and depressive feelings affecting the frequency of IM. Although compulsive use of instant online communication may occur at the expense of real-life social interactions, there was no evidence of its association with increased loneliness.

Intense internet use (i.e., 3 or more hours per day), as opposed to frequency (i.e., use on 6 days per week) was associated with a two to 3.5 fold increase in reporting DSM-IV (*Diagnostic and Statistical Manual of Mental Disorders, Fourth Edition*) symptoms of major depression among adolescent males and females respectively [33]. Further, youths with greater depressive symptomatology were more likely to talk with strangers and disclose personal information online. Unfortunately, the data were cross-sectional thus it could not be determined whether depressive symptoms predated online activity or vice versa. The significance of intense rather than frequent internet use is intriguing, and suggests that it may be prolonged, more immersive online activity that is associated with psychosocial vulnerability. Examined together, the foregoing longitudinal studies yielded patterns consistent with the poor-get-poorer model (e.g., individuals with fewer social resources prior to internet use are less likely to benefit socially from online activity), even as several cross-sectional investigations have failed to replicate this relationship [34–36].

Online sexual activity, or cybersex, is another broad area of research on internet use and youth adjustment. Cybersex refers to an array of online sexual activity associated with internet usage and may include: viewing erotic or pornographic images online; uploading or forwarding images or text descriptions of oneself or one's sexual partner; interacting with sex workers employed by particular websites; interacting with anonymous partners through blogs, chat rooms, etc.; meeting potential sexual partners for offline contacts; and violating interpersonal boundaries by initiating unwanted sexual contacts through email, social networking sites, and other internet forums [37]. A more restrictive definition of cybersex refers to a sequence of visual or textual exchanges with a partner for the purposes of sexual pleasure, frequently culminating in masturbation [38,39]. This form of cybersex therefore resembles sexting but occurs via computer rather than cell phone, and is defined by the primary aim of sexual gratification.

Forms of cybersex are thus diverse, and range from solitary acts, to consensual interactions, to coercive contacts [39]. The first generation of studies of online sexual behavior emphasized its pathological aspects, including its criminal, deviant use [40]. Others have suggested that cybersex may serve as a form of sexual expression that ranges along a continuum from curiosity to obsessive involvement, and may be linked to larger problems with social isolation, and possible paraphilia [41].

Most available research, however, has focused on cybersex among adults, with the majority of data on online sexual behavior among adolescents focused on internet-based sex crimes. Contrary to popular press coverage, the reality of internet-initiated sex crimes is different and more complex than the archetypically frightening, so-called cyberpredator [42]. In fact, the proportion of sex crimes with juvenile victims committed by offenders who use the internet to meet victims is relatively small [43]. For example, in 2006, there were an estimated 615 arrests for sex crimes involving online meetings between offenders and adolescent victims, in contrast with 28 226 arrests for all sex crimes against teen victims during the same time frame [42].

Interestingly, available data suggest the particular vulnerability of adolescents to internet-based sex crimes when compared to children [43]. By early adolescence (i.e., ages 12 to 13), youth internet users' general understanding of the social complexity of the internet matches that of adults [44]. However, as youths mature and gain online experience, their internet use grows more interactive [45], which puts them at greater risk than less-experienced youths, who may use the internet in more simple, less interactive ways. Indeed, youths aged 15 to 17 years were more prone to take risks involving privacy and contact with unknown people when compared to 12- to 15-year-olds [46], and, among girls, being older (i.e., 14 to 17 years) rather than younger (i.e., 10 to 13 years) predicted the formation of close online relationships with strangers [47].

The most widely cited and nationally representative data on online sexual behavior among US adolescents, both voluntary and unwanted, come from the First and Second Youth Internet Safety Surveys (YISS-1 and YISS-2) [47,48], and the National Juvenile Online Victimization (N-JOV) study [49]. The YISS-1 and YISS-2 surveys examined patterns of online sexual behavior among US adolescents in two nationally representative, independent samples of internet users (ages 10–17) by telephone survey. The N-JOV study describes the incidence and dynamics of internet-initiated sex crimes in which online offenders were arrested by law enforcement, as well as characteristics of victims and offenders in a nationally representative sample of law enforcement agencies.

Examined overall, this research group has argued that publicity about online "predators" who use the internet to gain access to young victims is largely inaccurate. Rather than featuring a pedophilic man with a history of sexual offenses, internet sex crimes are more likely to fit a model of statutory rape, with an adult who openly seduces, meets, and develops a relationship with an underage teenager rather than a forcible sexual assault or pedophilic child molestation (for a review, see ref. [43]). In the majority of cases, child victims are aware that they are conversing online with adults, with only 5% of offenders in the N-JOV study pretending to be teens when they met potential victims online [50]. Offenders rarely deceived victims about their sexual interest, with sex discussed online and most victims meeting offenders in person with the expectation of sexual activity. In the N-JOV study, 73% of victims who had in-person sexual encounters with offenders did so more than once.

Maladjusted youths were more likely to report forming close online relationships with individuals whom they do not know. Greater maladjustment (i.e., a composite variable including high levels of depressive symptoms and peer victimization) among male and female adolescents was associated with a greater likelihood of forming close online friendships or romances online with strangers [47]. Alienation from parents was also present for male and female youths, manifested among females as high levels of conflict with parents, and among males as low levels of communication.

In addition to online sexual predation, the First and Second Youth Internet Safety Surveys provide important information about a range of online sexual behaviors among a representative sample of US youth. These surveys describe the prevalence of unwanted sexual solicitations (i.e., requests by adults to engage in sexual activities, sexual talk, or to give personal sexual information); online sexual harassment (threats or other offensive behavior but not sexual solicitation, sent online to youths or posted online about youths for others to see); and unwanted exposure to pornography.

The percentage of internet-using youths who reported unwanted sexual solicitations significantly decreased between 2000 and 2005, from 19% to 13% [48]. These decreases were not, however, observed among Black and Hispanic youths, as well as youths who lived in lower income households (although the small sample sizes in these groups could account for this finding). However, despite this overall decrease in sexual solicitations, youths were 1.7 times more likely to report aggressive solicitations. Factors associated with receiving more aggressive solicitations included being female, using chat rooms, using the internet with a cell phone, talking and sending personal information to individuals met online, discussing sex online, and past experience of offline physical or sexual abuse [51]. Higher rates of unwanted sexual solicitation were also observed among youths who had recently engaged in non-suicidal self-harming behavior [52].

In contrast to overall rates of sexual solicitation, the number of youths who reported online harassment significantly increased during this same period, from 25% to 34% [53]. Online harassment may be best understood as "cyber-bullying," which may or may not be of a sexual nature [9]. The use of online activity to threaten, harass, or otherwise publicly humiliate peers is a pernicious related trend although beyond the scope of this chapter.

Unwanted exposure to pornography increased between the YISS-1 and YISS-2 studies among internet-using teens, particularly among 10–12-year-olds, 16–17-year-olds, boys, and White, non-Hispanic youths [54]. Youths seeking pornography were overwhelmingly more likely to be male, with one-quarter of all males reporting at least one intentional exposure to pornography in the previous year (as opposed to 5% of females) [54]. Older youths (i.e., 14–17 years old) were more likely to report intentionally seeking out pornography – ages during which it is developmentally appropriate to be sexually curious. Older youths also favored online as opposed to offline exposures, with the authors concluding that concerns about large numbers of young children accessing pornographic material online may be overstated.

Differences were observed between youths who reported intentional exposure to pornography, regardless of the online or offline source [54]. Youths who sought pornography were more likely to cross-sectionally report delinquent behavior and substance use in the previous year. Online seekers were more likely to report clinical symptoms associated with depression and lower levels of emotional bonding with their caregiver. Although pornography-seeking is unlikely to have caused these associations, these differences merit additional research to parse out the temporal sequencing, and better characterize youths for whom pornography use corresponds with greater vulnerability.

One concern about online activity among teens is the sharing of personal information that may render youths vulnerable to sexual exploitation. Data from the YISS-1 and YISS-2-surveys suggest that these risks are more nuanced. One popular form of online self-disclosure occurs via online journals, which are also known as blogs. Almost one in five youth internet users (ages 12–17) have created their own online journal or blog, which amounts to approximately four million adolescents. Older girls (aged 15–17) are most likely to blog [55]. Youths who blogged were more likely than other youths to post personal information online, and were at increased risk for online harassment, regardless of whether they had interacted with others online. However, bloggers were no more likely than non-blogging youths to interact with people they met online and did not know in person. Interestingly, it was youths who interacted with people they met online, regardless of whether or not they blogged, who had higher odds of receiving online sexual solicitations; posting personal information did not contribute to risk. These data suggest that it is youths who interact with people they do not know online who are at greatest risk of being sexually solicited, independent of their blogging status or even how much personal information they disclosed.

A related aspect of online risk is sending sexual pictures online. A nationally representative survey of US youths indicated that 4% of youths (ages 12–17) reported an online request to send a sexual picture of themselves in the previous year (i.e., 1 out of 25 youth; $n = 65$); only one of these youths complied with such a request. Factors associated with receiving a request resembled those already reviewed: being female, of Black ethnicity, having a close online relationship, engaging in sexual behavior online, and experiencing sexual or physical abuse offline [56].

Examined together, the results of the YISS-1 and YISS-2 surveys describe a changing landscape of exposure to sexual activities online, with sexual solicitations decreasing for most groups although solicitations were more aggressive, and rates of online harassment and unwanted exposure to pornography increasing. This research group suggests that concern about large numbers of young children seeking out pornography via the internet may be overstated, with results also suggesting greater levels of emotional challenge among youths who seek pornography online. Of particular concern, aggressive solicitations (i.e., attempts to make offline contact with youths through telephone, in person, or via regular mail) did not change among any subgroup of youths. This is especially worrisome given that these kinds of contacts are the most likely to evolve into crimes although only among youths who choose to interact with adults online.

Available data suggest that a majority of youths who engage in online sexual relationships do so knowing that they are corresponding with an adult who is interested in sexual contact. Because the internet is best understood as a mode of risk transmission rather than a creator of risk, it is critical to identify which youths are more vulnerable to this form of risk transmission [43]. Data from the YISS-1 and YISS-2 surveys and the broader psychological literature suggest important leads that future research should consider.

First, adolescents (ages 14–17) appear more vulnerable to online sexual behaviors as opposed to younger children (ages 10–13) [46,50]. Data from the N-JOV study indicate that 99% of victims of internet-initiated sex crimes were 13–17 years old; none were younger than 12 [50]. This is a considerably more restricted age profile than for conventional offline child molestation, which includes a large proportion of victims younger than age 12 [57]. Youths most vulnerable to online requests for sexual pictures include those who are female, are of Black ethnicity, or have a history of offline sexual or physical abuse. A greater risk of online sexual solicitations was associated with discussing sex online and interaction with unknown individuals; minority status (i.e., Black and Hispanic); more frequent chat room interaction; greater personal disclosure; and depressive symptoms [51,56]. Of course, these associations are all cross-sectional, and conclusions cannot be made about whether these factors led to risky online behavior or vice versa. Further, the majority of data are based on two nationally representative studies and the same research group; more research is needed.

It is critical for the next generation of research to consider *how* factors such as minority status, age, and a history of maltreatment confer online sexual risk. These data suggest the value of a developmental psychopathology perspective on matters of online sexual risk in order to best inform preventive efforts as well as clinical practice. Developmental psychopathology is a conceptual frame that departs from unidimensional causes of disorder and asserts the role of prior adaptation on future adaptation [58,59]. This perspective suggests understanding online sexual risk relative to an adolescent's broader developmental context, according to which early experiences of maltreatment and abuse render youths longitudinally more vulnerable to revictimization across the lifespan [60,61]. The fact that a history of abuse, depressive symptoms, and deliberate self-harm is associated with online sexual behavior suggests the ways in which cumulative psychosocial adversity offline may affect online risk.

In addition to online sexual behavior, the near universality of cell phone ownership among US adolescents has introduced a portable form of digital electronics with its own possible sexual applications.

SEXTING AND THE CELL PHONE: PREVALENCE, MEANING, AND CONSEQUENCES

The term sexting (i.e., the exchange of sexually explicit images via cell phone between minor teens [7]) has captured linguistically an evolving interface between technology and adolescent sexual behavior, with extensive media coverage suggesting a popular interest in both. A cursory survey of headlines from articles about sexting suggests both alarm and intrigue, with sexting called "shockingly common" [62] and a "disturbing new teen trend" [63]. Frequent media coverage about sexting, coupled with scarce reliable data about it, prompted a *Wall Street Journal* columnist opine, "Which is epidemic – sexting or worrying about it?" [64].

At the forefront of popular and scholarly interest in sexting are the potentially serious legal consequences for youths and the possible incongruity between these consequences and the behavior itself [65]. It is illegal under federal and state child pornography laws to create, possess, or distribute explicit images of a minor, and although these laws were drafted to address the adult exploitation of minors they do not exempt minors who create and distribute their own images via sexting. Thus, youths who take and exchange sexual images of themselves or others via a cell phone may be subject to the same laws designed to curb the distribution of child pornography among adults.

In response, some US state legislatures are now considering laws that reduce the charges – from felonies to misdemeanors – for creating or exchanging explicit images of minors by text. In 2009, for example, the Vermont and Utah state legislatures downgraded the penalties for minors and first-time sexting "perpetrators." At least 14 states are now considering legislation that

would differentiate minors who engage in sexting from adult pornographers (for a review of legislative reform by state, see ref. [66]). Some states are considering whether juvenile sexting should be a separate category, similar to status offenses (such as truancy or running away), which are typically heard in juvenile court. In March 2010, the first federal appellate opinion in a sexting case recognized that a prosecutor had "tried to enforce adult moral standards" in leveling charges of child pornography distribution against an adolescent for sexting [66].

These efforts at legislative reform highlight the lack of consensus about the nature of youth-produced sexual images, its function, and its meaning to involved youths, and what represents the most appropriate response (e.g., educational, psychological, legal). In this sense, youth produced sexual images are the most recent catalyst for discussions about the nexus among adolescents, technology, and sexual behavior. The question of whether sexting represents a normative aspect of adolescent sexuality in a technologically complex era, and/or a harbinger of atypical sexual development remains an open question, with no longitudinal data currently available to provide guidance. At this writing, sexting and its consequences have been primarily discussed in the popular press, and the published evidence to help consider these questions is extremely limited.

It is important to consider sexting relative to contemporary patterns of cell phone use among US youths. Recent data suggest that cell phone texting has become the preferred form of basic communication between adolescents and their friends even ahead of cell calling [67]. Approximately 75% of 12- to 17-year-olds now own cell phones, which represents an increase from 45% in 2004. While other forms of communication among teens have remained steady between 2006 and 2009 (e.g., instant messaging, social networking sites, email, landline phone, face-to-face talk) the frequency of texting alone continues to climb. The frequency of text-messaging among teens is compelling: half of surveyed teens send 50 or more text messages a day, or 1500 texts a month. One in three youths sends more than 100 texts a day, or 3000 texts a month.

The economics of texting have also changed in recent years, with unlimited texting plans the new norm among adolescents [67]. This has affected trends in text messaging and sexting. Three in four cell phone users have unlimited texting plans and only 13% of teen cell phone users pay per message. These figures raise questions about parental involvement in adolescents' cell phone use and texting given that over one-half of teen cell phone users are part of family plans, which almost always a parent pays for entirely. Indeed, two-thirds of teens living in households with annual incomes of $50 000 or more report that their parent pays for their cell phone. Among adolescents living in households with annual incomes less than $30 000, only 31% are on a family plan that someone else pays for. Among this group, 15% reported prepaid plans that someone else has purchased, and 12% indicate paying for prepaid plans entirely on their own. Black teens living in low-income households are the most likely to report prepaid plans that they pay for themselves. The majority (i.e., 98%) of parents report that a major reason their child has a cell phone is to facilitate communication with them no matter where the teen is. These data suggest that parents and teens may have different perspectives about the primary purpose of the adolescent's cell phone, with teens' use of the phone for a broader range of activities, each with important developmental aims (e.g., safety, social, sexual).

Given the near universality of cell phone ownership among adolescents, what do teens report about the frequency and function of sexting? Three national surveys exist on attitudes and behavior related to sexting; none are peer-reviewed sources. The first survey was collected from online respondents and sponsored by The National Campaign to Prevent Teen and Unplanned Pregnancy and CosmoGirl.com ("Sex and Tech" survey [68]). This was not a nationally representative sample (with 73% Caucasian/White) but its estimates have been cited in the popular press ever since. Twenty percent of teens reported sending or posting nude or semi-nude pictures or videos of themselves online. Sexually suggestive messages (i.e., via text, email, IM) were even more common, with 39% of teens sending such messages. Around one-third of adolescent females and males reported that someone had shared a 'sext' message originally meant for someone else (25% and 33%, respectively). "Fun or flirtation" was cited as the main reason teens send sexually suggestive content by text or email (60% of teens). A large proportion of youths (40%) reported sending sexual material as a "joke," and 40% of females endorsed doing so to "feel sexy." Twelve percent of teen girls felt "pressured" to send sexual images.

A nationally representative phone survey in 2009, sponsored by the Pew Internet & American Life Project ("Teens and Sexting" [69]), reported lower prevalence rates. Only 4% of surveyed youths (ages 12–17) reported sending sexually suggestive nude or nearly nude images of themselves to someone else via text messaging. Fifteen percent of cell phone-owning teens reported that they received such images from someone they know. Older teens (i.e., 17-year-olds) reported more frequent sending of sexts (8%) as well as receiving (30%). Survey data indicated that youths who pay their own cell phone bills are more likely to send sexually explicit images: 17% of teens who pay for their cell phone, as compared to 3% of those who do not pay their own bill or contribute a portion of the cost.

Focus group data suggested three scenarios for sexting: exchange of images between two romantic partners; exchanges between partners that are shared with others outside the relationship; and exchanges between people not yet in a relationship, where at least one person hopes to be [69]. Generally speaking, these data are methodologically limited (e.g., low response rates; self-selection biases), although they may be more representative than other popular surveys that have yielded higher estimates.

Finally, a 2009 phone survey conducted by MTV and the Associated Press was designed to evaluate "digital abuse" among a geographically representative sample of US teens [70]. Although participation was invited randomly, there are likely (unreported) self-selection biases that inform study results. Estimates were similar to those in the "Sex and Tech" survey, with 24% of teens (ages 14–17) reporting some involvement in sexting. One in ten youths reportedly shared a naked picture of themselves by cell phone, with white females more likely to share pictures of themselves, and males more likely to circulate images of someone else. Sexually active youths were twice as likely to engage in sexting than those who were not sexually active. Participants in this survey reported complex opinions about sexting, with respondents describing the behavior as "hot," and "trusting" as well as "uncomfortable" and "slutty."

The one peer reviewed study on youth- produced sexual images among U.S. teens found that approximately 6% of surveyed youth reportedly received sexually explicit images by cell phone. These data suggest that earlier, non-peer reviewed surveys likely overestimated the behavior [71]. Empirical research on the topic is essential to identify reliable prevalence estimates of sexting as well as the youths most vulnerable to its various forms of misuse (e.g., bullying, coercion). In addition to data on prevalence and frequency, information is needed on its meaning, effects and correlates for youth. For example, qualitative data is needed on how teens regard the experience of sexting relative to their emerging sexuality. Does the behavior correlate with other risk factors for early sexual initiation or exploitation, or does a normative discourse about sexting exist for some youths that reflects "identity play" rather than psychopathology? Is it sexting itself or its social and legal consequences that are associated with potential harm? In terms of phenomenology, can comparisons be made between exhibitionist behavior and sexting naked images of oneself? If so, what accounts for these differences? Future research is required to consider these possibilities.

SOCIAL NETWORKING SITES

An estimated 14 million youths in the U.S. (ages 12–17 years) used social networking sites (SNSs; i.e.,

Facebook and MySpace) in 2006, with estimates likely higher today [72]. Like text messages, sexting, and cybersex, SNSs facilitate new patterns of virtual and offline interaction. SNSs allow members to create a personal web profile that may include text, images, and audio. The possible role of SNSs in sex crimes against adolescents is a long-held concern [73–75], and emerging data provide information about the veracity, nuance, and possible overstatement of such concerns.

Arrest data from a nationally representative sample of US law enforcement agencies indicated that although a number of internet sex crime arrest cases involved SNSs in some way, SNSs do not seem to present risk in and of themselves, or a greater risk than other interactive online venues (e.g., chat rooms) [42]. The largest number of SNS-related arrests involved law enforcement acting in an undercover capacity, with the majority of these cases initiated in chat rooms (82%). (The SNS aspect was a profile created by police under the guise of a teen as a site for the suspect to view pictures of the "victim.")

Further, arrests with some SNS nexus represented an extremely small proportion of adolescent SNS users overall: 14 million youths had an SNS profile during the study period, with arrests for the 503 cases that involved juvenile victims representing an extremely small proportion of the broader class of teen users. Potential risks certainly should not be ignored, but these data indicate that concern about SNSs should not supersede that regarding other venues, particularly chat rooms.

Another way in which SNSs inform adolescent sexual development is the shaping of social norms among youths, with implications for sexual behavior. Given that national debates about appropriate sexual education remain politically contentious and largely unresolved [76,77], researchers have argued that media (e.g., television and music videos) have collectively come to serve as a sexual "superpeer." This includes media that model sexually risky behavior that may not be condoned in the teen's own peer culture but that may nonetheless substantially affect sexual attitudes and behavior [78]. Indeed, longitudinal research has demonstrated that sexually explicit media are not inert; they can significantly affect the sexual attitudes and behaviors of certain youths [78]. Greater exposure to sexually explicit material online has been longitudinally associated with more permissive attitudes toward uncommitted sexual exploration among teens [79,80]. Arguably, the internet represents the current generation's sexual superpeer par excellence, especially for vulnerable youths.

Content analysis of randomly selected MySpace profiles has documented frequent references to alcohol use [81], and focus group data suggest that teens typically interpret these references as actual use, regardless of whether displayed alcohol references correlate with actual consumption [82]. These data suggest that SNSs provide a novel conduit for social norms that prior research has shown influence adolescent sexual behavior. Specifically, perceived peer norms (i.e., the perceived proportion of peers who have had sex) affect adolescent sexual behavior (for a review, see ref. [83]), suggesting the possibility that online sexual content in SNSs could facilitate the same.

An early writer on the psychology of internet use emphasized factors (termed the internet's "Triple A Engine") that may facilitate problematic online sexual behavior among vulnerable users (i.e., affordability, anonymity, accessibility) [84]. The vastly more interactive, immediate, and sensorily engaging nature of the internet is likely to create a more intense immersion than that of television, and potentially amplify the impact of a superpeer.

These factors – affordability, anonymity, accessibility [84] – are also implicated in how internet use may become problematic or compulsive for adolescents [31], whether due to overuse, unsafe online interactions, and/or detrimental effects on functioning in real time. Currently, the psychiatric and psychological literature has emphasized the concept of addiction to describe the effects of internet misuse among adolescents. Whether problematic internet behavior should be conceptualized as an addiction remains controversial; however, it is being considered by the DSM-V committees [21].

INTERNET ADDICTION AMONG ADOLESCENTS: A CRITICAL REVIEW

Reports of "computer dependent" people [85] and "technological addiction" [86] first appeared in the 1990s, with the latter described as "non-chemical addiction involving human-machine interaction." Interestingly, reports of various kinds of out-of-control sexual behavior (e.g., "hypersexuality," cybersex, so-called sexual addiction) also emerged during this period [87], with both sexual and internet addiction largely unresolved concepts. A series of papers [19,88,89] asserted internet addiction as an emerging clinical presentation, and suggested the use of DSM-IV criteria for pathological gambling to diagnose so-called internet addiction – criteria based on DSM-IV's category of impulse-control disorders not elsewhere classified [90].

The DSM-V committee has considered a new diagnostic category tentatively labeled "Behavioral and Substance Addictions" that would include substance abuse disorders, impulse-control disorders, and those currently described by the category of impulse-control disorders not otherwise classified (e.g., internet addiction, pathological gambling, kleptomania). These behavioral and substance-based forms of addiction are conceptually blended due to similar phases in the two classes of disorder: increased arousal before the act; gratification; decrease in arousal; and subsequent guilt and remorse [91].

The concept of behavioral addictions remains controversial [92] although the National Institute on Drug Abuse considers behavioral addictions relatively "pure" models of addiction since an exogenous substance does not contaminate their presentation [23,93]. Problematic internet use can show features similar to excessive substance use, including withdrawal phenomena, tolerance, and negative consequences [21]. Others have argued that terms like withdrawal are more metaphorical given that putative physiological indicators comparable to those with substance dependence have not been identified [27].

Like many forms of psychopathology among adolescents, the downward application of adult-based diagnostic criteria can be problematic given important developmental differences. The matter of problematic internet use may be even more complex given the near universality and social acceptability of the activity itself, and an equivocal evidence base among adults. Against this backdrop, the phenomenon of problematic internet use is associated with many names, including compulsive computer use, pathological internet use, and internet dependency. Even these terms vary in whether computers or the internet is primary, and qualifiers such as compulsive and dependence also cause clinical confusion. Because internet misuse is typically comorbid with numerous conditions [94,95], it is critical to evaluate whether an additional set of criteria are necessary [96].

Research has begun to consider to what extent problematic internet experiences are extensions from conventional mental health disorders as opposed to distinct problems. Cluster analysis among adults suggests initial support for the idea that problematic internet use is an extension of problems that predate internet use, with this modality introducing new dimensions such as increased severity and frequency [97]. Indeed, no clusters evaluated were characterized by online or offline problems only, suggesting complex associations between the two that future research should disentangle, especially as this manifests among teens.

Correlates of internet addiction in youths have been more widely studied in Asian samples, with research suggesting an association with depressive symptoms, lower self-esteem, poor family function [98–100], and aggressive behaviors [101]. Gender effects are equivocal, with several studies reporting a male preponderance in internet addiction among adolescents [23], the increased vulnerability of females [102], or no gender differences [96].

The concept of internet addiction (and related terms) is increasingly applied to adolescent populations

without established criteria or standardized assessments. Even in the absence of these critical tools, adolescents may be susceptible to problematic internet use based on the foregoing review of vulnerability and risk, as well as adolescents' unique vulnerability to addictive behaviors more generally. For example, the immaturity of the frontal cortical and subcortical monoaminergic brain systems is hypothesized to underlie adolescent impulsivity [103]. On the one hand, this neurodevelopmental process may adaptively enhance the learning drive, but on the other hand it may facilitate vulnerability to addiction in vulnerable adolescents [104]. Researchers argue that it is this combination of enhanced vulnerability and the sheer popularity of the internet, especially modalities such as IM with a more highly addictive potential, that engender risk for the development of compulsive online behaviors [31].

Even as problematic internet use lacks a diagnostic home, available data suggest important associations between it and certain forms of clinical risk. Compulsive online activity is prevalent among some youths [15,105,106], and the foregoing review has highlighted the effects of the internet on certain teens. Given the available research base, it may be premature to apply the label of "internet addiction" to adolescents although there is likely a subset of vulnerable teens for whom some version of the construct will apply. Even if risk is limited to a minority of adolescents, problematic internet behavior may amplify preexisting vulnerabilities and result in significantly negative consequences; this may be particularly dramatic in cases of online activity given the possible legal nexus. Future research that employs standardized measures and empirically derived diagnostic criteria [107] is required on US adolescent samples.

INTEGRATION AND SUMMARY

In considering the effects of technology on adolescent sexual behavior, we emphasize that the adolescent population in general is very heterogeneous, and we cannot yet draw firm and unambiguous conclusions about these topics. Because of this heterogeneity, psychopathology among adolescents is often not clearly defined, and the interaction of any possible diagnoses or syndromes with technology use will also confound assessment.

In addition, this review has emphasized the dearth of available data on the relationship between emerging technologies and adolescent sexual behavior despite extensive coverage and alarm in the popular press. Given the foregoing heterogeneity and limited extant data, it is critical for mental health professionals to be as data driven as possible in rendering opinions about individual adolescents. Professionals must furthermore be aware of the limitations of available data and how these may inform their conclusions. We therefore urge caution in rendering conclusive opinions at this point, as these may be detrimental to an individual adolescent as well as to the population at large. Unequivocal conclusions are likely to be misleading and uninformative, with potentially damaging conclusions to individual youths, as suggested by the case vignette that began this review.

These caveats notwithstanding, available research on the relationship between adolescent sexual behavior and electronic technologies suggests several important themes. First, the nexus of technology and adolescent sexuality is an evolving one, with internet use and misuse as one element of a larger, rapidly changing constellation. Indeed, new technology and its applications within adolescent culture evolve faster than peer-reviewed study, which represents a key limitation to research in this area.

Second, in light of concern that research on adolescent sexuality emphasizes a "risk-centric" perspective [77,108], future research on adolescents and technology should engage questions beyond those of harm to how they inform the evolution of sexual identity and desire among teens. For example, how do youths themselves describe the effects and meaning of technologies such as the internet and cell phone on their interpersonal relationships (e.g., with friends, family, romantic partners)? Do technologies afford a safe means of sexual exploration for certain teens, and if so, for whom? Such questions require qualitative data that may stand on their own as well as inform future quantitative investigation.

Rather than merely a passive store of information, the internet is also a conduit for socialization [80,109], which has critical implications in the domain of sexual behavior. The immediacy and anonymity of internet communication (particularly via IM and within chat rooms) may unhook emotion and relationships from sexual behavior, to the possible detriment of an adolescent's emerging sexual self. Similarly, research should differentiate between the broader issue of internet addiction/misuse and the emerging effects of novel technology on adolescent sexuality – in other words, the importance of understanding the range of developmental functions for which these technologies may become shorthand.

Third, the concept of "addiction" or compulsive internet use may have merit for a small proportion of teens, but a focus on the broader effects of this technology on adolescent sexual behavior is also required. The current emphasis on addiction has eclipsed these related developmental questions, which future research should help expand.

Examined overall, the empirical literature on online behavior among US teens suggests that youths vulnerable to other forms of psychosocial risk (e.g., maltreatment and abuse; depressive symptomatology; self-harm) are more likely to engage in higher-risk online activity (e.g., interactions with unknown individuals online; self-disclosure around sexual topics). Further, research suggests that it is not merely the disclosure of information online that is associated with offline risk, but *interaction* with unknown individuals. These converging results, despite their correlational limitations, underscore the importance of a developmental psychopathology perspective on future research in this area.

Additional research is required to help evaluate the concept of problematic internet use among adolescents as well as define who may be most vulnerable. However problematic internet use is defined, it has been associated with various forms of maladjustment (e.g., low self-esteem, depressive symptoms, aggression). This suggests that the internet may amplify pre-existing difficulties for a proportion of adolescent users, and for others it may represent an independent manifestation of psychological troubles. The role of real-time online communication (i.e., IM) has been uniquely associated with compulsive internet use among teens, a replicated finding that may help inform future research.

Currently, available data on adolescent sexual behavior and technology use are largely cross-sectional; no long-term prospective data exist on how internet use affects sexual behavior across developmental time. Such data are especially needed to help determine for whom internet misuse during adolescence may be a harbinger of future maladjustment (sexual or otherwise), and/or to what extent it represents a normative dimension of contemporary adolescence. In the absence of such data, caution is highly recommended in drawing conclusions about an individual youth given the elasticity of change during this developmental period and the limited state of available research.

References

1. Feyerick D, Steffen S. 'Sexting' lands teen on sex offender list. CNN Justice, 2009. Available from: http://articles.cnn.com/2009-04-07/justice/sexting.busts_1_phillip-alpert-offender-list-offender-registry?_s=PM:CRIME.
2. Prieto B. 'Sexting' teenagers face child porn changes. *Orlando Sentinel*, 2009. Available from: http://articles.orlandosentinel.com/2009-03-08/news/orl-asec-sexting-030809_1_sexting-face-child-porn-charges-nude-photos.
3. Brunker M. 'Sexting' surprise: Teens face child porn charges. msnbc.com, 2009. Available from: http://www.msnbc.msn.com/id/28679588/print/1/displaymode/1098/.
4. Richmond R. 'Sexting' may place teens at legal risk. *New York Times* 26 March 2009. Available from: http://gadgetwise.blogs.nytimes.com/2009/03/26/sexting-may-place-teens-at-legal-risk/?pagemode=print.

5. 'Sexting' shockingly common among teens. CBS News, 11 February 2009. Available from: http:www.cbsnews.com/stories/2009/01/15/national/main4723161.shtml.

6. Lewin T. Rethinking sex offender laws for youth texting. 3/20/10 URL (consulted on 3/22/10): http://www.nytimes.com/2010/03/21/us/21sexting.html?pagewanted=all

7. Lenhart A. Teens and sexting: How and why minor teens are sending sexually suggestive nude or nearly nude images via text messaging. *Pew Internet & American Life Project* 2009.

8. National Campaign to Prevent Teen and Unplanned Pregnancy. Sex and Tech: Results from a survey of teens and young adults. Available from: www.TheNationalCampaign.org/sextech.

9. Kowlaski RM, Limber SP, Agatson PW. *Cyberbullying: Bullying in the Digital Age*. Malden, MA: Blackwell Publishing, 2008.

10. Kaye R. How a cell phone picture led to a girl's suicide. 10/7/10 URL (consulted on 10/7/10): http://articles.cnn.com/2010-10-07/living/hope.witsells.story_1_photo-new-school-year-scarves?_s=PM:LIVING

11. Lenhart A, Arafeh S, Smith A, Macgill AR. Writing, technology, and teens. Washington, DC: Pew Charitable Trusts, 2008. Available from: http://www.pewinternet.org/~/media//Files/Reports/2008/PIP_Writing_Report_FINAL3.pdf.pdf.

12. Cole JL, Suman M, Schramm P, *et al.* UCLA Internet Report. Surveying the digital future. UCLA Center for Communication Policy, 2003. Available from: http://www.digitalcenter.org/pdf/InternetReportYearThree.pdf.

13. Lenhart A, Madden M, Hitlin P (2005) Teens and technology. URL (consulted on 6/14/10): http://www.pewinternet.org/Reports/2005/Teens-and-Technology.aspx

14. Chou C, Hsiao MC. Internet addiction, usage, gratification, and pleasure experience: the Taiwan college students' case. *Comput Educ* 2000;**35**:65–80.

15. Johansson A, Gotestam KG. Internet addiction: Characteristics of a questionnaire and prevalence in Norwegian youth (12–18 years). *Scand J Psychol* 2004;**45**:223–229.

16. Black DW, Belsare G, Schlosser S. Clinical features, psychiatric comorbidity, and health-related quality of life in persons reporting compulsive computer use behavior. *J Clin Psychiatry* 1999;**60**:839–843.

17. Caplan SE. Preference for online social interaction: a theory of problematic Internet use and psychosocial well being. *Commun Res* 2003;**30**:625–648.

18. Morahan-Martin J, Schumacher P. Incidence and correlates of pathological Internet use among college students. *Comput Hum Behav* 2000;**16**:13–29.

19. Young K. Internet addiction: The emergence of a new clinical disorder. *CyberPsychol Behav* 1998;**1**:237–244.

20. Ha JK, Yoo HJ, Cho IH, *et al.* Psychiatric comorbidity assessed in Korean children and adolescents who screen positive for Internet addiction. *J Clin Psychiatry* 2006;**67**:821–826.

21. Block JJ. Issues for DSM-V: Internet addiction. *Am J Psychiatry* 2008;**165**:306–307.

22. Byun S, Ruffini C, Mills JE, *et al.* Internet addiction: Metasynthesis of 1996–2006 quantitative research. *CyberPsychol Behav* 2009;**12**:203–207.

23. Shaw M, Black SW. Internet addiction: definition, assessment, epidemiology and clinical management. *CNS Drugs* 2008;**22**:353–365.

24. Hur MH. Demographic, habitual, and socioeconomic determinants of Internet addiction disorder: An empirical study of Korean teenagers. *CyberPsychol Behav* 2006; **9**:514–525.

25. Yen J, Yen C, Chen C, Ko C. Family factors of Internet addiction and substance use experience in Taiwanese adolescents. *CyberPsychol Behav* 2007;**10**:323–329.

26. Bancroft J. Sexual behavior that is "out of control": A theoretical approach. *Psychiatr Clin N Am* 2008;**31**:593–601.

27. Pies R. Should DSM-V designate "internet addiction" a mental disorder? *Psychiatry* 2009;**6**:31–37.

28. Turkle S. Always on/Always-on-you: The tethered self. In: Katz JE (ed.), *Handbook of Mobile Communications Studies*. Cambridge, MA: MIT Press, 2008; pp. 121–137.

29. Kraut R, Patterson M, Lundmark V, *et al.* Internet paradox: A social technology that reduces social involvement and psychological well-being? *Am Psychologist* 1998;**53**:1017–1031.

30. Kraut R, Kiesler S, Boneva B, *et al.* Internet paradox revisited. *J Soc Issues* 2002;**58**:49–74.

31. van denEijnden RJ, Meerkerk G, Vermulst AA, *et al.* Online communication, compulsive Internet use, and psychosocial well-being among adolescents: A longitudinal study. *Dev Psychol* 2008;**44**:655–665.

32. Meerkerk GJ, van denEijnden RJ, Vermulst AA, Garretsen HF. The compulsive Internet use scale (CIUS): Some psychometric properties. *CyberPsychol Behav* 2009;**12**:1–6.

33. Ybarra ML, Alexander C, Mitchell KJ. Depressive symptomatology, youth Internet use, and online interactions: a national survey. *J Adolesc Health* 2005;**36**:9–18.

34. Gross EF. Adolescent Internet use: What we expect, what teens report. *J Appl Dev Psychol* 2004;**25**:633.

35. Gross EF, Juvoven J, Gable SL. Internet use and well-being in adolescence. *J Soc Issues* 2002;**58**:75–90.

36. Sanders CE, Field TM, Diego M, Kaplan M. The relationship of Internet use to depression and social isolation among adolescents. *Adolescence* 2000;**35**:237–242.

37. Southern S. Treatment of compulsive sexual behavior. *Psychiatr Clin N Am* 2008;**31**:697–712.

38. Cooper A, Delmonico DL, Griffin-Shelley E, *et al.* Online sexual activity: an examination of potentially problematic behaviors. *Sex Addict Compuls* 2004;**11**:129–43.

39. Daneback K, Cooper AM, Mansson SA. An Internet study of cybersex participants. *Arch Sex Behav* 2005;**34**:321–328.

40. Cooper AM, Scherer CR, Boies SC, Gordon BL. Sexuality on the Internet: from sexual exploration to pathological expression. *Prof Psychol* 1999;**30**:154–164.

41. Leiblum SR, Sex and the net: Clinical implications. *J Sex Educ Ther* 1997;**22**:21–27.

42. Mitchell K, Finkelhor D, Jones LM, Wolak J. Use of social networking sites in online sex crimes against minors: An examination of national incidence and means of utilization. *J Adolesc Health* 2010;**47**:183–190.

43. Wolak, J, Finkelhor D, Mitchell K. Online "predators" and their victims myths, realities, and implications for prevention and treatment. *Am Psychologist* 2008;**63**:111–128.

44. Yan Z. What influences children's and adolescents' understanding of the complexity of the Internet? *Dev Psychol* 2006;**42**:418–428.

45. Livingstone S, Bober M, Helsper EJ. Active participation or just more information? Young people's take-up of opportunities to act and interact on the Internet. *Inform Commun Society* 2005;**8**:287–314.

46. Wolak J, Mitchell KJ, Finkelhor D. Escaping or connecting? Characteristics of youth who form close online relationships. *J Adolesc Health* 2003;**26**:105–119.

47. Finkelhor D, Mitchell KJ, Wolak J. Online victimization: a report on the nation's youth. Alexandria, VA: National

Center for Missing & Exploited Children Bulletin (#6-00-020), 2000.

48. Wolak J, Mitchell KJ, Finkelhor D. Online victimization of youth: 5 years later. Alexandria, VA: National Center for Missing & Exploited Children (#07-06-025), 2006.

49. Wolak J, Mitchell KJ, Finkelhor D. National Online Victimization Study (N-JOV): Methodology report. Crimes Against Children Research Center, 2003. Available from: http:www.unh.edu/ccrc/pdf/jvq/CV72.pdf.

50. Wolak J, Finkelhor D, Mitchell KJ. Internet-initiated sex crimes against minors: Implications for prevention based on findings from a national study. *J Adolesc Health* 2004;**35**:424.e11–424.e20.

51. Mitchell KJ, Finkelhor D, Wolak J. Youth Internet users at risk for the most serious online sexual solicitations. *Am J Prev Med* 2007;**32**:532–537.

52. Mitchell KJ, Ybarra ML. Online behavior of youth who engage in self-harm provides clues for preventive intervention. *Prev Med* 2007;**45**:392–396.

53. Mitchell KJ, Wolak J, Finkelhor D. Trends in youth reports of sexual solicitations, harassment and unwanted exposure to pornography on the Internet. *J Adolesc Health* 2007;**40**:116–126.

54. Ybarra M, Mitchell KJ. Exposure to Internet pornography among children and adolescents: A national survey. *CyberPsychol Behav* 2005;**8**:473–486.

55. Mitchell KJ, Wolak J, Finkelhor D. Are blogs putting youth at risk for online sexual solicitation or harassment? *Child Abuse Neglect* 2008;**32**:277–294.

56. Mitchell KJ, Finkelhor D, Wolak J. Online requests for sexual pictures from youth: risk factors and incident characteristics. *J Adolesc Health* 2007;**41**:196–203.

57. Snyder HN. *Sexual Assault of Young Children as Reported to Law Enforcement: Victim, Incident and Offender Characteristics*. Washington DC: US Department of Justice, 2000.

58. Cicchetti D, Rogosch FA. A developmental psychopathology perspective on adolescence. *J Consult Clin Psychol* 2001;**70**:6–20.

59. Schwartz MF. Developmental psychopathological perspectives on sexually compulsive behavior. *Psychiatr Clin N Am* 2008;**31**:567–586.

60. Finkelhor D, Ormrod RK, Turner H. Revictimization patterns in a national longitudinal sample of children and youth. *Child Abuse Neglect* 2007;**31**:479–502.

61. Raj A, Silverman, JG, Amaro H. The relationship between sexual abuse and sexual risk among high school students: Findings from the 1997 Massachusetts Youth Risk Behavior Survey. *Matern Child Health J* 2000;**4**:125–134.

62. CBS and Associated Press. 'Sexting' shockingly common among teens: Latest case involves three teen girls in PA who sent nude pics to three boys. 1/15/09 URL (consulted on 2/28/10): http//www.cbsnews.com/stories/2009/01/15/national/main4723161.shml.

63. Joffe-Walt C. 'Sexting': A disturbing new teen trend? npr, 11 March 2009. Available from: http://www.npr.org/templates/story/story.php?storyId=101735230.

64. Bialik C. Which is epidemic – sexting or worrying about it? *The Wall Street Journal* 8 April 2009. Available from: http://online.wsj.com/article/SB123913888769898347.html#printMode.

65. Weins WJ, Hiestand TC. Sexting, statutes and saved by the bell: Introducing a lesser juvenile charge with "aggravating factors" framework. *Tennessee Law Rev* 2009;**1**:77.

66. Sacco DT, Argudin R, Maguire J, Tallon K. Sexting: Youth Practices and Legal Implications. Berkman Center for Internet & Society, Harvard University, 2010. Available from: http://cyber.law.harvard.edu/sites/cyber.law.harvard.edu/files/Sacco_Argudin_Maguire_Tallon_Sexting_Jun2010.pdf.

67. Lenhart A, Ling R, Campbell S, Purcell K. Teens and mobile phones. Pew Internet & American Life Project, 2010. Available from: http://pewinternet.org/Reports/2010/Teens-and-Mobile-Phones.aspx

68. National Campaign to Prevent Teen and Unplanned Pregnancy. Sex and Tech: Results from a survey of teens and young adults. 2009. Available from: http://www.TheNationalCampaign.org/sextech.

69. Lenhart A. Teens and sexting. Pew Internet & American Life Project, 2009.

70. Associated Press–MTV. A Thin Line: Digital Abuse Study. Knowledge Networks, 2009. Available from: http://www.athinline.org/MTV-AP_Digital_Abuse_Study_Full.pdf.

71. Mitchell KJ, Finkelhor D, Jones LM, Wolak J. Prevalence and characteristics of youth sexting: a national study. *Pediatrics* 2012;**129**:1–8.

72. Lenhart A, Madden M. (2007) Social networking websites and teens: An overview. Pew Internet & American Life Project, URL (consulted on 6/15/10): http://www.pewinternet.org/pdfs/PIP_SNS_Data_Memo_Jan_2007.pdf.

73. Angwin J, Steinberg B. (2006) "News Corp. goal: Make MySpace safer for teens." The Wall Street Journal Online, URL (consulted 3/15/10): http:online.wdj.com/Article/SB114014309410176595.html.

74. Associated Press (2006) "MySpace.com subject of Connecticut sex-assault probe," Fox News Network, URL (consulted 3/15/10): http://www.foxnews.com/story/0,2933,183709,00.html.

75. Bahrampour T, Aratani L. Teens' bold blogs alarm area schools. *The Washington Post* 17 January 2006. Available from: http://www.washingtonpost.com/wp-dyn/content/article/2006/01/16/AR2006011601489.html.

76. Ehrhardt AA. Our view of adolescent sexuality: A focus on risk behavior without the developmental context. *Am J Public Health* 1996;**86**:1523–1525.

77. Diamond LM, Savin-Williams RC. Adolescent sexuality. In: Lerner RM, Steinberg L (eds), *Handbook of Adolescent Psychology*, Vol. **I**, 3rd edn. Hoboken: John Wiley & Sons, Inc., 2009; pp. 479–523.

78. Brown JD, Halpern CT, L'Engle KL. Mass media as a sexual super peer for early maturing girls. *J Adolesc Health* 2005;**36**:420–427.

79. Brown JD, L'Engle KL. X-rated: sexual attitudes and behaviors associated with US early adolescents' exposure to sexually explicit media. *Commun Res* 2009;**36**:129–151.

80. Peter J, Valkenburg PM. Adolescents' exposure to sexually explicit Internet material and sexual satisfaction: A longitudinal study. *Hum Commun Res* 2008;**35**:171–194.

81. Moreno MA, Briner LR, Williams A, et al. A content analysis of displayed alcohol references on a social networking site. *J Adolesc Health* 2010;**47**:168–175.

82. Moreno MA, Briner LR, Williams A, Walker L, Christakis DA. Real use of "real cool": Adolescents speak out about displayed alcohol references on social networking websites. *J Adolesc Health* 2009;**45**:420–422.

83. DiClemente RJ, Salazar LF, Crosby RA. A review of STD/HIV preventive interventions for adolescents:

Sustaining effects using an ecological approach. *J Pediatr Psychol* 2007;**32**:888–906.

84. Cooper A. Sexuality and the Internet: Surfing into the new millennium. *CyberPsychol Behav* 1998;**1**:181–187.

85. Shotton M. The costs and benefits of "computer addiction." *Behav Inform Technol* 1991;**10**:219–230.

86. Griffiths MD. Internet addiction: Internet fuels other addictions. *Student Brit Med J* 1999;**7**:428–429.

87. Schwartz MF, Berlin FS. Preface to special issue on sexually compulsive behavior. *Psychiatr Clin N Am* 2008;**31**:xi–xii.

88. Young K. *Caught in the Net: How to Recognize the Signs of Internet Addiction and a Winning Strategy for Recovery*. New York: John Wiley & Sons, Inc., 1998.

89. Young K. Internet addiction: Evaluation and treatment. *Student Brit Med J* 1999;**7**:351–352.

90. American Psychiatric Association. *Diagnostic and Statistical Manual of Mental Disorders, Fourth Edition*. Washington, DC: APA Press, 2004.

91. Hollander E, Allen A. Is compulsive buying a real disorder, and is it really compulsive? *Am J Psychiatry* 2006;**163**:1670–1672.

92. Griffiths M. Sex on the Internet: Observations and implications for Internet sex addiction. *J Sex Res* 2001;**38**:333–342.

93. Holden C. Behavioral addictions: Do they exist? *Science* 2001;**294**:980–982.

94. Caplan SE. Relationships among loneliness, social anxiety and problematic Internet use. *CyberPsychol Behav* 2007;**10**:234–242.

95. Ko CH, Yen JY, Chen CS, Chen CC, Yen CF. Psychiatric comorbidity of Internet addiction in college students: an interview study. *CNS Spectr* 2008;**13**:147–153.

96. Fu K, Chan WSC, Wong PWC, Yip P. Internet addiction: prevalence, discriminant validity and correlates among adolescents in Hong Kong. *Brit J Psychiatry* 2010;**196**:486–492.

97. Mitchell KJ, Finkelhor D, Becker-Blease KA. Classification of adults with problematic Internet experiences: Linking Internet and conventional problems from a clinical perspective. *CyberPsychol Behav* 2007;**10**:381–392.

98. Ko CH, Yen, JY, Yen CF. Factors predictive for incident and remission of Internet addiction in young adolescents: A prospective study, *CyberPsychol Behav* 2007;**10**:545–551.

99. Yen JY, Ko CH, Yen, CF, *et al.* The comorbid psychiatric symptoms of Internet addiction: attention deficits and hyperactivity disorder, depression, social phobia, and hostility. *J Adolesc Health* 2007;**41**:93–96.

100. Yen JY, Yen CF, Chen CC, *et al.* Family factors of Internet addiction and substance use experience in Taiwanese adolescents. *CyberPsychol Behav* 2006;**10**:323–329.

101. Ko C, Yen J, Liu S, *et al.* The associations between aggressive behaviors and Internet addiction and online activities in adolescents. *J Adolesc Health* 2009;**44**:598–605.

102. Leung L. Net-generation attributes and seductive properties of the Internet as predictors of online activities and internet addiction. *CyberPsychol Behav* 2004;**7**:333–348.

103. Casey BJ, Jones RM, Hare TA. The adolescent brain. *Ann N Y Acad Sci* 2008;**1124**:111–126.

104. Chambers RA, Taylor JR, Potenza MN. Developmental neurocircuitry of motivation in adolescence: A critical period of addiction vulnerability. *Am J Psychiatry* 2003;**160**:1041–1052.

105. Kaltiala-Heino R, Lintonen T, Rimpela A. Internet addiction? Potentially problematic use of the Internet in a population of 12–18 year-old adolescents. *Addict Res Theory* 2004;**12**:89–96.

106. Nichols L, Nicki R. Development of a psychometrically sound Internet Addiction Scale: A preliminary step. *Psychol Addict Behav* 2004;**18**:381–384.

107. Ko C, Yen J, Chen C, *et al.* Proposed diagnostic criteria of Internet addiction for adolescents. *J Nerv Ment Dis* 2005;**193**:728–733.

108. Wright MT. Beyond risk factors: Trends in European safer sex research. *J Psychol Hum Sexuality* 1998;**10**:7–18.

109. Greenfield PM. Developmental considerations for determining appropriate Internet use guidelines for children and adolescents. *Appl Dev Psychol* 2004;**25**:751–762.

39

The Therapeutic Community for the Adolescent Substance Abuser

Gregory C. Bunt[1] and Virginia A. Stanick[2]

[1]*Department of Psychiatry, New York University School of Medicine; Daytop Village, Inc., New York, NY, USA*
[2]*Daytop Village, Inc., New York, NY, USA*

INTRODUCTION

The therapeutic community (TC) model originated in the 1940s, when British psychiatrist Maxwell Jones and others introduced a community framework into the treatment of inpatients with severe personality disorders [1]. In contrast with other models, in which professionals were exclusively responsible for all aspects of treatment, early psychiatric therapeutic communities were operated as milieus in which all participants were "expected to contribute to the shared goals of creating a social organization with healing properties" [2]. Therapeutic interventions were redefined to include more than isolated, formally scheduled, protocol-driven exchanges between staff and patients. The milieu in its entirety – all members, behaviors, and interactions – was viewed as germane to the therapeutic process and its results.

The drug-free residential TC for individuals with chemical abuse and dependence developed independently of other established public healthcare models, including the psychiatric community milieu noted above. Although the latter possessed marked similarities in philosophy and approach, addiction-focused TCs were primarily influenced by Alcoholics Anonymous (AA) and other concepts related to chemical abuse/dependence. TCs evolved out of weekly "free association" meetings of AA members struggling with severe addictions, into a distinctive encounter group process, eventually moving to a relatively well-differentiated form of residential community with a culture committed to self-help concepts [3]. Fundamental principles of the TC model, established in the United States

in the late 1950s and continuing to evolve and operate to the present, include [3]:

1. The assumption that "the power to change primarily resides within the individual and is activated through his or her full participation in the peer community."
2. Use of self and communal control to modify addictive behaviors and build more constructive behavior patterns.
3. Use of a hierarchical, often autocratic family-structured model that promotes emotional connection, provides opportunities for vertical mobility within the organizational structure, and pursuit of status and privileges as a prime source of social rewards.
4. Emphasis on group processes directed at raising the individual's self-awareness of negative personality features and behaviors through their impact on others (e.g., problems with authority, impulse control, low self-esteem, manipulative or self-defeating behaviors).
5. Use of group persuasion to elicit absolute personal honesty, self-disclosure, and commitment for self-change.

The above principles were supported by a foundation comprising what might be considered a TC-specific "culture." Some key elements of that culture were techniques and methods that served and reinforced the above-noted principles. The lexicon of TCs, likewise, reflected both the ideology and methods of the TC milieu. Dye *et al.* [4] described classic, "traditional" TCs

Clinical Handbook of Adolescent Addiction, First Edition. Richard Rosner.
© 2013 John Wiley & Sons, Ltd. Published 2013 by John Wiley & Sons, Ltd.

as "characterized by confrontational group therapy, treatment phases, a tenure-based resident hierarchy, and long-term residential care."[1]

Early TCs were staffed almost exclusively by individuals who had "risen through the ranks" in the treatment environment. Given the nature of TC methods and operations, having primary focus on community membership and individuals' roles within that context, this was a logical outgrowth of the underlying philosophy. The hierarchic structure of the TC itself, in which participants' attitudes, behaviors, and contributions to the community determined their position within the program, assumed that as "seniority" developed, so did capacities to mentor, serve as a model to others, live by the principles of the TC, and apply insight. The TC's unique culture, its relatively heavy emphasis on experiential learning, and participative demonstration as the main vehicle for determining individuals' status in TC systems, virtually required that the TC itself serve as the primary training ground. Thus, it was such that the lifeblood of intervention delivery in a TC setting was provided by those who "came from treatment," in the strictest sense implying *TC-based* treatment.

Many TCs have worked closely from the outset with public officials, clergy, and health and social service professionals, and have come to be significantly influenced by traditional fields of education, medicine, psychiatry, law, religion, and social sciences. Professionals in medicine, social work, education, and other fields now complement the traditional TC staff of individuals in recovery from addictive disorders who historically have comprised the framework of most TC programs. The latter serve as role models, lifestyle "coaches," stalwart sources of peer support, and reliable authorities to the TC client. Many TCs now provide a full continuum of care, and have developed into fully recognized service agencies preparing clients for reintegration into society at large, as evidenced by progressively increased public funding for TC clinical and administrative operations, calling for compliance with various forms of regulatory requirements and external oversight.

THE THERAPEUTIC COMMUNITY MODEL OF ADDICTION TREATMENT

Outlined below are some essential components of the TC model and practice, as documented by De Leon, one of the foremost authorities on the TC modality applied to addictive disorders [3,5].

1. *View of the disorder:* Chemical dependence is viewed from a broad perspective on the individual's psychological status and lifestyle. Drug problems are seen primarily as problems of "the person, not the drug" [3]. Drug abuse is a disorder pervasively affecting cognition, behavior, mood/psychiatric status, physical health, occupational performance, and social functioning.

2. *View of the person:* Drug use patterns, while obviously significant, are viewed as secondary or symptomatic of disordered or inadequate functioning in more general terms. Individuals are described with parameters of behavior, attitude, affect, and social patterns often associated with substance abuse (e.g., poor frustration tolerance/impulse control, low self-esteem, problems with authority and responsibility, unrealistic expectations, difficulty expressing affect, manipulation, guilt, and cognitive deficits.

3. *View of recovery:* Goals of treatment are not exclusively focused on abstinence from drugs and alcohol, but radical changes in lifestyle and identity essential to sustained recovery. Recovery is conceptualized as a "developmental process of social learning" in which self-help and mutual peer-help are crucial components [3].

4. *View of right living:* To promote more productive alternatives to behaviors frequently displayed by addicted persons, part of TC programming centers on inculcation of beliefs, values, and precepts deemed by the model as essential to self-help, personal growth, social learning, recovery, and healthy living. Among those are honesty, awareness of the present moment, personal responsibility, a moral code, a work ethic, belief that "self" and "behavior" are separable (i.e., *people* are essentially "good," even though their behaviors may be judged as "bad," "harmful," etc.), embracing change, learning to learn, economic self-reliance, community involvement, and good citizenship.

As indicated by its name, the primary therapeutic setting, agent of change, and method of the TC is the community of peers and staff. The "community as method" approach, that is, "purposive use of the peer community to facilitate social and psychological change in individuals," distinguishes the TC from other therapeutic modalities [5]. While formalized interventions have a significant role in TC-based treatment, these are perhaps less compartmentalized in the TC than in other forms of treatment. In addition, as indicated earlier, specific methods of intervention within the TC may differ from those of other models. The TC approach

---

[1] Detailed description of that material is outside the focus of this chapter; one recommended text for readers desiring more extensive information on this and related topics is: George De Leon *The Therapeutic Community: Theory, Model, and Method;* New York, NY: Springer Publishing Co., 2000, frequently referenced here.

views the total organization, its members, interactions, and functions as the primary medium in which the therapeutic process takes place.

All activities in the TC, both scheduled and naturally occurring, are viewed as opportunities for therapeutic change in lifestyle and identity. Equally, all community members have potential roles as agents of therapeutic change through their relationships, daily interactions, participation in group work, mutual support, role modeling, public disclosure of experiences, and inculcation of norms and values that protect physical and psychological safety of the community. As such, in the early history of TC practices, "boundaries" among sectors of the TC were less defined than in other service delivery systems. Thus, distinctions between those on the giving and receiving end of services (i.e., clients and staff) were relatively blurred. That seems a natural, logical outgrowth of the early foundation of TCs, in which staff almost exclusively consisted of those who had "risen through the ranks," having themselves progressed through the phases of TC treatment. Since TCs have professionalized and come to be accepted as more mainstream (albeit still on the "intensive-treatment" part of the spectrum), however, the concept of boundaries has grown much closer to a match with that of other ("agent/recipient") systems.

Another source of therapeutic material within the TC arises from social and work structures and systems. Organization of chores, tasks, and management roles predicated by daily operations of the facility provide naturalistic opportunities for skill development, self-examination, and behavior change. Learning goes beyond specific skills training to foster adherence to generic principles such as orderliness of procedures and systems, accepting supervision and authority, courtesy, and acting as a responsible community member with whom others are interdependent.

Aligned with the above system of hierarchy and social order, is the fact that most TCs have traditionally devised and followed a "phase" or "stage" format of treatment. While there are individual variants, TC treatment usually consists of three identifiable stages:

1. *The induction stage,* a period in which each new resident is assimilated into the community, promoted through a focused orientation process, maintains relative isolation from the environment outside the TC, begins moderated participation in all therapeutic activities, and crisis intervention if needed. This stage commonly lasts 1–3 months.
2. *The primary* or *core stage,* primarily devoted to developmental rehabilitation, socialization, personal development, and psychological and behavioral awareness and change. The exposure regarding values and culture of the TC ("right living," citizenship,

ethics, self-motivation/discipline, etc.) continues in this post-induction "main" phase, at a greatly intensified level. This primary treatment, in practice, moves toward objectives such that residents demonstrate greater insight into their problems, personal characteristics, and behaviors, as well as growing self-esteem and capacity for personal disclosure. As they progress through this active phase of the TC, residents begin to accept more self- and community responsibility, and become fully trained participants, if not facilitators, of TC group processes. This stage commonly ranges from 3 to 12 months; however, for younger groups or those with special needs, it may be abbreviated to last 5 to 7 months.

3. *The re-entry phase* is reached when residents begin to prepare for return to independent living. In this phase, residents begin separation from active TC treatment and reintegration into the larger community. They begin applying to the outside world what was learned in primary treatment, and work to create for themselves occupational, home, and relationship environments and situations that are conducive to recovery. Depending on individual circumstances, this phase may take place in a facility separate from the original TC setting (often closer to the individual's permanent home), or on an outpatient basis. Therapeutic activities focus on adjustment to community living, and center around practice of daily living and problem-solving skills. After completing the residential re-entry stage, graduates may be referred to outpatient aftercare services, which may be operated by the original TC, a separate provider, or in the form of community-based self-help, recovery support fellowships (12-Step groups, etc.). Former residents are encouraged to stay in contact with the TC and to "give back" to others what they have received from their peers and staff, through direct, participative activity with the TC, or through extending skills they have acquired into the larger community.

The TC structure with its criterion-based phases, highly defined hierarchy, functions, and roles also provides rich potential for experiences of success and progression by virtue of one's own efforts. These features may serve to modify the often quite narrowed view of addicted individuals, regarding the nature and value of "reward." The TC's emphasis on human interaction and its power and value, creates a context within which intangible, non-concrete reinforcers (praise, recognition, status, social exchanges) may come to be seen as having greater valence, where previously, in the throes of chemical abuse/dependence, there may have been almost exclusive focus on concrete, physical items (drugs, money, etc.). In effect, then, opportunities to learn to value social reinforcement contingencies may be enriched by this type of environment; in turn that capacity to perceive a greater array of events as rewarding may be carried forward and facilitate greater gains in a number of areas.

As may be inferred by the above description of the TC model, philosophy, and culture, many aspects of TC operations could be considered distinctive. In fact, substantial research has documented factors that constitute basic elements of a TC model, and gave rise to development of instruments to measure adherence to those elements (by organizations self-identified as TCs). "Generic" TC characteristics noted by De Leon and colleagues [3,5–10] include:

1. Adherence to a "TC perspective."
2. Treatment approach and structure (on the part of the operating agency) congruent with the TC modality.
3. Use of "community as therapeutic agent" (i.e., "community as method").
4. Relative emphasis on education and work activities.
5. Presence of "formal therapeutic elements" consonant with fairly universal TC methods shared among identified TCs (specific styles of group sessions, use of any TC interactions as material, etc.).
6. Therapeutic "process," i.e., the complex interaction between TC intervention methods with individuals' self-perceived and outwardly observed changes in lifestyle, thought, and behavior [3]. (Eloquently described details of the "process" concept may be found in De Leon [3], pp. 367–379.)

That line of investigation has yielded measurement tools to quantify "fidelity" to the above-noted essential elements of TC operations (i.e., the "Survey of Essential Elements Questionnaire" [9–11]). This has led to research regarding relative concordance of a given TC, or set of TCs, with that set of empirically documented TC characteristics and "core technology" deemed to be at the crux of the model and its application [4]. Previous research provided evidence of validity and applicability of indices of adherence to established TC methodology. There is some recent evidence that fidelity may be a significant influence on treatment outcome, suggesting that, "attention should be placed on the importance of implementing the TC drug abuse treatment model with high fidelity," particularly with "younger clients" [12].

Thus, we have a substantial historical context in which the TC model has survived, thrived, and evolved, while demonstrating capacity to retain critical components of its foundation. Throughout the extensive history of the TC movement, there have been radical changes in system-level factors affecting TC operations (growth of the managed care industry, a series of shifts in public regulatory focus, altered funding priorities,

developments in overlapping areas such as psychotherapy, etc.). Irrespective of such changes, the TC model has continued to yield results indicating it is efficacious, "particularly for certain subpopulations that may be difficult to reach through other treatment methods" [4]. (We might suggest that the model's efficacy is not "particularly" more effective for "difficult to reach" populations; but point out instead that this model may have efficacy that is *robust enough to evoke positive outcomes* in a range of populations including, but not limited to, subgroups in which other models have not shown remarkable promise.)

Despite extensive history that has evolved a distinctive methodology and culture, many TC systems have elected to incorporate relatively recently developed approaches (e.g., cognitive-behavioral therapy, motivational interviewing techniques) into their repertoire of intervention strategies. Such initiatives are often governed by a given TC organization's definition of "best practices," and often derive from empirically supported "evidence-based practices." Adoption of speculative, "new," and experimental treatment practices is probably a less-than-popular concept in most TC organizations. TCs have a long history beginning with what at the time was fairly radical "milieu-therapy" concepts, and have evolved a well-studied and relatively well-defined set of TC-based methods. Thus, there may be a surprisingly "conservative" outlook toward taking on untested, theoretical methods, without being able to appraise the value of a given technique or theory by examining data that derive from its study. On balance with that, however, is the survival and reputation of the TC model, as a unique, rigorous method that is well studied and efficacious, as well as the fact that *with evidence,* TCs may carefully consider and adopt additional, newly developed methods, with view that "whatever works" may be worth an investment, as long as it is in keeping with established TC practices and philosophy.

THE MODIFIED TC APPROACH

There has been considerable success in efforts to adapt the TC model to a range of subpopulations, including the homeless, mentally ill chemical abusers, clients with "co-occurring disorders," methadone-maintained individuals, correctional facility inmates, women, and adolescents [6,11,13–17]. The Treatment Communities of America (TCA), generally considered the primary professional association for TCs, with over 600 organizational affiliates throughout the United States and Canada, provides a listing of "special needs populations" served by member organizations. Those include pregnant and post-partum drug-addicted women, individuals with HIV/AIDS and hepatitis C, mentally ill substance abusers (including individuals with chronic and persistent mental illness), criminal justice populations, the homeless, the physically handicapped, gang-involved individuals, adolescents, the elderly, veterans, and mothers with children [17].

In the last 20 years, with increasing frequency, "modified" TCs (MTCs) have arisen. MTCs are based on the more traditional TC prototype; specialized services or structural alterations are adopted in order to reap the advantages of the model with populations for which the most narrowly defined TC practices may not be ideally suited. Variations in design/practice may be cultural or nationalistic, as in adaptations that have given rise to migration of the TC model to some 65 countries worldwide [18]. Most germane here, an MTC design may accommodate the needs of specific target populations. Applied to the latter, parameters noted to be most frequently subject to modifications are program structure, intensity, availability of "tailored services," and degree to which staffing patterns include proportionally more professionals than would be the case in a "standard" TC treatment environment [4].

Given a caveat of sorts, that MTC treatment outcomes may be significantly tied to fidelity in implementing critical aspects of the model (e.g., correlation between "implementation fidelity" and outcome measures with strongest impact on younger clients), there is also evidence that effective "balances" may be achieved, between some threshold level of authenticity (fidelity) and modifications deemed necessary for specific populations [12]. Dye et al. documented differential effects of six factors derived from the Survey of Essential Elements Questionnaire (SEEQ), which were identified as "core TC principles and structures," namely:

1. "TC Perspective," most prominently capturing established points of TC philosophy such as "right living" and "community as method" [4].
2. "Hierarchy," i.e., a progressive, multilevel system of client and staff roles.
3. "Clients as Therapists," whereby peer interactions regarding therapeutic goals are relatively heavily emphasized.
4. "Work as Therapy," focus on either formal educational activities or employment (working within the TC or outside of it).
5. "Aspects of the Program," comprising structural elements that determine programming (specific activities and manner in which they are carried out), such as various meetings, therapeutic group formats, use of a phase or stage system, and codified "house rules" that define behavioral expectations, extents/limits of privileges, etc.
6. "Disciplinary Actions," i.e., defined forms of sanctions for rule violations.

Further, Dye et al. studied a large sample of randomly selected organizations self-identified as TCs, in part to investigate levels of adherence to the above-defined core TC elements by programs defined as "modified" along several parameters [4]. Those MTCs included: (i) gender-specific programs (vs the standard mixed-gender TC); (ii) client age range (i.e., adolescent-only or mixed-age programs vs standard adult-only TC); (iii) provision of integrated care for co-occurring disorders; (iv) staffing characteristics (i.e., proportion of professionally trained staff, ratio of counselors in recovery to those with no addiction history); and (v) variations on (traditional) long-term residential level of care, including exclusively outpatient, short- and long-term residential, and mixed levels of care. Overall, adoption of various MTC approaches was not found to significantly impact upon adherence to the above-described key elements that comprise the "core technology" of the TC model [4]. Thus, it appears that a variety of MTCs can be designed for specialized subpopulations, while successfully adhering to essential practice elements of the established TC model.

THE ADOLESCENT-SPECIFIC MODIFIED TC

Progressively, adolescents have come to represent, at any given time, roughly 20–25% of the total of TC admissions [19,20]. Some organizations have opened TC facilities that are exclusively designed for adolescents, and tailored specifically to the needs of their younger residents. In reference to adolescent-specialized programming, Dye et al. reported that MTCs designed to accommodate adolescents were found overall to adhere to the essential TC elements with fidelity at essentially the same level as that of traditional, adult-only TCs [4]. Of note is the fact that significant effects of age-group-related modifications were found in adolescent-only TCs, in two of the above-outlined elements: "Work as Therapy" and "Disciplinary Actions." (There was also a single element in "Aspects of Program" that stood out, to be discussed below.) With the former element, there was significantly less emphasis on work, relative to TCs serving adults, while significantly more emphasis was found in the area of disciplinary actions. The greater emphasis on disciplinary action was a finding in common among TCs with exclusively adolescent programs, women's programs, and those serving co-occurring psychiatric and substance abuse disorders.

Regarding the above distinguishing features, or deviations from classic TC elements, found in adolescent-specific TCs, we concur with Dye et al. in interpreting those results, as well as in speculation regarding how these distinctions may have come about [4]. First, the differences in degree of emphasis on work and disciplinary actions, between exclusively adolescent TCs and those serving adults, may be age-congruent reflections of population developmental stages and needs, rather than modifications of the TC model per se. The adolescent population as a whole, at least in Western cultures, is directed toward completing developmental processes, including educational attainment, physical maturation, social skills, formation of values and core identity, etc. In parallel, one of the accepted hallmarks of adolescence, "limits testing," usually calls for creation of structure by rules, behavioral guidelines, and consequences. Thus, as is almost inevitable, adolescent programming that considers such factors might predictably emphasize mechanisms to handle violations.

Another more global comment on the above, regarding the finding-in-common among adolescent, women's, and dual-diagnosis programs and greater emphasis on the element of "Disciplinary Action," is as follows. While this emphasis may seem counterintuitive, at least in programming for both women and co-occurring disorders, this may be seen in a less "draconian" light if, as posited by Dye *et al.*, it reflects heightened application of "behavior modification" principles by such programs [4]. These authors also incorporated investigation of TC methodological factors, in this instance to clarify whether or not behavior modification was used as an alternative to the more traditional, in fact virtually iconic, technique in TCs, of frequent use of confrontational therapy techniques. This was deemed by Dye *et al.* to fall within the area of "Aspects of Program" as alluded to above [4]. While in TCs for women and those with co-occurring disorders, this proposition appeared to be at least partially supported, there was actually a *contrasting* finding in adolescent-only TCs, where "disciplinary action" (perhaps with behavior modification techniques at the foundation) had greater-than-traditional programmatic emphasis, *so, also, did the use of confrontational intervention styles.*

Proposing conclusions about program-development mechanisms that gave rise to the above would probably be grossly overstepping the boundaries of data available to date. However, without venturing that far, we can observe based on findings such as the above, in the context of earlier investigations that documented the feasibility and efficacy of adolescent-focused MTCs, that: (i) the TC model is a viable, potentially useful treatment option for adolescents, and (ii) exclusively adolescent MTCs seem to have developed characteristic features that match well with developmental challenges of this subgroup [15,20].

The above, quite appropriately, includes the following specific features:

1. There can be TC structure with fidelity to the classic "reference" model.
2. For adolescent-only MTCs, there is less emphasis on vocational pursuits, either in the sense of "work-as-therapy," or in the intensity of focus on employment-directed activities. In place of work as a priority, the focus may be on attainment of developmental milestones, such that adolescent TC participants may have optimized probability of reaching adulthood with the improved status of addiction recovery, physical development, basic educational attainment, life skills, ties with more positive peer influences, and productive values. Ideally, educational resources can be woven into MTC program structure, with cognitive level-appropriate basic or remedial education available on site or in TC-based facilities. In some locations, MTC-based academic work can be accredited with local public education systems, so school credits can be earned by completion of coursework while in residence in an adolescent MTC.
3. There is the possibility of an integrated system in which behavior modification principles may be applied, with specific methods of delivering "consequences" and well-defined *forms* of consequences for various levels of rule-violation; and this can be interwoven with relatively liberal application of confrontational intervention strategies. This, of course, does not presume exclusive use of this triad of techniques, in the absence of a strong, well-implemented TC, with key elements providing the main context. However, this combination of MTC characteristics in adolescent TC environments may be of particular advantage to the population under discussion.

The reasoning behind the above suggestions is as follows. Experience with adolescents, developmental theory with some empirical support, and knowledge of the particular subgroup(s) of adolescents most frequently seen in the MTC setting, indicate, like a truism, that this is a distinctively challenging group. Hser *et al.* found that adolescents treated in TCs, compared to peers in outpatient programs, had higher rates of prior drug abuse treatment experience, more severe problems, and were more likely to have a criminal justice history [21]. Even with these challenging features at baseline, TC-treated adolescents demonstrated positive outcomes in drug use, psychological adjustment, school performance, and reduction in criminal activities. Outcomes for adolescents referred through probation to TCs versus those referred to group homes of equivalent size and duration, indicated that both groups had marked improvements in areas of drug use, criminal behavior, and measures of psychological functioning 3 months into these placements. However, on extended follow-up, the TC group maintained and/or demonstrated further improvements in problem areas assessed; those placed in group homes showed regression. This is evidence in support of the efficacy of the TC approach, per se, as opposed to other "restrictive environment" settings or intervention systems to which troubled, potentially criminally involved adolescents may be referred.

Of note is the fact that planned lengths of stay may vary markedly across TC operations, ranging from around 3 months up to over 1 year in some cases. It seems that more than length of stay, *treatment completion* and *post-treatment peer group influences* may be stronger predictors of adolescent TC outcomes, at least on extended follow-up [15]. Again, this indicates that entering a different environment, in-treatment absence of former peers, living with greater structure, etc., is by no means sufficient to evoke lasting behavioral improvement with this group of adolescents. Rather, experiences such as assimilation of TC principles, attainment of behavioral, social, and community skills to warrant advancement, and emulation of positive role models apparently are critical. These transformations of any given adolescent are supported within the MTC system hierarchy, by progressing through a set of community-determined "hurdles," ultimately achieving completion status, within a community practiced in accurately assessing attitudes and behaviors of its own members. In the case of adolescents, sometimes this process occurs with the input of others in a more extended network than might be seen with adults in TCs (e.g., adult peer-counselors, professional staff, involved educators, family members, juvenile justice representatives, etc., as well as "peers" in the traditional TC sense).

Nonetheless, the above process of progressive advancement toward a goal does occur in the adolescent-tailored MTC, in a fashion similar to that in traditional adult TCs. As above, length of TC "exposure" is less critical than the adolescent's level of "buy-in" while actively in residence in the MTC [22]. Given the particular stages of development and behavior that are typical in adolescence (or virtually *stereotypical,* even in "average," normally developing, relatively untroubled adolescents), some features of which seem to be heightened in those likely to be TC candidates, the treatment-related tasks of building engagement, commitment, and overt motivation, that is, the "buy-in", may need particular attention. This may be brought about by the nature, structure, and expectations of the TC/MTC model itself, applied to the characteristic features of an adolescent

population, perhaps intensified by subgroup characteristics found in adolescents with substance use disorders.

By the time most members of the adolescent MTC population actually reach a given MTC for admission, they are very likely to bring with them a litany of problems, at levels of severity that far outstrip those found in other sectors of the adolescent population. As noted earlier, they are likely to have previous treatment histories often in a progressive, stepwise fashion, beginning with lower levels of treatment intensity, greater problem severity, and greater probability of involvement with criminal activities. This group is likely to have become developmentally "derailed" and may have done so at an earlier age than peers whose problems are less severe.

Experience with adolescents in general, that is, the "normative" expectations applied to this group as a whole, indicates that this group is distinctive in character and behavior. "Questioning, exploring, and risk-taking" are expected – even, to a certain level, *desirable* – as normal parts of adolescent development [23]. The hope, for any given individual, is that he or she will successfully complete this phase of development, with sufficient resilience to emerge into adulthood with few serious or lasting consequences. Even at best, parts of the experience of adolescence are tumultuous; demands and challenges are greater than at earlier stages, while relevant cognitive and psychosocial mechanisms may be taxed or overwhelmed in efforts to surmount them. As would be expected with adolescents as a group, by adult-determined standards, questioning or ignoring others' credibility, mistrust or insecurity in relationships, risk-taking, and a strong element of denial can all be commonly observed [23]. With the social, cultural, and physiological effects of drug abuse, such characteristic elements of adolescence can be seen as intensified.

While symptoms of chemical abuse/dependence in adolescents parallel those of adults, they manifest in ways that are "emotionally, behaviorally, attitudinally, and chronologically more developmentally specific" [23]. Morrison astutely observed that only in relatively recent times have healthcare professionals recognized the disease of chemical dependence in the adolescent population, due to that group's lack of display, in most cases, of pathognomonic signs that appear in adults [23]. In addition, "the more entrenched denial, that is, delusional, system in adolescents is another factor that affects the identification and recognition of symptoms" [23]. This is compounded by adolescent versus adult differences in societal expectations (employment, self-support, relationships, etc.), as well as "larger systems of enablers" found amid the social network and support structure of adolescents [23].

Compounding the above is the profound effect of the peer-associate network in adolescents. The influence of peers' behavior regarding drug use has been found to be a major factor that can predict the likelihood of drug use in individual members of an extended network [21]. This is very much in keeping with standard expectations about adolescents as a group: peer relations become paramount in adolescence; they are likely to exert a more profound influence on the behavior, choices, tastes, and (eventually) teen-years development than any other single factor. (Of course, surrounding factors such as earlier developmental experiences, genetics, parental behavioral influences, etc., are not without effect, but peer-focused axioms of adolescence continue to be supported by data [24–29]. Similarly, the influence of peers "may serve to amplify the effects of interventions," which has hopeful implications, but also indicates that the effect of peers is pervasive enough that it works on multiple axes (i.e., both negatively and positively) [27].

By the time an adolescent arrives for treatment admission in an MTC, it is likely that he or she has previous treatment experience (with less than ideal outcomes, thus the impetus for an MTC referral). That adolescent also may have some background of socialization in criminal behavior, and is likely to have a peer group with considerable influence that may act to reinforce problem-related behaviors and attitudes that operate as treatment barriers. Congruent with the above-outlined information, in addition, it is probable that treatment motivation and "readiness" in this subgroup are low [30].

The above factors begin to describe a situation in adolescents who become MTC candidates and adolescents who abuse drugs as a more general group. This subgroup, harmonious with the "normative" questioning of previously influential authority, may desire to appear "tough" or impervious to being affectively touched or impacted by others. There is a probable history of plentiful reinforcement of denial, escalated problem severity, possibility of consequences, and as observed, in general less physical/health-related sequelae of chemical abuse than in older groups [23]. There may as a result be markedly low levels of problem recognition in this group – a "thick" form of denial. This returns to the salience of the distinctive character of MTCs for adolescents discussed above.

The "triad" of distinctions between adolescent MTCs and other MTC operations (with traditional TC characteristics as "standards"), consists of the following:

1. reported emphasis on "Disciplinary Actions;"
2. in part, at least, attributable to enhanced application of behavior modification principles; and
3. greater (than other MTCs) use of confrontational therapy techniques.

Given the thick form of denial, reinforced by an extended period of enabling by parents and other adults, and the pronounced influence of peers prior to entering the MTC, recognition of problems/consequences of drug abuse and correlated treatment motivation may be very challenging, especially in the early stage, for most adolescent MTC participants.

A behavioral approach, with principles of TC "Disciplinary Actions" attached, may be much needed such that some measure of order may be brought to the chaotic behavioral ground presented by a group of adolescents who have substantial histories, by the time they reach the MTC, of behavioral problems in many areas. There is often a desire to keep denial intact and to continue to avoid facing uncomfortable affect and self-concept issues that may have contributed to the chemical abuse. In the interrelated context of low levels of motivation/readiness to change, in order to penetrate these barriers, confrontation may be one of only a few viable options [31].

Within a TC (MTC) structure, confrontational therapy applied to adolescents may serve two major purposes. First, it may be needed initially as a "wake-up call" to the newly admitted, still heavily denying, posturing, "cooler-than-thou" adolescent. TC-style confrontation allows for observations of an individual's behavior within the TC to be described by others present in the community; and the implications and ways in which that behavior deviates from TC standards of acceptability to be presented. Those who have experienced the types of confrontational therapy that are frequently practiced in the TC/MTC can attest to the fact that the atmosphere of such a group is not one that allows anyone present to "sit back" or remain unengaged. Especially for adolescents who are quick to jump to their own defense, the nature of confrontation of this sort is that, at the very least, it is *engaging*. Part of the engaging quality of the "encounter group" (in classic TC terminology) may be the evocation of that defensiveness. The escalation of anxiety, stress, and increased vigilance evoked by confrontation may serve to shake the certainty of a previous entrenched position and increase motivation to change.

In addition, this group process, unlike prior treatment experiences, most often concludes with some resolution, if not full, at least substantial, of the issues that have been raised, along with encouragement from other TC members, for progress, and willingness to receive feedback on positive aspects of the individual's behavior. This allows participants to complete these sometimes very intensive sessions with the experience of closure and social reinforcement.

At the same time, this process enables the foundation of new relationships with more productive role models, who are "senior" to the individual. Their credibility can be established by both their accurate reflection of behavioral observations and potential consequences, and their depiction of their own histories, as "relatable" role models. Although it has been observed that additional research is needed in the area of peer influences in treatment, it is probably not a quantum leap to assume that peer relationships are for adolescents some of the most critical influences on outcome [31]. Available evidence suggests that both close and extended peer networks have significant influences on adolescents' drug use patterns, that peer relationships in adolescent TC settings may significantly impact upon the treatment experience, and that such relationships may be agents of tension and stimulus for TC treatment material [25,32]. A related comment is that as a result, adolescent MTCs should have staffing and programming equipped to accommodate those elements [32]. In fact, we would venture, such MTCs should *anticipate* such events, and assume they will be utilized as part of the therapeutic process inherent in a TC, with skilled staff who can make full use of such opportunities. Further, post-treatment peer group characteristics and treatment completion status have been reported to be the most significant factors related to outcome status on long-term follow-up in adolescent TC participants [15]. Adolescents' peer group characteristics and perception of counselor's skills while in treatment have also been found to be predictive of length of stay in treatment [33].

The above points highlight the potential impact of MTC peers on adolescents, both in treatment and beyond. Transformations in peer networks may be fostered by MTC stays, such that new, hopefully more productive, less deviant, more supportive peers may be integrated with and ideally replace those influential in the past. Given already established experiential knowledge and a growing body of empirical evidence about the profound importance of peer influences in behavioral choices, this may be critical to sustaining MTC-assisted changes in behavior, attitude, and lifestyle for adolescents [34].

By the time most adolescents reach the point of referral to a TC level of care, they may already have developed a spectrum of social, psychological, educational, and vocational problems along with substance abuse and criminal behaviors that may have provided initial impetus for treatment admission. The motivation for change is far from ideal in many substance abusers; however, this is intensified in adolescence by the natural historical shift from childhood to adulthood with adolescence awkwardly sandwiched between the two, as the intensely uncomfortable "transition period." While this period is "normally" turbulent at best, many adolescent substance abusers are not "at their best" by the time they come to the attention of a practitioner. This group display a tendency even greater than their adult counterparts, to deny the costs of their behavior, display what sometimes appears to be tolerance or indifference to cycles of failure, and are frequently both thoroughly socialized to and captivated by drug-related and "street" lifestyles. Arrival at the point of referral at quite a young age indicates problematic substance abuse at an earlier age than the average "experimenting" teen. This fact is related to stalled development of psychosocial, cognitive, and interpersonal skills, among an array of other developmental functions.

Although "community as method" remains a core principle of MTC treatment of adolescents, the following modifications would be considered standard accommodations for the age, developmental stage (or arrest thereof), and specific habilitative needs of adolescents, in contrast to the "standard" adult TC population [3,20].

Treatment Goals

Lifestyle and identity change are common objectives in the population of adult residents; TC treatment for adolescents is designed to facilitate normative lifestyle and identity development. Principles of normal development presume that some experimental, non-conformist, and perhaps risk-taking behaviors are part of adolescence; however, within certain limits of safety, average adolescents demonstrate sufficient maturity and resilience to prevent extreme expressions and potentially harmful long-term consequences.

Staff-Peer Relationships

In adult TCs, residents with more time in treatment mentor or supervise "younger" residents, with professional staff as secondary agents. Staff in adolescent MTCs are more active in supervising, evaluating, and guiding adolescent residents. Many adolescent MTC residents have extensive histories of negative experiences with authority figures. Adults who demonstrate credibility and consistency, and who create a rational, supportive, but appropriately corrective milieu, are critical to adolescent MTC treatment. They provide physical and emotional safety and positive role models, helping adolescent residents to learn skills to interact more productively with rational authority figures. The success of program staff in shaping adolescents' behavior is dependent in large part on clearly established, consistently enforced, meaningful rules. Over time, this measured exercise of specified guidelines and consequences can counterbalance adolescents' earlier experiences with adult figures who were less than ideal, or even pathological, influences. Recovering staff members provide a unique parental role model for successful recovery. Because of the need for greater staff presence, the staff-resident ratio is usually higher in adolescent than in adult treatment.

Work Structure

Adolescent TC residents spend a large part of their day in school, working to complete high-school coursework and studying for equivalency diplomas. Adult TC residents' daily job functions provide therapeutic opportunities. For adolescents in MTCs, classroom experience is both educational and therapeutic. Teachers often function dually, as instructors and as treatment team members. This extends the field of learning experiences to the MTC-related classroom, helping to reduce negative, self-defeating behaviors in a setting where, in the past, there may have been a residue of failure and disengagement. In addition to academic remedial or maintenance work, adolescent MTC residents are also assigned job functions appropriate to the age and capacities of adolescents. Assigning a job function compatible with an individual's skill is critical in this population, to provide the potential for successful experiences as an antidote to self-stereotyping cycles of failure common to young residents.

Family Involvement

The adolescent's substance abuse and behavioral problems are often interwoven with family dynamics, and as noted previously, in many cases denial and low motivation may be perpetuated by parents, siblings, extended family, and peers [30]. Many adolescent MTC residents will return home after treatment. Thus, integrating the adolescent's family members into the treatment process is critical to sustaining desired long-term outcomes [33]. Family-focused programming frequently comprises both therapeutic and educational components. Often the adolescent MTC resident is not involved in family work until later phases of treatment.

In meetings and seminars, family members learn about the nature of drug abuse, its prevention and treatment, and important developmental issues. Family groups may assist members to identify their own behavior patterns and personal contributory issues, provide opportunities to improve parent-child interactions, teach communication skills, and assist with identification of problems and solutions. Enlisting, engaging, and maintaining family members in the adolescent's treatment process is a challenging pursuit. Many families have reached "the end of the rope" with a given adolescent, and/or there may be estrangement, difficulties with underlying family patterns

and dynamics, or existence of substantial problems in adults; any of these factors may be barriers to family engagement. On the other hand, successful work with an adolescent's family unit, from a systems perspective, may be a key to clinical success [35–38].

Planned Treatment Duration

The recommended treatment stay is on average shorter for adolescents than for adults, usually ranging from 3 months ("short-term") to 12 months ("long-term"), with individual recommended times dependent on each individual's circumstances. For adolescents with relatively intact families, or families who have become solidly engaged in the treatment process, re-entry to the home environment may be somewhat expedited. Residents coming from highly dysfunctional, chaotic, or high relapse-potential homes may ultimately choose more distance from home, and remain in the MTC to prepare for an independent living situation. The length of stay may also be influenced or determined by a court system, juvenile justice officials, or another branch of the criminal justice system.

THE ADOLESCENT CLIENT PROFILE

Therapeutic communities typically admit a client population that comes with a multitude of problems that were precipitated or exacerbated by substance abuse and addiction. The following section presents the adolescent client profile as it has been recorded by Daytop Village over the past three decades. Daytop is the oldest and one of the largest TC organizations in the United States, and has, along with Phoenix House, Samaritan Village, Odyssey House, Walden House, Integrity House, and many other influential programs, contributed to the evolution of the TC model and its current status, and as such may be considered representative. Founded in 1963, Daytop consisted of one small facility in New York. The organization has developed in the interim into a network of comprehensive programs providing a continuum of care with capacity for 1000 residents in a variety of live-in TC/MTC programs, and approximately 2000 outpatient clients enrolled at any given time. (Despite integration of outpatient services into the TC, this chapter focuses on the traditional residential TC.) Initially, Daytop treated adolescents within its largely adult population. Today, adolescents receive age-specific services in separate facilities. This is illustrative of the general trend in TCs, whereby a special need in the TC population is recognized, a system may make various programmatic and administrative

Table 39.1 Characteristics of adolescent clients admitted to Daytop Village residential treatment center from 1980 to 2009.

	1980 (%)	1990 (%)	2000 (%)	2009 (%)
Adolescent proportion of population	32	16	26	20
Age at admission:				
<15 years	7	3	7	3
15–18 years	61	54	76	66
19–20 years	32	44	17	31
Average age at admission	18.09 years	18.44 years	17.25 years	17.3 years
Male/female ratio	68/32	85/15	87/13	81/19
Ethnic distribution:				
White	70	64	32	34
African-American	17	14	41	36
Hispanic	13	17	25	24
Highest grade achieved:				
1–8th grade	18	19	28	25
9–11th grade	58	52	54	61
12th grade or higher	24	29	18	14
Criminal Justice status:				
CJ involved	43	50	75	70
CJ mandate to treatment	20	16	49	47
Other referral sources (CJ excluded):				
Self/family	62	65	31	26
Social services	7	7	6	5
Other treatment program	2	11	13	8
Other	9	1	1	1
Drug use history:				
Primary marijuana use	21	27	81	82
Primary alcohol use	24	27	6	4
Primary cocaine use	5	12	5	1
Primary crack use	1	18	<1	<1
Primary heroin use	19	12	6	2
General marijuana use	38	63	96	95
General alcohol use	78	85	73	41
General cocaine use	22	25	18	8
General crack use	2	29	4	<1
General heroin	19	12	6	8
Average age of first general use:				
Marijuana	12.75 years	13.56 years	12.98 years	13.49 years
Alcohol	12.7 years	12.95 years	13.21 years	13.9 years
Previous drug treatment	3	17	64	69
Mental health history upon admission:				
Ever diagnosed with mental illness	0	2	5	27
Ever treated for mental illness	0	3	9	26
Ever hospitalized for mental illness	0	0	4	20
Suicide attempts	23	10	8	10

accommodations to that subgroup; then often separate, specialized programs are created specifically to serve that group.

Table 39.1 presents admission data for adolescent clients admitted to Daytop residential treatment in the years from 1980 to 2009, demonstrating notable changes in the adolescent client population. Data are based on admissions to Daytop's New York programs, which represent the largest sector of the organization's service population.

Adolescent Proportion

The proportion of young residents under the age of 21 years has decreased over the past three decades, from close to one-third to a relatively stable proportion that constitutes roughly one-fifth of all residential clients.

Age

On average, adolescent residents are somewhat younger upon admission to treatment currently than they were in the 1980s. The majority of adolescent clients are in the age range 15–18 years.

Gender

The number of female adolescents admitted decreased over the period 1980 to 2000; recent increases may be due to special outreach efforts designed to engage young women in need of treatment. All female adolescents receive treatment in one co-ed Daytop adolescent facility, allowing them to "gain strength in numbers" and address gender-specific issues they have in common.

Ethnicity

The vast majority of Daytop adolescent residents in the 1980s were white, but that proportion has changed over time. Progressively, the number of African-American and Hispanic adolescents increased during the 1990s; in 2000, the number of African-American clients was 2.5 times, and the number of Hispanic clients twice that in 1980. The ethnic distribution among Daytop residents reflects regional characteristics of New York City and surrounding counties; client populations in other areas may be expected to present a different ethnic breakdown.

Education

The slightly younger age of adolescent residents today compared with 30 years ago has been correlated with lower school grades achieved at the time of admission. Despite grade levels achieved, and 17 being the average age, actual academic performance levels of adolescent admissions on average remain lower than grade or age expectations. According to educational assessment scores, approximately 28% of adolescents entering treatment are performing at the 8th-grade level or lower. Sixty-four percent score at the 9th- to 11th-grade level, and 8% are at the 12th-grade or above. Girls generally have entered treatment with less schooling: 48% are at or below the 8th-grade achievement level, 43% are between 9th and 11th grades, and 10% have achieved 12th grade or higher. Of concern is the fact that Daytop adolescent admissions have shown a trend toward increasing academic impoverishment. The portion of the adolescent population achieving 9th- to 12th-grade status has diminished since the 1990s, and the percentage of adolescents at or below 8th-grade achievement level at intake has risen, in recent years comprising one-quarter or more of the adolescent population admitted.

Criminal Justice Status

In 2004, four of five, or 1.9 of 2.4 million US adolescents in the criminal justice system (CJS) had chemical abuse or dependence problems when arrested; in many cases these problems were directly or indirectly related to the crimes committed [39,40]. According to the 2004 National Center on Addiction and Substance Abuse at Columbia University (CASA) report, fewer than 4% of those juvenile offenders received substance abuse treatment during incarceration or upon release [41]. However, progressively more collaborative systems integrating the CJS and treatment have yielded steadily increased numbers of juvenile offenders referred for treatment. This development is reflected by CJS involvement in the Daytop adolescent population, which has almost doubled since 1980. Over the last 20 years, reports of recent CJS involvement have risen to roughly four of five adolescent admissions. Adolescents receiving mandated treatment as part of a sentencing requirement, by drug or family courts, probation, or other authorities, have more than doubled. Mandated treatment has in general grown in judicial application, as a method to divert those eligible for such sentences from incarceration. The adolescent population here seems illustrative of that. Further, according to these figures, presently more than half of all adolescent residents face the possibility of legal consequences if they do not complete treatment.

Referral Sources

Self and family referrals to treatment have precipitously decreased since the 1990s. At the same time, referral of court-mandated clients increased markedly. Referrals by other treatment programs, often based on their assessment of a given client's need for more intensive treatment, account for roughly 10% of referrals, while referrals from other types of social service agencies have remained relatively stable over the years, at levels slightly lower.

Drug Use History

Marijuana has historically been the most widely used illicit drug among adolescents [42]; national studies of adolescent clinical populations have found marijuana to be the most frequently reported drug of choice [43,44]. Similarly, Daytop adolescent primary and general marijuana use outstrips rates of other drug use; in recent years more than four out of five adolescent residents have entered treatment due to primary abuse of this drug. This, however, is a very different picture from the 1980s. At that time, marijuana, alcohol, and heroin were reported as primary drugs at similar rates, and many more clients reported general use of alcohol than of marijuana. Over the intervening years, adolescent heroin use steadily declined, while cocaine and crack cocaine use peaked in the late 1980s and early 1990s. Both primary and general crack use have declined since then, most recently reaching levels that could be considered negligible compared to earlier points in history, as well as compared to contemporary use of other substances. General cocaine use has declined since the mid-1990s, and primary cocaine use among adolescents is consistently at a relatively low level.

For marijuana and alcohol, the two drugs most frequently used by report of adolescent residents presently, the average age of their first use has varied, potentially indicating changes in patterns of accessibility. Of note also is that first use of marijuana is, on average, reported to be at a slightly younger age than that of alcohol. This raises interesting points of speculation regarding the driving forces in operation. We might speculate that alcohol prevention campaigns and early education about risks from alcohol may have succeeded to some degree. In an opposite direction, perhaps concurrent popular folklore regarding "weed" makes marijuana appear more "mainstream," less risky, and more appealing, although, again, this is only at a speculative level and suggests material for further investigation.

Only a small minority of adolescents in 1980 reported any previous drug treatment. However, that statistic has steadily reversed, so that over time an increasing proportion of the population admitted to TCs reported prior treatment experience. Recently that figure has approached 70%, indicating perhaps that referrals of adolescents to treatment have become more common, and that there may be a progression of referrals, such that a given individual, similar to adults, may first be referred to less intensive treatment modalities, and arrive at the door of an adolescent MTC having not obtained long-term success with lower intensity programs.

Mental Health History

National estimates have assumed that up to 75% of adolescent substance abusers have a comorbid mental health problem, with conduct disorders, affective disorders, and attention-deficit/hyperactivity disorder

(ADHD) cited as the most prevalent among them [43,44]. Previously diagnosed mental illness reported for Daytop adolescents reflects only clients' awareness of any major mental illness with which they have been diagnosed, and is thus much lower. However, reported diagnosis rates have steeply increased from 0% in 1980 to 27% in 2009. Based on the observation of Daytop's mental health staff and an unpublished survey conducted among Daytop adolescent residents ($n = 181$), approximately 40% of annual admissions present with psychiatric comorbidity that warrants evaluation and enhanced treatment, which may include medication and/or psychotherapy. In the Daytop survey, 40% of the adolescents reported having been prescribed psychotropic medication at some time in their lives, and around 33% of the adolescent population are currently prescribed psychotropic medication, such as Zoloft, Paxil, or Prozac. An additional 30–40% of adolescent residents have been previously diagnosed with or show symptoms of ADHD. These numbers are discrepant with the admission reports of previously diagnosed conditions, indicating that there may be many adolescents with comorbid disorders that are undetected and unaddressed as they attempt to navigate through educational, medical, criminal justice, and other significant systems.

Fortunately, the rate of suicide attempts reported in this adolescent population has decreased from almost 1 in 4 in 1980 to a relatively stable rate of around less than 1 in 10 adolescents in the years from 1990 to the present.

SUMMARY

The original therapeutic community model has been successfully modified to accommodate a number of subpopulations with special needs and characteristics, including adolescents with chemical abuse/dependence and a host of correlated problems. TC admission statistics indicate that the adolescent TC population constitutes a group with a variety of psychological, behavioral, social, and educational dysfunctions that may increase vulnerability to substance abuse and criminal justice involvement. Most come to be admitted to TCs with prior treatment episodes, and are assessed to be in need of intensive and comprehensive treatment. Affiliation with a peer-focused milieu appeals to the adolescent need for identification with peers; however, ideally the TC offers a more constructive peer group than was experienced previous to index treatment in the TC setting. TCs also offer adolescents alternative models of adult authority, which are often in stark contrast to prior experiences with adults. The daily schedule, social structure, and well-defined expectations and consequences found in the TC provide ample opportunity for adolescents to practice skills to effectively cope with affect, emotional trauma, and social pressures. The TC environment provides experiences that support and promote development of age-appropriate capacities for problem-solving and goal achievement. Throughout their stay in the TC, adolescents receive opportunities, both structured and naturally occurring, to practice these skills with immediate support and consistent feedback. Despite challenges inherent in treatment of the adolescent population, the TC modality has been found to be adaptable to this population, and has demonstrated efficacy in reducing substance abuse, criminal involvement, psychosocial problems, and ideally improvements in adolescent TC residents' self-esteem, coping, and academic and vocational achievement.

References

1. Jones M. *The Therapeutic Community: A New Treatment Method in Psychiatry*. New York: Basic Books, 1953.
2. Rapaport RN. *Community As Doctor*. London: Tavistock Publications, 1960.
3. DeLeon G. *The Therapeutic Community: Theory, Model, and Method*. New York: Springer, 2000.
4. Dye MH, Ducharme LJ, Johnson JA, Knudsen HK, Roman PM. Modified therapeutic communities and adherence to traditional elements. *J Psychoactive Drugs* 2009;**41**:275–283.
5. DeLeon G (ed.). *Community as Method: Therapeutic Communities for Special Populations*. Westport: Praeger, 1997.
6. DeLeon G, Sacks S, Staines G, McKendrick K. Modified therapeutic community for homeless mentally ill chemical abusers: Treatment outcomes. *Am J Drug Alcohol Abuse* 2000;**26**:461–480.
7. DeLeon G, Sacks S, Staines G, McKendrick K. Modified therapeutic community for homeless mentally ill chemical abusers: Emerging subtypes. *Am J Drug Alcohol Abuse* 1999;**25**:495–515.
8. Melnick G, DeLeon G, Hiller ML, Knight K. Therapeutic communities: Diversity in treatment elements. *Subst Use Misuse* 2000;**35**:1819–1847.
9. Melnick G, DeLeon G. Clarifying the nature of therapeutic community treatment: The survey of essential elements questionnaire (SEEQ). *J Subst Abuse Treat* 1999;**16**:301–313.
10. DeLeon G, Melnick G. *Therapeutic Community Survey of Essential Elements Questionnaire (SEEQ)*. New York: Community Studies Institute, 1993.
11. Sacks S, McKendrick K, Sacks JY, Cleland CM. Modified therapeutic community for co-occurring disorders: single investigator meta analysis. *Subst Abuse* 2010;**31**:146–161.
12. Johnson K, Pan Z, Young L, *et al*. Therapeutic community drug treatment success in Peru: a follow-up outcome study. *Subst Abuse Treat Prev Policy* 2008;**3** (26).
13. Edelen MO, Tucker JS, Wenzel SL, *et al*. Modified therapeutic community for homeless mentally ill chemical abusers: Treatment outcomes. *Am J Drug Alcohol Abuse* 2000;**26**:461–480.
14. Welsh WN. Inmate responses to prison-based drug treatment: a repeated measures analysis. *Drug Alcohol Depend* 2010;**109**:37–44.
15. Jainchill N, Hawke J, DeLeon G, Yagelka J. Adolescents in therapeutic communities: One-year posttreatment outcomes. *J Psychoactive Drugs* 2000;**32**:81–94.
16. Coletti DS, Huges PH, Landress HJ, *et al*. PAR Village: Specialized intervention of cocaine abusing women and their children. *J Fla Med Assoc* 1992;**79**:701–705.
17. Edelen MO, Tucker JS, Wenzel SL, *et al*. Treatment process in the therapeutic community: Associations with retention and outcomes among adolescent residential clients. *J Subst Abuse Treat* 2007;**32**:415–421.
18. Treatment Communities of America. Website: http://www.therapeuticcommunitiesofamerica.org/.
19. Bunt GC, Muehlbach B, Moed CO. The therapeutic community: An international perspective. *Subst Abuse* 2008;**29**:81–87.
20. Jainchill N. Therapeutic Communities for Adolescents: The same and not the same. In: DeLeon G (ed.), *Community as Method: Therapeutic Communities for Special Populations*. Westport, CT: Praeger, 1997; pp. 161–177.
21. Hser Y, Grella CE, Hubbard RL, *et al*. An evaluation of drug treatments for adolescents in four US cities. *Arch Gen Psychiatry* 2001;**58**:689–695.
22. Zhang Z, Friedmann PD, Gerstein DR Does retention matter? Treatment duration and improvement in drug use. *Addiction* 2003;**98**:673–684.
23. Morrison MA. Addiction in adolescents. In: Addiction Medicine [Special Issue]. *Western J Med* 1990;**152**:543–546.
24. Ali MM, Dwyer DS. Social network effects in alcohol consumption among adolescents. *Addict Behav* 2010;**35**:337–342.
25. Ali MM, Amialchuk A, Dwyer DS. The social contagion effect of marijuana use among adolescents. *PLoS ONE* 2011;**6** (1): e16183; doi: 10.1371/journal.pone.0016183.
26. Ali MM, Dwyer DS. Estimating peer effects in adolescent smoking behavior: a longitudinal analysis. *J Adolesc Hlth* 2009;**45**:402–408.
27. Clark A, Loheac Y. It wasn't me, it was them! Social influence in risky behavior by adolescents. *J Health Econ* 2007;**26**:763–784.
28. Lundborg P. Having the wrong friends? Peer effects in adolescent substance use. *J Health Econ* 2006;**25**:214–233.
29. Simons-Morton B, Chen RS. Overtime relationships between early adolescent and peer substance use. *Addict Behav* 2006;**31**:1121–1223.
30. Etile D. The moderating effect of peer substance use on the family structure-adolescent substance use association: quantity versus quality of parenting. *Addict Behav* 2005;**30**:963–980.
31. Melnick G, DeLeon G, Hawke J, Jainchill N, Kressel D. Motivation and readiness for therapeutic community treatment among adolescents and adult substance abusers. *Am J Drug Alcohol Abuse* 1997;**23**:485–506.
32. Nathan S, Foster M, Ferry M. Peer and sexual relationships in the experience of drug-dependent adolescents in a therapeutic community. *Drug Alcohol Rev* 2010;**29**:419–427.
33. Foster M, Nathan S, Ferry M. The experience of drug-dependent adolescents in a therapeutic community. *Drug Alcohol Rev* 2010;**29**:531–539.
34. Evans N, Gilpin E, Farkas AJ, Shenassa E, Piere JP. Adolescents' perception of their peers' health norm. *Am J Public Health* 1995;**85**:1064–1069.
35. Battjes RJ, Gordon MS, O'Grady KE, Kinlock TW. Predicting retention of adolescents in substance abuse treatment. *Addict Behav* 2004;**29**:1021–1027.

36. Griswold KS, Aronoff H, Kernan JB, Kahn LS. Adolescent substance use and abuse: recognition and management. *Am Fam Physician* 2008;**77**:331–336.

37. Venza J. Treating the adolescent and their family in the therapeutic community: A parallel process. TCA NEWS, Therapeutic Communities of America website feature. Available from: http://www.therapeuticcommunitiesofamerica. org/ (accessed February 2011).

38. Weidman A. Family therapy and reductions in treatment dropout in a residential therapeutic community for chemically dependent adolescents. *J Subst Abuse Treat* 1987;**4**:21–28.

39. Hubbard RL, Craddock SG, Flynn PM, Anderson J, Etheridge RM. Overview of 1-year follow-up outcomes in the Drug Abuse Treatment Outcome Study (DATOS). *Psychol Addict Behav* 1997;**11**:261–278.

40. Hser Y, Grella CE, Hubbard RL, *et al.* An evaluation of drug treatments for adolescents in four US cities. *Arch Gen Psychiatry* 2001;**58**:689–695.

41. National Center on Addiction and Substance Abuse at Columbia University (CASA). *Criminal Neglect – Substance Abuse, Juvenile Justice and the Children Left Behind*. Research report. New York: Columbia Press, 2004.

42. Johnston LD, O'Malley P, Bachman J. *Monitoring the Future: National results on Adolescent Drug Use. Overview of Key Findings, 2002*. Bethesda, MD: US Department of Health and Human Services, 2003.

43. Grella C, Hser Y, Joshi V, Rounds-Bryant J. Drug treatment outcomes for adolescents with comorbid mental and substance abuse disorders. *J Nerv Ment Dis* 2001;**189**: 384–392.

44. Tims FM, Dennis ML, Hamilton D, *et al.* Characteristics and problems of 600 adolescent cannabis abusers in outpatient treatment. *Addiction* 2002;**97**:46–57.

40

Treatment Issues for Youths with Substance Abuse in Juvenile Detention

Eraka Bath,[1] Le Ondra Clark,[2] and Julie Y. Low[3]

[1] Department of Psychiatry, UCLA Neuropsychiatric Institute, Los Angeles, CA, USA
[2] California State Senate, California State Capitol, Sacramento, CA, USA
[3] New York Medical College, New York, NY, USA

PREVALENCE OF SUBSTANCE USE AMONG JUVENILE OFFENDERS

The prevalence of mental health problems among youths is growing at an alarming rate. According to the 2001 Surgeon General's Report on Children's Mental Health, 1 in 10 youths in the United States suffers from mental illness severe enough to cause some level of impairment. However, in any given year, only about one in five youths receives mental health services [1]. Equally concerning is the rate of substance use among youths. A study of 12th-graders revealed that close to half (48.2%) had used illicit drugs at some point in their lives, and 22% reported use in the month prior to the study [2]. Data from youths, ages 12 to 17 years old, who participated in a national study by the Substance Abuse and Mental Health Services Administration (SAMHSA) showed that the substance abuse disorder rate for youths was 8%, but for those youths who had resided in a juvenile detention facility, the rate was 23.8% [3]. Of those detained, around 9% indicated current use of any illicit drugs, and 7.6% met criteria for substance abuse or dependence. Adding to the concern, the results from the 2009 Monitoring the Future study showed that the proportion of youths using any illicit drug had risen over the previous two years, and youths involved with the juvenile justice system had the highest rates of substance abuse and dependence [4]. In light of these statistics, an examination of the substance use and mental health problems of youths in juvenile detention facilities is warranted.

PREVALENCE OF JUVENILE DETAINEES WITH SUBSTANCE USE DISORDERS

The rate of youth involvement with the juvenile justice system is staggering. According to Puzzanchera and Sickmund, more than 31 million US youths were under juvenile court jurisdiction in 2005 [5]. More than 104 000 juveniles are held in juvenile placement facilities on a given day, either awaiting trial in detention centers or having been placed in residential facilities after being adjudicated delinquent [6–10]. Many others are supervised by juvenile probation officers after referral to the juvenile court. Over 60% of these youths are from racial or ethnic minorities [6]. Notably, the most recent annual estimates from the US Department of Justice show that of the approximately 2.4 million juvenile arrests each year, more than 203 000 are for drug charges [8,11]. Given these findings, a review of the substance use patterns and risk factors for substance abuse among youths involved with the juvenile justice system is needed.

On many levels, the relationship between adolescent substance abuse and delinquency is straightforward. It is well established that substance use is associated with increased risk for delinquency and higher rates of recidivism; reducing adolescent substance abuse reduces juvenile crime [12]. In many jurisdictions the majority of juveniles who enter the justice system are substance users, and research indicates that adolescent substance use is strongly associated with chronic and violent

Clinical Handbook of Adolescent Addiction, First Edition. Richard Rosner.
© 2013 John Wiley & Sons, Ltd. Published 2013 by John Wiley & Sons, Ltd.

delinquent behavior, which can persist into adulthood. Juvenile drug use is also strongly linked with other risk factors that increase delinquency. These include poor health outcomes, familial conflict, and deterioration in social, academic, and psychological functioning [12]. The rates of substance abuse in the juvenile justice system are significantly higher than in the general population, and this is particularly true for youths who are detained. The data for 2006 showed that among young offenders who were detained, 56% of boys and 40% of girls tested positive for drugs [13]. One study found that about one-half of both male and female juvenile detainees met criteria for a substance use disorder [8].

It is important to note that while many young offenders may test positive for illicit drugs and have problematic drug-related behaviors, not all young offenders require formal substance abuse treatment. This is especially true given the paucity of available treatment slots relative to the high level of need. Staff ratios in detention facilities (mental health clinicians to young offenders) highlight this gap even further. One study found that while approximately one in three young offenders taken into custody was in need of substance abuse treatment, there were only enough treatment slots for one in six of these young offenders. Better screening to identify young offenders who need formal substance abuse treatment is necessary. To meet the high volume of treatment needs, most facilities rely on drug education as the most common form of substance abuse intervention, yet this has been found to be largely ineffective in reduction of substance abuse [6].

TYPES OF SUBSTANCES USED

It has been established that substance use is a concern for youths, and especially problematic for youths who have been involved with the juvenile justice system. Roberts *et al*. examined a sample of 4175 youths from Houston. Alcohol and marijuana were found to be among the most popular substances abused by adolescents, with a higher prevalence of abuse or dependence among males compared to females [14]. For youths within the juvenile justice system, around one-half met clinical criteria for alcohol or other drug disorders [15]. A study by Deas looked at data from multiple surveys and reported that alcohol was the most commonly abused substance among adolescents, and associated with abuse or dependence of illicit drugs such as marijuana [16]. A 2006 study funded by the Office of Juvenile Justice and Delinquency found that of a sample of 1829 detained youths, 28.3% of 13-year-olds, 51.3% of 14–15-year-olds, and 54.4% of male youths aged 16 years and older

had a substance use disorder. Of the female participants, 30.5% of 13-year-olds, 45.8% of 14–15-year-olds, and 52% of youths aged 16 years and older had a substance use disorder [8]. Another study of 1742 detained juveniles found that 77.3% of participants reported using any substance over the past year, and 90.1% reported lifetime use [11].

While marijuana has been cited as the most widely used illicit drug for youths in general, substance use patterns for youths who have had involvement with the juvenile justice system indicate concurrent use of multiple substances [2,8]. In a study examining the drug use and related perceptions of 292 young offenders, nearly 25% had used drugs from nine or more drug groupings. Alcohol (94.8%), analgesics (94.5%), and nicotine (92.4%) were the drugs most used, with 86.6% having used cannabis, 53.3% stimulants, 48.5% inhalants, 40.5% hallucinogens, and 25.8% narcotics. The major reasons given for use were: wanting to feel good, curiosity, and boredom [17].

Nationally, while the use of methamphetamine ("ice," "crystal," "glass," "tina") has been on the rise and associated with delinquent and non-law-abiding behavior, studies that examine the clinical and judicial outcomes of young offenders who abuse methamphetamine are limited. Whereas most of the existing literature focuses on young adults, aged 18–26, crystal methamphetamine use is increasingly becoming a concern for the juvenile justice system. Western states in particular continue to struggle with the consequences of methamphetamine use. In January 2008, the Idaho Meth Project released the results of its Statewide Meth Use & Attitudes Survey, which indicated that young people in that state continue to be at grave risk from methamphetamine abuse [18]. There are innumerable adverse psychiatric and medical effects from methamphetamine use, including but not limited to mood disturbances, psychosis, irritability, cognitive impairment, cardiovascular problems, hyperthermia, and convulsions [19–21]. Methamphetamine use also has a very high correlation (even in comparison to other illicit substances) with high-risk behavior, including risky sexual behavior, violence, crime, and interaction with law enforcement. More specifically, methamphetamine use was also associated with concurrent illicit drug use such as marijuana, cocaine/crack, hallucinogens, and pain relievers [21,22], and with previous criminal justice system involvement such as probation [21,23] and prior arrests [22]. High rates of criminal behaviors (previous arrests, drug sales, violence) have been found among methamphetamine treatment clients [24] as well as in non-random community samples of methamphetamine users [25,26].

CO-OCCURRING CONDITIONS

The high rate of substance use among youths involved with the juvenile justice system is startling, and the findings about the co-occurring conditions that these youths are at risk for are equally disturbing. Estimates provided by both state and local juvenile justice facilities throughout the United States indicate that juvenile offenders have significant mental health treatment needs. A study by the Virginia Department of Juvenile Justice showed that more than 40% of males and almost 60% of females in detention homes were in need of mental health services; more than 7% of males and more than 15% of females had urgent mental health treatment needs [27]. Epidemiological studies estimate that between two-thirds and three-quarters of detained youths have one or more psychiatric disorders, and more than 15% of detained youths have major mental disorders (e.g., affective disorders, psychosis) and associated functional impairments [8–10]. A growing body of research suggests that many of these youths meet criteria for at least one mental disorder and that at least one in five has a serious mental disorder, often coupled with a co-occurring substance use disorder [28,29]. Also concerning is the fact that racial or ethnic minorities, females, and homosexual youths are most vulnerable to mistreatment and mismanagement among those suffering from mental health and substance abuse problems [30].

Research indicates that substance use disorders and behavioral disorders (conduct disorder, oppositional defiant disorder, and attention-deficit/hyperactivity disorder) are most common among adolescents in the juvenile systems [8,31]. One study found that almost one-half of males and females detained in Cook County had a substance use disorder, and 60% of these youths had mental health disorders [8]. Furthermore, among this same population, 30% of females and 20% of males with any substance use disorder had significantly higher odds of having a comorbid mental disorder, especially among those who used alcohol or marijuana [31]. For most of these youths, the diagnoses of both mental disorder and substance use disorder occurred during the same year. Deas found that the number of comorbid diagnoses was greater for adolescents with substance dependence, rather than substance abuse, and this trend was more pronounced for those with four or more comorbid diagnoses [16]. Roberts *et al.* also reported that adolescents with comorbidity had increased odds of functional impairment. This is an important finding, which supports the salience of recognizing the risk factors contributing to substance use among this population [14].

RISK FACTORS FOR SUBSTANCE USE DISORDERS

Multiple studies have investigated features associated with substance abuse in juvenile offenders. A large body of research has clearly shown that substance abuse in juveniles is associated with a significant range of problems, including academic difficulties, mental health and medical issues, peer relationship difficulties, and involvement with the juvenile justice system [32]. Poor grades, school truancy, and early termination of education are correlated with juvenile substance abuse. Cognitive and behavioral problems associated with alcohol and drug use may also interfere with academic performance [33]. Among adolescents in the justice system, data also suggest that substance use is higher in individuals who possess impulsive characteristics compared to their non-impulsive counterparts [34]. Comorbid substance abuse problems and psychiatric diagnoses are associated with worse outcomes, poorer quality of life, and increased recidivism among juvenile delinquents [8,35].

The unmet need for mental health and substance abuse services for detained youths has drawn considerable attention to the risk factors that predispose youths to substance abuse. Court-involved youths with disabilities appear to be at the greatest risk for treatment failure. Youths with criminal behavior, from low-income and minority backgrounds (two-thirds of youths with disabilities are poor minority children), those not attending school or educational programs (youths with learning and behavioral disabilities have the greatest rate of school dropout), and those who have psychological or learning problems have the poorest outcomes [36]. Typically, male youths with less family involvement and a family history of substance use have greater risk of abusing substances and involvement in the juvenile justice system. The combination of these risk factors indicates that the juvenile justice system must employ practices to address the complex needs of youths who are served by their systems.

SCREENING AND ASSESSMENT OF SUBSTANCE USE DISORDERS IN DETAINED YOUTHS

Screening

Given the high prevalence of young offenders with some degree of substance use, every adolescent should receive screening for the presence of substance use disorders at the time of arrest or upon entering a detention facility. Considering the concordance of mental health and substance use disorders, all adolescents who are receiving mental health treatment also warrant screening for substance use disorders. Screening for substance use disorders and their potential associated problems should also be routine practice for probation staff, who often are the first point of contact with law enforcement for youthful offenders, and who may have discretionary power to grant diversion to treatment programs.

The Substance Abuse and Mental Health Services Administration (SAMSHA) Center for Substance Abuse Treatment (CSAT) protocol recommends that substance use screening and assessment activities begin as early as possible during the youth's contact with the juvenile justice system, preferably within the first 24 hours. Additionally, it is recommended that youths receive ongoing screening and assessment at different stages (intake, pre-, and post-adjudication) while under jurisdiction of the juvenile justice system [37].

Screening is the critical preliminary step in determining whether a youth may or may not have problematic drug use. Utilization of screening tools that are targeted and brief (less than 30 minutes, and ideally 10–15 minutes) is essential given the time constraints and staffing issues that pose ongoing challenges for many detention facilities. The ideal screening tool is brief, simple, and developmentally and age appropriate. The screening tool should also provide a broad assessment, and be sufficient at extracting potential warning signs such as academic decline or new-onset truancy that would warrant further assessment from the evaluator.

Although a detailed review of the different inventories is beyond the scope of this chapter, examples of youth screening instruments include the following [37]:

- Adolescent Drinking Index (ADI)
- Adolescent Drug Involvement Scale (ADIS)
- Drug and Alcohol Problem (DAP) Quick Screen
- Drug Use Screening Inventory–Revised (DUSI-R)
- Personal Experience Screening Questionnaire (PESQ)
- Problem Oriented Screening Instrument for Teenagers (POSIT)
- Rutgers Alcohol Problem Index (RAPI)
- Teen Addiction Severity Index (T-ASI)

SAMSHA recommends that screening and assessment efforts should be explored through five categories: preliminary screening, risk assessment, drug testing/urinalysis, psychosocial assessment, and comprehensive assessment. During the preliminary screening, identification of acute intoxication and withdrawal, suicidality, and any other immediate medical or psychological needs is of primary concern.

Selecting screening tools that can be easily used by both clinical and non-clinical staff (such as probation staff) is especially important given the limited resources that characterize most detention facilities. One principal goal of the screening process is to triage the level of substance abuse and determine whether a more formal and comprehensive assessment is warranted. Additionally, effective screening enables the evaluator to begin to explore the presence of the myriad associated legal, academic, family, and social problems that are common to young offenders with substance use problems. Developing a baseline understanding of the presence of any of these issues will assist the evaluator in determining the degree and severity of substance use and accordingly determine the need for more comprehensive assessment.

Assessment

The comprehensive assessment is the second step in the trajectory of substance use disorder evaluation and management. The goal of the comprehensive assessment is to elicit more in-depth information that can facilitate the development of an appropriate treatment plan and determine the level of care required to implement the plan.

Additional tasks for the evaluator are to analyze the interplay between the substance use disorder and any associated mental health conditions. Identification of co-occurring mental health disorders is critical. Determining the degree to which each disorder interferes with functioning helps shape the treatment plan. Failure to identify and effectively treat co-occurring mental health disorders can limit the viability of treatment interventions.

One particular challenge is that while the DSM-IV-TR (*Diagnostic and Statistical Manual of Mental Disorders, Fourth Edition, Text Revision*) gives clear criteria for many disorders in childhood and adolescence, the diagnostic criteria for substance use disorders were developed with adult bias and norms. To date, there is no diagnostic classification in the DSM-IV-TR for evaluating the frequency, intensity, and duration of substance use problems in children and adolescents. Despite the fact that many youths fail to meet the specific DSM-IV-TR criteria for diagnoses of substance abuse or substance dependence disorders, they continue to have problematic substance use that interferes with day-to-day functioning across multiple life domains. The lack of specific child- and adolescent-driven criteria for the diagnostic classification of substance use disorders also highlights the importance of using standardized structured or semi-structured instruments during the assessment process. The distinction between diagnosing substance use problems in

Table 40.1 Frequency of substance usage over time.

Type of Substance	Never	AGE AT FIRST USE	1 YEAR AGO	PAST YEAR	PAST MONTH	PAST WEEK	DAILY USE	AMOUNT USED EACH TIME
Tobacco								
Alcohol								
Marijuana								
Cocaine/crack								
Inhalants								
Amphetamines								
Hallucinogens								
Tranquilizers								
Opiates								
Prescription drugs								
Over-the-counter								
Other								

the child and adolescent population versus the adult population, further underscores the importance of gathering additional data regarding functioning in other domains to assist in determining the severity of the problems.

Examples of commonly used instruments for the evaluation and comprehensive assessment of substance use disorders in children and adolescents are listed below [37].

- Adolescent Drug Abuse Diagnosis (ADAD)
- Adolescent Diagnostic Interview (ADI)
- Adolescent Self-Assessment Profile (ASAP)
- The American Drug and Alcohol Survey (ADAS)
- The Chemical Dependency Assessment Profile (CDAP)
- Comprehensive Adolescent Severity Inventory (CASI)
- Hilson Adolescent Profile (HAP)
- Juvenile Automated Substance Abuse Evaluation (JASAE)
- Personal Experience Inventory (PEI)
- Prototype Screening/Triage form for Juvenile Detention Centers
- The Texas Christian Inventory Prevention intervention Management and Evaluation System (TCU/PMES)

As a general rule, interviews with adolescents regarding substance use should, in any setting, be performed without the parents present. For a variety of reasons, many adolescents tend to under-report and minimize their substance use. Parental presence during this

sensitive interview encounter may hinder the dialog and potential disclosure even further. Many clinicians approach the task of evaluating the presence of a substance use disorder in this population haphazardly, often with limited and vague questioning that barely skims the surface. Questions like "Do you ever use drugs?" are overly simplistic and run the risk of eliciting false negatives from young offenders who may be wary of disclosing illegal activity to an evaluator. While asking about every category of substance may seem tedious, it is the only way to obtain accurate information about the adolescent's degree of substance involvement. Table 40.1 is designed to provide the clinician with a blueprint for exploring the components of commonly abused substances in the adolescent population.

Many clinicians who work in detention facilities face the challenge of acting as a "double agent." While clinicians ethically are bound to the "first do no harm" duties inherent in the doctor-patient relationship, providing care in correctional settings places implicit demands on clinicians to balance confidentiality with public safety and reports to court, attorneys, and other correctional staff. While probably unaware of the complexity and nuances of these dynamics, many adolescents may identify their clinicians in these settings as part of the authoritarian power structure and therefore may have difficulty in establishing a therapeutic rapport. It is recommended that clinicians review and establish the limits of confidentiality during the assessment. It is important to ensure that sufficient rapport has been established with the youth and his or her family. Questions about substance use should be asked in neutral tone and embedded into the overall assessment. Youths are

Table 40.2 Additional questions for the evaluation of substance use disorders.

Areas of concern	Additional information to be explored
Determining the context of use	Who is it used with? Where is it used? At what times is it used? How is the substance obtained?
Perceptions about the benefits of use	What feelings does it give? What do you like about it?
Insight about the negative consequences of use	Have you had problems in school? Have you had problems in your relationships with family and/or peer groups?
Attempts to control use	Have you ever tried to cut down or limit your use? Has anyone been concerned about your drinking or other drug use or suggested cutting down? Have you ever told someone that you don't have a substance use problem but at the same time you questioned yourself that maybe you do have a problem?

apt to be more candid in a non-judgmental atmosphere. The tasks of completing paperwork and broaching specific topics may need to be two different events as pacing of the interview questions is important. After obtaining basic information regarding the type of substances used and their frequency and duration of use, it is important to methodically obtain additional data on other contextual factors of use. Table 40.2 provides suggestions as to other relevant topics to be explored in the assessment interview.

While parental presence is not indicated during the actual individual screening and assessment interview with the minor, parental input as a source of collateral information is essential. Many adolescents have limited appreciation of the various difficulties they may have been having, and how these difficulties may be impacted by substance use. Similarly, parents are often able to provide a wealth of historical and contextual data that may assist the evaluators in determining the severity and

presence of onset behaviors. The participation of parent (s) and/or caregiver(s) in the comprehensive assessment process also represents a valuable opportunity to provide psychoeducation about the associated consequences of substance use, and potential areas and warning signs to which they should be attentive in the future. Parents and caregivers are vital partners in the treatment and rehabilitation process. Therefore, increasing their competency and knowledge in this area can further optimize the viability of treatment interventions.

TREATMENT APPROACHES

Since most detained juveniles with substance abuse issues have an array of other challenges, any effective intervention must be multi-targeted, integrated, and coordinated in order to have lasting impact. Thus, recent research has focused on developing comprehensive programs that simultaneously target a constellation of social and psychological issues, instead of attempting to address them in isolation from one another.

Differences Between Community-Based Treatment and Institutionally Based Treatment

It may seem to be a logical assumption that most of the substance abuse programs utilized for juveniles in detention environments would be equivalent to programs that are effective in the outpatient environment [38]. However, the population of juvenile detainees has unique needs and characteristics related to the origins of delinquent behavior, as well as the distinctive environment of the detention facility itself. Therefore, because of the special needs of both the population and the detention facility, community-based programs must be tailored to reflect the differing reality and circumstances in the correctional setting.

While shifting the effective programmatic treatment models from the outpatient clinic-based setting to the detention-based setting makes sense on some levels, the different environments demand that the clinical interventions be modified to compensate for challenges inherent in each setting. For example, in a detention center, an adolescent may not have the family and community support generally required to facilitate his or her substance abuse recovery. He or she may be contending with educational deficits or delays, and social and familial isolation. An effective substance abuse program in the detention environment must therefore consider and compensate for these factors that may predispose the adolescent offender to continued substance abuse. Only programs that address multiple social and systemic factors while treating substance abuse will ultimately be effective for this population.

Although it is logistically possible to offer some of the components of effective community, evidence-based practices to the detention environment, research surveys have found that the most effective community practices are often not provided in detention facilities. Furthermore, even if they are offered, the services are frequently not accessed by the adolescents in detention. One study compared substance abuse treatment of juvenile offenders in the community versus in an institutional setting. In this study, the authors found that there were significant differences in the implementation of effective evidence-based practices between community and institutional settings. Institutional settings implemented fewer evidence-based practices than did the community-based programs. Community programs were more likely to have staff qualified to provide substance abuse treatment, involve families in treatment, and assess their treatment outcomes. Institutional programs were more likely to provide comprehensive services. Interestingly, both settings were found to have programs that were not developmentally organized, a characteristic that has been shown to be crucial to effective treatment of children and adolescents. The researchers also found that a connection between the treatment setting and non-criminal justice facilities was associated with higher levels of evidence-based treatment [39].

Access to, and continuation of, treatment services by juvenile detainees are two critical elements related to substance abuse interventional success in the juvenile justice population. A research group surveyed facilities in the institutional and community correctional systems, such as residential facilities, local jails, community correctional offices, and detention centers. Across all of these settings, "drug and alcohol education" was the most frequently offered substance abuse intervention (73% of facilities), but the least intensive approach. Across this survey of 141 juvenile institutional and community correctional facilities, the second most common treatment intervention was brief (1–4 hours), weekly substance abuse group counseling, an intervention that 40% of the facilities provided. Thirty-two percent of facilities offered relapse prevention treatment, and 21% offered case management. Approximately only 20% of facilities provided more intensive treatment, comprising 5–25 hours each week, with 18% offering a segregated treatment community model [40].

Many detained youths do not avail themselves of the substance abuse treatment provided. In the aforementioned study, only 13% attended the brief group counseling, and just 1% were engaged in the more time-intensive treatment. These low percentages should be interpreted against the high prevalence of substance abuse disorders in this population. The study also found that both prevalence and access to substance abuse services were highest in residential detention facilities, as contrasted with community correctional centers such as jails, detention centers, and probation offices. Residential facilities were the most likely settings to provide effective substance abuse treatment when long term (90 days). The duration of treatment was much briefer in jails and outpatient settings [40].

The authors of this study point out that they found comparatively high rates of substance abuse treatment offered in long-term residential facilities and lower rates of provision in jails, detention centers, and probation offices, the latter group being the sites where juveniles are first introduced to the juvenile justice system. Although research has demonstrated that the most effective treatment interventions are those that are provided in the early stages of delinquency, the fact that most interventions are received in the latter stages of a juvenile's passage through the juvenile justice system is problematic [41].

This study also revealed that there are significant differences in aftercare referrals to substance abuse services depending on the type of setting in which the adolescent is housed. Assessment of the critical factor of re-entry care after release from detention showed that 51% of substance-abusing juveniles were referred to a community treatment provider at discharge. This referral percentage was 31% when a juvenile was released from jail. Post-discharge substance treatment appointments were made for 55% of juveniles in residential facilities while appointments were made for only 24% of juveniles released from jail [40]. The above findings indicate that although youths released from detention centers are highly vulnerable to relapse and recidivism, they receive fewer referrals to much needed substance abuse follow-up and aftercare treatment.

Evidence-Based Substance Abuse Treatment in the Correctional Setting

The identification and deployment of effective, evidence-based substance abuse treatments in the correctional setting is crucial. Research and consensus reports on evidence-based practices for the treatment of substance abuse disorders in juvenile correctional facilities have identified specific elements found to be critical to treatment success [42].

These components include appropriate initial substance abuse screening and assessment techniques, systems integration, treatments that utilize cognitive-behavioral and family-based modalities, and the employment of a developmentally informed perspective. Other evidence-based practices for this population are the use of effective motivation, engagement, and retention techniques; graduated sanctions and incentives for program non-compliance or adherence; and the use of standard risk assessment tools. Additional evidence-based components include drug testing, treatment for a minimum of 90 days, family involvement in treatment, diagnosis and treatment of comorbid disorders, and comprehensive treatment integration by qualified staff. Finally, there should be fluid and consistent re-entry services upon discharge from detention and a multi-system continuing service plan, along with assessments of treatment outcomes [43].

Studies have also demonstrated that among detained juvenile offenders, several factors were associated with greater recovery from substance abuse. These factors included increased integrity of treatment implementation, long duration of treatment, focus on development of interpersonal skills, and family education and involvement [44].

Specific forms of intensive treatment have been studied to determine their effect on preventing antisocial behavior and substance abuse. Multi-systemic therapy (MST) has been demonstrated to reduce the rates of arrests, psychiatric symptoms, and drug use in a population of juveniles with serious antisocial behavior [45]. Multi-systemic therapy targets the risks for antisocial behavior that reside in the adolescent, his or her family, and the larger environment of his or her home. A meta-analysis demonstrated that adolescents treated with MST functioned 70% better than youths treated with other interventions, resulting in lower rates of criminal activity, truancy, and substance use. These beneficial effects appeared to be sustained for 4 years after treatment [46]. Functional family therapy (FFT) and multidimensional treatment foster care programs have also been shown to reduce delinquent behaviors in a juvenile population with psychiatric and substance abuse disorders [47].

Multivalent, systemic treatment approaches to substance abuse in the juvenile offender population have been examined, including the Reclaiming Futures project, which is currently underway at multiple sites across the United States. It is based on a theory of change that states that the entire community must be restructured and reorganized to solve the problem of drug abuse in the juvenile justice population. The project is "defined as a team of professionals, relevant systems, and community members who provide comprehensive, individualized substance abuse treatment and related services to youth within the juvenile justice system." This approach prioritizes "mobilizing a wide range of resources across every sector of the offender's life, as well as relevant

programs" [47]. The interventions exist on every level, from the adolescent, to the juvenile justice facility, to the wider community.

When taking the multi-system approach to substance abuse treatment delivery in this population, another necessary step is to evaluate the characteristics that predispose a correctional facility to adopt evidence-based practices of substance abuse treatment, as well as the characteristics that lead to substance abuse treatment prioritization. Certain characteristics of correctional facilities have been shown to predict their adoption of evidence-based substance abuse treatments. These traits include positive organizational structure, positive organizational climate, open administrator attitudes; training opportunities for staff; adequate funding; and system network interconnectivity [48]. One study found a correlative link between a facility administrator's high prioritization of substance abuse treatment versus other detention programs, and the amount of evidence-based substance abuse programs employed in that facility [49]. Other findings show that greater program staff turnover and older age of the substance program are correlated with worse treatment outcomes in this population [50].

Evidence-Based Treatment Modified to Optimize its Efficacy in the Correctional Environment

Multidimensional Family Therapy (MDFT) is an effective, family-focused dual diagnosis program that addresses adolescent substance abuse and comorbid emotional and delinquency problems, and serves as one example of one treatment modified for optimum efficacy in the correctional environment [51]. This model, which combines substance abuse treatment, family systems therapy, and individual therapy, has been shown to be effective for adolescent substance abuse [52].

One study linked the MDFT program with other targeted interventions modified for the juvenile detained population. This two-stage study, which followed juveniles during their detention and also after their release from custody, included a prevention program for sexually transmitted diseases (STDs), including HIV, as well as an "in-detention module" to intensively monitor for any criminal behavior along with focused therapeutic effort toward the possibility of behavioral change. The STD arm of the intervention was included on the premise that substance-using juvenile offenders are at high risk of infection by HIV and other sexually transmitted diseases.

Each juvenile was assigned a therapist who was in charge of targeting all three arms of this intervention, substance use, HIV/STD risk, and criminal behavior, with the therapist remaining in that role until 4 months after release, with the addition of family therapy, STD prevention, and case management. Therapists in this program work "simultaneously in four interdependence treatment domains – the adolescent, parent, family, and extrafamilial (domains)" [53]. In each of these areas, there are three stages – building a foundation for change, facilitating change in the juvenile and family, and solidifying the changes, "launching" the family into the greater world. To these aims, the MDFT therapists attended school and court hearings with the juvenile and family.

Compared to a control group receiving "enhanced services as usual," the MDFT-Detention to Community (DTC) study participants demonstrated superior treatment enrollment and retention (a major issue with most substance abuse programs for adolescents), and more satisfaction with the treatment, as expressed by the juveniles and their families. This model also demonstrated greater cross-system professional collaboration between the substance abuse treatment provider and the juvenile justice system.

With organized coordination, this study was structured to link substance abuse treatment in detention centers with this population's special need for post-detention community reintegration [53]. The study researchers described the program as requiring "consistency of effort between the clinician and family and stakeholders from juvenile probation, the public defender's office, state attorneys, and juvenile court judges to support youths' treatment participation, reduce recidivism, retain the youth in the juvenile system, and avoid or delay transfer to the adult system" [53].

For any sustainable, cross-system, MDFT-based intervention, the challenges are numerous, as this type of program requires funding to support robust connections between systems, and requires adequate staffing and available time for personnel to comprehensively monitor the juvenile as the transition is made from detention to the outside environment. The greater degree of cross-system communication and integration is one of the essential ingredients for successful substance abuse treatment with detained juveniles, as compared with children and adolescents in the community.

FUTURE CONSIDERATIONS

Despite the many federal mandates for improving mental health, substance abuse treatment, and outcomes for detained young offenders, numerous challenges remain that limit the implementation of evidenced-based treatment models for this population in the detention setting. Among those challenges is the minimal staffing level of mental health professionals in these settings. Unfortunately, the staff-to-patient ratio is such that the viability of many of the more intensive multimodal and multi-disciplinary treatment models, which have demonstrated good efficacy, is limited. Additionally, because many youths have unpredictable lengths of stay and can be transferred amongst different facilities once they are detained, disruption in the continuity of care poses an even greater challenge to the implementation of long-term treatment for those with substance use disorders. Although limited in its efficacy, the mainstay of detention-based treatment is the model that combines stabilization and management of acute intoxication/withdrawal states with group-based programs that provide drug education. Using more of a medical model and shifting the focus to discharge and aftercare planning *prior* to a minor's re-entry to his or her community is critical. Once a minor is released, barriers to accessing meaningful mental health and substance abuse aftercare in the community are significant and necessitate action. Sadly, many young offenders experience significant lag times between release and their first follow-up appointment. This period before accessing services is a key intervention time, when newly released youths are particularly vulnerable. Suggested alternate approaches to consider include extending the focus toward long-term management of substance use disorders throughout the range of judicial placements, with an emphasis on identifying appropriate treatment referrals prior to release and linkage to community-based drug treatment programs immediately upon release.

References

1. US Public Health Services, Office of the Surgeon General. *Report of the Surgeon General's Conference on Children's Mental Health*. Rockville, MD: US Department of Health and Human Services, 2001.
2. Johnston LD, O'Malley PM, Bachman JG, Schulenberg JE. Teen marijuana use tilts up, while some drugs decline in use. National Press Release. Ann Arbor, MI: University of Michigan News Service, 2009.
3. Substance Use and Mental Health Services Administration. *Substance Use, Abuse, and Dependence Among Youths who Have Been in Jail or a Detention Center. National Survey on Drug Use and Health Report*. Rockville, MD: Substance Abuse and Mental Health Services Administration, Center for Substance Abuse Treatment; Office of Applied Studies, 2004.
4. Johnston LD, O'Malley PM, Bachman JG, Schulenberg JE. *Monitoring the Future: National Results on Adolescent Drug Use*. Bethesda, MD: US Department of Health and Human Services, National Institutes of Health, National Institute on Drug Abuse, 2009.
5. Puzzanchera C, Sickmund M. *Juvenile Court Statistics 2005*. Washington, DC: US Department of Justice, Office

of Justice Programs, Office of Juvenile Justice and Delinquency Prevention, 2008.

6. Sickmund M. *Juveniles in Corrections*. Washington, DC: US Department of Justice, Office of Justice Programs, Office of Juvenile Justice and Delinquency Prevention, 2005.

7. Snyder HN. *Juvenile Arrests 2000*. Washington, DC: US Department of Justice, Office of Justice Programs, Office of Juvenile Justice and Delinquency Prevention, 2002.

8. Teplin LA, Abram KM, McClelland GM, *et al*. Psychiatric disorders in youth in juvenile detention. *Arch Gen Psychiatry* 2002;**59**:1133–1143.

9. Teplin LA, Abram KM, McClelland GM, *et al*. Detecting mental disorder in juvenile detainees: Who receives services? *Am J Pub Health* 2005;**95**:1773–1780.

10. Wasserman GA, McReynolds LS, Lucas CP, *et al*. The voice DISC–IV with incarcerated male youths: Prevalence of disorder. *J Am Acad Child Adolesc Psychiatry* 2002;**41**:314–321.

11. McClelland GM, Elkington KS, Teplin LA, Abram KM. Multiple substance use disorders in juvenile detainees. *J Am Acad Child Adolesc Psychiatry* 2004;**43**:1215–1224.

12. VanderWaal CJ, McBride DC, Terry-McAElrath YM, VanBruen H. *Breaking the Juvenile Drug-Crime Cycle: A Guide for Practitioners and Policy-makers*. Washington, DC: US Department of Justice, Office of Justice Programs, National Institute of Justice, 2001.

13. Chassin L. Juvenile justice and substance use. *Future Child* 2008;**18**:165–185.

14. Roberts R, Roberts C, Yun X. Comorbidity of substance use and other psychiatric disorders among adolescents: Evidence from an epidemiological survey. *Drug Alcohol Depend* 2007;**88**:513–516.

15. National Center on Addiction and Substance Abuse at Columbia University. *National Survey of American Attitudes on Substance Abuse VX: Teens and Parents*. New York: National Center on Addiction and Substance Abuse at Columbia University, 2010.

16. Deas D. Adolescent substance abuse and psychiatric comorbidities. *J Clin Psychiatry* 2006;**67**:18–23.

17. Howard J, Zibert E. Curious, bored and wanting to feel good: The drug use of detained young offenders. *Drug Alcohol Rev* 1990;**9**:225–231.

18. Idaho Meth Project. *Statewide Meth Use and Attitudes Survey*. Palo Alto, CA: The Meth Project Foundation, 2008.

19. National Institute on Drug Abuse. Methamphetamine use and addiction. NIDA research report. Bethesda, MD: National Institutes of Health, 2006. Available from: http://drugabuse.gov/researchreports/methamph/methamph.html.

20. National Institute on Drug Abuse. InfoFacts: Methamphetamine. Bethesda, MD: National Institutes of Health, 2010. Available from: http://drugabuse.gov/infofacts/methamphetamine.html.

21. Iritani BJ, Hallfors DD, Bauer DJ. Crystal methamphetamine use among young adults in the USA. *Addiction* 2007;**102**:1102–1113.

22. Wu LT, Schlenger WE, Galvin DM. Concurrent use of methamphetamine, MDMA, LSD, ketamine, GHB, and flunitrazepam among American youths. *Drug Alcohol Depend* 2006;**84**:102–113.

23. Substance Abuse and Mental Health Services Administration. *Results from National Survey on Drug Use and Health Findings*. Rockville, MD: Substance Abuse and Mental Health Services Administration, Office of Applied Studies, 2005.

24. Brecht ML, O'Brien A, vonMayrhauser C, Anglin MD. Methamphetamine use behaviors and gender differences. *Addict Behav* 2004;**29**:89–106.

25. Sommers I, Baskin D, Baskin-Sommers A. Methamphetamine use among young adults: Health and social consequences. *Addict Behav* 2006;**31**:1469–1475.

26. Semple SJ, Grant I, Patterson TL. Female methamphetamine users: Social characteristics and sexual risk behaviors. *Women Health* 2004;**40**:35–50.

27. Virginia Joint Commission for Behavioral Health Care. Studying treatment options for offenders who have mental illness or substance abuse disorders; Senate document 25. Virginia State Crime Commission and Virginia Commission on Youth, 2002. Available at: http://leg2.state.va.us/DLS/h&sdocs.nsf/a762cd2685f84d7a85256f0300531 96e/5f89aeb84aa01eba85256bc1004544fd?

28. Cocozza JJ, Shufelt JL. *Juvenile Mental Health Courts: An Emerging Strategy*. Delmar, NY: National Center for Mental Health and Juvenile Justice, 2006.

29. Grisso T. *Double Jeopardy: Adolescent Offenders with Mental Disorders*. Chicago: University of Chicago Press, 2004.

30. Hubner J, Wolfson J. *Handle With Care: Serving the Mental Health Needs of Young Offenders; Annual report*. Washington, DC: Coalition for Juvenile Justice, 2000.

31. Abram KM, Teplin LA, McClelland GM. Comorbid psychiatric disorders in youth in juvenile detention. *Arch Gen Psychiatry* 2003;**60**:1097–1108.

32. Crowe AH, Bilchik S. *Drug Facts*. Washington, DC: Office of National Drug Control Policy, 1998.

33. McCluske C, Krohn MD, Lizotte AH, Rodriguez ML. Early substance abuse and school achievement: An examination of Latino, White, and African American youth. *J Drug Issues* 2002;**32**:921–943.

34. Turner AP, Larimer ME, Sarason IG, Trupin EW. Identifying a negative mood subtype in incarcerated adolescents: Relationship to substance use. *Addict Behav* 2005;**30**:1442–1448.

35. Abrantes AM, Brown SA, Tomlinson KL. Psychiatric comorbidity among inpatient substance abusing adolescents. *J Child Adolesc Subst Abuse* 2003;**13**:83–101.

36. Hird S, Khuri E, Dusenbury L, Millman R. Adolescents. In: Lowenson J, Ruiz P, Milman R, Langrod J (eds), *Substance Abuse: A Comprehensive Textbook*. Baltimore, MD: Williams & Wilkins, 1996.

37. Winters, KC. Treatment improvement protocol (TIP) series 31: Screening and assessing adolescents for substance use disorders. DHHS Publication No. (SMA) 99-3282. Rockville, MD: Substance Abuse and Mental Health Services Administration, Center for Substance Abuse Treatment, 1999.

38. Becker SJ, Curry JF. Outpatient interventions for adolescent substance abuse: A quality of evidence review. *J Consult Clin Psychol* 2008;**76**:531–543.

39. Henderson CE, Young DW, Jainchill N, Hawke J, Farkas S, Davis RM. Program use of effective drug abuse treatment practices for juvenile offenders. *J Subst Abuse Treat* 2007;**32**:279–290.

40. Young DW, Dembo R, Henderson CE. A national survey of substance abuse treatment for juvenile offenders. *J Subst Abuse Treat* 2007;**32**:255–266.

41. Butts JA, Mears DP. Reviving juvenile justice in a get-tough era. *Youth Soc* 2001;**33**:169–198.

42. Drug Strategies. *Bridging the Gap: A Guide to Drug Treatment in the Juvenile Justice System*. Washington, DC: Drug Strategies, 2005.

43. Henderson CE, Taxman FS, Young DW. A Rasch model analysis of evidenced based treatment practices used in the juvenile justice system. *Drug Alcohol Depend* 2007;**93**: 163–175.

44. Lipsey MW, Wilson DB. Effective intervention for serious juvenile offenders. In: Loeber R, Farrington DP (eds), *Serious and Violent Juvenile Offenders*. Thousand Oaks, CA: Sage Publications, 1998; pp. 313–345.

45. Henggeler SW, Cunningham PB, Picrel SG, *et al.* Multi-systemic Therapy: An effective violence prevention approach for serious juvenile offenders. *J Adolesc* 1996;**1**:47–61.

46. Curtis NM, Ronan KR, Borduin CM. Multisystemic Treatment: A meta-analysis of outcome studies. *J Fam Psychol* 2004;**18**:411–419.

47. Cuellar AE, Markowitz S, Libby AM. Mental health and substance abuse treatment and juvenile crime. *J Ment Health Policy* 2004;**7**:59–68.

48. Aarons GA, Sawitzky AC. Organization culture and climate and mental health provider attitudes toward evidence based practice. *Psychol Serv* 2006;**3**:61–72.

49. Henderson CE, Taxman FS. Competing values among criminal justice administrators: The importance of substance abuse treatment. *Drug Alcohol Depend* 2008;**103** (S):S7–S16.

50. Dowden C, Latimer J. Providing effective substance abuse treatment for young-offender populations: What works! *Child Adolesc Clin N Am* 2006;**15**:517–537.

51. Liddle HA, Rowe CL, Dakof GA, *et al.* Multi-dimensional family therapy for young adolescent substance abuse: Twelve-month outcomes of a randomized controlled trial. *J Consult Clin Psychol* 2009;**77**:12–25.

52. Waldron HB, Turner CW. Evidence-based psychosocial treatments for adolescent substance abuse. *J Clin Child Adolesc Psychol* 2008;**27**:238–261.

53. Liddle HA, Dakof GA, Henderson C, Rowe C. Implementation outcomes of Multidimensional Family Therapy – Detention to community: A reintegration program for drug-using juvenile detainees. *Int J Offender Ther* 2011;**55**:587–604.

Section Seven

Forensic Considerations

Edited by Robert Lloyd Goldstein

41

Forensic Psychiatry for Adolescent Psychiatrists: An Introduction[1]

Richard Rosner

Forensic Psychiatry Residency Program, New York University School of Medicine;
Forensic Psychiatry Clinic, Bellevue Hospital Center, New York, NY, USA

There is increased public concern about violent youth, and increased political pressure to have juvenile offenders tried in adult courts. Many of the adolescents in the juvenile justice system and in the adult criminal justice system suffer from mental disorders. The interests of adolescent psychiatrists and forensic psychiatrists converge in the assessment and management of troubled teenagers. In order that adolescent psychiatrists may function more effectively on those occasions when they are asked to work in forensic settings or to collaborate with specialists in forensic psychiatry, this chapter will provide adolescent psychiatrists with an introduction to forensic psychiatry – including an explanation of how it differs from therapeutic psychiatry, a four-step conceptual framework for understanding how forensic psychiatrists approach their work (i.e., how to think like a forensic psychiatrist), and an example of how the conceptual framework may be applied to the assessment of whether a teenage defendant is competent to stand trial.

DIFFERENCES BETWEEN FORENSIC PSYCHIATRY AND THERAPEUTIC PSYCHIATRY

"Forensic psychiatry is a subspecialty of psychiatry in which scientific and clinical expertise is applied to legal issues in legal contexts embracing civil, criminal, correctional or legislative matters; forensic psychiatry should be practiced in accordance with guidelines and ethical principles enunciated by the profession of psychiatry" (ref. [1], p. X). This is the definition initially adopted by the American Board of Forensic Psychiatry, Inc. and subsequently adopted by the American Academy of Psychiatry and the Law. Whereas clinical psychiatry is directed to therapeutic issues in healthcare contexts, forensic psychiatry is directed to legal issues in legal contexts. Because the ends of the law differ from the ends of healthcare, forensic psychiatry differs from clinical psychiatry.

In the healthcare context, a relationship exists between the examining clinical psychiatrist (doctor) and the person (patient) who is the focus of his or her examination. In the legal context, there is often no doctor-patient relationship between the examining forensic psychiatrist and the person (defendant/appellant/claimant/litigant) who is the focus of the examination. Because there is no doctor-patient relationship, the forensic psychiatrist has an ethical obligation (and often a legal obligation) to clarify for the examinee the nature of the forensic examination (i.e., at minimum, by whom he or she has been employed, what the legal purpose of the evaluation is, that no confidentiality of communications exists, and that the forensic psychiatrist is not necessarily concerned with doing what will be of assistance to the person being examined). This ethical obligation to clarify the nature of the forensic examination is important because, regardless of who has paid for the physician's time and skills, most people have come to expect that a physician is going to help them, that a physician will keep their communications in confidence, and that a physician's primary concern is the best interests of the patient.

[1]Introduction to Forensic psychiatry for adolescent psychiatrists. Previously published as "Forensic Psychiatry for Adolescent Psychiatrists: an Introduction" in Adolescent Psychiatry, Volume 24, Analytic Press, Hillsboro, NJ, 1999, and reprinted her with their kind permission.

Forensic psychiatry is not unique in medicine in having obligations in addition to, or other than, the welfare of the individual as a patient. All physicians have a societal obligation to report gunshot wounds and child abuse to the proper legal authorities. To ensure the scientific integrity of their work, research psychiatrists may properly withhold potential treatments from patients in a study's control group and may conceal during the course of the study which patients are receiving a placebo as opposed to the active drug. Administrative psychiatrists may properly place the interests of a healthcare system as a whole above the interests of an individual healthcare consumer. Military psychiatrists may have an obligation to maintain the fighting capacity of a soldier rather than the safety of that particular soldier. In all of these fields, psychiatrists must be aware of the limitations of their commitment to the person they examine and of their ethical obligation to reveal those limitations.

Forensic psychiatrists must be able to present their clinical and scientific knowledge effectively in legal contexts. That may entail testimony and cross-examination. In a court, the issue is not the sincerity of the psychiatrist; it is whether he or she can support their opinions with relevant facts sufficient to compel the assent of the majority of rational persons. Much of clinical medicine remains an art rather than a science. The courts may require that forensic psychiatrists reveal to what extent their opinions are based on science and to what extent they are not. For many clinicians, it is uncomfortable to be obliged to explain the exact database from which their opinions are derived, the exact scientific literature that supports the inferences they make from their database, and the logical process of reasoning by means of which they reach their opinions. Unlike some overly compliant patients, the courts demand that doctors demonstrate that they actually have knowledge and have correctly applied that knowledge – not merely that they are honest and benevolent. Physicians for whom this type of logical rigor is an attractive challenge, rather than a daunting confrontation, will enjoy forensic work.

THE FOUR-STEP APPROACH TO FORENSIC PSYCHIATRY

In order to organize their consideration of practical problems in their subspecialty, forensic psychiatrists use a four-step conceptual framework:

- What is the exact legal issue?
- What are the exact legal criteria for the issue?
- What data are relevant to the legal criteria?
- What reasoning process has led to the forensic psychiatric opinion?

Legal Issues

The range of issues that confront forensic psychiatrists is extensive. In civil law cases there are, for example, conservators and guardianships, testimonial capacity, competence to make a will, personal injury litigation, competence to make a contract, and disability determinations (for social security, worker's compensation, and private insurance coverage). In family law and domestic relations law there are, for example, divorce, child custody, spouse abuse, child abuse, child neglect, elder abuse, termination of parental rights, and delinquency. In criminal law, examples include: competence to confess, competence to stand trial, competence to waive representation by counsel, competence to enter a plea, not responsible by reason of insanity, diminished capacity, diminished responsibility, and guilty but mentally ill. In legal regulation of psychiatry, examples include: treatment over objection, voluntary hospitalization, involuntary hospitalization, confidentiality, the right to refuse treatment, competence to consent to treatment, competence to authorize do-not-resuscitate orders, malpractice, and ethics.

Legal Criteria

The various forensic psychiatric issues are presented in various legal contexts. To the surprise of many citizens, there really is no such thing as "the Law" in the United States. Rather, there are 51 different legal contexts and 51 different sets of law. Each state, as well as the federal government, has its own constitutional laws, its own legislated laws, its own judge-made case laws, and its own administrative laws. The legal criteria that will determine how any of the various forensic psychiatric issues will be decided differ according to which of the 51 legal contexts the specific case at hand will be considered in. This matter of different legal criteria for any single forensic psychiatry issue is not initially easy to grasp.

By way of analogy, consider the clinical psychiatry issue of whether a patient meets the diagnostic criteria for schizophrenia. The diagnostic criteria in the various editions of the *Diagnostic and Statistical Manual of Mental Disorders* (DSM–I, DSM–II, DSM–III, DSM–III–R, and DSM–IV) may be different. Whether a patient meets the diagnostic criteria for schizophrenia will depend on which diagnostic criteria are used. Analogously, consider the forensic psychiatry issue of whether a patient meets the legal criteria for not guilty by reason of insanity (NGRI). The legal criteria in Washington, DC, Virginia, New York, and Michigan, for example, may be different. Whether a defendant meets the legal criteria for NGRI will depend on which jurisdiction's legal criteria are used.

Relevant Data

No matter how complete a forensic psychiatry report may be in other respects, it will be of no value if it does not contain information relevant to the legal criteria for the specific issue. In the same way that the diagnostic criteria determine what data are relevant to resolve a particular diagnostic issue, the legal criteria determine what data are relevant to resolve a particular legal issue. If the clinical psychiatric report does not contain information relevant to the diagnostic criteria, there will be no data upon which to decide the diagnostic issue; if the forensic psychiatric report does not contain information relevant to the legal criteria, there will be no data upon which to decide the legal issue.

For example, consider the legal issue of competence to make a will. The law usually will include some variation of the criteria that the person making the will (i) should know what a will is, (ii) should know the nature and extent of his/her property, (iii) should know who are the "natural heirs of his/her bounty," and (iv) should know that he/she is making a will. Unless the forensic psychiatrist has asked questions directed to these legal criteria and has included the data in his or her report, the court will not be able to decide whether the person was competent to make the will.

Reasoning Process

The basic model of reasoning in forensic psychiatric reports is to state (i) the legal criteria for the issue; (ii) the data relevant to the legal criteria; and (iii) the conclusion. For example:

1. A person is mentally competent to make a will if he knows what a will is, knows the nature and extent of his property, knows the natural heirs of his bounty, and knows that he is making a will.
2. Mr John Doe knows what a will is (e.g., he said, "A will is a legal instrument to ensure that, after my death, my property is distributed in accordance with my wishes"), knows the nature and extent of his property (e.g., he said, "I own my home and have $257,000 in savings and securities"), knows the natural heirs of his bounty (e.g., he said, "My natural heirs are my wife and my son"), and knows that he is making a will (e.g., he said, "This document I'm signing is my last will and testament").
3. Therefore, Mr John Doe is mentally competent to make a will.

This four-step conceptual framework for forensic psychiatry is not merely a convenient method of structuring the data in forensic reports and testimony. It helps forensic psychiatrists to organize and focus their thinking, facilitates communication about cases, and makes sure that the essential forensic psychiatric matters have all been appropriately addressed.

A PRACTICAL EXAMPLE: ASSESSMENT OF AN ADOLESCENT'S COMPETENCE TO STAND TRIAL

Legal Issue

In applying this four-step conceptual framework, the forensic psychiatrist who receives a request to evaluate an adolescent for competence to stand trial would first clarify if that was the only legal issue or issues that need to be addressed. For example, a single teenager could have several forensic psychiatric legal issues under consideration: At the time of the alleged offense, was the teenager not criminally responsible by reason of mental disease or mental defect? At the time that he was arrested, was the teenager mentally competent to confess to the police? Is he suffering from a mental disease or mental defect that makes him more likely to be a danger to the public if he were to be granted bail? At the present time, is the teenager mentally competent to stand trial? At the present time, is the teenager mentally competent to enter a plea to the charges against him? At the time he will be sentenced, will the teenager be competent to abide by the terms of probation, and/or will he be competent to be incarcerated in prison? If this is a capital case, is he suffering from a mental disease or mental defect that renders him incompetent to be executed? The referring attorney, court, or probation officer should be able to advise the forensic psychiatrist regarding exactly which issue or issues need to be considered.

Legal Criteria

After the legal issue or issues to be considered have been clarified, the forensic psychiatrist must determine what the legal criteria are for each of the issues that must be decided. For example, if the issue is competence to stand trial, the legal criteria will include some variation on these questions: Does the teenage defendant have the capacity to understand the charges against him? Does the teenage defendant have the capacity to assist in his own defense? Does the teenage defendant suffer from a diagnosable mental disease or mental defect? If the teenage defendant lacks the capacity to understand the charges against him or lacks the capacity to assist in his own defense, is that lack of capacity due to his diagnosable mental disease or mental defect? The forensic psychiatrist needs to know both the legislated criteria and how the courts have interpreted the criteria in prior cases. The referring attorney or the court should be able to provide the forensic psychiatrist with (i) the legislated statute establishing the criteria for competence to stand trial in the particular state or the federal jurisdiction, and (ii) the prior judge-made case-law decisions establishing how the court has interpreted the legislated statute establishing the criteria for competence to stand trial in the particular state or federal jurisdiction.

Relevant Data

After the forensic psychiatrist has determined the legal criteria and how the court has interpreted them, he or she is in a position to obtain the legally relevant information. For example, in an evaluation of a teenage defendant's competence to stand trial, the forensic psychiatrist would need to ask the adolescent questions such as these: What crime are you accused of having committed? Do you have an attorney? What is your attorney supposed to do for you? What is the district attorney supposed to do in your case? What is the judge's job in a court case? What does a jury do in a court case? What is a plea bargain? What plea have you entered, if any? What are the consequences of being found guilty? What happens if you are found not guilty? In addition, the forensic psychiatrist would have to evaluate the adolescent's capacity to rationally understand such questions and their answers (as contrasted to the teenager providing mere rote responses) and the adolescent's capacity and motivation to assist in his or her own defense. If the teenage defendant demonstrates a lack of capacity to understand the charges he or she faces, or to assist in his or her own defense, the forensic psychiatrist needs to determine if the teenager is suffering from a diagnosable mental disease or mental defect. If the adolescent defendant has a demonstrated lack of capacity to understand the charges or to assist in his or her defense and also has a diagnosable mental disorder, then the forensic psychiatrist must evaluate whether the lack of capacity is directly caused by the mental disorder or if it has some other cause (e.g., lack of familiarity with the legal system, coming from a foreign nation, willful oppositionalism, sociopolitical motivation).

Reasoning Process

Forensic psychiatrists must organize their data in a logical manner to support their opinion. For example:

1. A person is competent to stand trial if he has the capacity to understand the charges against him and the capacity to assist in his own defense.
2. Mr John Doe, a 16-year-old male defendant, has the capacity to understand the charges against him (he

said that he was charged with "rape, forcing a girl to have sex with me against her will") and the capacity to assist in his own defense (he said that he had an attorney and that the job of his attorney was "to help me, to defend me in this case, to protect my rights;" that the job of the district attorney was "to convict me, to get me sent to prison," that the job of the judge was "to keep things fair in the courtroom, to pass sentence if I'm found guilty;" that the job of the jury was "to decide if I'm guilty or not guilty;" that he would "go to prison for a long time" if he were found guilty and that he would "go free" if found not guilty; that a plea bargain meant "guaranteed less lime in prison than if convicted at trial, in exchange for pleading guilty instead of going to trial;" and that he had "not decided yet" whether to enter a plea of guilty). He demonstrated no diagnosable mental disorder.
3. Mr John Doe is competent to stand trial.

There is no such thing as a single, comprehensive forensic psychiatric evaluation. There is only a series of individually focused specific forensic psychiatric assessments. Each specific forensic psychiatric issue would be addressed in a similar systematic method. For each individual issue, the legal criteria would be set forth, the legally relevant data would be obtained, and a logically structured opinion would be offered.

CONCLUSION

It is impossible to condense all of forensic psychiatry into a brief discussion. This presentation has been designed to provide adolescent psychiatrists with an introduction to forensic psychiatry – including an explanation of how it differs from therapeutic psychiatry, a four-step conceptual framework for understanding how forensic psychiatrists approach their work (i.e., how to think like a forensic psychiatrist), and an example of how the conceptual framework may be applied to the assessment of whether a teenage defendant is competent to stand trial. To learn more about forensic psychiatry for adolescent psychiatrists, see Rosner [2,3] and Rosner and Schwartz [4].

References

1. American Academy of Psychiatry and the Law. *Membership Directory*. Bloomfield. CT: AAPL, 1998; p. X.
2. Rosner R. *Principles and Practice of Forensic Psychiatry*. New York: Chapman & Hall, 1994.
3. Rosner R. *Textbook of Adolescent Psychiatry*. London: Edward Arnold, 2003.
4. Rosner R, Schwartz H. *Juvenile Psychiatry and the Law*. New York: Plenum, 1989.

42

Ethical Considerations in Adolescent Addiction

Robert Weinstock

University of California Los Angeles, Los Angeles, CA, USA

INTRODUCTION

Ethical considerations require special care in the assessment and treatment of adolescent patients in general and even more so in those patients with addiction problems. In adolescent patients with addiction problems, the problems and considerations of both adolescence and addictions arise and require consideration and sometimes can present special challenges, as well as some special problems of patients with both. This chapter will consider many of these aspects, as well as some complex dilemmas that can arise and require thought and assessment by every practitioner. Ethical guidelines are helpful and can assist in resolving most everyday problems. But such guidelines, although sufficient for ordinary situations, can provide only the beginning of any such analysis in more complex situations, since guidelines can conflict and may require resolution of these conflicts by practitioners themselves. Also, ethical guidelines are the minimum considerations in an ethical analysis. They represent the minimum (the floor) of ethical analysis and not the maximum or ceiling (aspirational ethical goals). That is because as with any guidelines, they reflect the consensus of a large number of professionals and are chosen to lend themselves to possible enforcement. But that does not end the debate since there are many ethical facets that might not be capable of enforcement or might be matters of disagreement. To say a practitioner is ethical because no guideline is violated is like saying a person is ethical and a good citizen if he or she does not violate the law. It might take much more than that to be an ethical good citizen. More than not committing a crime is needed. The same is true with professional ethics.

Legal considerations are relevant for ethics but are not determinative. Attorneys should not be consulted to make clinical decisions or determine what is clinically ethical. Instead, practitioners themselves need to determine the most ethical course of action. Since the law itself can be complicated and subject to more than one interpretation, an attorney should be asked how to do what is indicated ethically within the constraints of the law. Too often clinicians just ask attorneys what to do. That is a mistake. Attorneys recommend the safest way to avoid legal liability. However, a clinician might be willing to risk minimal legal liability in order to do what is best for a patient. Additionally, if the attorney represents an institution for which a clinician also works, the attorney may not make the clinician the highest priority. That is because the institution is a "deeper pocket" with much more money at stake. As a result, an attorney might sacrifice a practitioner in order to protect the institution. For example, the attorney and institution might be willing to settle a case in a way that conceded liability of the practitioner and for a settlement that requires a report to the National Data Bank rather than fight a case in which the practitioner does not think liability is warranted. The interests of the institution and practitioner may not coincide. It might be best for an institution to minimize possible significant damages and settle for a lesser amount while admitting liability by a practitioner, who in reality may have had a bad outcome but was not negligent.

Also, the law and ethics are not the same. Usually it is ethical to follow the law, and a legal requirement should be a defense to any ethical complaint. But there are rare instances in which it might still be ethical and even heroic to violate the law, if the law is rigid and if following the law too narrowly might result in harmful consequences for all involved. An example might be child abuse reporting. The law in most jurisdictions allows for no flexibility or judgment by a clinician, most likely out of concerns that clinicians might not make protection of the public the predominant consideration. In rare instances, a clinician might be more effective in stopping abuse than an overworked state agency or a punitive clinical justice system though the clinician risks serious legal consequences if a required report is not made to the requisite state agency. Another example might be a refusal to reveal confidential information in a legal case even if ordered by a judge. The clinician risks contempt of court and jail time, but it is not necessarily an unethical decision. It might even be possible for the legal system to get the information in a way that does not betray patient confidences or it may just be cumulative evidence. Such a request could be made by the clinician to the court, but the judge could deny the request to respect privilege out of convenience and order the information to be provided. Failure to provide that information may be highly ethical even if not legal. Additionally, there are many ethical requirements not enforced by the law. Many are not even enforced by the organizations that promulgate them or for that matter anybody else. That does not mean though that a good ethical practitioner should not follow those guidelines, and in fact should try to go beyond them in an effort to do the most ethical thing in complex situations.

In the assessment and treatment of adolescents with substance abuse disorders, there are two complex areas in which ethical dilemmas can arise and often do. This chapter will explore some of these areas and provide recommendations on how to navigate these complexities.

CONFIDENTIALITY

Confidentiality is an ethical requirement, sometimes also required by law. In contrast, privilege is the ability to keep relevant information out of a legal setting because society values more highly the need for keeping the communication between certain parties privileged than it does revealing this relevant information in a legal setting. There is a need to keep the communications between a doctor and a patient confidential, in order for patients in general to trust doctors well enough to share sensitive, embarrassing information. That is more important than revealing the information in a specific case. If the information is not relevant or the prejudicial value outweighs the probative value, it should be possible on that basis alone to exclude the information. The need for confidentiality applies to substance-abusing adolescent patients at least as much as any patient.

There are special considerations in treating adolescent patients. Parents ordinarily pay for treatment and may feel like they are entitled to know what is going on with the adolescent. Parents are likely also to have a legal right to the adolescent's medical records. Ordinarily, in the treatment of adolescents, a therapist will work out an understanding with the parent that most things will be kept confidential with a few exceptions. For example, an exception will be made if the adolescent becomes a serious danger to himself or others. Sometimes an exception is made for drug abuse in a patient where that is one of the main problems. This issue comes to the fore when the treatment is of an adolescent substance abuser. It is essential to consider and address this issue at the outset of treatment and again if treatment developments lead to a need to change the original agreement. Sometimes, if the parents already know of the substance abuse, it might be best that they know if the adolescent starts to reuse. At other times, if the problem is not too out of control, maintaining confidentiality from the parent might be preferable. Also, treatment of adolescents differs from treatment of adults, insofar as involvement of the parents directly in the treatment commonly is an integral part of the treatment. Nonetheless, it is important that everybody be clear what will be shared with the family. Ordinarily, adolescents should be involved in and told about decisions to share information with the family. When the family shares information, they should be told if the therapist thinks it may be necessary to share the information with the patient. In many instances, it is better to have a social worker deal with the family, in order to avoid many of the confidentiality problems and potentially conflicting roles. In other instances, the family dynamics are essential parts of the problem, and it is best that the family be directly integrated into the treatment. HIPAA laws may provide additional protection.

In the legal area, the parameters may be clearer, but even here there are ambiguities. Just because the government sometimes pays for treatment does not mean that adolescents should be deprived of the confidentiality afforded other patients. Adolescent substance abuse almost always is illegal. Even with legal substances like alcohol and cigarettes, they are illegal for adolescents since they are underage. Additionally, there are special federal legal protections for confidentiality of treatment records of patients treated for substance abuse. Accordingly, even though the substance abuse might be a crime in some jurisdictions, therapists are legally required to keep the information confidential. Thus the law in these cases reinforces ethical confidentiality obligations. An exception might be in a type of legal diversion program to avoid punishment in which treatment is mandated, and there is an initial understanding that certain types of information will be shared. In treating adolescent substance abusers though, the legal aspects can get complex, and might require consultation with an attorney, since parents may be entitled to some information about the treatment of their adolescent child. An agreement about this understood by both the adolescent and the parent at the outset of treatment, generally is the best clinical and ethical way to address such situations.

Drug treatment also is an area in which federal law requires additional confidentiality not required for other kinds of treatment. Thus, it is important to know whether any exceptions to confidentiality are forbidden by law before violating confidentiality. It may require consultation with an attorney or even a ruling by a judge to determine this. The legal parameters of confidentiality with adolescents with addictions can be more complex than the treatment of adolescents with other problems or adults with addiction problems. Although doing the ethically "right" thing clinically may generally be the best thing legally too, it is important that any actions at least be informed by the law, so a practitioner makes an informed decision about the legal risks.

Law May Complicate Confidentiality for Adolescent Drug Treatment

There are federal and state legal requirements that can be complicated and differ from state to state. It is important to be aware of a state's legal requirements in your jurisdiction. For those who receive federal funding and must comply with federal rules, federal regulations prohibit disclosing any information to parents without a minor's written consent (if the minor acting alone under applicable state law has the legal capacity to apply for and obtain alcohol or drug abuse treatment) (42 C.F.R.§ 2.14). However, a provider or program may share with parents, if the individual or program director (if it is a program) determines that three conditions are met: (i) the minor's situation poses a substantial threat to the life or physical well-being of the minor or another; (ii) this threat may be reduced by communicating relevant facts to the minor's parents; and (iii) the minor lacks the capacity because of extreme youth or a mental or physical condition to make a rational decision on whether to disclose to his parents (42 C.F.R.§2.14). For providers who do not have to follow the federal rules, state law applies.

For example, in California under state law, if a parent or guardian consents for a minor's drug or alcohol treatment, "the physician [must] disclose medical information concerning the care to the minor's parent or legal guardian upon his or her request, even if the minor child does not consent to disclosure, without liability for the disclosure" (Cal. Family Code § 6929(g)). California state law holds that when a minor consents for his or her own drug or alcohol treatment, a healthcare provider is not permitted to share records with a parent or legal guardian without the minor's written authorization. At the same time, California state law requires healthcare providers to involve the minor's parent or guardian in the treatment plan, if appropriate, as determined by the professional person or treatment facility treating the minor. The professional person providing care to the minor must state in the minor's treatment record whether and when the professional attempted to contact the minor's parent or guardian, and whether the attempt was successful, or the reason why it would not be appropriate to contact the minor's parent or guardian in the opinion of the professional person (Cal. Family Code § 6929(c)). Involving parents in treatment will necessitate sharing certain otherwise confidential information; however, having them participate does not mean parents have a right to access *all* confidential records. Psychiatrists in California should attempt to honor the minor's right to confidentiality to the extent possible, while still involving parents in treatment.

CONFLICTING DUTIES AND RESPONSIBILITIES

There are situations in which the doctor may wear two hats with different and potentially conflicting responsibilities. It is important for both the doctor and patient to be clear about these conflicting duties. First, all therapists have reporting duties that sometimes can go counter to a patient's welfare. Child abuse reports may protect the adolescent, but they could also cause harm to the adolescent if the family realizes the adolescent was the source of the information and uses punitive measures against the adolescent, including things like failure to pay for school. Also, if the adolescent is the abuser against a younger adolescent with something like consensual sex, if the jurisdiction requires filing a child abuse report, that could lead to harm to the adolescent, especially since the adolescent is in treatment that could address the issue. It could even lead to the adolescent leaving treatment. There also are Tarasoff-type obligations that require therapists in some jurisdictions to protect potential victims from the actions of a patient. Most of the time, there is no ethical or clinical problem since stopping a patient from doing something dangerous would protect the patient from serious consequences arising from a dangerous action, as well as protecting a potential victim. However, if a therapist elects to warn the potential victim and the police because the therapist regards that as the best way to avoid liability, that action sometimes can cause harm to the adolescent patient. Ethically, a better way to protect the potential victim likely is possible. Almost all jurisdictions provide for such an option.

The issue can arise if the therapist is treating several members of an adolescent family individually, as well as in family therapy. The problem can arise if the needs of the individual family members conflict and the therapist needs to decide whose needs should be given primacy. Problems can also arise if a family member wants information kept confidential from another family member. Additionally, it would be next to impossible for a therapist not to consider the confidential information when advising the family. It is a reason why this area of potential conflicts of interest is best avoided, unless there are other overriding reasons to do it and each family member is aware of the drawbacks, but still wants to do this because of perceived advantages such as confidence and trust in the specific therapist. If the family dynamics are the primary focus of treatment, the same therapist may be the best option. Otherwise, separating the roles usually is preferable.

EMPLOYMENT BY OR CONSULTATION TO SCHOOLS AND COLLEGES

The most common role conflict situations arise in school or college settings. They arise because the needs of the school and adolescent substance-abusing patient have a strong potential to lead to conflict. An obvious concern is that the school will not want drugs being used in school or given or sold to other students. Accordingly, issues of confidentiality or lack of it need to be addressed at the outset of treatment and as a general issue with the school, if the doctor works for the school. Otherwise, serious misunderstandings can arise. The same issues can arise in college, although colleges might be more ready to respect confidentiality in these situations because the college students are older and there is less need to have a protective environment. The conflict is clearest when the issue is whether the adolescent should be dismissed from the school. It can make a difference at what point the doctor gets involved with the adolescent. There also is the reality that drug use and abuse is common in schools, despite policies against their use.

If the doctor is in a treatment situation, it should be clear whether things like drug use by the adolescent are confidential. Considering how common drug use is, it would be difficult to see how an adolescent could be treated meaningfully without such confidentiality. If there are disciplinary actions against a student for drug use in the school, then it is especially important to clarify the role of the doctor and whether duties are primarily to the student or school. Even in a hospital setting, such conflicts can arise. If drug use is not permitted on a unit, the doctor might discharge the adolescent, and put the need to keep the hospital ward drug free over the needs of the adolescent patient.

If the adolescent commits an act of serious violence on a hospital ward, most hospital doctors will put the needs of the hospital first and even call authorities to press charges. That might be appropriate, but it would be dishonest to claim either to the patient or oneself that it always is to the benefit of the adolescent.

The situation can be most complex in high school, when there can sometimes be no tolerance for drugs. Usually psychiatrists are not employed by high schools, but other mental health professionals are. Also, to whom does a psychiatrist owe a duty if a consultation is requested by and paid for by the school and drug use by the adolescent is one of the questions? These are not simple questions, but what is clear is that the psychiatrist has an ethical responsibility to make clear to the adolescent at the outset the limits to confidentiality, so that the adolescent does not reveal things to a psychiatrist under the mistaken belief that something is confidential when it is not. That would be a betrayal of trust. Additionally, if the word got around, other adolescents would have good reason not to reveal sensitive material to the psychiatrist, thereby limiting the ability of the psychiatrist to help either the adolescent or to be of any assistance to the school requesting a consultation.

CRIMINAL JUSTICE SYSTEM

Problems arise in the criminal justice system because psychiatrists have duties to the institution that conflict with and can take precedence over responsibilities to the adolescent. Confidentiality therefore cannot be fully assured. The best way to approach this is to clarify any limitations to confidentiality at the outset of treatment, so there are no misunderstandings consistent with professional ethical guidelines. The criminal justice system also has values different from other treatment settings. For example, an escape may be considered worse than a suicide.

INFORMED CONSENT

Informed consent requires the capacity to weigh the risks and benefits of a proposed treatment. The law also establishes minimal ages required to give informed consent, as opposed to the actual capacity of a specific adolescent to give informed consent. That is because it would be too difficult practically to assess each adolescent individually for capacity to give informed consent. It is easier to establish a somewhat arbitrary cut-off point legally that comes close to the actual age of a specific adolescent's capacity. This age also recognizes adolescent immaturity and impulsivity that might not show itself in a simple cognitive test. Many states have age 18 as the legal cut-off point for giving informed consent. For adolescents below that age, consent must be obtained from a parent or legal guardian. There are exceptions made for things like emancipated minors. Even if not required legally, it usually would be wise to obtain the assent of the adolescent for most treatments and explain the risks and benefits to the adolescent nonetheless. Assent is similar to consent in someone lacking the legal capacity to give informed consent even though a specific individual might in fact have that capacity. At the very least, some type of assent by the adolescent can be helpful.

Many states make exceptions to what a caregiver who is a relative can consent to on behalf of an adolescent. For example, in California, if the minor is 14 years of age or older, no surgery may be performed upon the minor without either the consent of both the minor and the relative who is a caregiver, or a court order, absent an emergency. The law therefore is requiring adolescent assent in this context. California law is even more restricted for the non-related caregiver, who can consent only to school-related treatment for the adolescent. Thus, it is important to know the law in a specific jurisdiction.

Exceptions often are made for consent in specific situations to treatment for things like pregnancy, abortion, counseling, and treatment for drug abuse. State laws differ in regard to consent for drug treatment, so it is necessary to know the law in your jurisdiction. For example in California, "A minor who is 12 years of age or older may consent to medical care and counseling relating to the diagnosis and treatment of a drug- or alcohol-related problem" (Cal. Family Code § 6929(b)). However, this statute does not authorize a minor to consent to replacement narcotic abuse treatment (Cal. Family Code § 6929(e)). State law also does allow a parent or guardian to consent to medical care and counseling for a drug- or alcohol-related problem of a minor when the minor does not consent to the care (Cal. Family Code § 6929(f)). In many states, adolescents independently can consent to drug treatment without parental consent.

It is especially important for a psychiatrist to give the welfare of the adolescent priority. For example, special care should be taken in research, and the psychiatrist most likely should not do it if an adolescent dissents, even if a patient or guardian gave consent for the research. Adolescent preferences regarding specific treatments ordinarily should be respected, despite parental preferences. Ideally, consent by the parent and assent by the adolescent should both be obtained. The psychiatrist has some additional ethical and legal fiduciary responsibilities to an adolescent's welfare beyond that required for adult patients.

ETHICAL GUIDELINES

Relevant ethical guidelines have been promulgated by the American Psychiatric Association (APA) [1], the American Academy of Child and Adolescent Psychiatry (AACAP) [2], the American Society of Addiction Medicine (ASAM) [3], and the American Academy of Psychiatry and the Law (AAPL) [4]. Only the APA enforces its ethical guidelines. The American Psychological Association (APA) has developed ethical guidelines for psychologists [5]. It is important to be aware of these guidelines, especially if a practitioner belongs to an organization like the APA that enforces its ethical guidelines. State Medical Boards also enforce ethics and sometimes can do so on an ad hoc basis. Ethical guidelines are only the starting point of an ethical analysis and are not the last word. Ethical guidelines represent a consensus of what the profession can agree are minimal ethical guidelines. They represent the floor of ethics and not the ceiling. To say a practitioner is practicing at the highest ethical standard because he or she has violated no ethical guideline is like saying a person is highly ethical if he or she has not violated the law. An ethical practitioner should try to go beyond minimal ethical guidelines in deciding the most ethical course of action.

Some ethical considerations can be considered aspirational because they are difficult goals to achieve and impossible to enforce because they would require getting into the mind of the practitioner to determine his or her intent. An example might be putting the needs of a patient above other considerations. Also, this is not absolute. Sometimes there are other overriding considerations, such as the needs of society if a patient is dangerous to others, the needs of an institution in a prison, school, or hospital, or the needs of the psychiatrist if a patient threatens the psychiatrist or refuses to pay the bill despite a number of efforts to make payment arrangements. In the latter situation, appropriate referral is needed ethically or to prevent charges of patient abandonment. In situations such as these, patient welfare needs to be balanced against other considerations. Depending on the seriousness of the specific actions by the patient, different courses of action would be appropriate. In the more complex situations requiring the weighing of a number of considerations, different appropriate actions may be chosen by different practitioners.

In ordinary practice situations, the appropriate ethical action could be determined readily by considering principles and guidelines like the ones described in this chapter. Some therefore advocate just following these guidelines. The problems arise in complex cases when guidelines conflict or there is no guideline. In such a situation, practitioners trying to act in the most ethical way must perform their own ethical analysis and try to balance the competing considerations for themselves. In difficult situations, consultation with other practitioners knowledgeable about ethics often is advisable.

Ethics is not the same as the law. Attorneys should not be asked what is ethical or even what to do. Instead, a practitioner should determine the best course of action on a clinical and ethical basis. Then an attorney should be consulted about how best to accomplish this result within the constraints of the law. Attorneys may think only in terms of what is best for the institution or the practitioner. Even these two considerations can lead to opposing courses of action. The practitioner may also want to give priority to patient welfare that might not be a priority for the attorney or the institution. Practitioners may consider a small liability risk worthwhile to do what is best for the patient. On rare occasions, a practitioner might even want to violate the law in the name of doing what is ethical for the patient. In such cases, practitioners need to be willing to risk legal consequences if they lose in their efforts to persuade authorities of the appropriateness of their actions. It always is ethical to follow the law, except if living in a highly unethical society like Nazi Germany. However, on rare occasions it might be even more ethical to do what is "right" even it violates a law.

ETHICAL PRINCIPLES

Beauchamp and Childress developed the Principles of Bioethics [6]. The principles are beneficence, non-maleficence, autonomy, and justice (equal distribution of resources). These are not the last word in bioethics since they can conflict with each other or with other considerations and are not universally accepted; but they remain a good start if one accepts these principles. Candilis et al. [7] have advocated for an approach of robust professionalism that involves consideration of differing, sometimes conflicting, roles exemplified by forensic psychiatry.

ETHICAL CONCERNS

Considerations can be complex in all patients with addictions. Adolescents are no exception. Although addiction is seen more frequently as a disease, it retains some moral approbation. Although it is readily accepted that psychotic patients have minimal control over decisions such as stopping psychotropic medication, the same is not true for decisions of addicted individuals to use their substance of choice [8]. In both situations there is denial and loss of control, but in both instances it is possible to make the opposing decision. These issues become relevant when questions of criminal responsibility arise.

FORENSIC ETHICS

Forensic psychiatric ethics can be complex because the law is devoted to quick resolutions of disputes. Medicine is devoted to helping patients. When these fields interface in forensic psychiatry, complex ethical dilemmas can arise. Weinstock [9] wrote an annotated bibliography reviewing ethical writings in this area. Appelbaum [10] and Rosner [11] have written on the ethical foundations of forensic psychiatry, and see forensic psychiatry as having an ethics of its own. Weinstock et al. [12] agree that forensic psychiatry is different but still believe traditional medical ethics retains a place and needs to be balanced against other factors. Hundert [13] describes an approach to resolving ethical issues that requires a practitioner to balance competing considerations. Since adolescent drug use usually violates the law, forensic psychiatrists frequently become involved in such cases. As such they need to consider the ethical complexities.

Usually, the ethical principles and guidelines discussed in this chapter are sufficient. In difficult situations, it can be more difficult. Books have been written on these issues by Candilis et al. [14] and Sadoff [15], which discuss how to approach the complex forensic role. These issues are relevant when treating and assessing adolescent substance abusers with legal issues. Adding in substance abuse to other forensic issues, just adds to the potential complexity of the dilemmas.

RESOLVING ETHICAL DILEMMAS

Ethics in treating and assessing adolescents with addictions necessitates taking into account both considerations of treating adolescents and those with substance abuse. If there are legal considerations, as often happens when illegal drugs are used, it is even more complex in that the law and the ethical requirements when interfacing with the law in forensic psychiatry, or even in treatment, need consideration when doing an assessment for legal purposes. There is no rule determining how to balance these or to which issue to give priority. More than one ethical decision may be legitimate, and decisions may vary with the specific factors in a case. That is why the ethical practitioner needs to teach him or herself to balance these considerations, since there is no overriding rule that can apply in every case.

The good thing though is that in most clinical situations the considerations do not conflict and the most ethical course of action can be readily determined by considering the aspects enumerated in this chapter. Only in the relatively rare complex situations do these considerations conflict. In such situations it often can help to consult with other practitioners who are knowledgeable about ethics and experienced in analyzing complex ethical dilemmas that arise in clinical and forensic practice with adolescent substance abusers.

References

1. American Psychiatric Association. *The Principles of Medical Ethics with Annotations especially Applicable to Psychiatry* [revised]. Washington, DC:American Psychiatric Association, 2009.

2. American Academy of Child and Adolescent Psychiatry. *Code of Ethics*. Washington DC:AACAP, 2009.

3. American Society of Addiction Medicine. *Public Policy Statement on Principles of Medical Ethics*. Chevy Chase, MD:ASAM, 1992.

4. American Academy of Psychiatry and the Law. Ethical Guidelines for the Practice of Forensic Psychiatry [revised]. Bloomfield, CT:AAPL, 2005.

5. American Psychological Association. *Ethical Principles of Psychologists and Code of Conduct*. Washington, DC: American Psychological Association, 2010.

6. Beauchamp Tl, Childress JF. *Principles of Biomedical Ethics*, 6th edn. New York:Oxford University Press, 2008.

7. Candilis PJ, Martinez R, Dording C. Principles and narrative in forensic psychiatry. Towards a robust view of professional role. *J Am Acad Psych Law* 2001;**29**:167–173.

8. Weinstock R. Moral capacities of psychotic and addicted individuals. In: Thomasma DC, Weisstub DN (eds), *The Variables of Moral Capacity*. Boston:Kluwer Academic Publishers, 2004; pp. 299–307.

9. Weinstock R. Ethics in forensic psychiatry – an annotated bibliography. *Bull Am Acad Psych Law* 1995;**23**:473–482.

10. Appelbaum PS. A theory of ethics for forensic psychiatry. *J Am Acad Psych Law* 1997;**5**:233–247.

11. Rosner R. Foundations of ethical practice in the forensic sciences. *J Forensic Sci* 1997;**42**:1191–1194.

12. Weinstock R, Leong GB, Silva JA. The role of traditional medical ethics in forensic psychiatry. In: Rosner R, Weinstock R (eds), *Ethical Practice in Psychiatry and the Law*. New York:Springer, 1990; pp. 31–51.

13. Hundert EM. Competing medical and legal ethical values: balancing problems of the forensic psychiatrist. In: Rosner R, Weinstock R (eds), *Ethical Practice in Psychiatry and the Law*. New York:Springer, 1990; pp. 53–72.

14. Candilis PJ, Weinstock R, Martinez R. *Forensic Ethics and the Expert Witness*. New York:Springer, 2007.

15. Sadoff RL. *Ethical Issues in Forensic Psychiatry. Minimizing Harm*. Hoboken, NJ:Wiley-Blackwell, 2011.

43

Informed Consent, Parental Consent, and the Right to Refuse Treatment

Jack A. Gottschalk[1] and Daniel P. Greenfield[2]

[1] Seton Hall University, Stillman School of Business, Livingston, NJ, USA
[2] Seton Hall University School of Health and Medical Sciences, Millburn, NJ, USA

While we will deal with the topic of informed consent to open this chapter, it must be recognized that the subject and the legal doctrines of consent and informed consent, together with ethical considerations, are interrelated and apply with equal vigor to the right to refuse treatment or to end treatment at once.

An added corollary is that of confidentiality; this concept has a very long history, and is perhaps best exemplified in the doctor-patient privilege. This privilege is recognized in every state, and prevents a doctor from providing testimony about any aspect of a patient's medical condition.

In the United States, the laws dealing with the confidentiality of medical information existed at the state level. Until the passage of the Health Insurance Portability and Accounting Act (HIPPA) [1] in 1996, virtually all laws dealing with the confidential nature of medical information were found at the state level. The confidential nature of medical information is now covered by the HIPPA provisions and, in fact, is a specific concern of those engaged in the development of the Electronic Medical Record (EMR) program that has been mandated by the US Department of Health and Human Services. Further, a key HIPPA provision focuses on the combined requirement for both consent and confidentiality.

Although cases of adolescent medical records confidentiality have often focused principally on the use of contraceptive information, physicians and other healthcare providers should be particularly aware of new laws, rules, and regulations that will principally emanate from the federal government as they may concern alcohol and drug addition treatment.

Our plan in the presentation of this chapter is to begin with a discussion of informed consent, then to follow that with an examination of adolescent refusal to provide consent to medical treatment, and finally to explore parental rights in terms of refusal to treatment by adolescents. Following these discussions, we will present a general summary of the chapter that is designed to be both easily digested and of practical value.

Finally, as a further assist to the reader, it should be noted that whenever we refer to medical treatment we are speaking about treatment of adolescents for alcohol and drug addiction issues. This treatment is, of course, the essential focus of this chapter.

A starting point for this discussion is to set out the definitions of both consent and informed consent, two separate and distinct doctrines. We then turn to explore the historical reasons that have led to current interest in this important area.

CONSENT

Definitions of Consent

Consent – sometimes called basic, general, or implied consent to differentiate it from the informed version – is simple to define. A visit to the doctor – in an ongoing doctor-patient relationship, when a patient has a cold or even to have blood taken as part of a normal physical examination – will not trigger the requirements that typically surround providing (on the patient's part) or acquiring (on the doctor's part) informed consent. The standard that applies in terms of consent in such a case is general in nature and requires essentially only that the patient understands why the doctor is doing what is required under the circumstances. As a result, the consent is said to be implied, with less elaborate or extensive information being provided as to, for example, what is being done to treat sneezing and a sore throat. This kind of general medical consent protects the physician from civil liability or, depending on the circumstances, from a charge of criminal assault.

From the physician's position, informed consent implies a significantly increased level of liability, namely that of negligence. From the patient's point of view, that can mean undergoing a treatment or procedure of some risk and for which the consent would not have been given if the extent of that risk had been fully made known before it was undertaken. Obviously, in a scenario in which the patient is an adolescent, the informed consent doctrine applies with certain well-defined exceptions. We will explore these exceptions along with the specific requirements involved in obtaining informed consent for an adolescent, and in deciding who can give it when dealing with an adolescent.

The Historical Background

What we now refer to as the patient's "Bill of Rights" includes the right to be provided with complete information as to medical treatments and procedures. This concept did not have its beginning in US hospitals or in doctors' offices in the United States. Instead, the initial (and dramatic) movement was generated as a direct result of the involuntary medical research that was carried out by the Germans and Japanese during the Second World War. Equally important to the rights of patients was the medical research conducted by the federal government at Tuskegee, Alabama, between 1932 and 1972, to study syphilis and its effects.

In the wake of the requirements that were developed from these two experiences, it was mandated that full information be provided to any patient undergoing medical research; the need for full disclosure and the accompanying requirement to achieve informed consent was extended to all medical patients. The movement to provide more information grew to include not only medical and other healthcare treatments and procedures, but also drugs and medical devices distributed on an interstate basis. Most states have enacted laws that require providing information to patients that will permit such medical consumers to make decisions relevant to their healthcare on the basis of informed consent.

The Elements of Informed Consent

There is no doubt that the doctrine of informed consent has strong roots in the competency of the individual providing it. In short and simple terms, informed consent cannot exist without competency. This point is again a

reminder (in terms of an adolescent's competency) of the adolescent connection and the focus of this chapter.

Whether consent is basic, implied, or informed, the situation and the circumstances under which the consent is being sought and provided are important to consider. Individuals in a doctor's office or in a hospital are often nervous, even fearful. The term "white coat syndrome" is not an empty one. This "syndrome" may result in a patient's consent to a treatment based on a level of fear and intimidation tantamount to duress. Additionally, faced with having to absorb a considerable amount of possibly confusing information in a short time while, perhaps, only half-listening to its presentation, the consent may be legally, but not mentally, effective. The ultimate determination of whether consent was given in such a situation is often a legal one, based on the standard of whether it is reasonable to believe that the patient understood the ramifications of the decision that was made.

Equally important, informed consent must be of a specific, not general, nature otherwise it is meaningless and may open up the healthcare provider to liability as a result. A good example is that the informed consent of a patient for an appendectomy does not mean the surgeon has permission to remove another organ. Doing so would go beyond the obtained consent. Today, the tort law principle that not many years ago was taught in law schools and known as the "good surgery rule," no longer applies. Under that rule, if a surgeon were performing an operation and saw another problem that could be surgically resolved, it could be done in the best interest of the patient. Obviously, this is no longer the case; appropriate preoperative consents must be written that are both clear and reasonable in scope.

There is no basis for doubt about the point that a positive relationship between the healthcare professional and the patient, either adolescent or adult, will help pave the way for the kind of effective communication necessary to generate informed consent. But it is equally true that such a relationship, often the result of years of doctor-patient contact (particularly in the case of primary care physicians and their patients), does not always exist. Despite these points, the necessary elements of information required for informed consent (concerning prospective treatment for which a formal consent must be obtained) include risk to life; ability to maintain employment or schooling; alternatives and treatment options; long- or short-term disabilities; insurance costs to include drug coverage; therapeutic factors; and any potential risks involved that may be incurred by not going forward with the recommended medical options or, in the alternative, hesitating to make a decision at a later date.

Having now discussed the essential part of *what* constitutes consent and, particularly, informed consent, we must inquire into the critical areas of *who* is considered capable, in a legal sense, of providing informed consent and of the applications of various exceptions to the informed consent doctrine as they are generally accepted.

One exception – perhaps the easiest to understand – is the emergency situation in which no possibility exists to obtain informed consent. This exception applies to both adults and adolescents. Other recognized exceptions include situations in which the medical risk is already known by the patient or where it is reasonably unforeseen, unlikely, or of such a nature as to be considered medically insignificant.

Adolescents and Informed Consent

As stated earlier in this chapter, informed consent and the capability of providing it are inexorably linked. Thus, there are special considerations in the law to deal with those individuals who, for one reason or another, are considered by the law as being incapable of meeting that standard. Among those groups of individuals are children, the mentally ill, the elderly, and those who are physically disabled in such a way that they are unable to communicate effectively. In each of those cases, if informed consent is required, a parent, guardian, or some other individual or agency, may provide the needed consent. Our focus here is broadly on children, and more specifically on adolescents; we will deal with them for obvious reasons as separate classifications.

The term "children" covers a very broad range of ages, from infancy to the age of 18. It is obvious that consequently, the younger the age of the child, the less capability that child has to provide consent, whether implied, expressed, or informed. In the final section of this chapter (dealing specifically with the subject of parental consent), we will explore the rights of parents and others who may be legal representatives of minors who are themselves incapable of providing or refusing consent in medical situations (including, of course, alcohol and drug addiction).

Consent with reference to the ability of children to provide it is largely based not only on age, but also on the emotional and intellectual level of the child in question. It can be argued, for example, that some children at the age of 10 are intelligent enough and possessed of sufficient judgment to make a decision regarding informed consent, whereas others of the same age are not. For this reason, efforts have been made in some states to stratify children, legally, by age group for consent purposes.

In Tennessee, for example, the doctrine of "the mature minor" has been accepted (that doctrine will be more fully explored here). As part of the doctrine, Tennessee courts have held that under the age of 7, in the absence of a statutory exception, parental, guardian, or judicial consent is always required. This is also the case of minors between 7 and 14 years of age. When dealing with an adolescent who is between 14 and 18 years old, there is a presumption of capacity to provide informed consent. The presumption is subject to challenge. Therefore, a physician may require parental, guardian, or other competent permission before providing treatment.

The Perceived and Accepted Need to Protect Children

As we continue to discuss the special considerations that exist in one form or another in US states and territorial jurisdictions, we must recognize the underlying social and public policy requirement to protect children. It is presumed that children cannot understand or appreciate many aspects of life and thus are unable to form judgments and make intelligent or, at least, competent decisions, including medical ones. One case decided in 2000 by the US Supreme Court clearly makes that point. While not directly relevant in terms of medical decision-making, the court majority opinion reads, in part, that "interest of parents in the care, custody and control of their children is perhaps the oldest of the fundamental liberty interests recognized by this Court." This case, Troxel vs. Granville, 350 U.S. 57 [2], will be referenced later in this chapter when we discuss the right of parents to refuse treatment for adolescents.

Over the passage of several decades, the concept has become eroded that children – most notably those between 12 and 18 years of age – must always require parental or other approval or guidance to make sometimes critical medical decisions. This fact brings us to review exceptions to the rule that parental or other such interventions are always required for all minor children – including adolescents for present purposes – to provide informed consent. We shall now discuss in some detail the basis for the exemptions from the parental or equivalent authority normally required to provide informed consent on behalf of a minor child, specifically, an adolescent.

Exceptions to the Rule

From this point forward in this section of the chapter, we will be discussing adolescents in a specific sense. Therefore, it is necessary to clarify the terms and the status of "adolescent" and "minor."

From a legal viewpoint, the term "adolescent" is rarely encountered, as opposed to that of "minor" or "juvenile." The latter refers to any individual with a chronological (not necessarily developmental) age up to 18 years. Having reached that threshold year of 18, individuals may vote, enlist without parental consent in the armed forces, enter into legally binding contracts, sue and bring suit in their own name, and be treated as adults as defendants in the criminal justice system. Despite the newly achieved status of legal maturity of some individuals, some states may prohibit an 18-year-old from purchasing alcoholic beverages or tobacco products until the age of 21 is reached.

The principal point here is that individuals below the age of 18, whether referred to as adolescents or minors, are considered by the law as being incompetent. They lack the capacity to make medical decisions, that is, to provide informed consent. However, there are some important exceptions to that rule. In fact, competency under the age of 18 is subject to rebuttal based on the proven intelligence and emotional development (and thus, judgment) of the minor. The specific legal exemptions refer to the "Mature Minor Doctrine," the status of "emancipated minor," and numerous laws that permit exceptions to the inability to provide informed consent, even in the absence of the minor's being emancipated or being recognized as a mature minor. As a general rule, depending on various state laws, minors who are married, or are members of the armed forces may be considered able to provide informed medical consent. We will now examine each of the major areas of exception.

The Mature Minor and Judicial Bypass

The Mature Minor Doctrine (above) is not recognized in all states. There is some resistance to it, largely based on the already-noted public policy grounds that the state has an essential interest in protecting minors in the absence of significant contrary evidence in individual cases illustrating that the minor does not require such protection.

In short, the individual who seeks the status of being a mature minor must show a level of maturity equal to that of an adult through a demonstration of judgment, intelligence, emotional stability, conduct, and demeanor when a medical decision is being made. These salient factors may be employed in an attempt to convince a physician or a court that an individual under the age of 18 is competent to make an informed medical consent decision.

We will more fully consider the concept of court intervention later in this chapter when the usual procedure for requesting that a court override parental refusal of a recommended medical treatment for a minor is discussed. In this context, the term "judicial bypass" has been used in cases dealing with abortion and Supreme Court cases, and has become linked to (i) the mature minor doctrine, and (ii) the right of an adolescent to have an abortion without parental consent. The use of judicial bypass allows the pregnant adolescent to seek court approval for the abortion procedure in those states where parental consent is necessary. Essentially, the result is a policy decision that the adolescent is then considered a mature minor for the narrow and specific purpose of being able to provide the informed medical decision for the abortion in the absence of parental consent.

The underlying question as to the constitutionality of a parental consent requirement arose as the result of a challenge to a Missouri law that required married women to have spousal consent and for minors to have parental consent for an abortion. The US Supreme Court dealt with the question in a case, *Planned Parenthood vs. Danforth* [3], decided in 1976. In the opinion of the Court in that case, the Missouri law was found unconstitutional, largely on the Fourteenth Amendment grounds. A line of cases followed relevant to the parental consent for an abortion issue. In the 1981 case of *H.L. vs. Matheson* [4], the Supreme Court held that where a state law required parental consent for an abortion, the parents should be advised of the abortion if such notification was possible. In 1983, the Court, in *Planned Parenthood vs. Ashcroft* [5], held that parental consent laws are constitutional if there is a judicial bypass procedure in place where the law exists. The line of relevant cases continued with the Court's decision in the 1990 case of *Hodgson vs. Minnesota* [6], which upheld Matheson, and with the 1992 case of *Planned Parenthood vs. Casey* [7]. While the latter case has been noted primarily because of the Court's continuing support of the *Roe vs. Wade* [8] decision on the right of a woman to have an abortion, it was also important because of the Court's ruling in support of parental consent.

While these cases deal specifically with the right of an adolescent to have an abortion, there seems little doubt that they will be cited for at least their persuasive value in the future in situations in which parental consent and adolescent rights collide with regard to other medical treatments; these may include those for addiction and alcohol.

The Emancipated Minor

The laws that provide for a minor to achieve emancipation vary widely from state to state. In general, the concept is that a minor who wishes to be free from parental control and supervision can go to the applicable court in his or her jurisdiction and file a petition seeking the status of emancipated minor. The reasons cited by the petitioner or applicant are limited only by the specific case. These reasons include facts showing, for example, that the minor is being abused or that possibly he or she is unable to live under the prevailing conditions in the parental home. Factors that can bolster such an application may include the petitioner's age (a

16-year-old will, e.g., have a stronger position, in most instances, than a 13-year-old) and may also include evidence showing that the petitioner has substantial and independent financial resources. Once the proper court approves the submitted petition, the emancipated minor may enter into contracts, conduct business, and act in virtually every manner as an adult who has reached the age of full legal responsibility.

The implications with respect to the law on informed consent and its relationship to these exceptions are clear. There is a substantial burden on the physician or other healthcare professional seeking informed consent when dealing with a mature minor, but less of a burden when seeking consent from an emancipated one. Except in an emergency situation (usually referred to as "therapeutic privilege" where consent is not an issue), the healthcare professional who accepts at face value the claim of a young person that he or she is emancipated has embarked on a perilous journey. If the claim is subsequently shown to be false, the probability of a lawsuit being filed against the medical care provider will be high and its ultimate success almost certain.

It is equally important for the physician or other healthcare professional always to remember the differences between the emancipated minor and the mature minor. The former has achieved a formal legal status based on the petition duly filed with an appropriate court and is therefore fully recognized as an adult by virtue of that judicial determination. The latter does not have this formal recognition or status.

Finally, there are situations in which minors, generally 12 years of age and older, may seek medical and other healthcare services on their own without the requirement for parental consent. These specific situations are provided for in the law and include treatment based on sexual assault; drug and alcohol counseling; treatment for a contagious disease; treatment for acquired immunodeficiency syndrome (AIDS); pregnancy care; care and counseling on the use of contraceptives and other birth control measures; mental health issues; and, of course, as we have discussed, abortion.

Summary: Consent

Questions and controversy continue to swirl around the issue of informed consent and minors. Court decisions and the passage of laws have failed to resolve many aspects of these issues (i.e., birth control measures; mental health issues; and as we have already discussed, informed consent and parental issues), thus leaving those having to deal with adolescent consent in somewhat uncharted or only partially charted territory. Beyond reference to existing law, the best general guidance is that physicians and other healthcare professionals must always remain focused on the goal of effective treatment and of providing patients – adults or adolescents – with all reasonable guidance and information needed for a truly informed consent.

Having now set out what we believe is valuable information that a modern healthcare professional should possess concerning the subject of medical consent, we will now proceed to an equally valuable discussion of dealing with the subject of the rights of adolescents to refuse medical treatment as well as the right to withdraw initially provided consent.

ADOLESCENTS AND THE RIGHT TO REFUSE TREATMENT

We opened this chapter with the observation that any realistic discussion regarding the right of an adolescent to provide informed consent for medical treatment purposes must also consider the equally important right of an adolescent to refuse medical treatment, either at the onset of treatment or at any subsequent time during the treatment.

While there may well be increased risks in a withdrawal of consent for treatment, in a situation without medical intervention, and by the treatment itself, the underlying consideration must concern what happens when the adolescent changes his or her mind and seeks to oppose the recommended medical care.

Once again, the applicable rules are found in two places: the law and medical ethics. Taking the latter first, medical actions must always be in the best interests of the patient. If competent, the patient is the final arbiter as to what is best for him or her.

Applicable Standards

The same standards already discussed concerning the right of competent adolescents to refuse or discontinue medical treatments, subject to the laws of the state where the physician practices, will usually be based on whether that state recognizes the mature minor doctrine – as a separate exception to the need for parental consent – so that the adolescent has been legally granted the status of an emancipated minor.

A competent minor may, of course, refuse medical treatment in some emergency situations, for example, a disaster where victims may be encountered and where treatment must be provided immediately. Such refusal would fall before the ethical requirement on the part of the physician to intervene despite the objections of the patient, regardless of age or status.

Thus, we repeat the critical point that readers should remember: In most states, there is a legal presumption (although it is subject to rebuttal) that anyone under the age of 18 is incompetent with regard to medical decision-making, either to provide consent, or to refuse or withdraw it.

In the final section of this chapter, we will examine the rights of parents to refuse medical treatment to their children. In this part of the chapter, the focus remains on the right of the adolescent child to refuse without having the consent of a parent or guardian to do so. The issue centers again around the historic interests of the state in its efforts to protect all of its citizens, including minor children, along with the perhaps equally strong and growing societal belief that every competent individual should be allowed both to refuse treatment initially as well as to end it. This latter point is best illustrated by the approved and widespread use of advanced medical directives that can be triggered by a parent, guardian, attorney-at-law, or any other individual who has been preselected by an adult to act if the selecting patient is unable to make a treatment or life-ending decision on his or her own. The use of such a directive is not solely for the informed use of an adult, but also for a mature or emancipated minor.

The desire of the courts in every state is constantly and continually to seek to effectively balance the need to protect individuals while at the same time respecting and acknowledging the rights of parents, the rights of minors, and the interests of the state – sometimes a daunting responsibility. When a minor is part of a case concerning the right to refuse medical treatment, the interest of the minor is always given the highest priority. When the minor can be considered as competent under the mature minor doctrine in those states that recognize that doctrine or when the minor is considered as being legally emancipated, the minor's rights are considered to be of a mature and competent adult. However, it must be remembered that the legislated laws and those laws created through judicial decisions are not uniform throughout the United States. In particular, the question of how far the rights of even a mature minor can extend into the realm of medically informed consent to receive and refuse medical – including critical and even life-saving medicine – care can only be determined by an examination of the laws concerning this subject on a "state by state" basis.

Summary: Adolescent's Right of Refusal

The guiding principle when dealing with an adolescent's right to refuse or to withdraw from medical treatment (including that recommended for drug and alcohol addiction) is that the underlying consent must be given (with the few stated exceptions) by the adolescent's parents or other legally appointed substitute. State law, either as passed by the legislature or set out in a court decision, provides the applicable rules for healthcare actions.

Having now set out a discussion on the rights (or the lack of such rights) of adolescents' consenting to, refusing, and withdrawing from treatment for addiction specifically and medical treatment intervention generally, our attention will now center on the rights of an adolescent's parent or parents to refuse medical treatment, and on how those parental refusals can be challenged.

PARENTAL RIGHTS TO REFUSE MEDICAL TREATMENT

The issue of the right of parents to deny or refuse medical treatment to a child has been present in our society for a long time. It is probable that the first major stories that gained public attention involved parental refusal on religious grounds, as best exemplified by the Jehovah's Witnesses (or "Witnesses"), a religious sect whose followers hold, among other beliefs, that blood transfusions result in blood impurities and are impermissible on religious grounds. Over the years, the same group has objected to injections of various types, including those considered generally recommended to prevent and treat diseases. The Jehovah's Witnesses, however, are not alone in the on-going issue over parental refusal and its social and legal arguments.

Obviously, situations in which the life of an adolescent is in danger represent the most dramatic types of cases. The same general principles apply when dealing with addiction to either drugs or alcohol and with the treatment necessary to deal with that problem.

In broad terms – and, once again, it bears repeating – the state, in recognition of the presumption that a minor is incompetent, feels a public policy obligation to shield the minor from harm. Thus, in any case in which a medical treatment is considered necessary when dealing with a minor, the medical professional (usually the physician) requires parental consent to proceed. In the event that consent is not provided, the assistance of an appropriate court is usually sought. It cannot be assumed, however, that the court will automatically step in and, acting in place of the parents (*in loco parentis*), override parental refusal. This point is illustrated by the US Supreme Court ruling in the 1944 case of *Prince vs. Massachusetts* [9], in which the majority opinion stated in part that " . . . parents may be free to become martyrs themselves. But it does not follow they are free, in identical circumstances, to make martyrs of their children before they have reached the age of full and legal discretion where they can make that choice for themselves."

In some states, as mentioned, adolescents may seek and receive medical treatment for drug and alcohol addiction without parental consent, thereby obviating any right in such states for parental refusal of such treatment. Furthermore, in some jurisdictions, although parental consent or the right to refuse consent may not exist, the law may require that parents be advised by the healthcare provider that the medical treatment is being provided.

Much of the debate and discussion with respect to the right of a parent to refuse adolescent medical treatment has focused on those cases in which the treatment is life-saving in character. It may be assumed that the decisions of courts in non-life-saving situations will be, to say the least, particularly difficult to predict in situations where the parental refusal is based on religious grounds.

In virtually all such cases, the already noted interest of the state in shielding a minor from harm, coupled by the traditionally accepted role of parents to act in the best interests of their children, is even more complicated by questions of importance arising under the federal constitution. In cases of a parental refusal on religious grounds, the exercise of religion clause in the First Amendment will inevitably arise. In other refusal cases, the Fourteenth Amendment, specifically its due process clause, may well be introduced in support of parental rights.

As a result of these conditions, it is difficult to easily set out controlling standards relevant to the refusal of parents to permit treatment of adolescents for addiction. Questions such as whether the treatment is life saving and how effective the treatment has proven to be, may conceivably affect the decision of a court in making a ruling about whether to override parental refusal of treatment. The answers to these questions, among others, have been used to create standards for court decisions in parental refusal cases for many years.

Obviously, there is a significant difference between the action of a parent to refuse consent to blood transfusions on religious grounds and a refusal to permit or to continue addiction treatment for an adolescent. We submit that a physician or, for example, a hospital will encounter far less of a hurdle in seeking court approval in the former case than in the latter. One 2007 unreported Virginia case is frequently used as a good example of successfully avoiding the tangle of interests that arise in parental refusal cases and how accommodations among and between the parties (i.e., the state, the parents, and the adolescent) may be resolved. In that case, a 4-year-old patient was diagnosed as suffering from leukemia and underwent treatment that included injections, oral medications, and chemotherapy. The parents became concerned about long-term side effects of the treatment regimen and attempted to discontinue treatment. The treating doctors opposed this idea and

sought to have the parents declared as unfit. A legal action was filed for that purpose. The matter was resolved through negotiations by which the doctors need to keep the parents informed of the treatment and involve them in all medical decisions.

Another unreported case (from 2004) involved a 16-year-old adolescent patient with Hodgkin's disease. Unhappy with the medical treatment that largely involved high doses of chemotherapy, the parents and adolescent embarked on a treatment that had long been rejected by the Food and Drug Administration (FDA). The doctors sought to have the parents charged with neglect. A court ruling to that effect was applied and the appellate court held that the alternative treatment could continue if monitored by a qualified medical expert.

Having noted the issues and problems that can arise when attempting to override a parent's refusal for addiction treatment, we must next explore the potential actions of a court after making a decision to override the parental refusal.

Court Actions

Once an appropriate court has weighed the alternatives and issues involved – always bearing in mind what is considered paramount to be in the best interests of the adolescent – the court assumes custody and thus stands in place of the parents (*in loco parentis*). Having assumed the place of the parents, the court will then appoint an individual – a guardian – who will agree to carry out the orders of the court. Unless it can be shown by relevant evidence that the adolescent has been neglected on grounds beyond the question of the medical treatment issue, the appointment in most cases will be a temporary one, and full custody of the adolescent will eventually be returned to the parents. Any actions of the court will be subject to proper appellate review, usually on an expedited basis.

The essential fact remains, however, that when a court ruling is sought on the question of overriding a parental refusal for medical treatment and where a balance between parental and children's rights is sought, the interest of the adolescent and those of the state can weigh more heavily than the parents' rights to refuse. As reviewed above with specific reference to the aforementioned *Troxel* case ruling, the rights of parents are not likely to be ignored during judicial decision-making.

CHAPTER SUMMARY

In this chapter, we have covered the historical background and guidelines of consent and informed consent with particular attention and application to the adolescent. In that regard, we also noted that adolescents are treated throughout the United States as being, in the eyes of the law and for reasons of long-term public policy, presumed to be incompetent although that presumption of incompetency is subject to rebuttal.

It was necessary, we believe, to show how rebuttal of this basic assumption usually arises through the application of either the mature minor doctrine – a creature of the law in some state jurisdictions – and through the statutory mechanism of the emancipated minor, a legal status that is available by application to the appropriate court in all jurisdictions.

In addition to discussing the elements of consent and, particularly, informed consent, we explored the question of adolescent competence and how it may be determined. We pointed out that what constitutes a minor is based on the laws of the individual jurisdictions. Chronological age considerations are issues separate and apart from the mature minor and emancipated minor exemptions.

We next explored the obviously related right of an adolescent to refuse medical treatment from its onset, as well as to withhold the initial consent as was provided, at a later time in the treatment regimen. Therefore, it must be borne in mind that refusal of medical treatment on the part of an adolescent (except under the emancipated minor laws, the mature minor doctrine, or under some other specific state law permitting such refusal) requires agreement of either a parent or guardian. In terms of minors generally, the lower the age of the minor, the greater the decision power of the parent or guardian to consent or refuse consent on behalf of the child. There is obviously a different standard relating to parental consent and decision-making when dealing with a newborn infant, as opposed to a 10-year-old child and to a 17-year-old adolescent.

SOME CLOSING THOUGHTS

While the essential points found in this chapter concern the law as it applies to adolescents and, in particular, the interrelated issues of informed consent, refusal of treatment, and parental refusal of treatment with regard to addiction problems with drugs and alcohol, there is an equally important aspect to consider in these issues, namely important ethical factors.

The relationship between the physician and the patient is not a static one. Indeed, this relationship has evolved over the passage of a relatively few years to the presently accepted view that discussions about medical care between a doctor and a patient, including the adolescent patient, are at the same time both a shared activity and a responsibility of both the doctor and the patient.

Today, for both medical and ethical purposes, it is incumbent on the physician to provide effective communication about treatments and health maintenance to a patient as part of the overarching requirement to provide informed consent, while seeking concurrently to place the needs of the patient at the highest plane of concern.

References

1. Public Law 104–191, Health Insurance Portability and Accounting Act of 1996 (1996).
2. *Troxel vs. Granville*, 350 US 57 (2000).
3. *Planned Parenthood vs. Danforth*, 428 US 52 (1976).
4. *H.L. vs. Matheson*, 450 US 398 (1981).
5. *Planned Parenthood vs. Ashcroft*, 462 US 476 (1983).
6. *Hodgson vs. Minnesota*, 497 US 417 (1990).
7. *Planned Parenthood vs. Casey*, 505 US 833 (1992).
8. *Roe vs. Wade*, 410 US 113 (1973).
9. *Prince vs. Massachusetts*, 321 US 158 (1944).

44

Third Party Liability for Supplying Adolescents with Illegal Substances

Daniel P. Greenfield[1] and Jack A. Gottschalk[2]

[1]Seton Hall University School of Health and Medical Sciences, Millburn, NJ, USA
[2]Seton Hall University, Stillman School of Business, Livingston, NJ, USA

In this chapter, using a case scenario as a springboard, we will (i) present an overview from a practical clinical perspective of the definition of "Third Party Liability" and aspects of it that might impact the practice of a clinical and adolescent mental health practitioner; (ii) expand on facts and their implications brought out in the scenario; and (iii) discuss a number of caveats and ways in which vicarious liability scenarios for the practicing child and adolescent mental health practitioner can be avoided or prevented, or the dangers from them minimized.

Additionally, because of the clear relevance to adolescent addiction, such topics as liability for sales of tobacco and illegal (CDS) substances to minors, the culture of street gangs ("Bloods," "Crips," "Latin Kings," among others) that promote drug use and drug dealing, and community and law enforcement approaches in dealing with adolescent substance abuse, will also be reviewed.

Last, readers are advised that we use the term "adolescent" in a clinical context, that is, an individual between the ages of 12 and 19 [1]. We recognize that the generally accepted age of what may be called "legal maturity" or "responsibility" is 18 years with statutory exceptions that, for example, concern the purchase of alcoholic and tobacco products.

THE SCENARIO

Consider the following scenario, from the perspective of a practicing female (adolescent) psychiatrist inexperienced in forensic issues, primarily in private practice affiliated with a public medical school.

> You are a practicing child and adolescent psychiatrist with about 20 years of treatment experience.

You receive a call on your personal cell phone at 3:00 am on a Sunday about an emergency involving a 17-year-old male clinic (i.e., not private) patient. The caller, a psychology intern "on call" at the hospital clinic where you teach and supervise, tells you that a raid by police based on a 911 call complaining of excessive noise resulted in the arrest of six adolescents 19 years of age or older, and the detention of seven others under that age. The police response to the usually quiet neighborhood led to the discovery of underage drinking of alcoholic beverages as well as drug possession and use. One of the younger children detained is a patient of a primary therapist (a licensed clinical psychologist) who works part-time at the clinic and who receives "informal supervision" from you. The psychologist was not on call that morning and her caseload was covered that weekend by the psychologist intern who called you. The party, raided by the police, was held at the home of the 17-year-old male whose psychotropic medication you supervise under the auspices of the clinic and whose parents were away from the house on a 2-week vacation. The only adult in the home was the male's 74-year-old grandmother, who had been left in charge by the male's parents. The male, an only child, had arranged the party without his grandmother's knowledge or permission. She had previously spoken to the boy's parents who had earlier refused permission for the party. The grandmother remained in her locked upstairs bedroom, cowering throughout the party until the police arrived.

Clinical Handbook of Adolescent Addiction, First Edition. Richard Rosner.
© 2013 John Wiley & Sons, Ltd. Published 2013 by John Wiley & Sons, Ltd.

About 20 minutes before the neighbor's complaint, an underage (17-year-old) partygoer who had been illegally drinking alcohol with the 17-year-old male host, had left the gathering in her parents' car that she had "borrowed" from them without permission. While operating the vehicle, she struck a young married couple on the sidewalk half a mile away from the site of the party. The female of the couple was in the third trimester of her second pregnancy. She sustained serious brain injury as a direct result of the accident and died while en route to the hospital. The male companion (her husband) suffered bilateral compound femoral fractures and a skull fracture and was in a critical condition by the time he was seen in the hospital emergency room. After her arrest, the driver's serum blood alcohol concentration was determined at the police station and recorded as being 179 mg/dL, which converts to 0.154%, well over the limit for a driving while intoxicated (DWI) charge.

If the above scenario were presented as part of a test question in a law school examination, the potential liability of a number of individuals for a variety of reasons could be posed. For example:

- With respect to the adolescent psychiatrist supervising the treating psychologist "informally" and monitoring, supervising, and prescribing medication, what liability, if any, might apply?
- With respect to the "on call" psychology intern, what liability, if any, might apply?
- With respect to the treating psychologist consulting to the clinic as an independent contractor and not an employee of the clinic or hospital, what liability, if any, might apply?
- With respect to the 17-year-old party host's 74-year-old grandmother, what liability, if any, might apply?
- With respect to the 17-year-old male's absent parents, what liability, if any, might apply?
- With respect to the 17-year-old party host, what liability, if any, might apply?
- With respect to the mental health clinic, staffed and managed by an outside group hired and contracted by the hospital, what liability, if any, might apply?
- With respect to the hospital that hired and contracted the mental health clinic to provide clinical services under the hospital's aegis, what liability, if any, might apply?
- With respect to the affiliated public (state) medical school that provided trainees and clinical faculty both for the mental health clinic and the affiliated hospital, what liability, if any, might apply?

- With respect to the state (the public entity) that sponsored and to some extend funded the medical school affiliated with the hospital, what liability, if any, might apply?
- With respect to the minor children present at the party and detained by the police, what liability, if any, might apply?
- With respect to the adult (age 18 or older) adolescents present at the party and arrested by the police, what liability, if any, might apply?
- With respect to the under-age female drunk driver who struck the young pedestrian couple, what liability, if any, might apply?
- Finally, with respect to the parents of the under-age female drunk driver who had not given permission to their daughter to operate the motor vehicle, what liability, if any, might apply?

Another hypothetical "third party liability" law school examination test question based on this same scenario could include naming the various types of liability that could potentially arise from this scenario. In the broad areas of civil liability, these include (i) strict liability; (ii) vicarious liability; (iii) host liability; (iv) parental liability; (v) contractual liability; and (vi) the *respondeat superior* doctrine, which generally arises from an agency-principal, employer-employee, or similar relationship. All of these will be discussed in further detail later in this chapter.

A CLINICIAN'S PRIMER ON LEGAL LIABILITY

Practically speaking, in the context of the above case scenario, the adolescent mental health practitioner needs to know that in the areas of "legal liability and negligence," several concepts might apply to potential liability in that practice. According to Spaulding [2] in his work entitled "Legal liability and negligence:"

- "Legal liability" is defined as "the liability of a party imposed by a court for their actions or inactions."
- "Torts" are "illegal or civil wrongs committed against people or organizations causing them a loss."
- "Intentional torts" are "willful acts or the willful failure to act when required to do so that causes injury to someone else."
- "Breach of conduct" is defined as "the lack of performance by a party to another to satisfy conduct that the parties agreed to."
- "Negligence" is defined as "the failure to exercise the required amount of care to prevent injury to others."
- "Absolute liability" or "Strict liability" is defined as "liability imposed on specific parties . . . which

obviates the need to prove fault in court" (in the area of medical negligence or malpractice, e.g., "sometimes, the act itself determines negligence." This would include such obvious cases as when a surgeon leaves an instrument in a patient's body during an operative procedure, resulting in serious consequences (*res ipsa loquitur*). The patient clearly finds it easy to prove the surgeon in this instance negligent in a malpractice suit.

- "Dram shop liability" holds "the seller of alcoholic beverages liable for drunken patrons" and the similar "host liability" holds the hosts – e.g., of parties in which alcoholic beverages are served and consumed – liable for the acts of their drunken partygoers.
- The "Family Purpose Doctrine" holds "parents responsible for the negligent acts of their children," and is an example of the broader category of "vicarious liability" in which one party is held liable for the actions (or inactions) of another.
- *Respondeat superior* ("let the master answer") is also a type of vicarious liability in which superiors, supervisors, and the like are held responsible for the actions (or inactions) of their subordinates.

Finally, in the context of an adolescent mental health clinical practice, the four elements of professional negligence (or malpractice), commonly know as the "Four Ds" [3], are:

1. Duty to treat a patient or client.
2. Dereliction of that duty or failure to perform that duty.
3. Damage – an injury or loss – that results from that dereliction.
4. Direct (or "proximate" or "causal") connection between the dereliction and the damage.

Without purporting to be a comprehensive analysis of the question of the potential tort liability of the supervising adolescent psychiatrist, the treating psychologist, the covering psychology intern, and so forth in the above scenario, in our experience, liability would apply as follows:

1. The adolescent psychiatrist might be considered liable for improper "informal" supervision of the treating clinical psychologist and for improper prescribing for the 17-year-old patient ("professional negligence" and *respondeat superior*).
2. The psychology intern might be identified as someone who allegedly failed to intervene – as an employee of the mental health clinic – with the 17-year-old male who had reportedly been drinking with the 17-year-old drunk female party-going driver ("professional negligence").

3. The treating psychologist, not on call at the time, might be considered as having failed to identify her 17-year-old male patient as having an alcohol problem, and as potentially giving alcohol to other underage friends and partygoers ("professional negligence").
4. The 74-year-old grandmother who would likely be scrutinized as the most directly responsible adult at the party in which the underage drinking took place ("host liability").
5. The absent parents, like the grandmother, would likely be identified as responsible adults ("family purpose doctrine") at the party in which underage drinking took place ("host liability").
6. The 17-year-old male drinking party host would likely face juvenile criminal charges for providing alcohol to his underage guests, as well as for "host liability" civil action.
7. The mental health clinic would likely be held liable for the alleged actions of its employees (*respondeat superior*).
8. The hospital that contracted for services with the mental health clinic, as with the clinic, would likely be scrutinized for the alleged liability of the clinic (*respondeat superior*).
9. The public (state) medical school – to the extent possible under applicable state and federal law – as with the clinic and hospital, would be liable for the alleged actions of the hospital (*respondeat superior*).
10. As with 7, 8, and 9, to the extent allowed by applicable state (and, possibly, federal) law, the state agency that sponsored, supervised, governed, and funded the other three agencies might be held liable (*respondeat superior*).
11. The minor children attending the party would likely face juvenile criminal charges to the extent that alcohol and/or drug use could be proven, and might be scrutinized about the extent, if any, to which they encouraged their fellow partygoers to drink and use drugs.
12. The adolescents (18 years of age and older) attending the party would likely face criminal charges applicable to their unacceptable behaviors there, and would likely be scrutinized about the extent, if any, to which they encouraged their fellow partygoers to drink and use drugs.
13. The drunk underage female licensed driver who struck the young pedestrian couple would very likely face criminal charges that may include driving while intoxicated (DWI) and vehicular homicide, along with civil liability actions arising from the accident.
14. The parents of the drunk underage female licensed driver would likely be in the same position as that of

the 17-year-old male partygoer's parents and, thus, responsible for their daughter's behavior under the ("Family Purpose Doctrine").

"AN OUNCE OF PREVENTION IS WORTH A POUND OF CURE"

Focusing first on the mental health professionals (the adolescent psychiatrist, the treating psychologist, and the covering psychology intern), we will now discuss ways in which these individuals might prevent or effectively deal with their potential liability in the above scenario. Several ways based on good common professional sense come to mind:

- *Document* all contacts with patients/clients, involved agencies, colleagues, administrators, and anyone else who might be part of such a scenario. Documentation must be explicit and detailed.
- *Be aware* of contractual relationships with agencies and of supervisory relationships with staff members.
- *Be sensible*, conservative and up-to-date in practicing mental health professions.

Turning to the agencies themselves (the mental health clinic, the hospital, and the state medical school), ways of preventing or, if necessary, dealing with potential liability in the context of this scenario will depend on applicable state and federal laws. A detailed discussion of these ways is beyond the scope of this chapter [4].

Concerning the potential liability of parents of the children in the above scenario – including the parents and grandmother of the 17-year-old male party-giver and the parents of the 17-year-old female drunk driver – their third-party liability is considerable. As a practical matter, after the incidents (the party and the motor vehicle accident) occurred, the damage had already been done. However, prior to those two events, such commonsensical and good child-rearing practices as communicating with children, setting limits on "acting out" behaviors (such as underage drinking), knowing the activities of children, encouraging positive activities, and others are all applicable preventive measures. Some of these will be discussed later in this chapter.

Finally, concerning the potential liability of the children involved in this scenario – underage, adult-age, and the two 17-year-olds in particular – the same may be said about them as about their parents. Positive and negative factors in this area – including the sale of tobacco products to minors; the culture of street gangs; community and school programs and strategies that discourage chemical dependency among children and adolescents; and positive law enforcement approaches to chemical dependencies in children and adolescents – will be discussed later in this chapter.

TOBACCO SALES TO MINORS

Consistent with public policy in recognizing the universally negative aspects of tobacco uses, the sale of tobacco products to minors is against the law in all jurisdictions of the United States including (recently) at the federal level.

Starting in 1933, with the passage of the 21st Amendment to the Constitution (which repealed the 18th Amendment prohibiting the sale of alcoholic beverages), the authority to regulate sales and distribution of alcohol was assigned to the individual states and territories of this country. Later, regulation of tobacco and tobacco products, and other psychoactive substances, came to be undertaken by the states and territories, with federal jurisdiction pertaining to areas of interstate interest and commerce (such as Department of Transportation regulations covering drug testing for interstate truckers and the national blood-alcohol concentration, or "BAC" of 0.08% for states that received federal highway funding). The principle of government regulation of potentially dangerous substances came to be an acceptable type of government control and regulation of citizens at various levels and in various jurisdictions [5].

In the case of tobacco sales to and tobacco use by minors, a great deal of regulation, and social and governmental study seems to demonstrate that the most successful form of tobacco use regulation is associated with high cigarette taxes and with significant penalties to sellers of tobacco products to minors. A survey in 2010 by the American Lung Association – an important not-for-profit research and watchdog organization in tobacco and related topics – showed, for example, a straight-line relationship between states with high excise tax rates on tobacco products and a decline in the rates of use of those products by minors [6]. Tobacco sales and use by minors have been declining throughout the country; this is a national trend demonstrated by surveys such as those reported by the federal Substance Abuse and Mental Health Administration. In this regard, as described in a newsletter of "Campaign for Tobacco-Free Kids," the "new federal FDA tobacco law, however, makes selling cigarettes to youths a federal offense for the first time (as of June 22, 2010) and establishes a strong federal-state system for stopping sales to kids" [7].

A full disclosure of the adverse health effects of tobacco and tobacco products is beyond the scope of this chapter. However, for present purposes, we emphasize the psychoactive and neuropsychiatric effects of tobacco products – especially cigarettes – on the developing and chaotic minds and brains of teenagers: Being a time of what has been characterized by some as "controlled craziness" – adolescence is not helped or stabilized by the sometimes stimulating, sometimes depressing, sometimes psychotogenic, and generally unpredictable effects of tobacco and tobacco products on those brains and minds.

"THE LITTLEST GANGSTA:" STREET GANGS IN CONTEMPORARY CULTURE

Consider the following scenario from a forensic psychiatric consultation/evaluation (C/E) done by the first-named author of this chapter:

> AB, a 14-year-old Hispanic female, presented with about 150 ("buck fifty") suture scars mostly on her torso and legs, with chronic pelvic inflammatory disease from multiple rapes (from the "sex-in" initiation process into her local gang) and with deformities in both knees, ankles, and her left temporal area (from the "beat-in" initiation process into her gang). The consultation/evaluation was court-ordered, in part, to assess the woman's competency to stand trial ("CST") status in connection with her alleged participation in a "beat-in" initiation by her gang of a 9-year-old boy seeking to join the gang. After a frustrating hour of attempting to achieve rapport, much less contact, with AB, the forensic consultation/evaluator psychiatrist simply gave up. She had been confronted by a wall of silence, alternating with such words as "love," "honor," "obedience," "loyalty," "respect," "courage," and many others, all providing an impenetrable shield to communication with the "gangsta."

Street gangs have been part of American culture for many years. Contemporary "supergangs" (with more than 1000 members) – the Bloods, Latin Kings, and Crips being probably the best known street gangs – began in California in the 1940s–1950s in their present "form." Other gangs (the "DeGraw Street Gang," "Back Street Gang," among many others) date back to the 1920s and even earlier (e.g., the New York City "Gopher Street Gang" from the 1800s). Some have been featured and glorified in films going back to the 1950s in such productions as *The Wild Ones*, and later in *West Side Story*.

While the relationships between organized crime and street gangs have been studied by sociologists and criminologists for many years, the practical usefulness and attraction of contemporary gangs lie in what they purport to offer to their prospective recruits: membership, camaraderie, sacrifice to a larger cause, a sense of belonging, false role models, financial success, friendship, drugs, security and protection, sex, unquestioned loyalty from fellow "gang bangers," a sense of continuity ("generational members"), and opportunities to act on aggressive impulses in ways that are socially acceptable to and are even valued by fellow members ("sexing-in" and "beating-in" are good examples). The sense of identification with, and loyalty to, fellow "bangers" is underscored and reinforced by what may be called symbols of membership: tattoos, hand signals, sports clothing, and coded baseball caps, graffiti, body markings and scarring, and various artifacts (knives, jewelry, and others). The cohesiveness, irreversibility, and military nature of typical gang members are conveyed by the following oath of membership sworn by "members" in the "NETA Association" gang:

> I swear to never violate the rules, regulations, and principles of the NETA Association. I understand that once violated, I have to accept the consequences for any of them. I will respect my leaders and will protect them so that the movement will always stand strong [8].

As a counterculture reminiscent of hippies, "flower children," and the like, gangs start out by satisfying the needs of their often disenfranchised and disadvantaged recruits – and gangs, especially "supergangs," do recruit in a variety of ways – and from a psychological/psychiatric perspective become surrogates for more conventional sources of well-being such as families.

With an estimated over 40 000 active and identified gang members in New Jersey now (an increase from 10 000 such members in 2003), and with over one million such members nationally – by one estimate – street gangs are a "growth industry" in the United States. They will likely continue to thrive, flourish, be dangerous, commit crimes in institutionalized ways, challenge the resources of law enforcement, and otherwise commit mayhem indefinitely.

No panacea for street gangs exists: Law enforcement directly both combats and works with at-risk youths; community organizations (such as religious-based initiatives, social service agencies, healthcare institutions, foundations, and others) make efforts to provide attractive alternative social programs to at-risk youths; governmental organizations and agencies at all levels also attempt to provide alternatives to street crime and street gangs for vulnerable and at-risk youths.

COMMUNITY-BASED PROGRAMMING

The ease with which drugs can be obtained, the price, the number of people using drugs, the violence on the border all show that . . . [we] need to rethink our responses to the health effects, the economic impacts, the effect on crime. We need to rethink our approaches to the supply and demand of drugs [9].

The traditional three-part approach to public health and preventive medicine consists of:

1. "Primary" prevention: reducing risk factors that predispose to active disease, such as elevated cholesterol, lipids, and blood pressure, and – in the behavioral area – cigarette smoking, drug and alcohol abuse, and life and lifestyles associated with excessive levels of stress.
2. "Secondary" prevention: treating active disease once it has occurred, such as treating heart disease with medications and various surgical interventions;
3. "Tertiary" prevention: rehabilitation for maximum recovery once the damage of the active disease has been done.

In concept, substance abuse prevention, intervention, and treatment lends itself to this tripartite model, and incorporates community-based, government, and formal professionally based biomedical treatment programs.

First, in *primary prevention* of substance abuse, risk factors may be considered social, behavioral, and medical/psychiatric, for present purposes. Non-medical and non-clinical prevention programs are found in this level of prevention. Examples of such programs at the "primary prevention" level include: school-based educational programs at the local level; larger and more extensive programs (the best example – admittedly controversial – is probably the international Drug Abuse Resistance Education, or DARE, program, which began in California in 1983 and which is currently present in over 40 nations); worldwide community-based law enforcement programs (such as the Police Athletic League, which provides athletic and related diversion programs for at-risk children and adolescents); hybrid approaches (such as the so-called "harm reduction" approach in which the elimination of substance abuse altogether is recognized as impossible and public health programs are undertaken – such as needle exchange programs to reduce the intravenous spread of HIV – to reduce harmful and adverse effects of substance abuse); approaches on the policy level (to reduce the supply and demand for drugs in the community); and community-based hybrid approaches (such as self-help recovery

programs – Alcoholics Anonymous (AA) and Narcotics Anonymous (NA) are examples. These work with affected individuals – addicts and alcoholics – and attempt to prevent further use or "relapse" to illicit substances). Volumes have been written, and scores of studies done about these "primary" prevention approaches to substance abuse and associated social psychology (such as gang membership) over the years: In our view, the "answer" for an effective approach or approaches in this area has not yet been found.

Second, in the *secondary prevention* of substance abuse, the user has begun the consumption of illicit substances, and has likely become engaged in associated dysfunctional behaviors, at least to some extent. "Secondary prevention" in this model equates with "treatment" in the biomedical model: *Medically*, measures include the use of hospitalization, detoxification, partial hospital (step-down) treatment, medications, and the like in attempting to interrupt and reverse the course of disease processes (such as hepatoxicity, CNS seizures, and so forth) caused by substance abuse; and *behaviorally* and *spiritually* there is use of psychotherapy, group therapy, self-help, recovery groups, psychotropic medications, and related such approaches to interrupt and reverse the behavioral decompensation process (such as compulsive drug use, robbery to support a drug habit, aggression, chronic intoxication, and other such phenomena) also caused by substance abuse.

Third, in *tertiary prevention* in the substance abuse context, medical and behavioral dysfunctions and treatment approaches converge. The overarching goal at this level of prevention – given and accepting that some irreversible damage has already been done – is to stabilize the abuser both medically and behaviorally and to prevent the worsening of the abuser's condition, to the extent possible. Some of the treatment approaches and modalities already mentioned – such as ongoing pharmacotherapy for chronic disease, and self-help recovery therapies – will continue to be used at this level of prevention.

Others, for individuals in poor health, will be used: long-term chronic disease hospitalization, chronic hemodialysis ongoing physical therapy (for chronic medical conditions), long-term psychiatric hospitalization, chronic use of psychotropic medications, and recurrent courses of electroconvulsive therapy (ECT) for chronic psychiatric/behavioral conditions.

While no single approach to adolescent substance abuse is a panacea, the concept of the three levels of prevention from the fields of public health and preventive medicine provides a useful framework and classification system for the many individual, medical, and community-based programs for substance abuse treatment.

CONCLUSION

Starting with the fairly discrete topic of "Third Party Liability for Supplying Adolescents with Illegal Substances," we have expanded that legally-based topic into discussions about what specific substances could represent "supplies" to adolescents and how they might be "supplied." We specifically discussed "Tobacco Sales to Minors," adolescents and gang membership, and community-based drug prevention and treatment programs.

These topics are all important sociocultural as well as individual psychological and psychiatric aspects of adolescent addiction. In our view, the reader should be aware of these topics and their implications in working effectively with "adolescent addicts."

References

1. American Academy of Child and Adolescent Psychiatry. Practice parameters for the psychiatric assessment of children and adolescents. *J Am Acad Child Adolesc Psychiatry* 1997;**36**:45.
2. Spaulding WC. Legal liability and negligence. Available from: http://thismatter.com/money/insurance/legal-liability.htm [accessed 27 February 2011].
3. Greenfield DP, Gottschalk JA. *Writing Forensic Reports. A Guide for Mental Health Professional*. New York: Springer, 2008; p. 144.
4. Department of Health and Human Services, Office of Inspector General (Kusserow RP). Youth and alcohol: laws and enforcement. Is the 21-year-old drinking age a myth? Department of Health and Human Services, 1992.
5. Wilford BB. *Drug Abuse: A Guide for the Primary Care Physician*. Chicago, IL: American Medical Association, 1981; pp. 251–253.
6. Berman J. Substantial reduction in tobacco sales to minors. USA Today, 2009. Available at: http://www.usatoday.com/news/health/2009-08-10-teen-smoking_N.htm.
7. Tobacco.org. Enforcing laws prohibiting cigarette sales to kids reduces youth smoking. Campaign for Tobacco-Free Kids; www.tobacco.org [accessed on 12 April 2011].
8. Presented as "Gangs 101", Detective J.E. Castellanos, New Jersey Gang Investigations Association Conference, Somerville, NJ, April 18, 2011.
9. Webb J, quoted in White DW, The future of the war on drugs, Charting a new course in the Commonwealth, Report of the Massachusetts Bar Association Drug Policy Task Force, 2008.
10. Mausner J, Kramer S, *Mausner and Bahn's Epidemiology: An Introductory Text*, Philadelphia, PA: W. Saunders, 1985; pp. 9–12.

45

Older Adolescents in Drug Court: Hammering the Revolving Door Shut

Laura A. Ward

Criminal Court of the City of New York, New York, NY, USA

INTRODUCTION

Since their inception in 1989, drug courts have provided treatment alternatives to incarceration in dealing with drug offenders. Some individuals need a hammer hanging over their head to reverse the course of their lives. Drug court is a substance abuse intervention model that operates within the criminal justice system, integrating social and legal services to adjudicate selected drug cases. It is a unique combination of mandatory drug treatment and the hammer of a prison sentence. This chapter will describe the objectives and inner workings of a drug court in the New York State Supreme Court in Manhattan, which deals with a mixed population of older adolescents (over age 16) and adults. Representative vignettes excerpted from cases involving younger members of this mixed population of drug offenders will be presented. (Juvenile drug courts, which are beyond the purview of this chapter, are now appearing in Family Courts in New York State. These courts deal with defendants up to the age of 16.)

ESTABLISHMENT AND OPERATION

The first drug court was established by former US Attorney General Janet Reno in Dade County, Miami, Florida, in 1989, when she was the local district attorney. Prisons in Florida were severely overcrowded. The state was facing the threatened loss of federal funds, if it failed to reduce its inmate population. In an effort to decrease the prison population and thus retain federal funds, Reno decided to divert defendants to drug treatment. Maryland and California were among the first states to follow Florida's lead and, over the next 20 years, drug courts were instituted throughout the country.

(There are now over 1800 drug courts in operation in all 50 states.) [1]

Since the early 1990s, there has been a dramatic increase in the number of drug arrests. Around the same time Reno was establishing the first drug court, arraignment courts in New York City were open 24 hours a day, 7 days a week. (A defendant is required to be brought before a judge to review the charges and either be released on his/her own recognizance or have bail set within a reasonable time after the arrest. The courts have defined "within a reasonable time" as within 24 hours of an arrest.) In Manhattan, there were three arraignments sessions. The first session ran from 9 a.m. to 5 p.m.; the second from 5 p.m. to 1 a.m.; and the third from 1 a.m. to 9 a.m. Two courtrooms operated between the hours of 9 a.m and 1 a.m., and one courtroom operated from 1 a.m. to 9 a. m. A judge sitting in one of these courtrooms during a single session could arraign between 50 and 150 defendants in a given shift, depending on the number of arrests that day, the speed of preparing the arraignment paperwork, and the production of the defendants.

An increasing number of the defendants arraigned each day in the 1990s were charged with possession or sale of narcotics or marijuana. Many other defendants were charged with crimes related to their drug addiction (e.g., they were charged with burglary, robbery, grand and petit larceny, and prostitution – crimes committed primarily to obtain money to buy drugs). Not infrequently, a variant of the following scenario would recur in a Manhattan arraignment court: a judge assigned to preside for 1 week in the arraignment courtroom could, on a Monday, take a plea to the crime of criminal possession of a controlled substance in the seventh degree, based on a defendant's possession of a crack

Clinical Handbook of Adolescent Addiction, First Edition. Richard Rosner.
© 2013 John Wiley & Sons, Ltd. Published 2013 by John Wiley & Sons, Ltd.

pipe or some other drug-related offense, and sentence the defendant to 3 days in jail. Thereafter, that same defendant could, and often would, appear before the same judge later in the week, charged with possessing drug paraphernalia or some other drug-related offense.

It became apparent to those in the Criminal Justice System in New York State that jail was not the answer to eradicate the drug epidemic. The judicial process seemed more like a revolving door, with the same defendants rotating in and out of the courtroom and jail. Eventually, the defendant's criminal activity was likely to escalate from a misdemeanor (with a maximum sentence of 1 year in jail) to a felony (with a sentence of more than 1 year).

The judicial system is adversarial in nature: prosecutors and defense attorneys are pitted against each other in a modern-day version of trial by combat. The prosecutor's role is to investigate criminal activity and charge defendants, to ensure that the guilty will be punished and sent to jail. Many long-time prosecutors support the old adage "don't do the crime, if you can't do the time." The defense bar works to keep defendants out of jail. The judge, in an effort to make sure both sides and the public receive a fair trial, presides over the battle between the prosecution and the defense as a rational arbiter of the truth-finding process. Although the legislature establishes sentencing guidelines, once a defendant pleads guilty or is convicted after a trial, it is the judge who determines the appropriate penalty. A sentence is supposed to (i) punish the defendant for his/her actions, (ii) rehabilitate the defendant, and (iii) deter others from committing a similar crime.

Thus, it is up to the court to fashion a sentence with these three potentially contradictory goals in mind. Once the defendant is sentenced, the case is essentially over in the mind of the trial court, unless the defendant receives a probationary sentence. In those instances, any violation of the terms or conditions of the defendant's probation is brought back to the attention of the sentencing judge, to determine whether the defendant should remain on probation or receive an incarceratory sentence.

Based on the soaring number of arrests and recidivism rates of drug offenders, it was obvious that the adversarial system and the sentences imposed were not rehabilitating these defendants or deterring their crimes. Radical measures were called for. In the 1990s, in an attempt to stop this revolving door of justice, Judith Kaye, the Chief Judge of New York State, decided to formally implement drug courts in the 57 counties of New York State. (Prior to this state-wide initiative, some individual District Attorney's offices scattered throughout New York had been offering drug treatment alternatives to incarceration on an informal basis [2].) Judge Kaye looked to the Dade County, Miami model, among others, to fashion New York State's drug courts. (During her 15-year tenure as

Chief Judge of the State of New York, Judge Kaye implemented other "problem-solving courts" as well, including mental health and community courts [3].)

The first New York State drug courts were established in 1995 and 1996, in Buffalo and Brooklyn, respectively. Initially, many district attorneys opposed the creation of these courts, arguing that the criminal justice system should not enter the "drug treatment business." Many judges refused to preside in these courts, arguing that they did not attend law school to become social workers. Some legal commentators suggested that drug courts compromised deep-seated legal values, by side-stepping the adversarial system and requiring judges to relinquish their traditional role [4].

In October 2009, the New York State legislature entered the fray and passed the Rockefeller Drug Reform Act [5]. This law not only decreased the previous draconian sentences for drug possession and sale, but also enabled judges to offer drug treatment to felony offenders without the consent of the District Attorney. (Prior to the enactment of the revisions to the Rockefeller Drug Laws, if the District Attorney did not agree to have a defendant placed in a drug treatment program as an alternative to incarceration, judges could only require drug treatment for defendants who were eligible for a probationary sentence. The Department of Probation would monitor the defendant's drug treatment.)

An effective drug court requires the prosecutor and defense lawyer to cast the adversarial system aside. In this unique setting, they must work together as a team, in an effort to get the defendant out of the revolving door of the Criminal Justice System. This is accomplished by giving the individual the tools to deal with his/her drug problem. The ultimate goal of the program is to assist the defendant to recover and become a law-abiding, productive member of society.

ASSESSMENT AND TREATMENT OPTIONS

In practice, the operations of the typical drug court follow a standard procedure. A defendant is identified either by the prosecutor or the defense attorney as an individual who could benefit from drug treatment. The initial assessment by the prosecutor is based on two elements: (i) a review of the defendant's criminal record, using his/her "rap sheet" (i.e., record of arrest and prosecution) as a guide; and (ii) an analysis of the defendant's role in the alleged crime.

Case Vignette #1

Mr A, a homeless male, is arrested for selling cocaine. The defendant has a history of misdemeanor drug, petit larceny, and trespassing arrests. The facts of the case currently before the court are as follows: an undercover officer approached the defendant and asked if he knew where the undercover officer could purchase some cocaine. The defendant took the undercover officer to another individual who, in exchange for pre-recorded buy money (i.e., money bearing pre-recorded serial numbers used by the undercover officer to make the drug purchase), gave the undercover officer two "twists" of crack cocaine (i.e., a small piece of crack cocaine packaged in cellophane with the top twisted tight).

After receipt of the drugs, the undercover officer gave the arrest team the prearranged sign that the sale had been completed. The arrest team approached the defendant and the other individual and arrested both of them. While waiting to be transported to the precinct for the booking process, the undercover officer confirmed the identification of the two perpetrators as the people from whom he purchased the drugs. Both are charged with the C felony of Criminal Sale of a Controlled Substance in the Fourth Degree. As a first-time felony offender, the defendant faces a sentence of up to $5\frac{1}{2}$ years of incarceration, followed by 2 years of post-release supervision. The prosecutor may believe that, based on the defendant's involvement in the crime and his criminal history, he would be an appropriate candidate for drug treatment. If the prosecutor arrives at that conclusion and the defendant is interested in an alternative to incarceration, he would be evaluated for drug treatment.

There are times when the defense lawyer may request drug treatment, based on what he/she knows about the client. For example, using a factual scenario similar to the one set out above, the defense lawyer seeks judicial diversion to drug treatment. The lawyer tells the court that her client has never had drug treatment and would benefit from the opportunity to confront his drug problem. Although the defendant had tested positive for heroin while previously on probation, he failed to attend the drug treatment program recommended by his probation officer. The defendant had, however, been in and out of methadone maintenance programs in the past (most drug courts require defendants to be detoxified off methadone). If the court agrees, the defendant is sent for drug treatment evaluation.

Depending on the resources available to the specific court, the defendant's evaluation may be conducted by a court-hired case worker, a probation or parole officer, a forensic psychiatrist or psychologist retained by the defendant, or a representative of a treatment program affiliated with the court. The evaluators are often Certified Alcohol and Substance Abuse Counselors. The evaluation is extensive. The goal of the clinical assessment is to determine if the defendant actually has an addiction to drugs and is not merely selling for profit, and to match the defendant to appropriate levels of care

and modalities of available substance abuse services. It is important for the defendant to understand that it is essential that he/she answers the assessment questions truthfully and does not tell the assessor what he/she thinks the assessor wants to hear or what he/she thinks will get him/her released. One way this is done is to have the judge tell the defendant, on the record, in open court:

I am sending you to be evaluated for a drug treatment program. It is essential that you answer all questions put to you honestly, because if you lie or tell us what you think we want to hear and we decide to put you into a treatment program based on your false answers, we would probably put you in the wrong program. This would cause you to fail because it was the wrong program. You would then end up doing your prison sentence. Do you understand?

The person conducting the assessment is trained to seek information by asking the defendant the same question in many different forms. The clinical assessment usually includes the following:

1. Defendant's demographics, i.e., name, present and former addresses, primary language, marital status, race/ethnicity, sexual preference, and contact information.
2. Diagnosis of the defendant's dependence, including identifying his/her drug or drugs of choice, frequency of use, and history of use.
3. Taking a urine or blood sample to test for the presence and/or level of drugs in the defendant's system.
4. A complete medical and psychological history of the defendant. In situations where the defendant has had previous hospitalizations, psychiatric care, or significant medical issues, the defendant executes a Health Insurance Portability and Accountability Act (HIPAA) waiver and prior psychiatric and medical records are obtained.
5. Sometimes a psychosocial examination report is prepared.
6. Copies of the defendant's documents, i.e., birth certificate, social security card, public assistance identification cards, passport, health insurance cards, immigration cards, driver's license, and employment identification, are obtained.
7. Educational background, including any vocational training.
8. Employment history.
9. Financial support, i.e., employment, family, and/or government assistance.
10. Veteran status.

11. Questions about the defendant's home environment, including with whom the defendant lives and the duration of this arrangement. In the best case scenario, the case worker performs a home visit to determine, in part, if the defendant lives in a drug-prone location.
12. A suicide risk assessment.

Once the clinical assessment is completed, copies of the assessment report are circulated to the prosecution, defense, and court. Thereafter the potential case manager meets with the prosecution, defense, and court, without the defendant present, to discuss whether or not the defendant should be accepted into an alternative to incarceration program. This decision is reached on an individualized case-by-case basis, taking into account the totality of relevant data that have been collected during the assessment process.

No one can predict the future with any degree of certainty, especially when dealing with an individual addicted to drugs. In determining whether or not the defendant is an appropriate candidate for an alternative sentence, the court must balance the interest of the defendant and that of the public. The court should consider not only the defendant's suitability for drug treatment, but also whether or not, upon release, he/she would pose an unacceptably high risk of absconding and continuing to engage in illegal activity, rather than remaining in treatment.

If the defendant is accepted into an alternative sentencing program, the court must not only create a treatment plan, but must also fashion an appropriate sentencing alternative. For example, a defendant may plead guilty to a felony and the promised sentence could be as follows:

> If you successfully complete the drug treatment program, you will be able to withdraw your previously entered guilty plea and your case will be dismissed. However, if you fail to complete the drug treatment program, your plea will stand and you will receive a sentence of two years in jail followed by two years of post-release supervision.

It is the better practice to make the jail alternative a higher sentence than the defendant would have received if he/she had refused drug treatment and either pleaded guilty or been convicted after trial. This gives the defendant a greater incentive to succeed at the drug treatment program and more to lose if he/she fails.

There are many reasons why a defendant fails treatment. He/she may be non-compliant with treatment or may be discharged from the program for bringing in contraband or otherwise violating the program's rules.

He/she may abscond from the treatment program, yet return voluntarily to court. He/she may abscond from the program and be returned to court involuntarily with a new arrest. The court is notified immediately if the defendant absconds from the program and a warrant is issued for his/her arrest on the previously entered plea of guilty. (It is regrettable and not uncommon for a defendant to be released from jail to an escort from a drug program and abscond as soon as he/she leaves the courthouse.) Accordingly, some courts have a two-tiered jail alternative, one sentence for failure in treatment and a longer sentence for situations in which the defendant absconds and fails to return voluntarily to court or is rearrested on new charges.

Unfortunately, although the defendant has undergone an extensive clinical assessment, hopefully conferred with his/her attorney and case manager, and been made to understand what will be expected of him/her while in drug court, most defendants really only hear "I am getting released." Such a defendant does not fully comprehend how difficult his/her participation in drug court will be. It is incumbent on the drug court judge, when taking the plea, not only to fulfill all the legal requirements of the plea, but also to try to make the defendant understand in no uncertain terms that drug court is different than any other court he/she may have previously experienced.

The New York State Court of Appeals has held that trial courts are not required to engage in any particular litany during an allocution to obtain a valid guilty plea in which a defendant waives a plethora of rights [6]. The following is a sample plea allocution:

Defense Counsel:	My client wishes to withdraw his previously entered plea of not guilty [the plea entered at arraignment] and enter a plea of guilty to the first count of the indictment, Criminal Sale of a Controlled Substance in the Third Degree.
Clerk:	Please raise your right hand. Do you swear or affirm that the statements you are about to give this court are the truth, the whole truth, and nothing but the truth?
Defendant:	Yes.
Court:	Did you hear what your attorney just said?
Defendant:	Yes.
Court:	Are you satisfied with the representation you have received from counsel?
Defendant:	Yes.

Court: Have you had enough time to discuss your plea and sentence with your attorney?

Defendant: Yes.

Court: Are you today under the influence of any drugs, medication, or alcohol that affects your ability to understand what is happening today?

Defendant: No.

Court: By pleading guilty you give up certain rights. These rights include, among other rights, your right to remain silent, your right to a trial, your right to have the People prove their case against you beyond a reasonable doubt, your right to confront witnesses and if you want to put witnesses on on your own behalf, and your right to make motions to suppress evidence and raise certain affirmative defenses. Do you understand the rights you are giving up by pleading guilty?

Defendant: Yes.

Court: Is anybody forcing you to give up those rights?

Defendant: No.

Court: In addition to the rights I have just listed, you are also giving up your right to appeal and in a moment you will be signing a waiver of your right to appeal. Had you gone to trial in this case and been convicted, you could have appealed your conviction, as well as your sentence, but by pleading guilty, I am requiring you to give up those rights as well. Do you understand?

Defendant: Yes.

Court: Is anybody forcing you to give up your right to appeal?

Defendant: No.

Court: Please sign the waiver.

Defendant: [Defendant complies.]

Court: Did anybody promise you any sentence other than the following: You will be placed into a drug treatment program. If you successfully complete that program, three things will happen. First, and probably most important to you at this moment, you will be permitted to withdraw your plea of guilty and the case will be dismissed. The second and third things are more important to me and will hopefully become equally as important to you. They are that you will be given the tools to deal with your drug problem and become a productive member of society. However, if you fail, and a defendant fails drug treatment because he/she just cannot stop using drugs, or leaves treatment without permission or authorization, gets rearrested, or gets discharged from drug treatment, you will receive a sentence of 3 years followed by 2 years post-release supervision. Any other promises made to you?

Defendant: No.

Court: Now, although we have agreed upon your sentence, I obviously cannot sentence you today. We have to see how you do in treatment. Quite frankly, I hope I never have to sentence you, because that would mean that you successfully completed drug court and your case was dismissed. But, should I ever have to sentence you, a pre-sentence report will be prepared. You will be interviewed for the report and asked a series of questions, including "are you guilty of these charges?" If you are unable to admit your guilt in the preparation of the report, you should not be pleading guilty here today. Do you understand?

Defendant: Yes.

Court: [To defense counsel] Did you have the required conversation with your client regarding immigration?

Defense Counsel: Yes. My client is a United States citizen.

Court: Before I formally take your plea, I want to make sure you understand what drug court entails. Drug court is different than any other court you may have experienced. In drug court, the defendant holds the key to his/her freedom. You will be released to a drug treatment program. That program will work with you to give you the tools to deal with your addiction for the rest of your life. You will also be required to participate in job training, have a place to live, and a means to support yourself, other than selling drugs in order to successfully complete drug court. This is a lot to do and it will be very hard. You will be coming to the court periodically and I will be receiving reports on your participation at the program. Your urine will be tested frequently. If the reports are good and you do not test positive for marijuana, alcohol, or any controlled substance, I will reward you. Rewards could include reduced program visits, reduced court appearances, or certificates of achievement. If your reports are bad, you will be sanctioned. Sanctions include being required to observe court and report on your observations, write an essay, increased program visits or court appearances, being sent to detox/rehab, lunch remand (remand means placed in jail without bail), or short jail sentences. So you can see that you control what happens to you. If you do what you are supposed to do, I can only congratulate you. But if you do not, I can punish you and that can include putting you in jail. Do not think this will be easy. But, if you do succeed it will be the best thing you have ever done for yourself and will prove that you can do anything you put your mind to. Any questions?

Defendant: No.

Court: You are pleading guilty to the first count of the indictment, which is charging you with the crime of Criminal Sale of a Controlled Substance in the Third Degree, in violation of Penal Law § 220.39. It is alleged that on or about May 3, 2010, in the City of New York, you knowingly and unlawfully sold a controlled substance to an undercover officer. Is that true?

Defendant: Yes.

Court: What was the drug?

Defendant: Cocaine.

Court: What borough were you in when you sold the cocaine?

Defendant: Manhattan.

Court: Are the People satisfied with the plea?

Prosecutor: Yes.

Court: Would the Clerk please enter the plea.

Once the plea is entered, the defendant is released and a date is set for the defendant to return with his/her lawyer for an update on how he/she is doing in treatment. Prior to the defendant's plea and release, the court fashions a treatment plan for the defendant. Treatment modalities include detoxification, outpatient treatment, intensive outpatient treatment, residential treatment, or some combination of modalities. For example, the defendant may be told he/she will be attending a residential treatment facility. While at the facility, the defendant will not only attend drug treatment sessions, but also high school classes and/or vocational training. Some treatment programs allow defendants to bring their dependent child(ren), under the age of 5, with them to reside at the program. This would apply to male or female defendants who have custody of the child(ren). (The day-care facilities at these programs rival any private day-care setting.) Finding the appropriate program for a defendant is easier said than done. Many addicted defendants are self-medicating and once they are detoxified off their drug of choice, it becomes apparent that they have an underlying mental disorder.

Case Vignette #2

It was observed that Mr B, after detoxifying from cocaine and prescribed pain medications, was wearing out his shoes. His outpatient program reported that he needed to have his shoes resoled constantly. When the defendant appeared before the court, the judge inquired about this. It took a great deal of prodding, but he finally disclosed that, after he stopped using drugs, he began to hear voices at night. The voices were telling him to do "terrible things." The defendant said that if he walked back and forth between 79th Street and 125th Street along a West Side avenue all night, he would not hear the voices. He was sent for a psychiatric examination and prescribed psychotropic medication to treat his psychotic disorder.

Many defendants have comorbid conditions, such as bipolar disorder, schizophrenia, and other major psychiatric disorders. There are very few available programs that adequately address mentally incompetent chemical addicted (MICA) defendants. There are also very few programs that cater to non-English-speaking defendants. There are no programs that deal specifically with gay, lesbian, bisexual, or transgender defendants. Accordingly, some defendants who are otherwise appropriate for drug court, may be denied the opportunity, simply because there is no treatment provider in the court's jurisdiction that can handle the defendant's complex needs. An addicted, transgender, Spanish-speaking, MICA defendant would likely be impossible to place.

Because long-term narcotic use not only ravages the mind, but also the body, defendants are often diagnosed with AIDS, HIV, and hepatitis C. In such cases, the court must find a facility that provides adequate medical care. (Long-term drug use may cause tooth decay. It is not uncommon for a defendant to have a history of numerous tooth extractions and fittings for dentures. Other defendants, although in need of eyeglasses, have never had enough money to purchase them and have never seen an eye doctor.) It is essential that the defendant's medical needs are addressed. If the defendant feels better physically, as well as mentally, he/she is more likely to succeed in drug treatment.

The court is consistently re-evaluating the appropriateness of a defendant's placement throughout his/her involvement with drug court. It is not uncommon for defendants to be moved from one program to another. For example a defendant may start in an outpatient program, but continue to test positive for his/her drug of choice. Rather than terminate the defendant from drug court and impose the jail alternative, the court may move the defendant to a residential treatment program. Another defendant may initially be placed in a short-term residential treatment program following his/her detoxification. However, at that point, it may be determined that he/she suffers from a mental disorder that is so severe that he/she requires a MICA program. In another scenario, a defendant may be sent to a residential program in one of the five boroughs of New York City, but he/she regularly leaves the facility without permission, misses treatment sessions, and continues to use drugs. Rather than terminate this defendant, the court may move him/her to a residential program in upstate New York, 100 miles away from the individual's stomping grounds.

ROLE OF THE DRUG COURT JUDGE

In most criminal courts, the only time the judge addresses the defendant directly is when he/she enters a plea or is sentenced. All other interactions are among the court, prosecutor, and defense lawyer. In this regard, drug court is completely different. In drug court, the judge interacts directly with the defendant at each court appearance. There is no single recommended judicial style. It is, however, important that the judge remains consistent in the messages that are conveyed to the defendant. The drug court judge receives progress reports before the defendant appears in court. It is essential that these reports are thorough, including information regarding the defendant's toxicology reports, program attendance and participation, any problems he/she might be experiencing, any successes he/she may have achieved, and anything else the program may want the court to specifically address with the defendant.

Many drug court judges say that by the time a defendant completes drug treatment, which can take anywhere from 1 to 6 years, the judge comes to know more about the defendant than the judge knows about members of his/her own family. The drug court judge has to balance his/her role as a caring authority figure and as a judge. He/she needs to gain the defendant's trust by acknowledging the challenges the defendant faces in dealing with his/her recovery. The judge should be a combination mother/father/cheerleader/teacher figure who attempts to motivate the defendant. For many of these defendants, this is the first time anyone has taken an interest in them, especially someone in a position of power and authority. Over time, it is interesting to observe how the dynamics change between the judge and the defendant. Some defendants test the judge by seeing how much they can get away with before they are sanctioned. Other defendants start out cautiously, unsure of how to respond to the judge. When the judge actually breaks through, it is apparent to all the observers in the courtroom. Many times, one will overhear a defendant refer to the judge as "my judge." When the judge praises the defendant for completing a phase in the program or getting a good grade on a test, one can see the defendant literally stand taller. When the judge chastises the defendant for breaking a rule at the program or missing a class, one can see the defendant's shoulders slump. All interactions between the defendant and the judge take place on the record in open court. Most courthouses designate a specific courtroom exclusively to hear cases involving defendants who are engaged in drug treatment. Thus, the audience is filled with similarly situated defendants and their families and friends. Communication between the judge and the defendant should be designed to affect the audience, as well as the defendant who is before the court.

Case Vignette #3

The defendant, Mr C, was addicted to marijuana. He had completed the 10th grade, but was only reading at a

3rd-grade level. Mr C was presently in an intensive outpatient program and attending school. The defendant had been in treatment for 3 months. Upon entering treatment, he tested positive for marijuana. Within 30 days, the defendant's toxicology reports were negative for marijuana. However, the most recent toxicology report was again positive for marijuana. The defendant denied smoking marijuana.

Court: Mr C, I was surprised to see you tested positive for marijuana. You had been testing negative for two months. I see you deny smoking marijuana. How do you explain this?

Mr C: I was visiting friends and they were smoking.

Court: Oh, so you are claiming that this is a contact high?

Mr C: Yes.

Court: Haven't you learned the concept of "People, Places, and Things" at the program?

Mr C: Yes.

Court: It is my understanding that that expression means that, in order to avoid using marijuana, you have to stay away from people who smoke marijuana, places where you can get marijuana, and doing things that make you want to use or make it easier to use marijuana. Is that right?

Mr C: Yes.

Court: So what were you doing hanging around with people who were smoking marijuana?

Mr C: I did not know they were smoking until I go there.

Court: Why did you stay?

Mr C: They are my friends.

Court: They may be your friends, but your friendship is going to get you in trouble. I have a problem with your story. In order for you to get a contact high you would have to be in a room that was so full of smoke you could barely see your friends. Is that what happened?

Mr C: [Silence from the defendant].

Court: I am really not as stupid as you think I am.

Mr C: [Interrupting the Court] I do not think you are stupid judge.

Court: If you were with friends who were smoking, then I am sure you had at least one hit off the blunt they probably had. I want you to think about what you did and in a few minutes I will ask you to tell me how you will avoid getting in situations like that again.

When the defendant's case was called again, he explained that, if he were ever to find himself with people who were smoking marijuana, he would leave immediately. The court then warned him that his next positive toxicology report would result in his transfer to an in-patient program. Although the defendant was clearly relieved that his sanction was not worse, the court put him on notice regarding the consequences, were he to continue to test positive. The audience saw that there are definite consequences for an individual's actions.

Case Vignette #4

In a similar situation, when his case was recalled, Mr D admitted to smoking marijuana. The court then praised the defendant for being truthful, telling him that the court could now trust his word, but also warning him that his next positive drug test would result in a remand. If the defendant tested positive again, the first remand might only be over the luncheon recess. The judge might say to him "I am going to remand you over lunch and then decide how long I will keep you in jail." After lunch, the defendant is brought back before the judge and the following colloquy may occur:

Court: How did you like lunch?

Mr D: I did not like it.

Court: I am going to release you today to return to the program. If you continue to use drugs you will be spending a lot more time in jail than just lunch. Do you understand?

Unsuccessful cases can be very frustrating for drug court judges. It can be extremely emotionally draining to deal with the problems of drug court defendants and judges are at risk to develop "burn-out." Specialized forums like drug court require a well-balanced judicial temperament to deal directly with this population and an openness to insights from the mental health field. The practice of therapeutic jurisprudence requires a change in the judge's role from dispassionate, disinterested magistrate to that of an interpersonally sensitive, concerned counselor [7]. "When a drug court judge steps down, it is not always possible to find a sufficiently motivated replacement. Without a highly motivated judge, the drug court approach simply does not work" [8].

COMPLIANCE AND FOLLOW-UP

Drug courts use urine testing as an objective measure of the defendant's compliance, and in some cases the testing serves to alert the court to his/her lack of motivation or readiness to engage in treatment. Testing positive repeatedly is a clear indication of treatment failure. Many defendants dispute the positive results of their urine tests. They claim, among other things, that the program mixed up the urine samples. Judges will often tell the defendant: "you want me to accept the tests when they show you are negative, but reject them when you test positive. Unfortunately, you cannot have it both ways." Other defendants try to "beat the tests." Although most programs supervise the collection of urine, sometimes a defendant is able to place a test tube containing another person's urine along the side of his leg and make it appear that the urine is coming from him.

Case Vignette #5

Mr E, who was concerned he was going to test positive for cocaine, his drug of choice, paid a person for her urine. When the toxicology report showed a positive result for heroin, Mr E disputed the result. Although the court seldom required a second test, it did in this defendant's case because the positive result was for a drug that was not his drug of choice. The court sent the urine sample out for further analysis, only to learn the donor was female. Mr E eventually admitted to his case manager that he had purchased another person's urine. On his way to court to see the judge, the defendant absconded. He was eventually returned on a warrant. He begged the court for another chance, but he had already committed numerous infractions while in treatment and it was clear to all involved that he was not committed to his recovery. Mr E was sentenced to jail.

Case Vignette #6

Not all drug court defendants are poor and uneducated. Some defendants are functioning addicts, successful people with white- or blue-collar jobs and families. One defendant, Ms F, was the daughter of a prominent New York lawyer. Ms F had a trust fund, which she depleted buying cocaine. The cooperative board of her apartment building was trying to evict her, because of the loud and destructive parties that were occurring on a nightly basis at her apartment. She was arrested for possession of cocaine with intent to sell. It was her first arrest. While she was being evaluated for drug court, her mother, dressed in a mink coat, appeared in the court audience to show her support for her daughter. The mother refused to pay her daughter's bail. Upon Ms F's release, she did not do well in treatment. She started in an intensive outpatient program, but continued to test positive for cocaine. The court was constantly warning her that her next positive test would result in a remand and transfer to a residential treatment facility. The first remand was over the luncheon recess. The second remand was overnight. Ms F was transferred to a residential program, but continued to obtain cocaine. The third remand was for 3 days. Eventually, Ms F was remanded for 2 months. When she was released from the 2-month remand, she told the judge "this time I will succeed." The very next week, Ms F was back before the court, once again testing positive for cocaine. After 2 years in drug court, it was apparent to the judge that Ms F was not ready to deal with her drug problem and that the bed she was taking up in the residential treatment facility should be made available to another defendant. The court sentenced Ms F to 1 year in jail. Her mother sent a note to the court, thanking the judge for trying to help her daughter.

Although many defendants have managed to navigate the complicated public assistance process (it should be noted that drug courts generally try to encourage defendants to get off public assistance), most of them have never been employed, lived in their own apartment, had a bank account, or received consistent medical, dental, and psychological care. Those who have obtained public housing may lose that housing based upon the pending drug case. Some drug court models treat only the defendant's addiction. Once the defendant has completed every phase of the residential and/or outpatient program, the defendant's case is dismissed. There are some drug court judges, however, who believe that merely treating the addiction is not enough. If all the defendant knew before entering treatment was how to buy and sell drugs, that is what the defendant may return to once his/her case is dismissed. In one tragic case, a defendant who had completed drug court was subsequently rearrested in an apartment where kilos of cocaine were being broken down for sale on the street. The defendant's drug court diploma (many drug courts have a formal graduation ceremony for those who successfully complete drug treatment) was lying among the drugs and paraphernalia. Fortunately, that defendant was the exception, rather than the rule. Before the defendant's case is dismissed, the court may require him/her not only to complete the drug treatment program, but also to obtain a high-school diploma (or pass a high-school equivalency exam) or vocational training and find a job and a place to live. A defendant who is given the tools to deal with his/her addiction, as well as a means of supporting himself/herself and a place to live in a non-drug-prone environment, has a better chance of succeeding on a long-term basis.

Case Vignette #7

The defendant, Ms G, was a mother of two with a crack/cocaine addiction. Her children were in the custody of foster care. She was in a residential treatment program for 6 months. Her progress report was good. She was attending the program, consistently testing negative for drugs, awaiting the results of her high-school equivalency exam, and was just accepted into a computer training program.

Court: Ms G, I have an excellent report. How was the exam?

Ms G: It was hard, judge.

Court: I know from previous reports how hard you studied and how hard you worked in class. If I remember correctly when you started in drug court you were only reading at a sixth grade level and your math was at a third grade level. It is quite an accomplishment that the program thought you were ready to take the test. Do you think you passed?

Ms G: I hope I passed. The math was real hard. If I don't pass, I plan to take it again as soon as possible.

Court: Tell me about the computer training program?

Ms G: They are going to teach me how to fix computers. And they said that once I finish the course they will help me find a job.

Court: How are your kids?

Ms G: The judge in family court is increasing my visits and said if I get out of treatment and find a decent place to live, he would consider giving me Carrie back and if that works I would get Jerome back.

Court: That's GREAT! It gives you something to work for. But you know that you have to do this, that is, work on your addiction, for yourself, not for the sole purpose of getting your kids back. I know you want your kids out of the system and back with you, but getting them back will be an added stress and stress is one of your triggers.

Ms G: I know that judge and I am talking about that a lot in group.

Court: Great! Let me know as soon as you get your test results, no matter what the results are. I'll keep my fingers crossed that you pass.

At the next court appearance, Ms G reported that she passed her test and received her high-school equivalency diploma. The court actually stood up and applauded for Ms G. That caused the entire audience, over 70 people, to also stand up and applaud. Needless to say, Ms G was beaming.

Despite uplifting, successful outcomes like the case of Ms G, drug court judges are quite aware that the road to recovery is often not a smooth one. The drug court model expects defendants to relapse. It is a great deal to ask of a defendant, who has spent years focusing only on how he/she will get money to finance his/her addiction, to go to group and individual treatment sessions, school and/or vocational training, and doctors' and other appointments.

Case Vignette #8

Mr H, a marijuana-addicted defendant, was consistently missing his appointments. In one month, the defendant missed or was late for 21 out of 30 appointments. The court asked him for an explanation. His response was that he overslept and, once he realized he would be late, often decided not to make the effort to go to the appointment. The court purchased an alarm clock for him and told him that now he had no excuse. At the first court appearance after Mr H had received the alarm clock, the court was informed he missed three group sessions in the last 30 days and was late for five other sessions, only a slight improvement. The court directed him to write an essay explaining what he would do to avoid being late. Thereafter the court had the following colloquy with him:

Court: I am sure if I told you that, if you attended all your appointments and arrived on time, you would receive a multi-million dollar home, a fifty thousand dollar sports car, one million dollars a year for life, and a sexy girlfriend, that you would not miss or be late for a single appointment. But what I am offering you has a greater value than all those things combined. I am offering you your freedom. If you continue to miss appointments without a valid excuse, for example, you were in the hospital, I will incarcerate you for one day for every appointment you miss and one half day for every appointment you arrive late. Do you understand?

At the next court appearance 2 weeks later, the progress report noted that Mr H. missed one appointment and was late for one appointment. The court remanded him for $1\frac{1}{2}$ days. Upon his release, Mr H looked tired, and told the court he was unable to sleep while incarcerated, because the jail was so noisy. He was told that his next missed appointment would result in 1 week in jail.

A month later, Mr H's progress report revealed that he had made it to all his appointments on time. The court praised him, telling him "I knew you could do it. That was not so hard, was it?"

HANDLING OF NON-US CITIZENS

From their inception, drug courts have been confronted with collateral problems related to immigration. Defendants who are in the United States illegally or hold resident alien cards or visas face a myriad of issues. Defendants who were brought to this country illegally by their parents, when they were infants, now face deportation to a country they never knew, based on their plea and participation in drug court. Treatment programs are denied funding for defendants who are in the country illegally. Thus, unless the defendant is able to pay for treatment (many programs offer a sliding scale based on ability to pay), he/she will be denied participation in drug court. Those defendants who hold resident alien cards or are in the United States on a work or tourist visa face mandatory deportation if charged with certain crimes, specifically violent or narcotics crimes, and could be deported if convicted of other crimes [9]. The problem with placing these defendants in jail pending or during treatment is that the Department of Homeland Security, Immigration and Customs Enforcement (ICE) is immediately notified of their arrest and may take the defendant into custody at any time during the proceedings.

Case Vignette #9

Ms I, a female defendant with an addiction to heroin and a history of mental problems, was accepted into drug court. In addition to the charge to which she pleaded guilty – selling cocaine to an undercover officer – the defendant had a lengthy rap sheet indicating over 30 arrests for petit larceny. Most of the petit larceny arrests were based on the defendant taking merchandise without paying for it from Macy's Department Store in Queens, New York. Ms I's parents were deceased, but she had siblings. Initially she was doing well in treatment. One day she was rearrested for petit larceny, again for taking merchandise from Macy's. While Ms I was incarcerated on the petit larceny case, the drug court judge was notified that ICE had taken her into custody. Apparently, Ms I had been brought to the United States from Poland

by her parents when she was an infant. She had no idea she was not a US citizen. She had never visited Poland after her parents had brought her to the United States. She did not speak or understand Polish and had no remaining relatives in Poland. Ms I was subsequently deported.

OUTCOMES

As noted at the beginning of this chapter, the very first drug court was established in Dade County, Miami, Florida, in an attempt to avert the threatened loss of federal funds, unless the severe overcrowding in the state's prison system was reduced. It was hoped that diversion of a number of drug offenders to treatment, instead of incarcerating them, would result in a reduction of the prison inmate population. Diverting a number of drug offenders to treatment might prove to be a "quick fix," an immediate short-term solution; however, from a long-term perspective, a more meaningful benefit would result if drug court programs proved to be a significant factor in reducing recidivism.

In the mid-1990s, the Manhattan Treatment Court (MTC), a drug court established to deal with first-time felony offenders, boasted an 82% success rate. This meant that 82 out of every 100 defendants who entered MTC successfully completed a drug program, obtained a job, found a place to live, received or had a high-school (or high-school equivalency) diploma, and were not rearrested within the five boroughs of New York for a period of 5 years following their completion of drug court. The MTC defendants ranged in age from 18 to 70 years, and their drugs of choice included marijuana, cocaine, crack, heroin, ecstasy, oxycodone, and alcohol. The success rate decreased to between 70% and 75% when the number of MTC participants whose sole drug of choice was marijuana increased. (Marijuana users tend to be younger, between the ages of 16 and 25 years old.)

Over the years, numerous studies have concluded that drug court programs throughout the country produced significant recidivism reductions, compared with conventional case processing [10,11].

For example, a study of six drug courts in New York State found that they generated an average 32% reduction in recidivism over the 1-year post-program period, and an average 29% reduction in recidivism over the 3-year post-arrest period. The study concluded that drug court graduation in itself was the "pivotal indicator" to predict avoidance of post-program recidivism [10].

When a graduation ceremony is held to commemorate defendants' successful completion of drug court, they invite their family, friends, and counselors. In addition, defendants currently participating in drug court attend the graduation. The court may designate one or more graduates to speak at the ceremony. There is seldom a dry eye in the house, as the graduates tell their stories. Parents speak of regaining custody of children, and children describe reconnecting with their family. Many defendants remain in contact with their case managers and the drug court judge after graduating. It is very rewarding for a judge to have a defendant who successfully completed drug court return years later just to say "hello" and "thank you."

Although the majority of defendants who pass through drug court successfully complete the program, some do fail. However, it may be that drug court has a positive impact even on those who failed. It has been reported that drug court may continue to exert a beneficial effect on those who fail to graduate. "Even offenders who do not succeed in drug court appear to be less criminally active than they were previously. This may be due to the benefits of treatment, or the supervision, sanctions . . . and specific deterrence of the drug court" [10]. It is difficult for the judge not to take the failures personally, to wonder "Did I fail to place the defendant in the correct program? Did I fail to motivate the defendant? Was it something I did or said that caused the defendant to fail?" The judge must bear in mind that, when all is said and done, it is the defendant who controls his/her future. It is the defendant who succeeds or fails, not the judge. Drug court gives the defendant the tools to successfully deal with his/her drug problem and become a productive member of society. It is the defendant who has to use these tools.

CONCLUDING REMARKS

The drug court model is a work in progress. Some courts are experimenting with treatment programs geared to specific drugs. (Currently, most drug programs do not separate addicts based upon their addiction. For example, a 17-year-old defendant who smokes marijuana may be placed in a program with 40-year-old heroin or cocaine users.) Other courts are separating defendants based on age. (For example, as noted above, juvenile drug courts are appearing in Family Courts in New York State for defendants up to the age of 16.) The criminal justice system is also establishing drug courts focusing on defendants who are veterans.

The National Drug Court Institute was established to expand and improve drug court programs, provide technical assistance and training, and promote data collection and research across drug court systems [12]. It does appear that drug court is doing a better job of hammering the revolving door shut, or at least slowing down the revolving door and enabling defendants to break the cycle and become productive members of society, than the traditional approach of incarceration.

References

1. Carey SM, Pukstas K, Waller MS, *et al. Drug Courts and State Mandated Drug Treatment Programs: Outcomes, Costs and Consequences.* Portland, OR: NPC Research, 2008.
2. Hynes CJ. Prosecution backs alternative to prison for drug addicts. *Crim Justice* 2004;**19**:122–146.
3. Berman G, Feinblatt J. *Good Courts: The Case for Problem-Solving Justice.* New York: The New Press, 2005.
4. Hoffman MB. The drug court scandal. *N Carolina Law Rev* 2000;**78**:1437–1534.
5. Criminal Procedure Law (C.P.L.) §§ 216.00 *et seq.* (7 October 2009).
6. *People vs. Moissett*, 76 N.Y. 2d 909, 910-911 (1990).
7. Rottman DB. Does effective therapeutic jurisprudence require specialized courts (and do specialized courts imply specialist judges)? *Court Rev* 2000;**37**:22–27.
8. Gebelein RS. *The Rebirth of Rehabilitation: Promise and Perils of Drug Courts.* Washington, DC: US Department of Justice, 2000.
9. United States Code Annotated (U.S.C.A.) § 1227 (23 December 2008).
10. Rempel M, Fox-Kralstein D, Cissner A, *et al. The New York State Adult Drug Court Evaluation: Policies, Participants and Impacts.* New York: Center for Court Innovation, 2003.
11. United States Government Accountability Office. *Adult Drug Courts: Evidence Indicates Recidivism Reductions and Mixed Results for Other Outcomes.* Washington, DC: GAO, 2005.
12. Office of National Drug Control Policy. National Drug Control Strategy: FY 2010 Budget Summary. The White House, Office of National Drug Control Policy, 2009. Available at: http://whitehousedrugpolicy.gov/publications/policy/10budget/ondcp.pdf.

46

Confidentiality and Informed Consent Issues in Treatment for Adolescent Substance Abuse

Robert Lloyd Goldstein

College of Physicians and Surgeons of Columbia University, New York, NY, USA

United States law generally requires parental consent before healthcare is rendered to minor children. Parents are presumed to act altruistically, in the best interest of their children, and to possess a level of experience, maturity, and judgment that minors have not yet attained, but that is needed to make decisions about medical treatment [1]. Notwithstanding this general principle, over the past 50 years, a number of exceptions to the parental consent rule have resulted in a steady expansion of the rights afforded to minors, whether by virtue of their legal status (see below for "Emancipated Minors" and "Mature Minors") or their medical condition and the type of healthcare service that is sought. In regard to the latter category, public health concerns often dictate that unrestricted access to treatment trumps parental rights. This would be the case for allowing minors to consent to treatment for sexually transmitted diseases (STDs), including AIDS, and other contagious, infectious diseases. In addition, US Supreme Court decisions have recognized minors' constitutional rights to privacy in regard to contraception and abortion [2–4]. Over the years, it sometimes has seemed that the growing list of exceptions to the general rule (of parents' control over their minor children's healthcare) threatens to swallow the rule. The list of condition-specific exceptions also includes pregnancy-related services, treatment for rape or sexual assault, mental health services, and treatment for substance abuse. This chapter will focus on confidentiality and informed consent issues in the treatment for adolescent substance abuse. It should be noted that confidentiality and informed consent fall under two distinct medico-legal rubrics in each jurisdiction. As a consequence, just because adolescents have the right to independently consent to treatment for substance abuse in a particular jurisdiction, it does not automatically follow that they will also be afforded confidentiality protection to prevent disclosure to their parents. (All references in this chapter to "adolescents" are meant to denote *adolescent minors*, which takes into account the fact that starting at the age of majority (which is at age 18 in 46 states and at age 19 or 21 in the others), individuals are legally adults in regard to the exercise of all their healthcare rights.)

CONFIDENTIALITY

Since the time of Hippocrates, confidentiality has been a cornerstone in the practice of medicine, an important prerequisite to encourage a patient to seek treatment and candidly reveal all the underlying facts and symptoms of his or her condition, in order to receive effective care [5]. Especially in the mental health field, confidentiality is essential, because "the inherently intimate nature of the patient's communications requires the inviolate security of an atmosphere of the utmost trust, confidence, and tolerance" [6]. This is no less true in the treatment of substance abuse, where the need for professional care under conditions of the utmost freedom from outside interference or intrusion is paramount.

Studies have found that a significant number of adolescents would be reluctant to seek or participate in treatment for their substance abuse if their parents had to be informed about or involved in the process [7,8]. Fear of disclosure often acts as a barrier to treatment, because of the adolescent's trepidation about embarrassment,

Clinical Handbook of Adolescent Addiction, First Edition. Richard Rosner.
© 2013 John Wiley & Sons, Ltd. Published 2013 by John Wiley & Sons, Ltd.

parental disapproval, and possible punishment. Without the promise of confidentiality, many adolescents would delay or be unwilling to seek urgently needed care at all. Because the alarming rise in adolescent substance abuse is a "major problem that incurs a large cost to society" [9], from a public policy standpoint, it becomes crucial to protect adolescent-clinician confidentiality, in order to facilitate and maximize utilization of treatment resources. The issue is further complicated by the important competing interest alluded to above, namely, the traditional rights of parents to protect their minor children, choose what is best for them, and control and consent to the healthcare they receive. This position would seem to be eminently reasonable, and many clinicians who work with adolescents agree that in general parental involvement and support is desirable and should be encouraged: "In the best of all worlds, teens and parents would work in partnership on decisions that could have a lifelong impact" [10]. Some conservative activists contend that the evolution of adolescent law in regard to consent and confidentiality issues serves to undermine parental authority and reflects "an increasing nonchalance about the sanctity of the family unit on the part of the government" [10].

Balancing the legitimate rights of parents and the emerging rights of adolescents continues to be a conundrum for policy-makers; but, in situations where adolescent concerns act as an impediment to seeking urgently needed care, most clinicians agree that encouraging access to treatment should take precedence over parental rights. Many professional organizations, including the Society for Adolescent Medicine and the American Academy of Child and Adolescent Psychiatry, recognize this reality and support the right of adolescents to consent independently with safeguards to protect their confidentiality [8]. The right of adolescents to consent, by itself, without assurance of confidentiality, does not provide a satisfactory solution to the problem. Yet this remains the state of the law in many jurisdictions, namely, that adolescents are authorized to consent to substance abuse treatment on their own, but cannot control access to their healthcare information and records by their parents. This chapter will attempt to elucidate how the labyrinthine network of US state and federal laws and regulations governing the confidentiality of adolescent substance abuse treatment attempts to resolve these complex issues.

INFORMED CONSENT

The doctrine of informed consent is based on the well-established legal premise that competent individuals, sufficiently informed and free from coercion, have the inviolable right to choose and consent to (or to reject) a proposed medical treatment for themselves [11]. The overarching deference that the law accords to individual autonomy in medical decision-making was articulated almost 100 years ago in the memorable words of Justice Cardozo: "every human being of adult years and sound mind has a right to determine what shall be done with his own body" [12].

Healthcare providers are required to disclose sufficient pertinent information that a patient would need to know, in order to make an informed and intelligent decision on whether to consent to the proposed treatment. The essential information that the clinician should disclose includes the following:

- the nature of the patient's condition (the diagnosis);
- the general nature of the contemplated treatment;
- the prospects of success (the benefits of treatment);
- the material risks involved;
- the benefits and risks of any alternative methods of treatment; and
- the risks of failing to undergo any treatment at all [11].

Although Cardozo's sweeping pronouncement on bodily autonomy specifically excluded adolescents from its scope, the law of adolescence has continued to evolve over the past century and, as discussed above, numerous exceptions to the traditional view (that minors are not competent to make treatment decisions) have been recognized by the law, based on adolescents' legal status (e.g., emancipated minors and mature minors) or on the nature of their condition (e.g., substance abuse, mental illness, or STDs).

There is convincing clinical evidence to support legal recognition of adolescent competency in the context of informed consent under certain circumstances. A number of studies have shown that adolescents as young as 14, when presented with various hypothetical medical scenarios, demonstrate a capacity, commensurate with that of adults, to make reasonable treatment choices and appreciate the benefits and risks of their choices [13,14]. Today, in the vast majority of US jurisdictions, adolescents have been granted the right to independently consent to substance abuse treatment [9].

One notable general exception to the doctrine of informed consent, as well as a specific exception to the requirement of parental consent, is when treatment of adolescents is necessary under circumstances that constitute an emergency. Under such exigent circumstances, after attempts to contact the parents and obtain their consent have been made, parental consent is presumed and the physician is allowed to treat the patient, according to his or her best judgment, without fear of liability. Some commentators advise that the physician obtain a concurring medical opinion ("the two physician rule"), if time permits, before providing treatment. Parents should be contacted as soon as they can be reached after treatment, and fully informed [15].

It behooves healthcare providers in this field to thoroughly acquaint themselves with the complex web of laws, both state and federal, that govern the treatment of adolescent substance abuse in the jurisdiction in which they practice.

THE ADOLESCENT'S LEGAL STATUS

Emancipated Minors

Adolescents are generally considered to be *emancipated minors* when certain conditions are met that indicate there is physical/psychological/economic separation from their parents [16]. Indicia of adolescents' emancipation generally include living apart from their parents, being self-supporting and managing their own finances, being married, or serving in the armed forces. In some cases, a minor may be declared emancipated by a court order. Pregnancy or parenthood confers an emancipated status in some states, but not in others. Generally, an emancipated minor can consent to all types of healthcare. When an emancipated minor consents to treatment, the healthcare provider is not permitted to disclose information to a parent without the minor's authorization.

Mature Minors

Mature minors are unemancipated minors whose level of cognitive development and maturity (based on the clinician's judgment and good faith assessment) enables them to make informed choices and understand the risks and benefits of treatment at a level equivalent to that of an adult. They demonstrate the capacity to make a reasonable choice and appreciate the nature, risks, and benefits of their choice in regard to a proposed treatment. A number of states have explicitly recognized the right of mature minors to consent to treatment for substance abuse, while others do not have a statutory law or any case law recognizing its application [17].

US STATE LAWS GOVERNING THE TREATMENT OF ADOLESCENT SUBSTANCE ABUSE

Surveying the thicket of state laws that govern the treatment of adolescent substance abuse in the United States, one finds wide variations and a lack of consensus. The vast majority of states (over 90%) authorize minors to independently consent to treatment for substance abuse [9]. In some states, the laws pertaining to minors' treatment for substance abuse are subsumed under the rubric of mental health services. A study by Weisleder highlighted the lack of consistency among the states in regard to the age at which minors are deemed capable of consenting to substance abuse treatment. Several states do not specify any age requirement. There is wide disparity among those states that do specify an age at which minors can begin to consent, ranging from 12 to 16 (with a modal age of consent of 14) [18]. In a later study, he investigated the state-by-state legislative history, where ascertainable, underlying the determination of a specific age at which adolescents would be considered competent to consent to confidential treatment for substance abuse. He found that only four states considered the scientific input of mental health clinicians before making a determination, while five states were mainly concerned with removing legal barriers to access to treatment [19].

It is relatively rare that state laws require mandatory disclosure to parents of health information pertaining to adolescent substance abuse treatment. The law in many states provides that adolescents' health information in this regard *may* be disclosed to parents, leaving it to the clinician to exercise good faith discretion in the matter, based on what is considered to be in the patient's best interest. In general, clinicians make an effort to encourage adolescents to inform and involve their parents in their treatment, where appropriate. However, parents do not have an absolute right to access their adolescent child's records. If the clinician determines in good faith that disclosure would be detrimental to the therapeutic relationship, or runs the risk of damaging the patient's relationship with his or her family, or even endangers the patient's physical safety or psychological well-being, then confidentiality would be maintained [1]. In some states, such as California, when an adolescent has independently consented to substance abuse treatment, the law explicitly prohibits disclosing information to the parents without the patient's written permission. Yet even under these circumstances, certain incongruities may result. For example, under California law, the provider is also required to contact the parents, *if appropriate* in the provider's judgment, to involve them in the adolescent's treatment plan. The California law explains that "involving parents in treatment will necessitate sharing certain otherwise confidential information; however, having them participate does not mean parents have a right to access all confidential records. Providers should attempt to honor the minor's right to confidentiality to the extent possible while still involving parents in treatment" [20].

It remains to be seen whether this elaborate balancing act is workable in practice or whether it renders the adolescent's right to consent to confidential treatment practically meaningless and serves to undermine his or her willingness to consent to treatment in the first place.

FEDERAL LAWS GOVERNING THE TREATMENT OF ADOLESCENT SUBSTANCE ABUSE

Federal Confidentiality Rules: 42 C.F.R. Part 2

As noted above, many adolescents will be reluctant to seek substance abuse treatment, if they know their healthcare information cannot be kept confidential from their parents. Assuring adolescents that their confidentiality will be protected is often the key factor in their decision to pursue treatment. US state law remains highly variable in this regard. Many states fail to take cognizance of this impediment and continue to allow parents broad access to adolescent treatment records (either by mandating disclosure or leaving the decision to the discretion of the provider). In sharp contrast, federal confidentiality rules, 42 C.F.R. Part 2, where applicable, address these concerns in an unequivocal manner and provide stringent bedrock protection of confidentiality for adolescent (as well as for adult) substance abuse patients:

> 42 C.F.R. Part 2 has been the bulwark, and indeed an essential precondition, to bringing people in need of substance use disorder care into treatment and keeping them there, to effectively coordinating their care, and to protecting them from discrimination [21].

In all of federal law, the most sweeping confidentiality rules to protect adolescents' substance abuse treatment records are provided by 42 C.F.R. Part 2, the regulations promulgated under the federal Public Health Service Act. These comprehensive federal rules encourage adolescents to seek substance abuse treatment and help ensure unimpeded access to the treatment they need, by going the furthest to guarantee their control over parental access to their substance abuse treatment information. In order for the adolescent substance abuse patient to qualify for protection under these federal confidentiality rules, two conditions must be met: (i) as a threshold issue, the applicable state law must allow the adolescent to consent to his or her own substance abuse treatment; and (ii) the healthcare provider must meet certain specified criteria, as set forth below. When these two conditions are satisfied, the adolescent patient is granted control over any disclosure:

> When state law allows adolescents to consent independently for their own substance abuse treatment, health care providers who must comply with the federal rules are generally prohibited by

the regulations from disclosing any information related to that treatment to parents without the adolescent's written consent [22].

Healthcare providers who *must comply* with federal substance abuse treatment confidentiality rules are those who meet the following two criteria set forth in 42 C.F.R. Part 2:

1. The individual, program, or facility is *federally assisted* (i.e., authorized, certified, licensed, or funded in whole or in part by any department of the federal government, such as programs that are tax exempt; receiving tax-deductible donations or any federal operating funds; or registered with Medicare).
2. The individual or program holds itself out as providing substance abuse diagnosis, treatment, or referral; or is a staff member at a general medical facility whose primary function is, and who is identified as, a provider of substance abuse diagnosis, treatment, or referral; or is a unit at a general medical facility that holds itself out as providing substance abuse diagnosis, treatment, or referral.

Providers who are federally assisted and also satisfy the second criterion above must follow the federal confidentiality rules, as well as state law. Providers who are not federally assisted or do not satisfy the second criterion do not have to follow the federal rules and are subject only to state law. Although healthcare providers are generally able to comply with both the federal and state confidentiality laws, in the event of a conflict, the law that most effectively protects confidentiality prevails. This generally means that the state law may be *pre-empted* and the provider must abide by the federal confidentiality rule, which explicitly states: "no State law may either authorize or compel any disclosure prohibited by these rules." The main exception to this provision (also set forth in 42 C.F.R. 42), allowing disclosure to parents without the patient's written consent, is when the provider determines that the following three conditions are met:

1. The minor's situation poses a substantial threat to the life or physical well-being of the minor or another.
2. This threat may be reduced by communicating relevant facts to the minor's parents.
3. The minor lacks the capacity because of extreme youth or a mental or physical condition to make a rational decision on whether to disclose to his or her parents.

HIPAA Privacy Rule

The federal personal privacy regulations issued under the Health Insurance Portability and Accountability Act of 1996 (HIPAA) are also known as the HIPAA Privacy Rule [23]. (The Privacy Rule's formal title is Standards for Privacy of Individually Identifiable Health Information.) The Privacy Rule establishes a national standard linking an individual's right to consent to healthcare and his or her ability to keep the health records confidential: when an individual provides consent for healthcare services, that individual generally has the right to control access to his or her medical information. However, the privacy regulations specifically exempt minors from this provision when it comes to controlling their parents' access to the medical information. On this issue, the Privacy Rule defers to state law that either requires, permits, or prohibits disclosure of health information about a minor to the parents. When state law explicitly requires parental access, the Rule requires providers to disclose the information; when state law explicitly permits but does not require parental access (or is silent on the question), the Rule leaves the decision whether or not to disclose to the discretion of the providers; when state law prohibits parental access without the minor's consent, the providers must comply with this restriction.

Critics charge that HIPAA poses significant risks to adolescent confidentiality. To all intents and purposes, it permits unfettered disclosure of substance abuse patient records, *without requiring prior patient consent*, to the full range of entities involved in healthcare payment and operations, including insurance companies and other healthcare providers. Furthermore, those entities are permitted to redisclose the records without restriction. However, when a substance abuse patient also qualifies for protection under the federal confidentiality regulations (42 C.F.R. Part 2), in that case the latter more stringent rule controls, in the event of any conflict with HIPAA. For example, if disclosure is permitted under HIPAA, but prohibited under 42 C.F.R. Part 2, in that situation the prohibition would control.

Even in jurisdictions where adolescent confidentiality is protected by law, there are a number of ways in which it may be inadvertently compromised. The HIPAA Privacy Rule attempts to address a number of these situations:

1. *Provider communications to the patient are received by the parents:* Adolescents typically reside with their parents and are vulnerable to this type of incidental leak of their protected information. The unsuspecting parents may learn that their child is in substance abuse treatment, when the provider leaves telephone messages or sends written communications intended for the patient, which are instead received by the parents. The Privacy Rule permits adolescents to request special privacy protections to try to avoid this type of inadvertent disclosure about their treatment to their parents. The Rule affords adolescents the right to control the manner in which the provider communicates with them, for example, by requesting that contacts be made via email rather than telephone, or at a location other than their own home. Although providers are required to accept such reasonable requests, the adolescent may have cause for concern that there is no fail-safe guarantee that such slip-ups will not occur [25].

2. *Private and public insurance practices:* Another situation that risks inadvertent disclosure of adolescent substance abuse treatment information involves administrative and billing practices of private insurers and Medicaid. "Economic reality rather than legal theory may determine the right to confidential information," when treatment is rendered to adolescent patients, who are typically financially dependent on their parents [24]. (California is the only state that allows adolescents to qualify for Medicaid coverage based on their own incomes, under its Medi-CAL program.) Insurance communications mailed to the parents, for the purpose of payment or healthcare operations – for example, Explanation of Benefits forms (EOBs) – do not require the adolescent patient's prior consent. These communications usually provide parents with a description of the services that were provided to their children and thereby may serve to negate whatever confidentiality protections were afforded to the adolescent by state or federal law. The Privacy Rule allows adolescents to request that an insurer restrict otherwise allowable disclosures or provide information by an alternate path, for example, by not sending benefit letters home. However, while insurance plans are generally required to consider such requests by adolescents, the extent to which they are likely to be honored remains problematic.

3. *Provider failure to implement office procedures and administrative safeguards to protect confidential adolescent records:* In the setting of a provider's busy office, it may be difficult to avoid inadvertent breaches of adolescent confidentiality. For example, providers may maintain adolescent health records that contain two different categories of information within the same file, that is, non-confidential health information (which parents can legally access) and confidential information (which should not be disclosed without the patient's

consent). The Privacy Rule requires that administrative, technical, and physical safeguards are implemented, in order to ensure that inadvertent disclosure of the adolescent's confidential healthcare information does not occur. This may be accomplished in a number of ways, for example, by carefully segregating the two types of information in different charts, writing sensitive information in code, or using different colored progress notes. The provider should appoint a "privacy official" to administer the office's policies and procedures to assure compliance with the Privacy Rule. There is a need to educate the staff about confidentiality issues and the special needs of adolescents. Appropriate training should be arranged for staff members who handle patient records and release of information [25].

Hippocrates or HIPAA?: Electronic Health Record (EHR) Systems and HIPAA

Some believe that, in this new age of rapidly evolving health information technology, HIPAA poses another risk to the confidentiality of adolescent substance abuse records. With the advent of interoperable networks linking multiple electronic health record (EHR) systems, a national health information highway is being developed, to facilitate the efficient collection, storage, and transfer of patient health records. While all agree that it is desirable to integrate substance abuse treatment information with the rest of the healthcare system, in order to enhance communication and coordination with other providers, a controversy is brewing about the best way to accomplish this goal. The focus of controversy is about how the confidentiality of substance abuse patients will be handled under the new system.

Some healthcare experts want to do away with or undertake the wholesale restructuring of 42 C.F.R. Part 2, which they view as a major barrier to the free flow of substance abuse treatment information to all parts of the healthcare system. They argue that the requirement of prior patient consent before disclosure is no longer workable under the new system. They call instead for adoption of the HIPAA approach, which authorizes the full flow of information to other entities (such as providers and insurers) for payment and healthcare operations *without* prior patient consent. These entities would then be able to redisclose the information (not only for healthcare use, but, since HIPAA bows to state laws mandating disclosure for a host of other purposes, also to law enforcement agencies and for litigation, e.g., divorce and child custody proceedings) [21].

Advocates for effective adolescent substance abuse treatment contend that adopting the HIPAA approach

would create unacceptable risks of eviscerating hard-won confidentiality protections already in place and undo much of the progress that has been achieved to remove barriers to care. Adolescent patients are likely to be alarmed about the unfettered disclosure of their substance abuse records throughout the system and be deterred from seeking treatment in the first place.

These advocates believe that communication and integration can be enhanced without changing or compromising the basic legal framework of confidentiality laws and regulations currently in place. They argue that the technology exists to facilitate the communication and integration of substance abuse treatment information without sacrificing patient confidentiality. According to them, this can be accomplished if EHR systems are constructed correctly and substance abuse treatment providers are given the necessary resources, technology, and technical assistance they need to participate. It remains to be seen whether or not the goal of integrating substance abuse treatment records into the envisioned nationwide health information network is achievable, without compromising the fundamental principles underlying federal confidentiality law and regulations (42 C.F.R. Part 2) [21]. The ultimate resolution of this controversy is likely to have a significant impact on adolescent access to substance abuse treatment in the future.

Clinical Vignette

Judy, a 16-year-old high-school student, lives at home with her parents in the state of M. Her out-of-wedlock pregnancy has greatly upset her parents, but they have started to calm down and accept the situation. Now 3 months pregnant, Judy considers seeking treatment for marijuana abuse at a hospital-based substance abuse clinic. (She receives care at a separate prenatal clinic at the same hospital and her obstetrician advised her that marijuana can cause premature birth or small birth size.) State law in M provides that minors may independently consent to treatment for substance abuse at age 15. However, state law in M also mandates that the parents of a minor receiving substance abuse treatment must be notified as soon as practicable in the course of treatment. Furthermore, pregnancy does not confer an emancipated minor status in M.

Judy wants to seek help for her substance abuse problem and is very concerned about the well-being of her baby. However, she is worried that if her parents learn about her marijuana abuse (on top of having recently learned about her pregnancy), it will be the last straw and they will become extremely angry at her. She is hesitant to seek treatment under these circumstances. She knows that under state law, disclosure must be made to her parents about her substance abuse treatment. The operative question is: does federal law apply? If it turns out that federal law does apply, then Judy's substance abuse treatment provider would follow the federal confidentiality rule (42 C.F.R. Part 2). The following analysis will determine this issue: (i) it is clear that the hospital is "federally assisted," since most hospitals meet this criterion, by virtue of either receiving federal operating funds, being registered for Medicare, or enjoying a non-profit status; (ii) it is also clear that the hospital's substance abuse clinic is a unit at a general hospital facility that holds itself out as providing alcohol or drug abuse diagnosis, treatment, or referral. Accordingly, the substance abuse clinic satisfies the criteria for providers who must follow federal law. As a result of the foregoing, federal law does apply (thereby pre-empting the state law's parental notification requirement) and the clinic is prohibited from disclosing any information about Judy's substance abuse treatment to her parents without her written consent. After the clinic apprises her of these confidentiality protections, Judy is greatly relieved and agrees to proceed with treatment. Determined to leave nothing to chance, Judy also arranges to pay for the treatment herself, out of her part-time job earnings, to avoid the possibility that her parents' health insurer might expose her substance abuse treatment by sending an E.O.B. form to her parents.

References

1. Vukadinovich DM. Minors' rights to consent to treatment: navigating the complexity of state laws. *J Health L* 2004;**37**:667–678.
2. *Carey vs. Population Services International*, 431 U.S. 678 (1977).
3. *Bellotti vs. Baird*, 443 U.S. 622 (1979).
4. *Planned Parenthood vs. Casey*, 505 U.S. 833 (1992).
5. Lloyd GER (ed.). *Hippocratic Writings*. Harmondsworth, UK:Penguin Books, 1978.
6. Goldstein RL. Psychiatric poetic license? Post-mortem disclosure of confidential information in the Anne Sexton case. *Psychiatric Ann* 1992;**22**:341–348.
7. Ford CA, English A. Limiting confidentiality of adolescent health services. What are the risks? *JAMA* 2002;**288**: 752–753.
8. Morreale MC, Stinnett AJ, Dowling EC (eds). *Policy Compendium on Confidential Health Services for Adolescents*, 2nd edn. Chapel Hill, NC:Center for Adolescent Health and the Law, 2005.
9. Smith DC, Boel-Studt S, Cleeland L. Parental consent in adolescent substance abuse treatment outcome studies. *J Subst Abuse Treat* 2009;**37**:298–306.
10. Boonstra H, Nash E. Minors and the right to consent to health care. *Guttmacher Report Public Policy* 2000;**3**: 1–5.
11. Prosser WL, Keeton WP. *The Law of Torts*. St Paul, MN: West Publishing, 1984.
12. *Schloendorff vs. Society of New York Hospital*, 105 N.E. 92, 93 (N.Y. 1914).
13. Scott ES, Reppucci ND, Woolard JL. Evaluating adolescent decision making in legal contexts. *Law Hum Behav* 1995;**19**:221–244.
14. Forehand LJr, Ciccone RJ. The competence of adolescents to consent to treatment. *Adolesc Psychiatry* 2004;**28**:5–27.
15. Schlam L, Wood JP. Informed consent to the medical treatment of minors: law and practice. *Health Matrix* 2000;**10**:141–175.
16. Batterman N. Under age: a minor's right to consent to health care. *Touro Law Rev* 1994;**10**:637–673.
17. Sigman GS, O'Connor C. Exploration for physicians of the mature minor doctrine. *J Pediatrics* 1991;**119**: 520–525.
18. Weisleder P. The right of minors to confidentiality and informed consent. *J Child Neurol* 2004;**19**:145–148.
19. Weisleder P. Inconsistency among American states on the age at which minors can consent to substance abuse treatment. *J Am Acad Psychiatry Law* 2007;**35**:317–322.
20. Cal. Family Code § 6929.
21. Legal Action Center. Confidentiality of alcohol and drug records in the 21st century. New York, 2010. Available at: http://www.scribd.com/doc/88295229/Confidentiality-of-Alcohol-and-Drug-Records-in-the-21st-Century-1-20-10.
22. Gudeman R. Federal privacy protection for substance abuse treatment records: protecting adolescents. *Youth L News* 2003;**24**:28–30.
23. 45 C.F.R. § 164.
24. Simon RI, Sadoff RL. *Psychiatric Malpractice*. Washington, DC:American Psychiatric Press, 1992.
25. Gudeman R. Adolescent confidentiality and privacy under the health insurance portability and accountability act. *Youth L News* 2003;**24**:31–36.

Saving Adolescents[1]

Richard Rosner

*Forensic Psychiatry Residency Program, New York University School of Medicine;
Forensic Psychiatry Clinic, Bellevue Hospital Center, New York, NY, USA*

The 2005 William A. Schonfeld Memorial Lecture

Core to the mission of the American Society for Adolescent Psychiatry (ASAP) are the tenets that adolescence is a critical developmental period that carries with it many psychosocial risks, and that treating adolescents effectively requires special knowledge and skills. The William A. Schonfeld Award of the ASAP honors the first president of the organization; the award is given to individuals recognized for their outstanding contributions to the field of adolescent psychiatry, as well as for their excellence and dedication to the clinical practice of adolescent psychiatry throughout the course of their career. This chapter is based on the author's presentation at the 2005 ASAP Annual Meeting, in which he summarized and synthesized four aspects of his life's work that are relevant to the mission of the ASAP, and which are conceptualized as ways of "saving adolescents:" (i) education and training in adolescent psychiatry; (ii) forensic psychiatry; (iii) addiction medicine; and (iv) moral philosophy.

EDUCATION AND TRAINING IN ADOLESCENT PSYCHIATRY

For the foreseeable future, there is likely to continue to be a gap between the mental health needs of teenagers and the number of practitioners available to meet those needs. Although efforts are being made to increase enrollment in the American Council on Graduate Medical Education (ACGME)-accredited residency programs in child and adolescent psychiatry, no one expects that those efforts will succeed soon in training sufficient

child and adolescent specialists to meet the current and immediately anticipated needs of teenagers in the United States. Saving adolescents will require that a large number of general psychiatrists take the time to acquire the knowledge and skills needed to help youngsters. The ASAP is in the forefront of the effort to attract general psychiatrists to work with teenagers. The ASAP has reorganized itself from being a federation of regional chapters into a unified national structure. The educational programs at our annual conventions provide a convenient route to obtain clinically relevant information about the diagnosis and treatment of adolescent mental disorders. Those general psychiatrists who wish to expand the size and scope of their practice by including adolescents can find in the ASAP the continuing medical education courses they need to address this underserved population of potential patients.

The ASAP's position on training in adolescent psychiatry has been consistent. Those persons who wish to work with both children and adolescents should be trained in child and adolescent psychiatry. Those persons who wish to work with adolescents and adults should not have to be trained in child and adolescent psychiatry, but should have the option of supplementing their general psychiatry training with additional training in adolescent psychiatry. For example, additional training in adolescent psychiatry can be obtained by taking elective clinical experiences in adolescent psychiatry during the general psychiatry residency. In the past, when the ASAP surveyed the ACGME-accredited child and adolescent psychiatry residencies, some of the latter (e.g., those that could not fill all of their positions) expressed willingness to offer 1 year of training in purely adolescent psychiatry. The ASAP's Accreditation Council on Fellowships in Adolescent Psychiatry, which I have been involved with since its inception,

[1]Saving Adolescents. Previously published as "Essays on Saving Adolescents", in Adolescent Psychiatry, Volume 30, Analytic Press, Hillsboro, NJ, 2008, and reprinted here with their kind permission.

developed and published criteria to evaluate the quality of the training offered in such 1-year adolescent psychiatry residency programs [1–3].

As an alternative pathway to formal residency or fellowship training, after graduation from a general psychiatry residency, additional training in adolescent psychiatry can be obtained by on-the-job training, by continuing medical education courses, and by self-guided systematic independent study. The ASAP-endorsed *Textbook of Adolescent Psychiatry* [3] and *Adolescent Psychiatry*, the ASAP's annual series of volumes, are useful components of a program of self-guided systematic independent study.

The American Board of Adolescent Psychiatry (ABAP), incorporated as an entirely separate organization from the ASAP, serves the important function of distinguishing between (i) those persons who claim to possess the knowledge essential to the care and treatment of adolescents and (ii) those persons who have objectively demonstrated that they possess the knowledge essential to the care and treatment of adolescents (by successfully passing ABAP's credentialing and examination processes).

Initially intended as a demonstration project, the New York Chapter of the ASAP cooperated with the ASAP's Accreditation Council on Fellowships in Adolescent Psychiatry to develop a one-semester training program, accredited for $25\frac{1}{2}$ hours of continuing medical education, for general and forensic psychiatrists who sought additional knowledge about adolescents and adolescent psychiatry. The course has subsequently been integrated into the forensic psychiatry residency programs offered at New York University Medical Center, New York Medical College, Albert Einstein College of Medicine of Yeshiva University, and the medical schools of Columbia and Cornell. The course has functioned as a model of how to integrate training in adolescent psychiatry into the curriculum of other psychiatric residency programs, without having to create freestanding residency programs in adolescent psychiatry per se. Graduates of the course have become members of the ASAP, have been certified by the American Board of Adolescent Psychiatry, and have become elected officers of both ASAP's New York Chapter and the ASAP's national organization.

FORENSIC PSYCHIATRY

The 1 March 2005 decision of the US Supreme Court in the case of *Roper vs. Simmons* is a dramatic demonstration of saving adolescents through the interface of adolescent psychiatry and forensic psychiatry. In that case, the Court ruled that the US Constitution prohibits the execution of a juvenile who was under 18 when the crime was committed. The ASAP was in the lead among the various medical amici curiae that submitted legal briefs to the US Supreme Court against the death penalty for adolescents in the Roper case. However, there are myriad opportunities in smaller, local, and individual legal cases where adolescent psychiatrists can create alliances with general and forensic psychiatrists and with attorneys to work together in saving adolescents.

From a public health standpoint, it is a curious fact that the city, state, and federal governments have no affirmative obligation to evaluate the mental health of teenagers at large in the community. However, the moment that a teenager is taken into custody by the police and held in detention, there is a governmental obligation to evaluate the mental condition of that teenager and to provide appropriate mental health care and treatment. In this manner, many youngsters who would otherwise never obtain a mental health evaluation are identified as in need of mental health (including substance abuse) services. Thus the juvenile justice system has become a *de facto* mental health system [4]. (This is true of the criminal justice system in general [5].) Unfortunately, the majority of general and forensic psychiatrists who work in the juvenile justice and adult correctional systems lack the knowledge and skills needed to evaluate and treat teenagers. Furthermore, in many instances there is a lack of continuity of care so that adolescents who are identified as in need of mental health services while in detention are not routinely and effectively referred to community-based mental health services upon their release from detention. Saving adolescents in detention, and promoting their post-detention care and treatment, will require an active alliance between the general and forensic psychiatrists who work in correctional and community-based settings and the adolescent psychiatrists who have the knowledge and skills needed to treat teenagers.

Even for adolescents who are not held in detention, there are opportunities for adolescent psychiatrists to cooperate with attorneys and forensic psychiatrists in saving adolescents. For example, when a juvenile is arrested the law requires that the police read the Miranda rights (the right to remain silent, the right to refuse to answer questions, and the right to be represented by an attorney) to him or her. But teenagers are vulnerable to witting and unwitting influence by the police that may undermine their ability to understand and assert their Miranda rights. Some adolescents who confess to criminal acts, who do not exercise their right to remain silent, who do not demand that an attorney be provided for them, may be incompetent to have waived their Miranda rights. Adolescent psychiatrists working with attorneys and forensic psychiatrists have a role to play in the evaluation of whether or not a particular adolescent was competent to have waived his or her Miranda rights, including whether or not a particular adolescent was competent to confess to a criminal act. In general, it is the obligation of a defendant in a criminal case to assert that he or she was not competent to have waived his or her Miranda rights. Not all attorneys and not all forensic psychiatrists know that teenagers may respond differently from adults to being informed of their Miranda rights. *Voluntariness* is the key legal criterion in determining whether or not a person's waiver of Miranda rights was valid. Teenagers may hear that they have the right to refuse to answer questions from the police and prosecutors, but may not understand or believe or be able to apply what they have heard to their own immediate reality. Teenagers may be unable to reconcile being told that they do not have to answer questions, on the one hand, and then being asked questions, on the other hand. One role of an adolescent psychiatrist is to bring these matters to the attention of attorneys or forensic psychiatrists, to raise the issue of a teenager's possible incompetence to have waived his or her Miranda rights.

Similarly, at a later stage of the criminal justice system's processes, a defendant may be examined to determine his or her competence to stand trial. That is, whether or not he or she "has sufficient present ability to consult with his lawyer with a reasonable degree of rational understanding – and whether he has a rational as well as a factual understanding of the proceedings against him" as set forth by the US Supreme Court in the case of *Dusky vs. United States* (1960). Attorneys and forensic psychiatrists, who are used to adult clients, may have difficulty communicating with teenagers, let alone evaluating their competence to stand trial. Teenagers may be unable to understand and apply abstract legal principles to the specifics of their own legal case. For example, that even if they have engaged in a criminal act, they are entitled to an attorney to represent them and defend them against the legal charges. An adolescent psychiatrist can *translate* communications between attorneys and their adolescent clients, to make sure that the words that are spoken by the attorney are genuinely understood by the adolescent defendant. The adolescent psychiatrist can discern that the teenager has only a factual, but not a rational, understanding of the proceedings against him or her, thus, that the teenager is not competent to stand trial.

While it is uncommon for a defense attorney to assert that a client is not criminally responsible due to mental disease or mental defect, at times it may be the only defense that is feasible. In many states, the defense of "not guilty by reason of insanity" is based on the American Law Institute's 1955 criteria: "A person is not responsible for criminal conduct if at the time of such conduct as a result of mental disease or mental defect he lacks substantial capacity either to appreciate the criminality of his conduct or to conform his conduct to the requirements of law" [6]. There is some question

as to whether or not adolescents generally (as compared to adults) have an impairment of their capacity to appreciate their conduct. Similarly, there is some question as to whether or not adolescents generally (as compared to adults) have an impairment of their capacity to conform their conduct to the requirements of law. By bringing to the attention of attorneys and forensic psychiatrists that a teenager may have known what he was doing, but may not have appreciated what he was doing, adolescent psychiatrists can make important contributions to saving adolescents within the juvenile and adult criminal justice systems.

Whether the issue is competence to waive Miranda rights, competence to stand trial, or insanity as a defense against criminal charges, saving adolescents may constitute excluding teenagers from inappropriate punishment, and diverting adolescents from the criminal justice system to the mental health system. To help save adolescents caught up in the criminal justice system by facilitating constructive alliances with attorneys and forensic psychiatrists, the ASAP has established liaisons with the American Academy of Forensic Sciences (AAFS) and the American Academy of Psychiatry and the Law (AAPL).

ADDICTION MEDICINE

Many of the teenagers who come to the attention of the criminal justice system are caught in the snare of substance abuse. While it is true that attorneys and forensic psychiatrists have much to learn from adolescent psychiatrists, it is equally true that adolescent psychiatrists have much to learn from specialists in addiction medicine and addiction psychiatry. By the time they have graduated from high school, the majority of teenagers have used an illegal substance. We are currently unable to predict reliably which youngsters will, and which will not, spontaneously and successfully resist the forces that lead from substance use to substance abuse to substance dependence. We are obliged to consider all teenagers as at risk for drug addiction and to develop our skills in the diagnosis and treatment of adolescents addicted to both legal and illegal drugs [7]. The public health risk of addiction to legal drugs needs to be stressed: more people will die from the effects of tobacco and alcohol than from the effects of all illegal drugs combined. The ASAP's Task Force on Adolescent Addiction has presented a major educational program to teach the essentials of addiction psychiatry to adolescent psychiatrists. Part of the contents of that program were published in volume 29 of the ASAP's annual series, *Adolescent Psychiatry*.

There are many reasons why substance use, abuse, and dependence are so common among teenagers. We live in a society that is metaphorically *addicted* to immediate gratification, turning for instant satisfaction to television, to computers, and to overconsumption of material goods. Apart from organized religion, what vision do we offer our youngsters as a counterweight to self-indulgent materialism? The success of programs based on spiritual values, such as Alcoholics Anonymous, is illustrative of the help these values offer in breaking free of addiction.

The Twelve-Step self-help model of Alcoholics Anonymous (AA) is the most widely available treatment for substance abusers. The separate self-help organizations modeled on AA include Narcotics Anonymous, Cocaine Anonymous, Marijuana Anonymous, Over-Eaters Anonymous, Gamblers Anonymous, and Survivors-of-Incest Anonymous. AA is a fellowship that offers a spiritual (rather than a religious) vision of the good life. The US government's report on Project Match, a research study under the auspices of the National Institute of Alcoholism and Alcohol Abuse (NIAAA), demonstrated that AA's style of Twelve-Step Facilitation Therapy works as well as cognitive-behavioral therapy or motivational enhancement therapy (the latter is based on motivational interviewing) [8,9]. AA helps substance abusers make the transition from self-destructive immediate gratification to societal-enhancing delayed gratification. AA gives its participants a vision of a life that is worth living; it is inspirational. As adolescent psychiatrists, we need to learn how to use the inspirational power of AA's spiritual fellowship to complement our scientific treatments to foster the growth and development of our patients. The idealism of youth, a feature of normal development, can be a powerful force for good.

Many psychiatrists have distrusted the AA approach and seen it as antagonistic. What makes some of our colleagues uncomfortable with AA is the very spirituality that is AA's strength. Perhaps we need to disentangle spirituality from religion, from mythology, from fairy tales. The word *spirituality* sounds uncomfortably similar to *spirits* and *sprites*. Words that sound similar do not necessarily refer to similar things. Spirituality is not about ghosts, angels, and demons. In secular terms, spirituality is about values. There is an initial and superficial resemblance between ghosts and values, neither of them is visible, neither of them is material, neither of them exists in the same way that a car or a house or a chocolate bar exists; but that is the end of the resemblances. The spiritual vision AA advances is set forth in the Twelve Steps of AA, shown in Table 47.1. Bowen and MacDougall [10] have noted that each of these steps corresponds to a specific value, which, although not explicitly stated, is nonetheless fundamental. The values associated with each step are also summarized in Table 47.1.

Twelve-step self-help groups like AA are ubiquitous, free, and effective for many adolescent substance abusers. In order to make intelligent referrals to these therapeutic resources, all adolescent psychiatrists who work with teenagers should be familiar with the 12 steps and with the specific values to which each step corresponds. When dealing with some teenagers, it is more effective to focus on the specific value associated with the step being considered. With other teenagers, it may be more effective to ask what relevant meaning the adolescent can find from his or her personal interpretation of the language of the step.

There are 12-step groups for agnostics, for atheists, and for secular humanists. The language of the 12 steps is meant to be inclusive, for example, the phrases "God as we understand Him" and a "power greater than ourselves" can refer to Nature, the cosmos, or any entity/concept that is not one's self, that is not as limited as one's self, and with which one can have a personal relationship (the Jewish existentialist, Martin Buber, wrote movingly about having a personal encounter with a tree).

MORAL PHILOSOPHY

We live in a time of anti-intellectualism, moral relativism, and *political correctness*, which makes many of us reluctant to assert and advocate for the values to which we adhere. However, we should not mistake every person's equal right to state his or her opinion, on the one hand, with every person's opinion being of equal worth, on the other hand. Those opinions that can be supported by facts and reasoned arguments are superior to those opinions that are not supported by facts and reasoned arguments [11,12].

Adolescents need moral guidelines. We must not abandon our adolescents to a wasteland, to the equally unacceptable poles of immoral materialism and irrational religion. We need to offer them a moral framework derived from sound principles and grounded on shared values. What are the values that we stand for? Insofar as we are citizens of the United States of America, we are advocates of legal equality (all persons are equal before the Law), and we are advocates of human rights (no one may be deprived of life, liberty, or property except by due process of law). Insofar as we are scientists, we are advocates of truth, honesty, and rationality. Insofar as we are physicians, based upon the traditions of medicine, we are advocates of non-maleficence (do no harm) and of benevolence (do good). Insofar as we are adolescent psychiatrists, we are advocates of respect for persons (including those impaired by mental disorders) and of fostering healthy human growth. In our commitment to

Table 47.1 Alcoholics Anonymous (AA) Twelve Steps and corresponding values.

Step	Statement[a]	Value[b]
I	"We admitted we were powerless over alcohol[c] and our lives had become unmanageable."	Honesty
II	"We came to believe that a Power greater than ourselves could restore us to sanity."	Hope
III	"We made a decision to turn our will and our lives over to the care of God as we understood Him."	Faith
IV	"We made a searching and fearless moral inventory of ourselves."	Courage
V	"We admitted to God, to ourselves, and to another human being that exact nature of our wrongs."	Integrity
VI	"We became entirely ready to have God remove all these defects of character."	Willingness
VII	"We humbly asked Him to remove our shortcomings."	Humility
VIII	"We made a list of all persons we had harmed, and became willing to make amends to them all."	Compassion
IX	"We made direct amends to such people wherever possible, except when to do so would injure them or others."	Justice
X	"We continued to take personal inventory, and when we were wrong promptly admitted it."	Perseverance
XI	"We sought through prayer and meditation to improve our conscious contact with God, as we understand Him, praying only for knowledge of God's will for us and the power to carry that out."	Spiritual awareness
XII	"Having had a spiritual awakening as the result of these steps, we tried to carry this message to alcoholics,[d] and to practice these principles in all our affairs."	Service

[a]Reprinted courtesy of Alcoholics Anonymous World Services, Inc.
[b]From White and MacDougall (2001) [10].
[c]Narcotics Anonymous says "powerless over addiction," Gamblers Anonymous says "powerless over gambling."
[d]Narcotics Anonymous says "addicts."

our shared values, we should not be reticent in offering ourselves as models for potential emulation by our patients.

Moral relativism undermines our confidence in our shared moral values. We are told that each culture determines its own morality; that there is no way to determine moral right and wrong outside of a specific cultural framework. In contrast, however, no one would say that each culture determines its own science; that there is no way to determine science outside of a specific cultural framework. If one culture said that the earth was round, and another culture said that the earth was flat, no one would accept that each culture was equally correct. Rather, we would insist that the different scientific assertions be tested to establish which was right and which was wrong. We use scientific techniques to test scientific assertions of facts. Some, but not all, scientific assertions can be tested by current scientific techniques. (Who can currently test whether anything existed before the Big Bang? Who can currently test whether or not String Theory is correct?) We hope science will advance so that, in the future, our scientific techniques will be able to test scientific assertions that cannot now

be tested. The same line of thinking applies to the evaluation of disagreements about morality as applies to the evaluation of disagreements about science. We should test moral assertions asrigorously as we test scientific assertions. We use philosophical techniques to test moral assertions. Necessarily, the techniques of philosophy are different from the techniques of science. Some, but not all, moral assertions can be tested by current philosophical techniques. We hope philosophy will advance so that, in the future, our philosophical techniques will be able to test moral assertions that cannot now be tested [13].

A literal belief in revealed truth as set forth in sacred texts (e.g., the Bible or the Koran), common in adherents to fundamentalist religions, also undermines our confidence in our shared moral values. This kind of narrow view holds that whatever God commands as set forth in the sacred text is good, and that whatever God forbids is bad. However, it is reasonable to ask, as a moral philosopher might: "Is what God commands good because God commands it; or is God commanding it because it is good?" This is a subtle but crucial distinction. If God commands us to do something because God knows that it is good because of sound moral principles and moral reasons, then it is not God's command that makes it good. If what makes something good is that God commands us to do it, it follows that if God told us to do the exact opposite thing, then that opposite thing would (by definition) be good.

Thus, either God is arbitrary (anything God commands is good, and its opposite would be good if God commanded us to do its opposite) or God has commanded us to do things that are good because of moral principles and moral reasons that are independent of God's commands. For most religious people, it is unacceptable that God is arbitrary. They share an interest in determining sound moral principles and sound moral reasoning with adherents to secular philosophy [13].

There have been many attempts to provide an objective, rational grounding for moral principles and moral reasoning. If adolescent psychiatrists are to save adolescents from America's current moral wasteland, the psychiatrists must have a basic understanding of the two leading philosophical theories of moral justification.

The first of these theories essentially says that the end justifies the means – what makes an action good is that its results are good. The most famous advocates of this position are the Englishmen Jeremy Bentham and John Stuart Mill. (For a fuller discussion of the views of these philosophers, see Rachels' *Elements of Moral Philosophy* [13].) As an initial introduction to moral reasoning, Bentham and Mill offer guidelines about what kinds of action one should pursue. They suggest that, given the choice between a variety of actions, one should always choose the action that leads to the greatest good for the greatest number of persons. Teaching adolescents to consider the long-term (as well as short-term) consequences of their potential actions is important. Teaching adolescents to consider the consequences of their potential actions on other people (as well as on themselves) is important. Bentham and Mill would have us teach adolescents to choose the course of action that produces the best long-term and short-term consequences for others and for themselves [13].

The second of these theories says that no one should do any action that he or she would not want any other similarly situated person to do in the same circumstances, that we should live according to universal rules that apply to all persons equally at all times. This position holds that the autonomy of all persons should be respected, that no person should be used merely as a means to someone else's ends. The most famous advocate of this position is the German Immanuel Kant. As an initial introduction to moral reasoning, Kant offers guidelines about what kinds of action should be avoided. It is important to teach adolescents that (in the absence of a morally relevant difference between oneself and everyone else) that what is permitted for oneself should be permitted for everyone, that no one is entitled to rights and privileges that he or she would not accord to all people. It is important to teach adolescents that people should not be manipulated, exploited, or used to attain whatever ends the adolescent is seeking, that all people should be respected [13].

CONCLUSION

Saving adolescents is not easy. Given the gap between the numbers of teenagers in need of services and the paucity of mental health personnel trained to address that need, it will be necessary to encourage general psychiatrists to obtain the knowledge and skills required to work effectively with youths. It is appropriate for adolescent psychiatrists to focus on high-risk groups – those in juvenile justice settings and substance abusers. It will be necessary to work with forensic psychiatrists and attorneys to use the justice system to reach troubled teenagers who would not usually seek mental health services on their own initiative. It will be necessary to work with specialists in addictions to learn how to diagnose and treat adolescents who suffer from comorbid illnesses such as mental disorders and substance abuse. It will be necessary to oppose materialism, relativism, and unintelligent religious authoritarianism. It will be necessary to teach sound moral principles, grounded in sound moral justification, to offer an alternative to blind self-indulgence and willful selfishness. We should not be reluctant to affirm our shared values. Who we are, and what we are, the models we offer of responsible, rational commitment to human well-being, may be our most important asset in our goal of saving adolescents.

Acknowledgments

The author was founding president of the Accreditation Council on Fellowships in Adolescent Psychiatry (ACFAP), a semi-autonomous component of the ASAP. During the author's tenure, ACFAP developed and published the Standards for Fellowships in Adolescent Psychiatry [1]. The ASAP-endorsed *Textbook of Adolescent Psychiatry* initially was proposed by ACFAP as an ASAP project [3].

The author participated in 26 graduate school courses in the departments of philosophy at New York University and Columbia University, with a concentration in ethics. He edited two editions of the book *Principles and Practice of Forensic Psychiatry* [14,15] and co-edited the book *Ethical Practice in Psychiatry and the Law* [12].

The American Society of Addiction Medicine certified the author in addiction medicine in 2004. During his tenure as president of the ASAP, he created ASAP's Task Force on Adolescent Addiction, arranged that approximately one-third of the scientific program at ASAP's annual convention was focused on adolescent addiction, and facilitated the publication of much of that portion of the program in volume 29 of *Adolescent Psychiatry*.

The Twelve Steps are reprinted with permission of Alcoholics Anonymous World Services, Inc. ("AAWS") Permission to reprint the Twelve Steps does not mean that AAWS has reviewed or approved the contents of this publication, or that AAWS necessarily agrees with the views expressed herein. A.A. is a program of recovery from alcoholism *only* – use of the Twelve Steps in connection with programs and activities which are patterned after A.A., but which address other problems, or in any other non-A.A. context, does not imply otherwise.

References

1. Rosner R. Report of the Accreditation Council on Fellowships in Adolescent Psychiatry. *Adolesc Psychiatry* 1997;**21**:389–407.
2. Rosner R. Education and training in adolescent psychiatry. In: Rosner R (ed.), *Textbook of Adolescent Psychiatry*. London:Edward Arnold, 2003; pp. 76–81.
3. Rosner R (ed.). *Textbook of Adolescent Psychiatry*. London: Edward Arnold, 2003.
4. Farmer EM, Burns BJ, Phillips SD, Angold A, Costello EJ. Pathways into and through mental health services for children and adolescents. *Psychiatr Serv* 2003;**54**:60–66.
5. Lamb HR, Weinberger IE. Persons with severe mental illness in jails and prisons: A review. *Psychiatr Serv* 1998;**49**:1094–1095.
6. American Law Institute. Model Penal Code, 1955. In: Rosner R (ed.), *Principles and Practice of Forensic Psychiatry*, 2nd edn. London:Edward Arnold, 2003; p. 214.
7. Rosner R. The scourge of addiction: What the adolescent psychiatrist needs to know. *Adolesc Psychiatry* 2005; **29**:19–31.
8. Project, MATCH Research Group. Project MATCH (Matching Alcoholism Treatment to Client Heterogeneity): Rationale and methods for a multisite clinical trial matching patients to alcoholism treatment. *Alcohol Clin Exp Res* 1993;**17**:1130–1145.
9. Project, MATCH Research Group. Matching Alcoholism Treatments to Client Heterogeneity: Project MATCH three-year drinking outcomes. *Alcohol Clin Exp Res* 1998;**22**:1300–1331.
10. White BF, MacDougall JA. *Clinician's Guide to Spirituality*. New York:McGraw Hill, 2001.
11. Rosner R. Ethical practice in the forensic sciences and justification of ethical codes. *J Forensic Sci* 1996;**41**:913–915.
12. Rosner R, Weinstock R (eds). *Ethical Practice in Psychiatry and the Law*. New York: Plenum, 1990.
13. Rachels J. *The Elements of Moral Philosophy*. New York: McGraw-Hill, 2003.
14. Rosner R. *Principles and Practice of Forensic Psychiatry*. London:Chapman & Hall, 1994.
15. Rosner R (ed.). *Principles and Practice of Forensic Psychiatry*, 2nd edn. London: Edward Arnold, 2003.

Index